INTERNAL MEDICINE

VOLUME 2

INTERDISCIPLINARY APPROACHES AND SPECIALIZED TOPICS IN INTERNAL MEDICINE

Dr. Ahmed Taha

ALLIED
HEALTH
PRESS

Internal Medicine Volume 2

Interdisciplinary Approaches and Specialized Topics in Internal Medicine

Author: **Dr. Ahmed Taha**

Allied Health Press
4164 Lakeshore Road
Burlington ON L7L 1A4
Canada
www.alliedhealthpress.com
Email: orders@arclereducation.com

ISBN: 978-1-77956-855-7

ABOUT THE AUTHOR

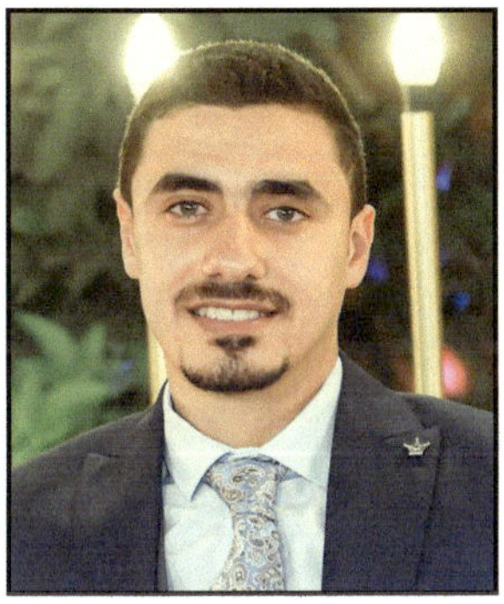

Dr. Ahmed Taha Abdel Sattar, MD, MBChB, is a distinguished graduate of Fayoum University with a GPA of 4 (Summa Cum Laude). Currently a Teaching Assistant in Ophthalmology at Fayoum University Hospital, he has over 14 peer-reviewed publications with 140+ citations and five years of experience in international medical publications. Committed to advancing medical knowledge and patient care, he mentors future healthcare professionals while providing compassionate care to patients.

Brief Table of Contents

1.	Internal Medicine for Dermatology	1
2.	Psychiatry and Behavioral Medicine	35
3.	Geriatric Medicine	71
4.	Internal Medicine for Oncology and Palliative Care	105
5.	Immunology and Allergy	139
6.	Tropical and Travel Medicine	173
7.	Genetics and Genomic Medicine	205
8.	Musculoskeletal and Orthopedic Medicine	239
9.	Obstetric and Gynecologic Medicine	273
10.	Critical Care and Emergency Medicine	305
11.	Internal Medicine for Clinical Nutrition and Metabolism	345
12.	Preventive Medicine and Public Health in Internal Medicine	379
	Index	413

Getting Started with This Book

Chapter Openers

A list of Chapter Outline is presented providing a brief Introduction to what will be covered in the chapter.

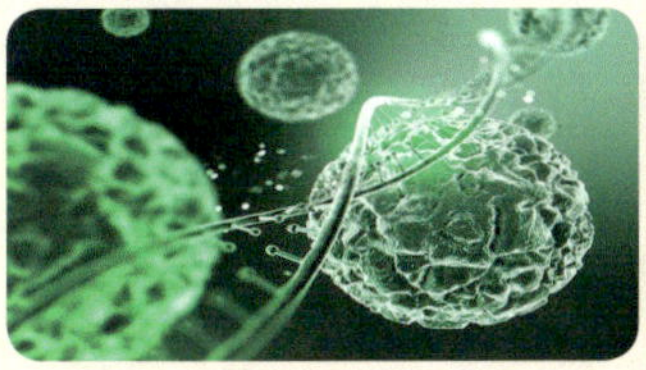

Introduction

Often referred to as the science of life, biology is a broad field of study aimed at comprehending the several kinds of life on Earth, from tiny creatures to sophisticated multicellular entities. Comprising several subfields, including molecular biology, ecology, and evolutionary biology, each of which advances our knowledge of living systems, this field clarifies the mechanisms controlling life events, including development, reproduction, and interaction with the surroundings, which is the central goal of biology. Moreover, biology fills in the void between the natural sciences and medicine by offering a necessary understanding of health, illness, and the interactions between organisms and their environments. Dealing with urgent global issues such as climate change, biodiversity loss, and new diseases depends on an awareness of these complex biological interactions, therefore highlighting the critical part biology plays in modern civilization. Fundamentally, biology explores and tests ideas about the living world using the scientific method. Through methodical observation and experimentation,

LEARNING OBJECTIVES

After studying this chapter, you will be able to:

1. Discuss the scientific method in biology;
2. Explain the cell theory;
3. Discuss the genetics and heredity;
4. Evolution and natural selection;
5. Focus on ecology and ecosystems;
6. Learn about human biology;
7. Evaluate the plant biology;
8. Explain the microbiology;
9. Focus on current trends in biology.

1.1. The Scientific Method in Biology

Learning Outcome

1. Describe the steps of the scientific method;
2. Focus on hypothesis formation;
3. Learn about experimental design.

Learning Outcomes

The beginning of each section of every chapter contains a set of Learning Outcomes that inform students of concepts they should understand. These outcomes help students understand what they should be able to do if they have mastered the material in that section.

Test Your Knowledge

Throughout each chapter, Test Your Knowledge cues you to note which topics have been covered and to self-test your understanding of the material presented.

Test Your Knowledge

1. Explain why correlation does not imply causation in scientific experiments.
2. How does the scientific method help reduce the influence of personal opinions in research?

Chapter Summary

The Summary Section appear at the end of each chapter and summarize main concepts covered throughout the chapter. These points provide key concepts in an engaging and meaningful way.

Summary

The investigation of biological principles highlights the importance of a comprehensive view of life by reflecting the intricate interactions that occur within living systems. The complexity of biology goes beyond individual species or systems, as this essay highlights; it also includes the interactions that mold ecosystems and affect biodiversity. Researchers can conduct in-depth analyses of metabolomic data using sophisticated technologies like MetaboAnalyst, which offer insights into the molecular mechanisms underlying these interactions. As demonstrated by the developments in MetaboAnalyst, for example, the integration of diverse omics data promotes a thorough understanding of metabolic pathways and helps identify important biological markers necessary for research on development and disease (Chong et al., 2018). Additionally, the phenomenon of ecological invasions is a key component of biological research and a vital field of study. The introduction of non-native species into unfamiliar habitats has significant ramifications and calls for multidisciplinary management strategies. Examining the origins and effects of these biological incursions, invasion science has become a crucial field that highlights the need to comprehend ecological dynamics and community interactions. As interest in biological invasions increases, new findings are emerging that put conventional ecological theories and practices to the test. The importance of incorporating various scientific viewpoints is shown by this developing discipline, which also highlights how invasive species shape ecosystems and advances our knowledge of ecological resilience (David et al., 2013). When taken as a whole, these discoveries from invasion science and metabolomics highlight the value of multidisciplinary biology research. Fostering cross-disciplinary collaboration and utilizing technological breakthroughs to improve our comprehension of intricate biological interactions are crucial as we look to the future of biological research. In addition to deepening our understanding of the complexities of life, this method lays the groundwork for tackling urgent environmental issues. Future studies can ensure the continued relevance of biology in a world that is constantly changing by acknowledging the interconnection of biological systems and opening the door to creative solutions that support sustainability and biodiversity conservation. We might imagine a thorough comprehension of life that serves both academia and society at large through ongoing investigation and integration of scientific knowledge.

Knowledge Assessment

The chapter includes material designed to review and reinforce each content. It includes Critical Thinking Questions to help test of your understanding of information presented in the chapter and Short answer Questions to review your understanding of the key concepts presented in the chapter.

Critical Thinking Questions

1. **Who is known as the "Father of Modern Biology"?**
   a. Aristotle
   b. Charles Darwin
   c. Gregor Mendel
   d. Louis Pasteur
2. **What is the basic unit of life?**
   a. Atom
   b. Molecule
   c. Cell
   d. Organism
3. **Which branch of biology studies the interaction of organisms with their environment?**
   a. Genetics
   b. Ecology
   c. Physiology
   d. Botany
4. **Which macromolecule is the main source of energy for living organisms?**
   a. Proteins
   b. Lipids
   c. Carbohydrates
   d. Nucleic acids
5. **DNA is primarily responsible for which function in living organisms?**
   a. Energy production
   b. Protein synthesis
   c. Storing genetic information
   d. Regulating body temperature

Short Answer Questions

1. What is biology, and why is it important to study biology?
2. What are the three main domains of life, and how are they different from one another?
3. Define homeostasis and give an example of how it works in living organisms.
4. What is the cell theory, and why is it fundamental to biology?
5. How do autotrophs and heterotrophs differ in the way they obtain energy?
6. What is the scientific method, and how is it applied in biological research?
7. Discuss how biology helps address global challenges such as climate change, disease, and food security.
8. Explain the levels of biological organization from the smallest unit to the largest. Provide examples at each level.
9. Describe the relationship between structure and function in biology, giving specific examples from cells or organs.
10. How has the discovery of genetics shaped our understanding of inheritance and variation among organisms?

Supplementary Materials

Key Terms: A list of key terms is given for quick reference

KEY TERMS FROM THIS CHAPTER

Annotation enrichment analysis	Biological structure	Cell
Cell theory	Cellular structure	Ecology
Ecosystems	Genetics	Human biology
Microbiology	Natural selection	Organism
Plant biology		

Further Resources: Recommendations for additional readings, websites, and multimedia resources.

References

1. Argelaguet, R., Velten, B., Arnol, D., Dietrich, S., Zenz, T., Marioni, J. C., Buettner, F., et al. (2018). Multi-omics factor analysis—A framework for unsupervised integration of multi-omics data sets. *Molecular Systems Biology, 14*. https://doi.org/10.15252/msb.20178124.
2. Bacher, S., Blackburn, T. M., Essl, F., & Genovesi, P. (2017). *Socio-Economic Impact Classification of Alien Taxa (SEICAT)*. https://core.ac.uk/download/286567949.pdf (accessed on 8th March 2025).
3. Barnett, R., Brace, S., Cucchi, T., & Dobney, K. (2013). *Divergent Evolutionary Processes Associated with Colonization of Offshore Islands*. https://core.ac.uk/download/20664364.pdf (accessed on 8th March 2025).

Detailed Table of Contents

List of Figures *xv*
Preface *xxi*

CHAPTER 1

Internal Medicine for Dermatology 1

Introduction **1**
1.1. The Role of Internal Medicine in Dermatological Conditions **5**
1.1.1. Common Dermatological Conditions with Internal Links 6
1.1.2. Systemic Diseases Manifesting as Skin Disorders 7
1.1.3. Importance of Comprehensive Patient History 8
1.2. Diagnostic Approaches in Internal Medicine for Dermatology **9**
1.2.1. Laboratory Tests and Their Relevance 10
1.2.2. Imaging Techniques in Dermatological Diagnosis 10
1.2.3. The Role of Biopsies in Internal Medicine 11
1.3. Treatment Modalities in Dermatology **12**
1.3.1. Pharmacological Treatments and Internal Considerations 13
1.3.2. Non-Pharmacological Interventions 14
1.3.3. The Role of Multidisciplinary Teams 15
1.4. Chronic Conditions and Their Dermatological Implications **16**
1.4.1. Diabetes and Skin Complications 17
1.4.2. Autoimmune Diseases and Dermatological Manifestations 17
1.4.3. Cardiovascular Health and Skin Integrity 18
1.5. Patient Management Strategies **20**
1.5.1. Importance of Patient Education 20
1.5.2. Follow-Up Care and Monitoring 21
1.5.3. Addressing Psychological Aspects of Skin Conditions 22
1.6. Emerging Research and Future Directions **24**
1.6.1. Advances in Dermatological Treatments 24
1.6.2 The Role of Technology in Dermatology 25
1.6.3 Future Trends in Internal Medicine and Dermatology 26
Summary **28**
References **30**

CHAPTER 2

Psychiatry and Behavioral Medicine 35

Introduction **35**
2.1. Historical Context of Psychiatry **38**
2.1.1. Evolution of Psychiatric Practices 39
2.1.2. Key Figures in Psychiatry 40
2.1.3. Impact of Historical Events on Psychiatric Approaches 41
2.2. Role of General Practitioners in Mental Health **42**
2.2.1. First Point of Contact for Patients 43
2.2.2. Integration of Mental Health Assessments 44
2.2.3. Collaboration with Mental Health Specialists 45

2.3. Common Mental Health Disorders in Internal Medicine 47
2.3.1. Depression and Anxiety Disorders 48
2.3.2. Substance Use Disorders 48
2.3.3. Stress-Related Disorders 49
2.4. Diagnostic Tools and Techniques 51
2.4.1. Clinical Interviews and Assessments 52
2.4.2. Standardized Screening Tools 53
2.4.3. Importance of Patient History 53
2.5. Treatment Approaches in Internal Medicine 55
2.5.1. Psychopharmacology 55
2.5.2. Psychotherapy and Counseling 57
2.5.3. Lifestyle Modifications and Support 58
2.6. Challenges in Integrating Psychiatry into Internal Medicine 59
2.6.1. Stigma Surrounding Mental Health 59
2.6.2. Time Constraints in Internal Medicine 61
2.6.3. Limited Resources and Training 61
Summary 63
References 66

CHAPTER 3

Geriatric Medicine 71

Introduction 71
3.1. Common Health Issues in the Elderly 75
3.1.1. Chronic Diseases Prevalent in Older Adults 76
3.1.2. Mental Health Challenges, Including Dementia and Depression 77
3.1.3. Mobility and Physical Health Concerns 78
3.2 Geriatric Assessment Learning Outcomes: 79
3.2.1. Comprehensive Geriatric Assessment Process 80
3.2.2. Tools and Methods Used in Assessment 81
3.2.3. Importance of Individualized Care Plans 82
3.3. Pharmacological Considerations 83
3.3.1. Polypharmacy and Its Risks 84
3.3.2. Age-Related Changes in Drug Metabolism 85
3.3.3. Strategies for Safe Medication Management 85
3.4. Non-Pharmacological Interventions 87
3.4.1. Role of Physical Therapy and Rehabilitation 87
3.4.2. Importance of Nutrition and Dietary Management 88
3.4.3. Social Engagement and Mental Stimulation 89
3.5. Palliative and End-of-Life Care 90
3.5.1. Principles of Palliative Care in Geriatrics 91
3.5.2. Advanced Care Planning and Decision-Making 92
3.5.3. Support for Families and Caregivers 92
3.6. Challenges in Geriatric Medicine 94
3.6.1. Barriers to Accessing Healthcare for Older Adults 94
3.6.2. Training and Education for Healthcare Providers 95
3.6.3. Ethical Considerations in Geriatric Care 96
Summary 98
References 101

CHAPTER 4

Internal Medicine for Oncology and Palliative Care 105

Introduction 105
4.1. Role of Internal Medicine in Oncology 108
4.1.1. Diagnosis and Treatment Planning 109
4.1.2. Management of Comorbidities 110
4.1.3. Coordination of Multidisciplinary Care 111
4.2. Principles of Palliative Care 112
4.2.1. Definition and Goals of Palliative Care 113
4.2.2. Distinction Between Palliative Care and Hospice Care 113
4.2.3. Importance of Symptom Management 114
4.3. Common Oncological Conditions 116
4.3.1. Types of Cancers Treated in Internal Medicine 117
4.3.2. Epidemiology and Risk Factors 117
4.3.3. Current Treatment Modalities 118
4.4. Challenges in Oncology and Palliative Care 120
4.4.1. Communication Barriers with Patients and Families 121
4.4.2. Ethical Considerations in Treatment Decisions 122
4.4.3. Resource Allocation and Access to Care 123
4.5. Advances in Oncology Treatments 124
4.5.1. Targeted Therapies and Immunotherapy 125
4.5.2. Role of Clinical Trials in Treatment Options 125

4.5.3. Impact of Technology on Patient Care 127
4.6. Integration of Palliative Care in Oncology 128
4.6.1. Early Involvement of Palliative Care Teams 129
4.6.2. Benefits of Holistic Patient Management 130
4.6.3. Case Studies Demonstrating Successful Integration 131
Summary 133
References 136

CHAPTER 5

Immunology and Allergy 139

Introduction 139
5.1. Types of Allergies 142
5.1.1. Food Allergies 143
5.1.2. Environmental Allergies 144
5.1.3. Drug Allergies 145
5.2. Mechanisms of Allergic Reactions 147
5.2.1. Role of IgE Antibodies 147
5.2.2. Histamine Release and Its Effects 148
5.2.3. Anaphylaxis and Severe Allergic Reactions 149
5.3. Diagnosis of Allergies 150
5.3.1. Skin Prick Tests 151
5.3.2. Blood Tests for Allergens 152
5.3.3. Patient History and Symptom Assessment 152
5.4. Treatment Options for Allergies 154
5.4.1. Antihistamines and Decongestants 155
5.4.2. Immunotherapy and Allergy Shots 155
5.4.3. Lifestyle Modifications and Avoidance Strategies 157
5.5. The Role of the Immune System 158
5.5.1. Innate versus Adaptive Immunity 158
5.5.2. Immune Response to Allergens 160
5.5.3. Tolerance and Sensitization 160
5.6. Current Research in Allergy and Immunology 162
5.6.1. Advances in Allergy Treatments 162
5.6.2. Genetic Factors in Allergies 163
5.6.3. The Impact of Climate Change on Allergy Prevalence 164
Summary 166
References 169

CHAPTER 6

Tropical and Travel Medicine 173

Introduction 173
6.1. Historical Context 176
6.1.1. Evolution of Internal Medicine 177
6.1.2. Development of Tropical Medicine 178
6.1.3. Impact of Travel on Disease Spread 178
6.2. Common Tropical Diseases 180
6.2.1. Malaria 180
6.2.2. Dengue Fever 181
6.2.3. Schistosomiasis 182
6.3. Preventive Measures 184
6.3.1. Vaccinations 184
6.3.2. Prophylactic Medications 185
6.3.3. Health Education and Awareness 186
6.4. Diagnosis and Treatment 187
6.4.1. Diagnostic Techniques 188
6.4.2. Treatment Protocols 189
6.4.3. Challenges in Treatment 190
6.5. Role of Travel Medicine 191
6.5.1. Pre-Travel Consultations 192
6.5.2. Risk Assessment 193
6.5.3. Post-Travel Follow-Up 193
6.6. Global Health Perspectives 195
6.6.1. Impact of Climate Change 196
6.6.2. Socioeconomic Factors 196
6.6.3. International Collaboration in Disease Control 197
Summary 199
References 202

CHAPTER 7

Genetics and Genomic Medicine 205

Introduction 205
7.1. Historical Background of Genetics 208
7.1.1. Key Discoveries in Genetics 209
7.1.2. The Human Genome Project 209

7.1.3. Evolution of Genetic Testing 210
7.2. Basic Concepts of Genetics 211
7.2.1. DNA Structure and Function 212
7.2.2. Genes and Alleles 213
7.2.3. Genetic Variation and Inheritance Patterns 214
7.3. Advances in Genomic Medicine 216
7.3.1. Next-Generation Sequencing Technologies 216
7.3.2. CRISPR and Gene Editing 217
7.3.3. Personalized Medicine and Targeted Therapies 219
7.4. Applications of Genomic Medicine 220
7.4.1. Disease Prevention and Risk Assessment 221
7.4.2. Treatment of Genetic Disorders 221
7.4.3. Pharmacogenomics and Drug Response 222
7.5. Ethical Considerations in Genetics 224
7.5.1. Genetic Privacy and Data Security 224
7.5.2. Ethical Implications of Gene Editing 225
7.5.3. Discrimination Based on Genetic Information 226
7.6. Future Directions in Genetics and Genomic Medicine 227
7.6.1. Emerging Technologies and Research 228
7.6.2. Potential for Curing Genetic Diseases 229
7.6.3. Global Health Implications and Accessibility 229
Summary 231
References 234

CHAPTER 8

Musculoskeletal and Orthopedic Medicine 239

Introduction 239
8.1. Anatomy of the Musculoskeletal System 242
8.1.1. Structure and Function of Bones 243
8.1.2. Role of Muscles and Tendons 244
8.1.3. Importance of Ligaments and Joints 245
8.2. Common Musculoskeletal Disorders 246
8.2.1. Osteoarthritis and Its Impact 247
8.2.2. Rheumatoid Arthritis and Treatment Options 248
8.2.3. Fractures and Their Management 249
8.3. Diagnostic Techniques in Orthopedic Medicine 251
8.3.1. Imaging Technologies: X-Rays, MRIs, and CT Scans 251
8.3.2. Physical Examination Methods 252
8.3.3. Laboratory Tests and Their Relevance 253
8.4. Treatment Modalities in Orthopedic Medicine 255
8.4.1. Non-Surgical Interventions: Physical Therapy and Medications 255
8.4.2. Surgical Options: Arthroscopy and Joint Replacement 256
8.4.3. Emerging Treatments: Regenerative Medicine and Stem Cell Therapy 257
8.5. Rehabilitation in Orthopedic Care 259
8.5.1. Importance of Rehabilitation Post-Surgery 259
8.5.2. Role of Physical Therapy in Recovery 260
8.5.3. Strategies for Preventing Re-Injury 261
8.6. Current Trends and Innovations in Orthopedic Medicine 263
8.6.1. Advances in Minimally Invasive Surgical Techniques 264
8.6.2. Use of Technology in Orthopedic Practice 265
8.6.3. Research on Biomaterials and Implants 265
Summary 267
References 270

CHAPTER 9

Obstetric and Gynecologic Medicine 273

Introduction 273
9.1. Historical Development of Obstetrics and Gynecology 276
9.1.1. Ancient Practices and Beliefs 277
9.1.2. Evolution of Medical Techniques 277
9.1.3. Key Figures in the Field 278
9.2. Major Areas of Focus in Obstetrics 279
9.2.1. Prenatal Care and Monitoring 280
9.2.2. Labor and Delivery Practices 281
9.2.3. Postpartum Care and Recovery 282
9.3. Major Areas of Focus in Gynecology 283
9.3.1. Routine Gynecological Exams 283
9.3.2. Management of Menstrual Disorders 284

9.3.3. Reproductive Health and Family Planning 285

9.4. Common Conditions Treated in Obstetric and Gynecologic Medicine 286

9.4.1. Pregnancy Complications 287

9.4.2. Gynecological Cancers 288

9.4.3. Hormonal Disorders 289

9.5. Advances in Technology and Treatment 291

9.5.1. Imaging Techniques in Obstetrics 291

9.5.2. Minimally Invasive Surgical Procedures 292

9.5.3. Telemedicine in Women's Health 293

9.6. Challenges in Obstetric and Gynecologic Medicine 295

9.6.1. Access to Care and Health Disparities 296

9.6.2. Ethical Considerations in Women's Health 296

9.6.3. Impact of Societal Attitudes on Care 297

Summary 299

References 302

CHAPTER 10

Critical Care and Emergency Medicine 305

Introduction 305

10.1. Historical Development of Critical Care 307

10.1.2. Evolution of Intensive Care Units (ICUs) 309

10.1.2. Key Milestones in Emergency Medicine 309

10.1.3. Impact of Technological Advancements 311

10.2. Role of General Practitioners in Emergency Situations 312

10.2.1. Initial Assessment and Triage 313

10.2.2. Stabilization of Patients 313

10.2.3. Referral to Specialized Care 314

10.3. Common Emergencies Encountered 316

10.3.1. Cardiac Emergencies 316

10.3.2. Respiratory Distress 317

10.3.3. Trauma and Injuries 318

10.4. Training and Skills Required for General Practitioners 319

10.4.1. Medical Education and Residency 320

10.4.2. Continuing Medical Education and Certifications 321

10.4.3. Practical Skills in Emergency Procedures 322

10.5. Challenges Faced by General Practitioners in Emergency Medicine 323

10.5.1. Resource Limitations in Rural Areas 324

10.5.2. Time Constraints and Patient Volume 324

10.5.3. Emotional and Psychological Stress 325

10.6. Integration of Technology in Emergency Medicine 327

10.6.1. Telemedicine and Remote Consultations 327

10.6.2. Electronic Health Records and Data Management 328

10.6.3. Use of Mobile Applications for Emergency Protocols 329

10.7. Case Studies and Real-Life Applications 331

10.7.1. Successful Emergency Interventions by General Practitioners 331

10.7.2. Lessons Learned from Emergency Scenarios 332

10.7.3. Impact of Emergency Medicine on Patient Outcomes 333

10.8. Challenges in Critical Care and Emergency Medicine 334

10.8.1. Staffing Shortages and Burnout 335

10.8.2. Access to Care and Health Disparities 336

10.8.3. Evolving Guidelines and Best Practices 337

Summary 338

References 341

CHAPTER 11

Internal Medicine for Clinical Nutrition and Metabolism 345

Introduction 345

11.1. Role of Internal Medicine in Patient Care 348

11.1.1. Comprehensive Patient Assessment 349

11.1.2. Development of Treatment Plans 350

11.1.3. Coordination with Multidisciplinary Teams 350

11.2. Nutritional Assessment Techniques 352

11.2.1. Dietary History and Food Frequency Questionnaires 353

11.2.2. Anthropometric Measurements 353

11.2.3. Biochemical and Clinical Evaluations 354

11.3. Common Nutritional Disorders 356

11.3.1. Obesity and Metabolic Syndrome 357
11.3.2. Malnutrition and Its Consequences 357
11.3.3. Diabetes Management and Nutrition 358
11.4. Therapeutic Diets in Internal Medicine 360
11.4.1. Role of Medical Nutrition Therapy 361
11.4.2. Specific Diets for Chronic Conditions 361
11.4.3. Evidence-Based Guidelines for Dietary Interventions 362
11.5. Impact of Lifestyle Modifications 364
11.5.1. Importance of Physical Activity 365
11.5.2. Behavioral Changes for Better Nutrition 366
11.5.3. Role of Patient Education and Support 367
11.6. Challenges in Clinical Nutrition 368
11.6.1. Barriers to Effective Nutritional Interventions 370
11.6.2. Cultural and Socioeconomic Factors 370
11.6.3. Addressing Patient Compliance and Motivation 371
Summary 373
References 376

CHAPTER 12

Preventive Medicine and Public Health in Internal Medicine 379

Introduction 379
12.1. Historical Context of Preventive Medicine 382
12.1.1. Evolution of Preventive Medicine Practices 383
12.1.2. Key Milestones in Public Health Initiatives 383
12.1.3. Impact of Historical Events on Current Practices 385
12.2. Role of Internal Medicine in Preventive Care 386
12.2.1. Preventive Screenings and Assessments 387
12.2.2. Chronic Disease Management Strategies 387
12.2.3. Patient Education and Counseling 388
12.3. Public Health Policies and Their Impact 390
12.3.1. Overview of Major Public Health Policies 391
12.3.2. Role of Government in Preventive Health 391
12.3.3. Community Health Programs and Initiatives 392
12.4. Preventive Medicine Strategies 394
12.4.1. Vaccination Programs and Their Importance 395
12.4.2. Lifestyle Modifications and Behavioral Interventions 395
12.4.3. Screening Guidelines for Various Populations 396
12.5. Challenges in Implementing Preventive Medicine 398
12.5.1. Barriers to Accessing Preventive Care 399
12.5.2. Socioeconomic Factors Affecting Health Outcomes 399
12.5.3. Resistance to Change in Patient Behavior 400
12.6. Future Directions in Preventive Medicine 402
12.6.1. Innovations in Technology and Health Monitoring 403
12.6.2. Integration of Genomics in Preventive Strategies 403
12.6.3. Collaborative Approaches in Public Health 404
Summary 406
References 409

Index 413

LIST OF FIGURES

Figure 1.1. The intersection of internal medicine and dermatology
Figure 1.2. Dermatology, a vital branch of medicine
Figure 1.3. The role of internal medicine in dermatological conditions
Figure 1.4. The exploration of common dermatological conditions and their potential links to systemic diseases
Figure 1.5. The intricate relationship between systemic diseases and skin disorders
Figure 1.6. A comprehensive understanding of diagnostic approaches
Figure 1.7. The implementation of advanced imaging techniques has revolutionized diagnostic practices
Figure 1.8. The treatment modalities utilized in dermatology
Figure 1.9. The non-pharmacological interventions represent a cornerstone of patient management
Figure 1.10. Chronic conditions often manifest with distinctive dermatological implications
Figure 1.11. Autoimmune diseases and dermatological manifestations
Figure 1.12. Cardiovascular health and skin integrity
Figure 1.13. Patient education serves as a cornerstone in the realm of internal medicine
Figure 1.14. Addressing psychological aspects of skin conditions
Figure 1.15. The field of dermatology has witnessed significant advances in treatment modalities
Figure 2.1. The internal medicine within the realms of psychiatry and behavioral medicine
Figure 2.2. The intricate relationship between psychiatry and behavioral medicine
Figure 2.3. The historical context of psychiatry
Figure 2.4. Key figures have significantly influenced the field's evolution and practice
Figure 2.5.A Psychiatrist motivating a patient
Figure 2.6. Primary care and mental health
Figure 2.7. The integration of mental health assessments within internal medicine
Figure 2.8. Collaboration with mental health specialists
Figure 2.9. Types of depression
Figure 2.10. Substance use disorders (SUDs) present significant challenges within the realm of psychiatry in internal medicine
Figure 2.11. The integration of diagnostic tools and techniques
Figure 2.12. Presentation of clinical interview
Figure 2.13. Gathering of patient history forms a foundational component of psychiatric assessment

Figure 2.14. Psychopharmacology plays a pivotal role in the treatment and management of mental health disorders

Figure 2.15. Types of psychotherapy

Figure 2.16. Stigma surrounding mental health in internal medicine

Figure 3.1. The field of geriatric medicine

Figure 3.2. The Definition of internal medicine is multifaceted

Figure 3.3. The aging population represents a significant demographic shift poised to reverberate through various facets of society

Figure 3.4. Common health issues in the elderly

Figure 3.5. Mental health challenges, including dementia and depression

Figure 3.6. The importance of geriatric assessment

Figure 3.7. Comprehensive geriatric assessment (CGA): An organized evaluation method to provide a multidisciplinary assessment of and care for the elderly

Figure 3.8. Cognitive-assessment for senior

Figure 3.9. Older adults receive tailored healthcare

Figure 3.10. Management plans for polypharmacy

Figure 3.11. Medication management tips for seniors

Figure 3.12. Physiotherapist for elderly care

Figure 3.13. Addressing the social needs of older adults

Figure 3.14. Palliative care

Figure 3.15. The support provided to families and caregivers plays a crucial role in the realm of geriatric medicine

Figure 3.16. Barriers to accessing healthcare for older adults

Figure 4.1. The integration of internal medicine into oncology and palliative care

Figure 4.2. An overview of oncology reveals a complex field dedicated to the study

Figure 4.3. The role of internal medicine in oncology

Figure 4.4. Management of comorbidities

Figure 4.5. The framework of palliative care is grounded in its holistic approach

Figure 4.6. The distinction between palliative care and hospice care

Figure 4.7. The management of common oncological conditions

Figure 4.8. The field of epidemiology plays a critical role in understanding the incidence

Figure 4.9. Challenges in the provision of palliative care

Figure 4.10. Ethical considerations in treatment decisions

Figure 4.11. The realm of oncology treatments has witnessed remarkable advancements over the last few decades

Figure 4.12. Role of clinical trials in treatment options

Figure 4.13. The integration of palliative care into oncology

Figure 4.14. Early involvement of palliative care teams
Figure 4.15. Diagrammatic presentation of the components of holistic care
Figure 5.1. Allergy and immunology
Figure 5.2. An overview of immunology and allergy
Figure 5.3. Hives on the back are a common allergy symptom
Figure 5.4. Food allergens
Figure 5.5. Common environmental allergens
Figure 5.6. Drug allergy
Figure 5.7. The role of immunoglobulin E (IgE) antibodies
Figure 5.8. Anaphylaxis represents one of the most severe forms of allergic reactions
Figure 5.9. Skin prick test
Figure 5.10. Blood tests for allergies
Figure 5.11. The treatment options for allergies are diverse
Figure 5.12. Immunotherapy has emerged as a pivotal treatment strategy for managing various allergies
Figure 5.13. Innate immunity versus adaptive immunity
Figure 5.14. The concepts of tolerance and sensitization
Figure 5.15. Sublingual immunotherapy (SLIT)–allergy relief without injections
Figure 5.16. The impact of climate change on allergy prevalence
Figure 6.1. The internal medicine for tropical and travel medicine
Figure 6.2. The significance of tropical and travel medicine extends beyond the mere treatment of diseases
Figure 6.3. Physicians conducting a clinical examination of a patient, demonstrating hands-on diagnostic evaluation
Figure 6.4. The increased global interconnectedness has significantly intensified the impact of travel on the spread of diseases
Figure 6.5. Malaria symptoms
Figure 6.6. Schistosomiasis, a parasitic disease caused by the *Schistosoma* species
Figure 6.7. Vaccinations play a crucial role in the field of internal medicine
Figure 6.8. Health education and awareness
Figure 6.9. The importance of diagnostic techniques in internal medicine
Figure 6.10. The multifaceted challenges in treating tropical and travel-related diseases stem from both biological and logistical barriers
Figure 6.11. Pre-travel consultations are a crucial component of travel medicine
Figure 6.12. Upon returning from international travel
Figure 6.13. The intersection of global health perspectives with internal medicine
Figure 6.14. The influence of socioeconomic factors on health outcomes

Figure 7.1. Definition of genetics and genomic medicine
Figure 7.2. Historical background of genetics
Figure 7.3. The Human Genome Project (HGP)
Figure 7.4. The principles of genetics
Figure 7.5. DNA structure and function in internal medicine
Figure 7.6. Genes and alleles serve as the fundamental units of heredity
Figure 7.7. Genetic variation and inheritance patterns
Figure 7.8. The advent of next-generation sequencing (NGS) technologies
Figure 7.9. CRISPR and gene editing
Figure 7.10. The transformative potential of genomic medicine
Figure 7.11. The treatment of genetic disorders
Figure 7.12. Pharmacogenomics and drug response
Figure 7.13. Genetic privacy and data security
Figure 7.14. Discrimination based on genetic information
Figure 7.15. Emerging technologies and research
Figure 8.1. Musculoskeletal medicine encompasses a broad spectrum of disorders affecting the musculoskeletal system
Figure 8.2. Musculoskeletal disorders encompass a wide range of conditions affecting bones
Figure 8.3. The structural composition of bones
Figure 8.4. The importance of ligaments and joints
Figure 8.5. Osteoarthritis and its impact
Figure 8.6. The management of fractures is a critical aspect of musculoskeletal and orthopedic medicine
Figure 8.7. Imaging technologies: X-rays, MRIs, and CT scans
Figure 8.8. Laboratory tests and their relevance
Figure 8.9. Non-surgical interventions: Physical therapy and medications
Figure 8.10. Emerging treatments: Regenerative medicine and stem cell therapy
Figure 8.11. The significance of rehabilitation following surgery in the realm of musculoskeletal and orthopedic medicine
Figure 8.12. Effective strategies for preventing re-injury in musculoskeletal
Figure 8.13. Current trends and innovations in orthopedic medicine
Figure 8.14. Advances in minimally invasive surgical techniques
Figure 8.15. Use of technology in orthopedic practice
Figure 9.1. The field of obstetric and gynecologic medicine
Figure 9.2. The historical development of obstetrics and gynecology
Figure 9.3. The evolution of medical techniques
Figure 9.4. Major areas of focus in obstetrics

Figure 9.5. Labor and delivery practices
Figure 9.6. Major areas of focus in gynecology
Figure 9.7. The management of menstrual disorders
Figure 9.8. Common conditions treated in obstetric and gynecologic medicine
Figure 9.9. Pregnancy complications can arise from a variety of sources
Figure 9.10. The topic of gynecological cancers
Figure 9.11. Hormonal disorders
Figure 9.12. Imaging techniques in obstetrics
Figure 9.13. Telemedicine in women's health
Figure 9.14. Challenges in obstetric and gynecologic medicine
Figure 9.15. Access to care and health disparities
Figure 9.16. The ethical considerations in women's health
Figure 10.1. Critical care encompasses a specialized area of medical practice
Figure 10.2. The historical development of critical care can be traced back to the early 20th century
Figure 10.3. Key milestones in emergency medicine
Figure 10.4. Medical personnel simulate emergency treatment
Figure 10.5. Initial assessment
Figure 10.6. Manually stabilize a patient's head
Figure 10.7. Doctors discussing the referral of the patient to specialized care
Figure 10.8. Types of cardiac emergencies
Figure 10.9. An illustration of a respiratory emergency
Figure 10.10. Briefing the staff on the emergency situation
Figure 10.11. Continuing medical education (CME)
Figure 10.12. Cardiopulmonary resuscitation (CPR) is being performed on a medical-training
Figure 10.13. High patient volume in emergency care
Figure 10.14. A lady doctor with psychological stress
Figure 10.15. Telemedicine and remote consultations
Figure 10.16. A clinical provider uses the Massive Transfusion Protocol mobile app to determine whether a trauma patient just admitted to the emergency room requires a massive blood transfusion
Figure 10.17. General practitioners (GPs) in emergency medicine
Figure 10.18. Impact of emergency medicine on patient outcomes
Figure 10.19. The phenomenon of staffing shortages in critical care and emergency medicine
Figure 11.1. Clinical nutrition and metabolism
Figure 11.2. Internal medicine plays a crucial role in patient care
Figure 11.3. A comprehensive patient assessment
Figure 11.4. Coordination with multidisciplinary teams
Figure 11.5. The nutritional assessment techniques

Figure 11.6. Anthropometric measurements
Figure 11.7. The prevalence of common nutritional disorders
Figure 11.8. The rising prevalence of obesity and metabolic syndrome
Figure 11.9. Diabetes management and nutrition
Figure 11.10. Therapeutic diets in internal medicine
Figure 11.11. Role of medical nutrition therapy
Figure 11.12. Evidence-based guidelines for dietary interventions
Figure 11.13. Lifestyle modifications play a pivotal role in managing various health conditions
Figure 11.14. Implementing behavioral changes to enhance nutrition
Figure 11.15. Challenges in clinical nutrition
Figure 11.16. Cultural and socioeconomic factors
Figure 12.1. Physician discussing a medical report with a patient during a consultation
Figure 12.2. The historical context of preventive medicine
Figure 12.3. Key milestones in public health initiatives
Figure 12.4. The role of internal medicine in preventive care
Figure 12.5. Chronic disease management strategies
Figure 12.6. Public health policies and their impact
Figure 12.7. One of the most significant responsibilities of the government in preventive health
Figure 12.8. The significance of community health programs and initiatives
Figure 12.9. The adoption of preventive medicine strategies
Figure 12.10. Vaccination programs and their importance
Figure 12.11. Lifestyle modifications and behavioral interventions
Figure 12.12. Challenges in implementing preventive medicine
Figure 12.13. Socioeconomic factors affecting health outcomes
Figure 12.14. Resistance to change in patient behavior
Figure 12.15. Future directions in preventive medicine
Figure 12.16. Integration of genomics in preventive strategies

PREFACE

The science of adult medicine extends well beyond treatment of isolated systems or organs; it demands a rich appreciation of how multiple disease processes and patient characteristics interact over the life course. Clinicians must integrate information from basic science, epidemiology, and clinical trials to tailor care plans that balance acute presentation with chronic health maintenance. Simultaneously, the shifting demographic composition of populations around the globe—greater longevity and variations in disease patterns—has enlarged the clinician's role to include decision-making about end-of-life care, rehabilitation, and optimization of quality of life.

Advances in diagnostic technologies, from imaging to molecular diagnostics, continue to transform practice. But the greatest challenge is applying these tools effectively: knowing when the next test will be helpful, integrating findings into the context of pretest probability, and balancing intervention risks with patient expectations. And as personalized medicine gains traction, this underscores the imperative of accounting for genetic, environmental, and social determinants to predict disease susceptibility and therapeutic responses.

Internal Medicine – Volume 2 builds on foundational principles, covering areas that intersect with allied disciplines and meeting the diverse needs of diverse patient populations. This volume offers brief, evidence-based summaries of subspecialty information, practical advice on interdisciplinary practice, and case-based commentaries to illuminate real-world clinical decision-making. Utilized sequentially or as a point-of-care quick reference, its organizational form enables both study and clinical consultation.

Chapter 1 presents the basics of adult dermatologic practice in internal medicine. Discussed are issues such as the evaluation of rash and pruritus, systemic conditions affecting the skin, and the management of chronic inflammatory dermatoses. Tips on biopsy techniques, topical versus systemic treatment, and referral to dermatology specialists are discussed.

Chapter 2 focuses on the management and diagnosis of mental and behavioral health disorders. It explains common disorders such as depression, anxiety, bipolar disorder, and psychosis with particular reference to evidence-based psychotherapeutic and pharmacological interventions. The chapter also addresses substance use disorders, risk assessment of self-harm, and integration of mental health care into the primary practice.

Chapter 3 discusses age-specific health concerns for older adults. Physiologic changes with age, multimorbidity, polypharmacy, and geriatric syndromes such as falls, frailty, and cognitive impairment are addressed. Comprehensive geriatric assessment, functional status assessment, and goals-of-care discussions are emphasized.

Chapter 4 addresses cancer and palliative care in the context of internal medicine. It addresses common oncologic presentations, principles of chemotherapy and immunotherapy, and recognition of treatment toxicities. The chapter also addresses symptom control techniques, communication skills for serious illness discussions, and interdisciplinary models for supportive and end-of-life care.

Chapter 5 covers immune-mediated and allergic diseases. Subjects include the clinical and pathophysiologic presentation of asthma, allergic rhinitis, drug hypersensitivity, and primary immunodeficiency. Diagnostic methods, such as skin testing and immunologic tests, are addressed, as are immunomodulatory therapy and desensitization protocols.

Chapter 6 offers tropical and travel medicine concerns for internal medicine practitioners. An in-depth discussion of the epidemiology and clinical management of conditions such as malaria, dengue, typhoid fever, and parasitic infestations is presented. Pretravel consultation, vaccine counseling, and post-travel screening recommendations provide practical advice for outpatient and inpatient practitioners.

Chapter 7 stresses the integration of genetics and genomics into daily practice. The chapter covers fundamental genetic principles, the interpretation of genetic test results, and genomic profiling to assess disease risk. The chapter illustrates the evaluation of inherited conditions, pharmacogenomics-guided prescribing by pharmacogenomics, and ethical concerns in genomic medicine through case examples.

Chapter 8 consolidates musculoskeletal and orthopedic presentations encountered by internists. They encompass evaluation of joint pain, soft-tissue injury, inflammatory arthritis, and bone metabolic disease. The chapter offers imaging interpretation strategies, nonoperative care, and referral indications for surgery.

Chapter 9 covers medical considerations during pregnancy and women's health. The care of chronic conditions such as hypertension, diabetes, and thyroid disease during pregnancy; obstetric complications such as preterm labor, placental pathology, and fetal growth restriction; and postpartum management are covered. Interdisciplinary practice with obstetrics and gynecology specialists is emphasized, as is counseling on reproductive health.

Chapter 10 covers critical care and emergency medicine principles relevant to the internist. The chapter covers the initial assessment of the critically ill patient, hemodynamic monitoring, fundamental mechanics of mechanical ventilation, and management of common emergencies such as acute coronary syndromes, sepsis, and respiratory failure. Emphasis is placed on the use of rapid decision pathways and coordination with emergency and critical care teams.

Chapter 11 covers clinical nutrition and metabolic disorders in adult care. Nutritional assessment techniques, the treatment of malnutrition, obesity, and metabolic syndrome are discussed. Specialized nutrition support—enteral and parenteral feeding—is also covered, as is the dietary intervention role in chronic disease care.

Chapter 12 presents preventive medicine and public health strategies for internal medicine. Key topics include screening guidelines for common chronic diseases, immunizations, behavioral counseling for health behavior change, and management of social determinants of health. The chapter highlights the internist's role in population health and multidisciplinary prevention programs.

This text is geared toward medical students, resident physicians, practicing internists, nurse practitioners, and physician assistants seeking an easy-to-reference but thorough resource for subspecialty topics. It is meant to aid exam preparation, clinical rotation, and daily patient care. Educators and allied health professionals will also welcome concise outlines and practical frameworks to support team-based approaches and improve health outcomes across diverse patient populations.

INTERNAL MEDICINE FOR DERMATOLOGY

1

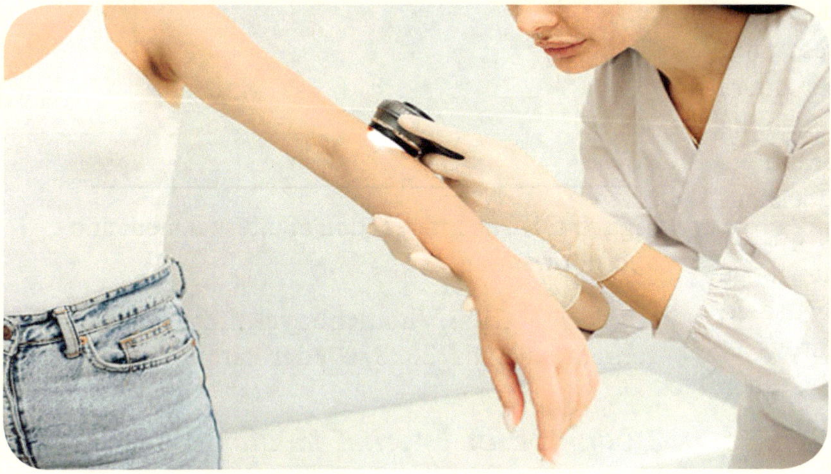

LEARNING OBJECTIVES

After studying this chapter, you will be able to:

1. Discuss the role of internal medicine in dermatological conditions
2. Explain the diagnostic approaches in internal medicine for dermatology
3. Focus on treatment modalities in dermatology
4. Describe the chronic conditions and their dermatological implications
5. Understand patient management strategies
6. Focus on emerging research and future directions

Introduction

In medicine, the intersection of dermatology and internal medicine has increasingly become a focus of study, addressing complex patient needs. Dermatology has traditionally been viewed as a distinct specialty, yet it frequently intersects with patients whose internal health conditions are closely reflected in their skin manifestations. Internal medicine provides a fundamental foundation of information on numerous systemic illnesses that dermatologists need to understand so they can properly diagnose and treat skin lesions that may represent more widespread underlying illnesses. This multidisciplinary approach not only serves the patient but also enables clinicians to devise holistic treatment regimens that address both skin and underlying disease. A profound knowledge of the human body from an internal medicine perspective equips dermatologists with the skills to make informed decisions, ultimately translating into improved patient outcomes. The evolving healthcare landscape has been significantly influenced by technological advances, particularly the embrace of artificial intelligence (AI) in healthcare environments. AI has emerged as a significant tool in healthcare, with the broad aim of improving patient outcomes and maximizing healthcare delivery. As healthcare organizations work to individualize patient care and improve population health, understanding the synergies between internal medicine and dermatology becomes essential.

The use of artificial intelligence in these disciplines enables the processing of enormous amounts of data, helping to produce more precise diagnoses and effective treatment plans. AI helps liberate healthcare providers by relieving them of mundane tasks, enabling them to have more meaningful interactions with patients and support complex decision-making, thereby improving the overall quality of care. A Strong internal medicine knowledge base can also help dermatologists to use AI more effectively in practice (Bekbolatova et al., 2024). Moreover, new technologies such as nanotechnology have been revolutionizing treatment processes, particularly in dermatology. The potential of nanotechnology in healthcare, particularly targeted therapy, is transforming traditional approaches to treating diseases, such as cancer.

By optimizing drug delivery and treatment efficacy, nanotechnology is a game-changing extension of patient care that in-house medical specialists must be aware of. This cross-disciplinary recognition enables dermatologists to consider holistic patient care, which could initiate revolutions in treating skin illnesses whose underlying causes are as yet unamenable to intervention. With continuous research revealing the synergy between these two fields, it is increasingly evident that integrating internal medicine and dermatology can lead to innovation for improving patient care and health outcomes (Chehelgerdi et al., 2023) (Figure 1.1).

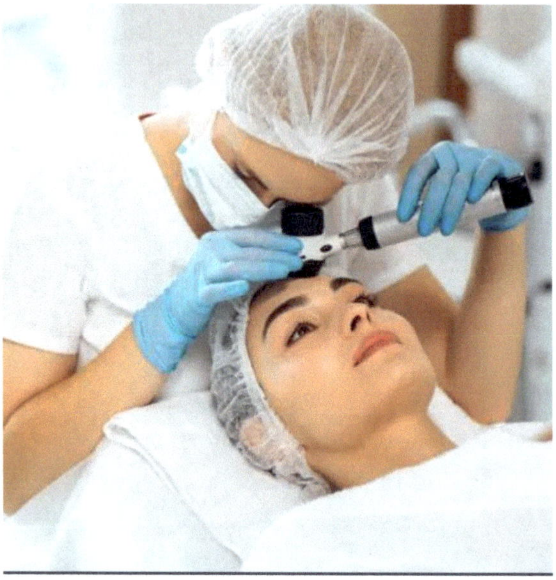

Figure 1.1. The intersection of internal medicine and dermatology.

Source: https://healthbayclinic.com/wp-content/uploads/2023/07/dermatology.webp.

Definition of Internal Medicine

The definition of internal medicine lies in its focus on the comprehensive treatment of adult patients, encompassing diagnosis, management, and prevention of a wide variety of diseases. internists, specialists in internal medicine, have expertise in both chronic and acute illnesses, providing detailed information regarding the body's various systems. This branch of medicine plays a fundamental role in multidisciplinary patient care, enabling collaboration with other disciplines such as dermatology. The internist's perspective is holistic, ensuring that underlying medical conditions that influence dermatological conditions receive adequate treatment and enhancing patient care significantly. This bridge between internal medicine and dermatology is needed, especially in evaluating skin illnesses with the potential for systemic implications or requiring multifaceted treatment, underscoring the necessity of an internal medicine background in dermatologic practice. In dermatology, the principles of internal medicine serve as a framework for interpreting complex dermatologic illness. These conditions have complex clinical presentations that need robust diagnostic skills to determine the underlying systemic etiology for dermatologic symptoms. For instance, cutaneous manifestations of systemic diseases such as lupus erythematosus or sarcoidosis require the services of internists to improve patient outcomes. The emergence of precision medicine, particularly in treating conditions such as atopic dermatitis, also illustrates the importance of integrating internal medicine into dermatological treatment paradigms. By employing deep assessments and biomarkers as determined by existing research, such as chemokine C-C motif ligand 17 analysis in atopic dermatitis, internists can optimize therapy regimens to address individualized patient needs, improving treatment efficiency and quality of life (Renert et al., 2021). In general, the prevailing significance of internal medicine is best seen in its utility to dermatology. There is an in-depth understanding of the pathophysiologic correlation between skin diseases and illnesses within the body, which is at the forefront of forcing the two fields to harmonize. With dermatologic complications becoming increasingly complex day by day, largely due to the rise in comorbidities and multifactorial causation, synergism between dermatology and internal medicine ensures a holistic approach to patient management. This integrated strategy enables disease prevention and tailors therapy regimens based on both general and dermatologic health. The Definition of internal medicine not only serves as the foundation of clinical practice but is also critical to the development of dermatology and to patient outcomes (Zuberbier et al., 2021).

Overview of Dermatology

Dermatology, a critical medical specialty, is focused on the investigation, diagnosis, and treatment of skin disorders, which significantly affect not only physical health but also patients' emotional and psychological well-being. Dermatology encompasses a wide variety of conditions, ranging from common conditions such as acne and eczema to complex conditions such as psoriasis and skin cancers. Given the skin's position as the body's largest organ, its various functions—varying from protective purposes, sensation, and heat regulation—it is crucial that dermatologists possess an extensive understanding of both internal and external factors affecting skin health. Also, the multidisciplinary nature of dermatology includes learning from immunology, pathology, and endocrinology. This integration is particularly relevant given the complex interplay between skin and internal diseases, with emphasis on the importance of dermatologists working in harmony with internal medicine specialists to provide effective patient care. The growing integration of technology and dermatology underscores the importance of incorporating new diagnostic methods and therapeutic approaches to enhance patient care. Most recently, artificial intelligence and deep learning have shown promise, particularly for early diagnosis of skin conditions such as vitiligo. Given that vitiligo is difficult to diagnose accurately due to its resemblance to other skin diseases, combining deep learning models can significantly improve diagnostic efficiency and accuracy. Utilizing models like Swin Transformer not only helps distinguish vitiligo of vitiligo from other hypopigmentation conditions but also offers better interpretability, which is essential for dermatologists tasked with making challenging decisions. Overall, the use of these technology tools underscores the need for dermatology to stay abreast of modern medicine, ensuring practitioners are equipped with the right tools to make accurate diagnoses and treat skin disorders effectively (Zhong et al., 2024). Additionally, dermatology incorporates key aspects of patient education and preventive medicine, which are components of internal medicine. Dermatologists are likely to be leaders in promoting healthy skin-related lifestyle habits, including sun protection, nutrition, and skin care.

Educating the patient about the risks of excessive sun exposure and the need for routine screening for lesions may lead to the early detection of malignancies, thereby supporting preventive care strategies. The discipline of dermatotherapy has also been expanded to encompass a wide range of interventions, from topical medications to advanced systemic therapies and phototherapy. This variety of options enables dermatologists to tailor treatments to individual patient needs, demonstrating the personalization of therapy in internal medicine. In this way, dermatology is not only a specialty that addresses skin diseases but also a dynamic contributor to health and well-being in the broader scope of medicine (Mergen et al., 2024) (Figure 1.2).

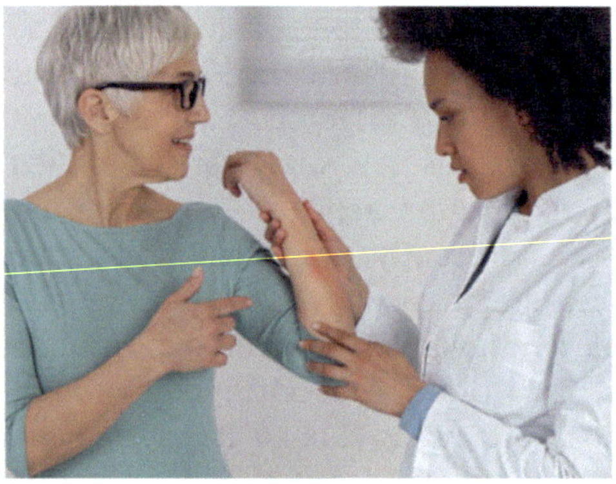

Figure 1.2. Dermatology, a vital branch of medicine.

Source: https://www.google.com/search?sca_esv=b0f9387028b0bfd0&sxsrf=AE3TifP-NwiTbTx4JavwmnGDixoVQh0KYQ:1751964469820&q=Internal+Medicine+for+Dermatology&udm=2&fbs=AIIjpHxU7SXXniUZfeShr2fp4giZ1Y6MJ25_tmWITc7uy4KIeioyp3OhN11EY0n5qfq-zENwnGygERInUV_0g0XKeHGJRAdFPaX_SSIJt7xYUfpm-75lA8Uar42yNWdqGuJlUAl_z5rxbQwJfseCgtKlK9ei0AWyXvoW1GpZmQ7JgAbwM0z2tYG_4RSbRyzyHcYz2pj6AZ4Q_AMYEQh-kh4YAtXa7uNJbA&sa=X&ved=2ahUKEwiz04ef8KyOAxWF1zgGHZ1rBREQtKgLKAF6BAgWEAE&biw=1517&bih=730&dpr=0.9#vhid=5eXwYR778p344M&vssids=mosaic.

Importance of Integrating Internal Medicine in Dermatology

The incorporation of internal medicine into dermatology significantly improves patient care through an integrated approach to diagnosis and therapy. Dermatological diseases often present as signs of systemic illnesses, and it is therefore imperative that dermatologists have a solid basis in internal medicine. For example, diseases such as lupus erythematosus or psoriasis might not necessarily be cutaneous in nature but can represent manifestations of underlying autoimmune or metabolic imbalances. This awareness allows dermatologists to collaborate with internists so that treatment plans address not only the cutaneous manifestations, but also any concurrent systemic consequences. By drawing on the knowledge gained in internal medicine, dermatologists can develop comprehensive treatment regimens that ultimately improve patient outcomes and maximize overall healthcare efficiency. Internal medicine and dermatology converge once more with the treatment of chronic illnesses that manifest through cutaneous changes. Research from large cohort studies, for instance, the Rotterdam Study, illustrates that cutaneous presentations are likely to occur alongside heterogeneous chronic disorders, e.g., diabetes, cardiovascular diseases, and hypertension. The Rotterdam Study has established significant correlations between the presence of skin illnesses and systemic markers of health, suggesting that cutaneous manifestations are predictors of underlying more serious disorders. Bringing internal medicine into dermatology equips dermatologists with the expertise to recognize such links and respond proactively. Not only does this integrative approach make it feasible for early diagnosis but also enables maximal opportunity to employ lifestyle or drug interventions that can treat both dermatologic and systemic conditions simultaneously. Additionally, newer technologies such as machine learning and deep learning in the healthcare sector warrant an integrated approach. These technological advancements are transforming how dermatologists process clinical data and detect patterns that can signpost broader systemic pathologies. While machine-learning algorithms can provide diagnostic insights, robustness issues and susceptibility to adversarial attacks highlight the utility of informed clinical judgment with internal medicine knowledge. Combining technology and a deep understanding of internal medicine makes it easier for dermatologists to navigate the complexity of patient care. With such sophisticated technologies in development, the integration of internal medicine and dermatology will be instrumental in ensuring safe, efficient, and patient-centered healthcare delivery, as noted in reports by researchers (Ikram et al., 2020; Qayyum et al., 2020).

1.1. The Role of Internal Medicine in Dermatological Conditions

Learning Outcome

1. Discuss the common dermatological conditions with internal links;
2. Explain the systemic diseases manifesting as skin disorders;
3. Focus on the importance of a comprehensive patient history.

Combining internal medicine and dermatology is critical to the complete care of many skin disorders. Internal medicine physicians are typically the first doctors to see patients with skin diseases, having access to early diagnosis and treatment of conditions that may have systemic implications. Psoriasis and eczema, for example, not only manifest on the skin but also indicate possible underlying metabolic or autoimmune illnesses. By recognizing the multifactorial nature of these diseases, internists can appropriately refer patients to dermatologists, enabling patients to access specialist treatment. Proper investigations by internists can also identify comorbidities that may complicate the treatment of skin disease and contribute to overall management planning for both skin and systemic disease. Lastly, this professional relationship between internal medicine and dermatology promotes integrated patient care that addresses not only the presenting skin symptoms but also general health issues. Beyond the diagnostic and referral proficiency of internal medicine, the management of chronic skin disease often involves multidisciplinary care. Internists are essential in coordinating care from several specialties, including endocrinology and rheumatology, where skin diseases are symptomatic of underlying health issues. For instance, conditions such as hidradenitis suppurativa and acne may require the services of several specialists to be treated appropriately. Internal medicine provides the basis for managing drugs and understanding how they interact, an aspect crucial when employing combination therapies used in dermatological management and other systemic treatments. Along with this, lifestyle modifications and education are also included in the treatment. Internists can advise patients about weight loss, smoking cessation, and dietary modification that will help the skin, along with overall health. Lastly, technological advancement at a rapid pace, particularly in artificial intelligence (AI), is revolutionizing internal medicine and dermatology to a great extent. The use of AI in clinics creates new opportunities to maximize diagnostic accuracy and therapeutic response. With advances in AI techniques, these can assist internists in detecting mild, easy-to-overlook dermatological disorders, enabling earlier intervention. Also, machine learning algorithms developed from deep learning make dermatoscopic image interpretation and clinical data easier to analyze, enhancing patient management streams. The application of AI in clinical practice not only makes diagnosis easier but also helps internists develop customized treatment plans according to the patient's profile. Therefore, the role of internal medicine in dermatological diseases is increasing, providing better patient outcomes through evidence-based and technology-based approaches (Esteva et al., 2021; Zuberbier et al., 2021) (Figure 1.3).

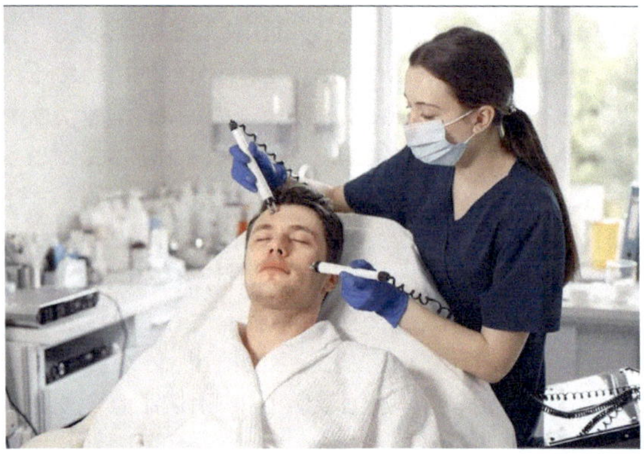

Figure 1.3. The role of internal medicine in dermatological conditions.

Source: https://lirp.cdn-website.com/af397b3f/dms3rep/multi/opt/Untitled+design+-+2024-07-16T103708.208-640w.png.

1.1.1. Common Dermatological Conditions with Internal Links

The dermatological and internal medicine interface is best represented by research on overlapping dermatologic conditions and their potential links to systemic disease. Eczema and psoriasis are clear examples of skin presentations that suggest the presence of occult metabolic or autoimmune disease. Psoriasis, which appears as red, thick, scaly lesions on the skin, has been found to be at high risk for cardiovascular disease, metabolic syndrome, and inflammatory processes. The inflammatory etiology of psoriasis would suggest a more systemic disease, highlighting the necessity for clinicians to intervene in the patient's overall health that extends beyond the skin's surface. This intersection of dermatologic and systemic health necessitates that the dermatology practice utilize a whole-system approach that incorporates dermatologic assessment alongside systemic disease screening to better serve the patient holistically. Eczema, a collection of inflammatory cutaneous diseases, is yet another prevalent dermatological condition that usually accompanies internal health issues. One can conclude that chronic eczema represents an atopic diathesis and, as such, is associated with asthma and allergic rhinitis, demonstrating how cutaneous afflictions may reflect sensitivities in the rest of the body. In addition, research into the microbiome has made it increasingly likely that imbalances of skin flora not only contribute to worsening eczema but also impact wider systemic illnesses such as metabolic disease and food allergy. This suggests that treating eczema effectively can have a snowball effect on patients' health and well-being, making it even more critical that dermatologists work extremely closely with other medical specialties. Lastly, this integrated management system emphasizes the need to acknowledge the intricately interrelated nature of skin diseases in internal medicine. The introduction of artificial intelligence (AI) into dermatological diagnosis holds promise for enhancing the detection and treatment of common skin diseases. Technologies based on artificial intelligence, designed to analyze medical images, have proven capable of detecting signs of diseases such as melanoma and other skin pathologies, thereby facilitating earlier diagnosis. Apart from that, large databases can be used to train AI algorithms that reveal correlations between skin state and systemic conditions, providing greater insight into how dermal conditions can serve as indicators of broader health conditions. With continued development in AI, it would reduce physicians' burden by optimizing diagnostic accuracy and speeding up treatment strategies for patients with chronic dermatological conditions. The technology benefits from combining the principles of internal medicine with dermatology practice, enabling a more comprehensive approach to patient care (Figure 1.4).

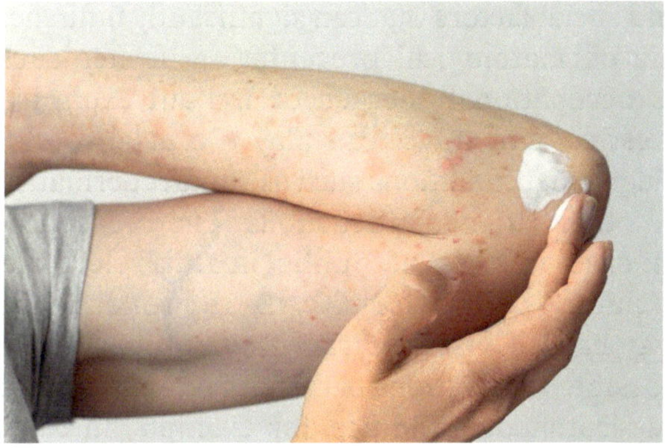

Figure 1.4. The exploration of common dermatological conditions and their potential links to systemic diseases.

Source: https://max-website20-images.s3.ap-south-1.amazonaws.com/Skin_Diseases_9e8c04488e.jpg.

1.1.2. Systemic Diseases Manifesting as Skin Disorders

The intricate interrelationship between systemic and skin diseases underscores the need for multidisciplinary approaches in internal medicine and dermatology. The majority of systemic diseases, such as autoimmune diseases and endocrine disorders, usually present initially as cutaneous manifestations. Skin, as the body's largest organ, is an important indicator of underlying systemic disease. For instance, vitiligo, which is depigmentation of body areas on the skin, can signify impairment of immunity or hormonal disturbance, as research emphasizes the significance of integrative treatment techniques in Ayurvedic medicine, which concluded that internal drugs together with external therapies can significantly influence the progression of disease and patient prognosis (Mulla, 2021). Understanding these associations not only aids in diagnosis but also guides effective treatment protocols that address both cutaneous manifestations and internal systemic illness. Pemphigus and pemphigoid are systemic immune diseases with severe cutaneous manifestations that often necessitate multidisciplinary medical intervention. These are illnesses that include the development of vesiculobullous lesions that can affect the skin and mucous membranes, leading to significant morbidity. Ocular surface involvement in these conditions ranges from mild irritation to severe complications, including vision impairment. Management must center on an interdisciplinary practice that unites dermatology, ophthalmology, and internal medicine to most effectively manage complications and optimize outcomes (Hansen et al., 2017). Integration is essential to adhering to carefully planned care that includes systemic treatments such as corticosteroids and immunosuppressants, which are necessary to manage inflammatory reactions and prevent damage to the skin and other affected organs. The recognition of systemic disease through dermatologic presentation underscores the importance of meticulous diagnostic evaluation and management planning.

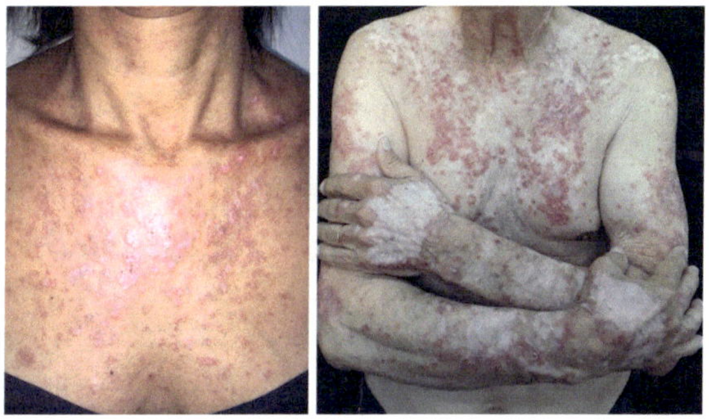

Figure 1.5. The intricate relationship b etween systemic diseases and skin disorders.

Source: https://static.elsevier.es/multimedia/03650596/0000009600000006/v2_202111180901/S036505962100204X/v2_202111180901/en/main.assets/gr2.jpeg.

Illnesses such as lupus erythematosus and psoriasis, for instance, affect not only the skin but also have systemic implications, including joint inflammation and organ dysfunction. Effective dermatologic management is more than the simple application of topical treatments;

incorporating systemic therapies to treat the underlying disease process is necessary. In dermatologically presented systemic disorders, recognition of pathophysiologic associations enhances treatment responsiveness and patient compliance. Additional clinical studies and research, particularly those measuring the impact of combined-modality treatment, are required to enhance further clinical practice in the management of skin-associated systemic diseases (Figure 1.5).

1.1.3. Importance of Comprehensive Patient History

A thorough patient history is the foundation of dermatology, as it can clarify the complexity of cutaneous disease that can be clinically indistinguishable yet pathophysiologically distinct. By obtaining complete historical data, clinicians can assess prior dermatologic illnesses, genetic skin diseases, and systemic illnesses that can affect the skin or manifest as cutaneous manifestations. For instance, the development of diseases such as multisystem inflammatory syndrome in adults poses clinical challenges, as skin symptoms overlap significantly with those of established dermatological diseases (Shaigany et al., 2020). Detection of these nuances relies on detailed patient histories that illuminate not only ongoing symptoms but also prior health events, leading to more accurate diagnoses and more effective treatment modalities. Additionally, a patient's history often includes environmental and social factors that can significantly influence the dermatological presentation. Issues such as occupational allergen or irritant exposure, lifestyle, and travel can play a crucial role in diagnosing conditions such as contact dermatitis or other cutaneous reactions. The recent rise in case reports of public health relevance, including those for COVID-19, reflects the way careful histories can provide insight into possible associations between systemic disease and cutaneous findings, for example, in cases simulating Kawasaki-like presentations in adults (Shaigany et al., 2020). In this way, awareness of these external influences through patient history enhances the physician's capacity to formulate effective therapeutic plans tailored to individual circumstances. Lastly, a good patient history not only enhances clinical understanding but also fosters a symbiotic doctor-patient relationship, which is very much a part of managing skin conditions. As soon as patients feel that their total histories are understood and appreciated, they are likely to engage in open communication about their complaints and therapeutic choices. This shared setting is helpful when considering both pharmacologic and non-pharmacologic treatment options, thereby providing a balanced approach to care. Specifically, using tools such as the SPIRIT Statement can help healthcare professionals design patient-centered clinical protocols, focusing on salient elements to improve dermatologist-patient relationships. This interplay of patient history and clinical practice ultimately results in improved patient outcomes for the dermatology practice.

Test Your Knowledge

1. Discuss the role of internal medicine in the diagnosis and management of systemic diseases with cutaneous manifestations.
2. Elaborate on the significance of comprehensive history-taking and systemic evaluation in the internal medicine approach to dermatological conditions.

1.2. Diagnostic Approaches in Internal Medicine for Dermatology

Learning Outcome

1. Focus on laboratory tests and their relevance;
2. Discuss the imaging techniques in dermatological diagnosis;
3. Explain the role of biopsies in internal medicine.

A systematic understanding of the diagnostic approaches in internal medicine for dermatology is essential to improved patient outcomes in the management of complex skin disorders. Integration with advancing medical technologies, e.g., molecular diagnostics and artificial intelligence, has revolutionized diagnostic approaches for dermatological disorders. For instance, the introduction of biomarkers enables better characterization of skin diseases, facilitating a more customized treatment approach. Such an approach aligns with the principles of precision medicine, which are most relevant in heterogeneous diseases like atopic dermatitis. Given the identification of specific biomarkers such as CCL17, physicians can stratify patients by clinical severity and predict therapeutic responses, thereby enhancing the compliance and efficacy of clinical interventions (Tiffany et al., 2023). In addition to biomarkers, the role of technology-based devices in diagnostic approaches cannot be underestimated.

The application of artificial intelligence, particularly large language models, to aid clinical decision-making has been established. Research has established that a large language model like ChatGPT scored at or near the passing score on the United States Medical Licensing Exam, underscoring its usefulness as an aid during medical education and practice. These models can potentially help clinicians review large datasets, provide differential diagnoses, and interpret lab results more efficiently (Tiffany et al., 2023). This technology is part of a broader trend of bringing computational assistance to dermatology, accelerating diagnostic speed without compromising accuracy. Lastly, the evolution of teledermatology has made it an indispensable diagnostic resource, particularly useful for expanding access to treatment and closing gaps in dermatologic care. Teledermatology enables dermatologists to remotely evaluate skin ailments using high-definition images and patient histories, cost-effectively. Not only does this overcome geographical limitations, but it also enhances patient compliance and convenience in follow-up treatment. Further, integrating teledermatology with traditional clinical assessments can lead to a more holistic understanding of a patient's condition when physicians use data on biomarkers and AI-based analytics. Overall, the combination of biomarkers, AI systems, and teledermatology is a synergistic advance in diagnostic methods, optimizing treatment in the field of internal medicine for dermatology (Renert et al., 2021) (Figure 1.6).

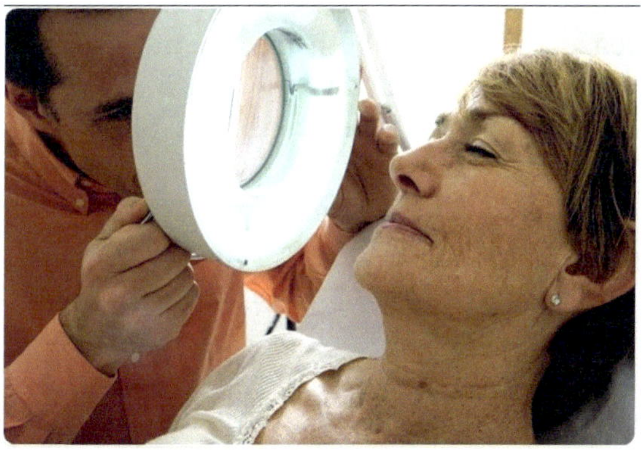

Figure 1.6. A comprehensive understanding of diagnostic approaches.

Source: https://www.news-medical.net/image-handler/picture/2016/10/Dermatology_Elderly_shutterstock_167925548.jpg.

1.2.1. Laboratory Tests and Their Relevance

In dermatology, laboratory investigations play a key role in the accurate diagnosis and treatment of many skin diseases. They allow clinicians to gather objective evidence that clarifies complex dermatologic processes, such as inflammation, infection, and malignancy. For instance, skin biopsies can provide histopathological data on psoriasis or skin cancers, enabling early and effective treatment interventions. Moreover, serological testing is helpful in detecting underlying systemic disease that manifests dermatologically, thereby allowing specific treatment to be instituted. Such tests enable dermatologists establish evidence-based management strategies, ultimately improving patient outcomes. The primary challenge in dermatology stems from the similarity of the presenting skin manifestations of different systemic diseases; hence, a multidisciplinary diagnostic approach is needed. Lab tests can differentiate between conditions that, on initial appearance, can look the same. For example, during the assessment of chronic urticaria, the presence of certain markers or antibodies can differentiate between autoimmune, physical, or idiopathicycc presentation of the disease and dictate both treatments as well as prognosis. As stipulated by newer guidelines, such as those for the treatment of urticaria, a deeper understanding of the biochemical mechanisms underlying skin reactions better equips physicians to prescribe personalized therapies, thereby improving patients' quality of life and clinical response (Zuberbier et al., 2021). Incorporation of novel laboratory tests aligns with newer therapeutic ideas, particularly for dermatological conditions with systemic implications. Inflammatory marker assays, either cytokines or specific antibodies, are more popular in laboratory and clinical studies. They are, for instance, useful not only for diagnosing chronic inflammatory disease but also for assessing therapeutic efficacy. Also, as evidenced in the management of anticoagulants for noncutaneous diseases, a structured approach based on test results can inform complex decision-making and optimize treatment plans (Steffel et al., 2018). This dynamic relationship between laboratory tests and dermatology underscores the crucial role they play in shaping the future of dermatologic medicine.

1.2.2. Imaging Techniques in Dermatological Diagnosis

In dermatology, the application of newer imaging techniques has revolutionized diagnostic work, improving the accuracy of assessing skin disease. Techniques such as dermoscopy, high-frequency ultrasonography, and reflectance confocal microscopy (RCM) are now irreplaceable for dermatologists. Dermoscopy is an extension of visual inspection that uses polarized or non-polarized light to observe subsurface anatomy and improve sensitivity in detecting malignant lesions. High-resolution ultrasonography provides clear images of the skin layers, enabling precise evaluation of conditions such as psoriasis or melanoma. These devices assist clinicians in making the right decisions, thereby reducing the need for invasive procedures in cases where a simple visual inspection is not sufficient. In contrast to the optimistic advances in imaging technology, problems concerning the accuracy of diagnosis and the standardization of these procedures exist.

A systematic review classifies the diagnostic performance of deep learning models applied to medical imaging as promising for dermatological assessment. While fusion with artificial intelligence is likely to enhance the performance of imaging equipment, there is a wide disparity in study designs and terminologies. Such heterogeneity can lead to biased perceptions of the efficacy of such models and thus call for universal reporting guidelines for dermatology. To address these challenges, researchers advocate for the development of artificial intelligence-specific EQUATOR guidelines that would detail protocols for reporting and assessing imaging devices' diagnostic accuracy, thus making them more reliable in clinical settings. Moreover, the future of dermoscopic imaging is likely to be influenced by emerging technologies and artificial intelligence. The use of machine learning and advanced analytics can potentially accelerate the diagnostic process, increasing the sensitivity and specificity of imaging modalities. By combining large datasets, machine learning algorithms can potentially enhance diagnostic criteria and enable the detection of skin cancers at an earlier stage. The impressive findings presented in studies assessing the diagnostic performance of deep learning across fields, including dermatology, point to the revolutionary capacities of such technologies (Tiffany et al., 2023). However, caution is necessary in the push for such integration to ensure that clinician training facilitates the interpretation of algorithmic assessments (Aggarwal et al., 2021). In light of the ever-evolving dermatological landscape, clinicians and scientists alike must be careful to objectively assess the value generated by these advanced imaging technologies (Figure 1.7).

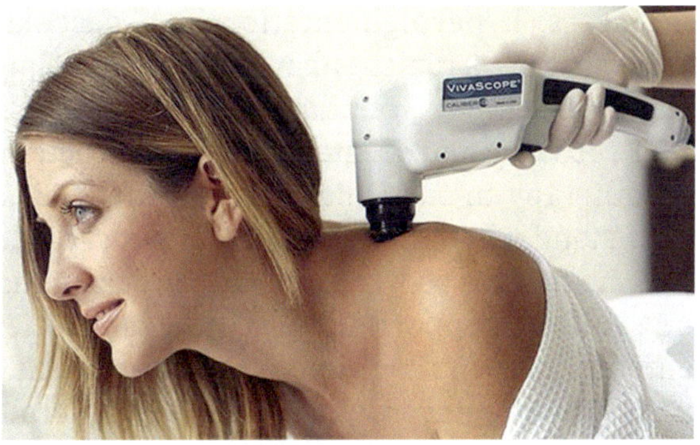

Figure 1.7. The implementation of advanced imaging techniques has revolutionized diagnostic practices.

Source: https://www.skincarenetwork.co.uk/wp-content/uploads/2018/05/scope-2.jpg.

1.2.3. The Role of Biopsies in Internal Medicine

In internal medicine, biopsies are an essential diagnostic tool, particularly in dermatology since skin lesions may indicate systemic disease. The utility of biopsies is not only in diagnosing skin disease; they can reveal occult pathology, such as malignancy or autoimmune processes. The scenarios seen in the General Medicine Unit of Ospedale del Mare illustrate the role of biopsies. For instance, patients with incorrect cosmetic skin conditions, such as spider lesions or suspicion of vasculitis, had their correct conditions—non-Hodgkin's lymphoma, for example—uncovered through large biopsies. This diagnostic precision not only shapes treatment plans but also enhances understanding of the interplay between dermatological presentations and internal diseases, underscoring the need for comprehensive diagnostic methods in internal medicine (Bologna et al., 2024). Besides their primary role in diagnosis, biopsies also provide critical prognostic information for the treatment of various conditions encountered in internal medicine. For example, in liver disease management, biopsies, despite their invasiveness, provide critical information on the degree of liver inflammation and fibrosis. This is most evident in non-alcoholic fatty liver disease (NAFLD), where differentiation between simple steatosis and non-alcoholic steatohepatitis (NASH) is essential. Non-invasive alternatives are more and more common; still, liver biopsies remain a gold standard that can guide the clinical pathway for the patients. Utilizing systematic diagnostic algorithms that involve biopsy results can guide treatment, particularly in determining the likelihood of progressing from NASH to cirrhosis or hepatocellular carcinoma (Awad et al., 2024). These considerations highlight the diagnostic and management role of biopsy, underscoring its irreplaceable value under challenging cases. Furthermore, biopsies may have a significant impact on research and educational aspects of internal medicine. As physicians encounter individual cases that fall short of usual diagnostic standards, these observations can stimulate enhanced awareness and ingenuity in diagnostic strategies. The interaction between skin and systemic disease, as evidenced by misdiagnoses in the clinic, underscores the need for continued education on biopsy methods and applications. Not only does such a comprehensive approach facilitate accurate diagnosis, but it also conveys the importance of what can seem like superficial signs of dermatologic disorders. This integration of biopsy data into broader clinical practice maintains the very collective expertise, ultimately advancing patient outcomes and facilitating a greater appreciation for internal medicine's complexity as it pertains to dermatology (Awad et al., 2024; Bologna et al., 2024).

Test Your Knowledge

1. Describe the diagnostic approach of internal medicine to a patient presenting with a generalized skin rash.
2. Explain the internal medicine-based diagnostic approach to cutaneous manifestations of autoimmune diseases.

1.3. Treatment Modalities in Dermatology

Learning Outcome

1. Discuss the pharmacological treatments and internal considerations
2. Explain the non-pharmacological interventions
3. Focus on the role of multidisciplinary teams

The treatment modalities employed by dermatology include a variety of techniques appropriate for addressing diverse dermatological conditions, an indication of multidisciplinary thinking regarding dermatological wellness. Topical agents, such as corticosteroids and retinoids, are the first-line therapy for widespread cutaneous inflammatory diseases such as eczema and psoriasis. They operate by regulating the inflammatory response and repair of the skin barrier. For the more complex conditions, treatments at the systems level, such as biologics and immunomodulators, are receiving more attention. These interventions target specific pathways in pathophysiologic processes and yield improved outcomes for patients when traditional therapies fail. The integration of individualized treatment regimens is paramount, as dermatologic diseases often have multiple etiologies and responses to therapy, requiring clinicians to be agile in their therapeutic strategies. Furthermore, advances in phototherapy and laser therapy have revolutionized the treatment of skin disorders, particularly those resistant to conventional modes of treatment. Laser technology, including pulsed-dye and fractional carbon dioxide lasers, offers novel treatments for conditions such as acne scars, hyperpigmentation, and vascular lesions. These therapies enhance skin remodeling without injuring surrounding tissue, resulting in faster recovery and greater patient satisfaction. Phototherapy, in particular narrowband UVB, is also a standard in the treatment of widespread skin illnesses like psoriasis and atopic dermatitis. The evidence supporting these new modalities demonstrates their efficiency, with patients' quality of life improving significantly from these chronic skin ailments, as evidenced by research. By adopting these new modalities, dermatologists can enhance the therapeutic ambiance within their clinic. The integration of machine learning and artificial intelligence into dermatologic treatment strategies is` making inroads as a new front, revolutionary in its potential to individualize care sufficiently. Recent incursions into deep learning algorithms demonstrate their capacity to handle enormous data sets, enhancing diagnostic accuracy and treatment planning. AI-based dermatology applications, for instance, can assist in detecting malignancies early enough to enable timely and effective interventions. Moreover, advances in computer vision can expand treatment options and improve clinical outcomes by enabling more accurate assessment of skin disease (Esteva et al., 2021). Their implementation, however, needs to be preceded by careful consideration of the effects on ethics and interprofessional cooperation between medical staff. By applying technological innovation alongside proven treatment modalities, dermatology can continue to transform and offer patients integrated care that addresses each patient's unique needs (Figure 1.8).

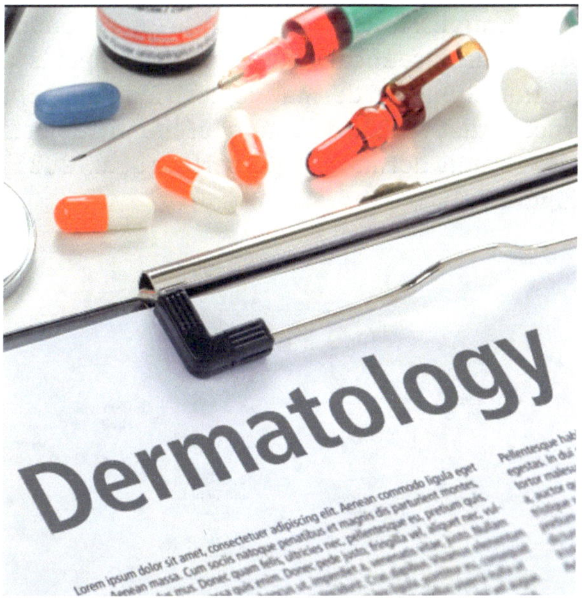

Figure 1.8. The treatment modalities utilized in dermatology.

Source: https://jivrajhealthcare.org/wp-content/uploads/2024/10/dermatology-treatment-in-ahmedabad.png.

1.3.1. Pharmacological Treatments and Internal Considerations

Pharmacologic management in dermatology thus necessitates a practical understanding of internal factors that can profoundly impact patient outcomes. Cutaneous disorders often have systemic elements, and their treatment accordingly necessitates coordinated care from specialists. A multidisciplinary approach, particularly with internal medicine, facilitates improved control of complex disorders that manifest cutaneous features. Evidence indicates that collaboration among these disciplines can improve diagnostic precision, leading to early intervention and treatment not only for skin conditions but also for related systemic health concerns (Borja et al., 2025). As medical care advances, fostering cross-disciplinary relationships remains critical to expanding treatment options and enabling optimal patient management in dermatology. Pharmacologic treatment regimens also need to address the potential metabolic and cardiovascular risks associated with dermatoses, such as psoriasis. A case-control study demonstrated the advantages of a multidisciplinary treatment strategy for psoriasis patients, including both dermatological symptom alleviation and decreased cardiovascular risk factors when primary care is shared between internal medicine and dermatology specialists (García-Malinis et al., 2024). Regarding not only cutaneous effects but also comorbidities, healthcare providers can develop coordinated treatment plans aimed at an integrative understanding of patient health. Therefore, combining dermatologic treatment with knowledge of internal medicine yields more effective management strategies tailored to each patient's needs. Systemic therapies, particularly immunomodulators and biologics, involve a carefully considered evaluation of the internal state of health, including laboratory examinations and cardiovascular risk factor assessment. Such pharmacotherapy can be severely toxic and compromise the overall well-being of the patients if not adequately monitored. Continual monitoring, through liaison with specialists in internal medicine, can guide adjustments of treatment regimens to reduce side effects and optimize therapeutic effectiveness. Education of the patient regarding lifestyle factors, such as dietary habits and physical exercise, also has a role in pharmacological management. By creating a model that encompasses both internal and pharmacological variables, medical professionals can optimize the efficacy of dermatological therapy and provide more holistic patient care.

1.3.2. Non-Pharmacological Interventions

In dermatology, non-pharmacological interventions are a mainstay of patient care, particularly for conditions such as urticaria. Unlike classical pharmacological treatments, these interventions target lifestyle modification and adjuvant therapies that maximize patient function. Examples are stress management strategies, including mindfulness and cognitive behavior therapy, which are increasingly recognized to alleviate symptoms of chronic urticaria. Their efficacy is often supported if used alongside integrative care approaches that consider not just the physical manifestations but also the psychological burden of skin diseases. The new international guidelines emphasize the priority of these support measures alongside evidence-based treatment measures, thereby validating their role in integrative patient care and chronic disease management (Zuberbier et al., 2021). Another promising non-pharmacological therapy in dermatology is the use of telemedicine, which is of very high significance in the face of the currently digitally reliant society. Telemedicine facilitates greater access to dermatology services, as patients can obtain consultations, follow-ups, and even educational resources from home. The approach not only adds convenience but also greater efficiency in healthcare. The research shows that telemedicine can deliver results comparable to, if not superior to, those of traditional face-to-face encounters, particularly in patient satisfaction and treatment adherence (Hashiguchi, 2020). Moreover, telemedicine erases the distance and accessibility hurdles posed by geography to healthcare and increases access for patients who may not be able to obtain the requisite dermatological care due to systemic disadvantages. Finally, dietary modifications and skin care habits are equally crucial in the management of dermatological disease through non-medical measures. Certain foods and allergens can trigger conditions such as urticaria or atopic dermatitis, so dietary interventions are a necessary component of management. The use of a personalized diet, perhaps with the help of a dietician, can make a significant difference to the skin and reduce flare-ups. Similarly, education on moisturization and soft-skin management may empower patients with the tools to maintain skin barrier function, which is crucial for preventing secondary infections or complications. Integration of these interventions with pharmaceutical interventions supports a multidisciplinary dermatological management process that enhances quality of life in subjects with chronic dermatosis (Zuberbier et al., 2021) (Figure 1.9).

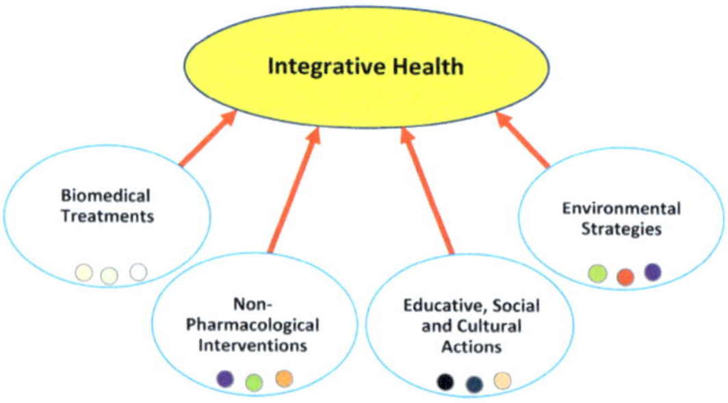

Figure 1.9. The non-pharmacological interventions represent a cornerstone of patient management.

Source: https://media.springernature.com/lw685/springer-static/image/chp%3A10.1007%2F978-3-030-60971-9_1/MediaObjects/499026_1_En_1_Fig1_HTML.png.

1.3.3. The Role of Multidisciplinary Teams

The use of multidisciplinary teams (MDTs) for the treatment of skin conditions is a clear example of how varied medical input can improve patient care. Because dermatological conditions often overlap with systemic disease, an interprofessional approach ensures effective treatment plans. For example, the coordinated care of psoriasis patients by both dermatologists and internal medicine professionals is highly beneficial. Such cooperation not only aims at dermatological symptoms but also at allied cardiovascular risk factors that are often overlooked in isolated treatment programs. The regular control of risk factors such as blood pressure and body mass index can be significantly improved by an MDT intervention. This association demonstrates how, through the exchange of knowledge across specialties, patient outcomes can be optimized through customized interventions, finally influencing the quality of care delivered in dermatology clinics (García-Malinis et al., 2024). In particular, the role of an MDT becomes crucial in complex cases where dermatological presentations are suggestive of systemic illnesses. Take, for example, the case of a young person presenting with Blue Rubber Bleb Nevus syndrome, where a complete assessment is needed beyond dermatological consultation. This involved significant internal complications such as anemia due to gastrointestinal bleeding, which required the expertise of gastroenterology and internal medicine experts, in addition to dermatology (Thomas et al., 2023). Multidisciplinary teams not only assist in identifying underlying conditions but also facilitate an integrated treatment approach. Coordination is especially critical in managing patients with rare or complex disorders, as all aspects of a patient's health are integrated to enhance patients' overall well-being. Additionally, establishing effective lines of communication among MDT members can lead to more streamlined processes, ultimately benefiting the patient. Ongoing case discussion, shared treatment planning, and collaboration on clinical resources foster a team culture that enables healthcare professionals to make informed group decisions. This model avoids disjointed care and enhances members' responsibility for patient outcomes. As in studies on the management of psoriasis patients, those treated by an MDT demonstrated improved health status, including reduced disease severity and enhanced cardiovascular parameters (García-Malinis et al., 2024). In summary, the contribution of multidisciplinary teams is paramount in providing integrative, patient-centered care, particularly in the complex realities of internal medicine and dermatology, where the intersection of physical and systemic wellness is central.

Test Your Knowledge

1. Discuss the various treatment modalities used in the management of chronic inflammatory skin diseases such as psoriasis and atopic dermatitis.
2. Explain the principles guiding the use of systemic therapies in dermatology, with emphasis on immunosuppressive and biologic agents.

1.4. Chronic Conditions and Their Dermatological Implications

Learning Outcome

1. Discuss the diabetes and skin complications
2. Focus on autoimmune diseases and dermatological manifestations
3. Understand cardiovascular health and skin integrity

Chronic illness characteristically presents with typical dermatologic manifestations, substantially modifying a patient's overall well-being and lifestyle. Cutaneous manifestations typically indicate incognito chronic illness, such as autoimmune disease, metabolic disorders, and systemic diseases. Conditions such as lupus erythematosus, for instance, induce cutaneous lesions that may be preceded by or accompanied by systemic symptoms. Also, diseases such as eczema and psoriasis affect not just the appearance of the skin but can be incapacitating and thus add to psychosocial impairment, which can exacerbate the already chronic conditions. Knowledge of these cutaneous manifestations is crucial for both dermatologists and internal medicine specialists, as early intervention can significantly influence patient prognosis by addressing not only the skin symptoms but also the underlying chronic diseases, thereby facilitating a more integrated treatment approach. The interconnection between dermatological manifestations and chronic diseases is also evident in the classification of urticaria as acute or chronic. New guidelines emphasize the importance of accurate diagnosis and personalized treatment regimens in chronic spontaneous and inducible urticaria, as these diseases can significantly impair a patient's quality of life and overall functionality (Zuberbier et al., 2021). Chronic urticaria, for example, can interfere with daily life, work performance, and even social conduct. Therefore, dermatologists are called upon to evaluate these patients not only on the basis of their cutaneous findings but also by understanding the nuances of their chronic illnesses. By applying evidence-based therapies and diagnostic approaches, dermatologists can provide comprehensive care for the multifaceted problems posed by chronic urticaria and its prevalence in broader health contexts. Advancements in machine learning and artificial intelligence have the potential to revolutionize the integration of dermatology and chronic disease management. There are emerging computer vision technologies, profound learning-based technologies, which are being found to be utilized in dermatology (Esteva et al., 2021). They can enhance diagnostic efficiency and treatment algorithms by identifying skin changes associated with chronic disease, thereby facilitating personalized medicine. For example, AI can be applied to identify early signs of skin cancer or to assess inflammatory skin disease that negatively affects health in chronic patients. As these technologies continue to evolve, they will help address some of the clinical problems dermatologists face, leading to better patient outcomes through improved surveillance and care for dermatological manifestations of chronic conditions, ultimately bridging the gap between dermatology and internal medicine (Figure 1.10).

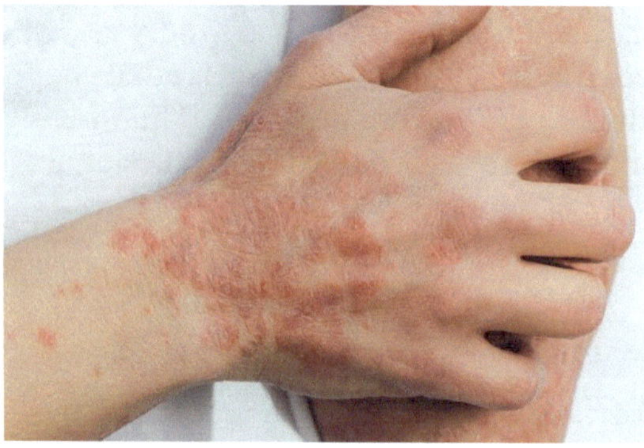

Figure 1.10. Chronic conditions often manifest with distinctive dermatological implications.

Source: https://drkumo.com/wp-content/uploads/2022/02/psoriasis-on-hands-chronic-skin-condition.jpg.

1.4.1. Diabetes and Skin Complications

Diabetes mellitus, with its resultant chronic hyperglycemia, significantly influences the skin, creating a myriad of associated complications that pose additional medical challenges. Diabetic skin lesions can manifest as xerosis, pruritus, and infection, as neuropathy and impaired circulation compromise the skin's integrity. The hyperglycemia also forms a substrate that supports bacterial and fungal infections, and there is therefore a clear indication for dermatologic evaluation and intervention. The development of diabetic cutaneous complications not only affects the quality of life but is also a marker for the systemic impact of the disease. Secondly, diabetic patients often present with conditions such as diabetic dermopathy and necrobiosis lipoidica, which are indicative of underlying metabolic dysfunction. Recognition of these cutaneous manifestations is helpful for clinicians, as they tend to indicate the overall level of glycemic control in patients and the likelihood of further complications. The solution also involves treating the psychosocial impact of cutaneous complications. Patients with visible skin diseases, such as those with diabetes, can be highly emotionally distressed, manifesting in a decreased sense of self-esteem and social retreat. These psychological states can exacerbate the disease process by stopping patients from continuing their diabetes management regimens or presenting themselves to obtain medical assistance in a timely fashion for skin issues. Thus, internal medicine doctors and dermatologists should adopt an integrated treatment model that not only mirrors the patients' physical health but also their psychological state. The integral model of care may include skin care advice and diabetes management training as part of an overall treatment plan. Moreover, overcoming psychological obstacles may empower individuals, enhancing compliance with treatment regimens and overall outcomes. In addition to conventional treatment modalities, new technologies such as telemedicine are becoming increasingly prominent as effective tools for the management of diabetic cutaneous complications. With telemedicine platforms, patients can receive proper consultation and follow-up without in-person visits, which can help fill gaps in health care access. This approach has shown promise across various specialties and may be of value in dermatologic practice by enabling faster diagnosis and treatment of diabetes-related dermatoses (Hashiguchi, 2020). Disparities in healthcare access and digital literacy must be reported, however, as they may detract from the value of telemedicine for some populations. Thus, while the incorporation of telemedicine promises to enhance diabetes management and treat skin complications, it must be implemented with careful consideration of equity and access to ensure that every diabetic patient benefits from these advancements.

1.4.2. Autoimmune Diseases and Dermatological Manifestations

Autoimmune illness is characterized by a pathological process in which the immune system is directed against the body's tissues, producing a wide range of clinical presentations. Skin manifestations are particularly prevalent in most autoimmune illnesses and are often important diagnostic clues. Systemic lupus erythematosus (SLE), for instance, can produce a distinctive butterfly rash, while scleroderma is indicated by skin thickening and changes in pigmentation. This correlation between systemic disease and cutaneous presentation underscores the importance of a comprehensive evaluation in dermatology practice. Not only do such correlations allow for early diagnosis, but they also allow for management interventions that consider both internal and external diagnoses, enhancing the quality of life for the patient. In addition, the pathophysiology of the dermatologic manifestations in autoimmune diseases involves immune dysregulation and inflammation. For example, psoriasis is a chronic autoimmune condition in which T cells invade the skin, leading to an exaggerated proliferation of keratinocytes and scaly plaques. Dermatomyositis, another autoimmune condition, presents with characteristic heliotrope rashes in the periocular area and a photosensitive, scaling rash over the trunk. These dermatological manifestations can be markers of incipient severe systemic involvement, including myopathy and malignancy, and highlight the central role that skin symptomatology plays in the comprehensive management of autoimmune illness. Early detection by these dermatological manifestations may permit intervention that averts hazardous sequelae. Management of autoimmune illness also extends beyond pharmacological treatments to include holistic regimens that address skin disease. Treatments may involve immunosuppressive medications that treat the underlying autoimmunity but also investigate such modalities as topical steroids and phototherapy to assist with alleviating skin symptoms.

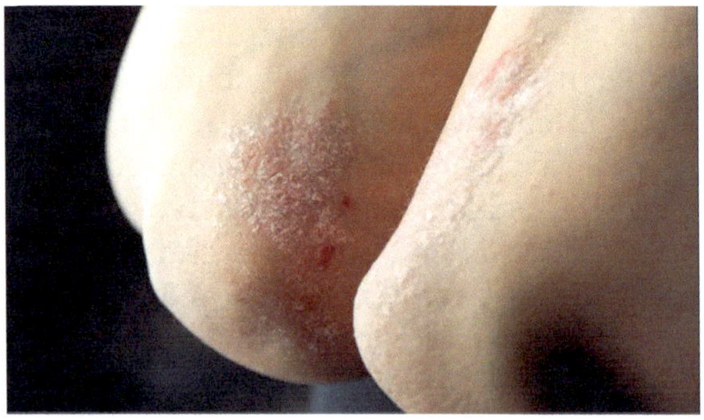

Figure 1.11. Autoimmune diseases and dermatological manifestations.

Source: https://images.everydayhealth.com/images/skin-beauty/psoriasis/9-autoimmune-diseases-that-affect-your-appearance-02-722x406.jpg?w=720.

Evolutions in targeted therapy and biologics over the past few years have dramatically changed treatment models for conditions such as chronic urticaria, prompting guidelines to update their evidence-based approaches to the management of this mast cell-mediated disease, which can profoundly impair quality of life (Zuberbier et al., 2021). In conditions such as atypical hemolytic-uremic syndrome, where complement dysregulation plays a role, novel treatment approaches point to the convergence of dermatological practice with internal medicine (Campbell et al., 2020). This combined view recognizes the necessity of dermatologists' interdisciplinary role in controlling complex autoimmune diseases (Figure 1.11).

1.4.3. Cardiovascular Health and Skin Integrity

The relationship between cardiovascular health and skin integrity is a multifaceted area of research that has attracted attention in dermatology research. Adequate circulation ensures the delivery of nutrients and oxygen to tissues, which directly impacts skin health and appearance. Dysfunctional cardiovascular health, typically characterized by hypertension and atherosclerosis, may lead to less-than-ideal blood flow. This decreased circulation can cause a myriad of skin conditions like delayed wound healing, skin aging, and increased infection susceptibility. With compromised dermal integrity, not only are the patients exposed to cosmetic woes but also severe health issues, placing the focus on treating cardiovascular aspects in dermatology. The role of systemic disease in dermal integrity cannot be overlooked either. Such chronic diseases as diabetes mellitus or chronic renal disease can exacerbate skin disease by damaging vascular function. For example, diabetes is well known to impair the skin's ability to regenerate through impaired circulation and elevated blood glucose levels, which also interfere with collagen production and skin elasticity. This endocrine disease demonstrates how internal physiological changes may manifest in the skin, leading to refractory problems such as infections or ulcerations that are difficult to treat. Solution-focused dermatologists need to adopt a solution-focused approach to patient management, recognizing that maintaining skin integrity can often be best achieved by addressing concomitant cardiovascular and systemic disease (Murugaiyan et al., 2022). New therapeutic modalities are now beginning to address the twin problems of cardiovascular and dermal health by exploring new approaches. New nanotechnology breakthroughs offer promising possibilities for more effective drug delivery, improving therapeutic response for skin ailments that are also associated with vascular health. Nanoparticles can be used to enhance drug delivery, enabling more targeted treatment of skin diseases caused by cardiovascular disorders. For example, nanomaterial formulations can enhance efficacy and absorption, thereby alleviating chronic skin conditions associated with compromised circulation, such as psoriasis and eczema. By employing such cutting-edge technologies, dermatology clinics can significantly enhance patient management and ensure skin integrity, ultimately bridging the gap that exists between dermatology and internal medicine (Harish et al., 2022) (Figure 1.12).

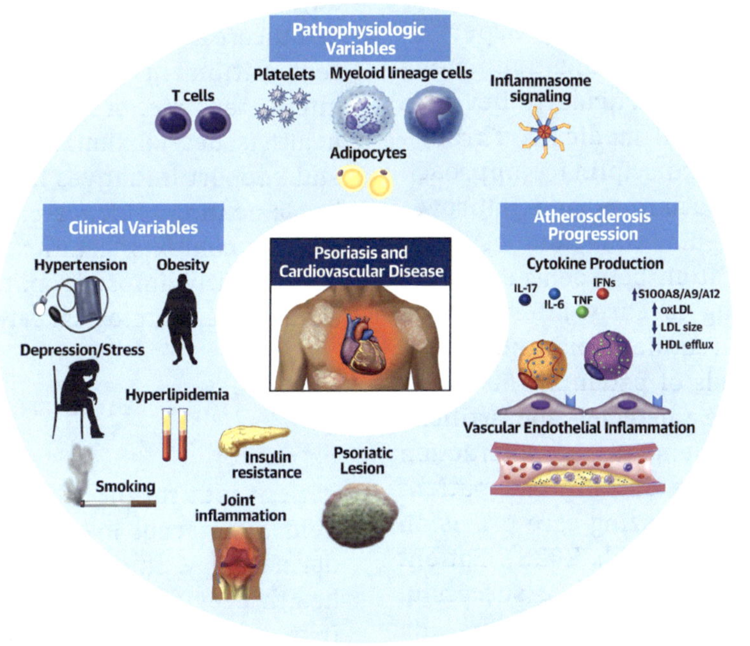

Figure 1.12. Cardiovascular health and skin integrity.

Source: https://www.jacc.rg/cms/asset/a10eecf8-8667-412b-966e-34c9761e4d45/fx1.jpg.

Test Your Knowledge

1. Discuss the cutaneous manifestations of chronic systemic diseases such as diabetes mellitus, chronic kidney disease, and chronic liver disease.
2. Evaluate the importance of dermatological findings in autoimmune and inflammatory chronic diseases such as systemic lupus erythematosus (SLE), rheumatoid arthritis, and inflammatory bowel disease (IBD).
3. How do these skin changes contribute to diagnosis, disease monitoring, and therapeutic decisions?"

1.5. Patient Management Strategies

Learning Outcome

1. Focus on the importance of patient education
2. Know follow-up care and monitoring
3. Understand addressing psychological aspects of skin conditions

In dermatology within internal medicine, practical patient management skills are vital for managing complex dermatology conditions that often overlap with conditions affecting the body at large. A key aspect of such skills is establishing coordination among interdisciplinary teams, particularly between dermatology and internal medicine. Through coordination, the multidisciplinary approach enhances diagnostic accuracy and improves patient outcomes. Regular consultations allow for better communication between healthcare professionals, leading to early interventions and a coordinated treatment plan adaptable to the individual needs of patients. The use of technology, such as telemedicine and artificial intelligence, can complement such interaction by enabling information sharing and patient monitoring, thereby optimizing care provision at multiple levels (Borja et al., 2025). Patient education is also a cornerstone of successful dermatological management programs. By educating patients about their conditions and potential treatments, clinicians can improve adherence to prescribed treatments and encourage active involvement in their disease care. Evidence-based education programs have been shown to increase patients' confidence in medical treatments and reduce the stigma commonly associated with healthcare for skin diseases. Moreover, awareness of the psycho-dermatological aspects of a patient's life—i.e., body image issues, and psychiatric impact—has a significant influence on treatment compliance and satisfaction with care. Patient education not only encourages patients but also creates a healthy support network in which health care professionals and patients can collaborate to adhere to treatment plans (Khanna et al., 2020). Lastly, determining the outcomes of varied patient management strategies is crucial to optimizing practices in internal medicine and dermatology. Prospective studies on the effectiveness of interdisciplinary collaboration and formalized patient education schemes are valuable for understanding what factors negatively or positively impact treatment outcomes. These findings will be used to inform subsequent management regimens and adjust the socio-economic determinants of healthcare access and provision. With increasing recognition in healthcare systems of the interdependence of systemic and dermatological health issues, maximizing resource distribution and support initiatives is of prime concern. By implementing evidence-based practice sensitive to local contexts, healthcare professionals can significantly improve patient outcomes and advance dermatological care (Borja et al., 2025).

1.5.1. Importance of Patient Education

Patient education is a cornerstone in the field of internal medicine, specifically within dermatology. Effective communication between health providers and their patients can result in a greater understanding of dermatologic disorders, adherence to treatment regimens, and ultimately in improved patient results. Informed patients about their conditions, signs, symptoms, and probable treatments, and become allies to their health care. This empowerment enables them to make informed decisions and adhere to suggested therapies to lower complication risks and enhance overall care satisfaction. Knowledge expansion via educational programs can also bridge gaps of health literacy found among different groups, ensuring equal access to medical care. Thus, integrating comprehensive patient education models into dermatological procedures is essential not only to address current problems but also to ensure long-term health maintenance. Besides, the use of new technologies, such as telemedicine, has revolutionized patient education in dermatology, providing scalable means to present vital information. Telehealth systems can provide visual materials, tutorial videos, and interactive guides tailored to the needs of specific patients. Most importantly, although telemedicine offers advantages in the delivery of educational content, digital illiteracy and health disparities may discourage disadvantaged groups from accessing these services, even when they need them most. Dermatologists must keep these differences in mind and work incrementally to create inclusive educational materials that serve diverse patient backgrounds. The implementation of telemedicine as a means to best utilize patient education enables the delivery of individualized advice promptly without the limitations of geographical location. The successful incorporation of technology ultimately can optimize the effectiveness of patient education in dermatology. In addition to education on their disease, patients must also learn the importance of adhering to prescribed therapies and recognizing side effects or complications. Understanding the likelihood of these adverse effects, especially with medications such as biologics or systemic agents, helps patients monitor their health more accurately. Indeed, education not only ensures compliance but also fosters an interactional climate in which patients feel valued and respected. When dermatologists effectively communicate the significance of routine follow-ups and the rationale behind maintenance therapies, patients are more likely to remain engaged over time. The implications of these strategies extend beyond individual care, as effective patient education contributes to better management of dermatological diseases across populations. Overall, the importance of patient education within dermatology cannot be overstated, since this lies at the root of both effective management and overall health literacy advancements capable of responding to the evolving healthcare delivery landscape (Figure 1.13).

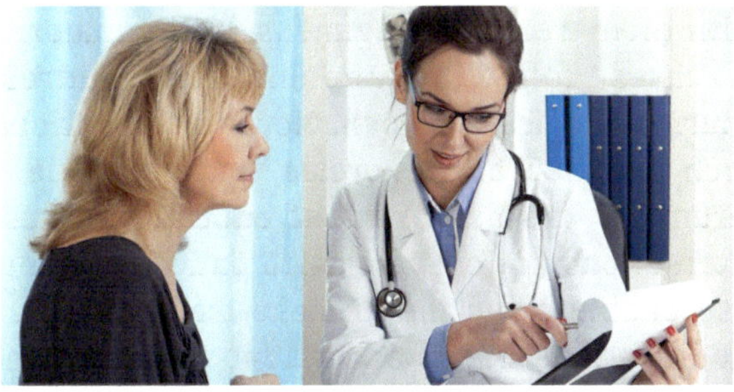

Figure 1.13. Patient education is a cornerstone of internal medicine.

Source: https://dermatology-innovation.com/wp-content/uploads/2024/05/patient-talking-to-doctor-instructions-1280x640.jpg.

1.5.2. Follow-Up Care and Monitoring

Successful management of dermatoses sometimes demands rigorous follow-up care and observation, particularly for patients with multifactorial or chronic diseases such as psoriasis. Multidisciplinary management, where dermatology and internal medicine collaborate, can significantly enhance patient outcomes. For instance, follow-up appointments allow medical teams to assess not only the cutaneous symptoms but also the associated comorbidities of skin diseases. This general monitoring will help detect cardiovascular risk factors, which are highly prevalent among psoriatic patients. Studies have established that collaborative follow-up care leads to better disease control and improvements in overall indicators of health, such as blood pressure and body mass index, as seen in collaborative models in clinics like the San Jorge University Hospital, where dermatology cross-refers between treatment methods (García-Malinis et al., 2024). Moreover, the implementation of routine follow-up regimens is important for ensuring patient adherence to therapies and lifestyle interventions. Follow-up allows frequent contact with an open forum where patients are encouraged to express problems with their treatment regimens. In the majority of cases, follow-up appointments address pharmacological and behavioral interventions, such as diet and exercise, and provide a forum for thorough patient education. These interactions not only facilitate patient care but also enable clinicians to make treatment plan modifications based on patient feedback and clinical improvement. The most recent guidelines established in 2023 emphasize the importance of individualized post-discharge follow-up care within the outpatient setting, emphasizing that productive monitoring practices contribute to improving quality-of-life outcomes as well as reduce the risk for complications among patients (Nehme et al., 2024). In addition to enhancing compliance among patients, rigorous follow-up care facilitates early detection of potential side effects of treatments, as treatments range from topical preparations to systemic immunotherapies. Monitoring is an essential tool for detecting complications or comorbidities in their early stages, thereby facilitating timely intervention. An active follow-up plan within the care of patients thereafter allows clinicians to mitigate risks, modulate treatment doses, and implement supportive interventions if necessary. Data from multidisciplinary clinics show that vigilant monitoring can significantly reduce the incidence of serious events, particularly among high-risk groups with metabolic syndromes. By optimizing follow-up care procedures, clinicians can enhance therapeutic effectiveness while improving skin condition stability and overall well-being in chronic dermatological patients (García-Malinis et al., 2024).

1.5.3. Addressing Psychological Aspects of Skin Conditions

The confluence of dermatology and psychology is critical since skin diseases tend to have severe psychological consequences, including depression and anxiety. People with visible skin ailments tend to have severe psychosocial disturbances, including stigma and social isolation, which further worsen the perception of their condition. Managing these psychological components is critical in dermatological practice to enhance overall patient outcomes. Psychodermatology, a new discipline combining psychological and dermatologic care, emphasizes the need to be sensitive to the emotional impact of skin diseases on patients. By incorporating mental health evaluations and interventions into dermatologic care, medical professionals can better support an integrated treatment plan that considers the patient's psychological status alongside physical symptoms, thereby increasing treatment compliance and patient satisfaction. Moreover, the early detection of the emotional burden associated with skin disease can lead to effective interventions that may prevent long-term psychological distress. Based on studies, patients with chronic skin diseases such as psoriasis and eczema are more prone to developing comorbid psychological disorders, thus underscoring the importance of routine screenings and psychiatric support. Collaboration between mental health specialists and dermatologists in an interdisciplinary environment is crucial to establishing a strong support network for patients. Not only does collaboration provide the support needed in psychological care, but it also enables frank discussions about the issues patients face. By successfully managing these psychological issues at the early stages of treatment, clinicians can assist patients with the intricacies of their conditions and enhance their quality of life. Finally, technology is becoming part of the healthcare system, particularly telemedicine, which offers new options for addressing the psychological needs of patients with skin disease. Telemedicine provides more flexibility and convenience in accessing mental health treatment, which can be very beneficial for individuals who are not comfortable with face-to-face consultations due to embarrassment or stigma. Because telemedicine has proven effective in providing care across various areas of medicine, including dermatology, the time has come to consider its role in offering mental health services alongside medical care. Regulatory uncertainty and varying degrees of digital proficiency pose obstacles. Still, the capacity to open up access to care can offer a means to meet gaps in mental health care, particularly for people who may not otherwise present themselves. This integration of dermatological care and psychological counseling through new service delivery has the potential to improve overall health outcomes, effectively meeting both the physical and mental needs of patients (Figure 1.14).

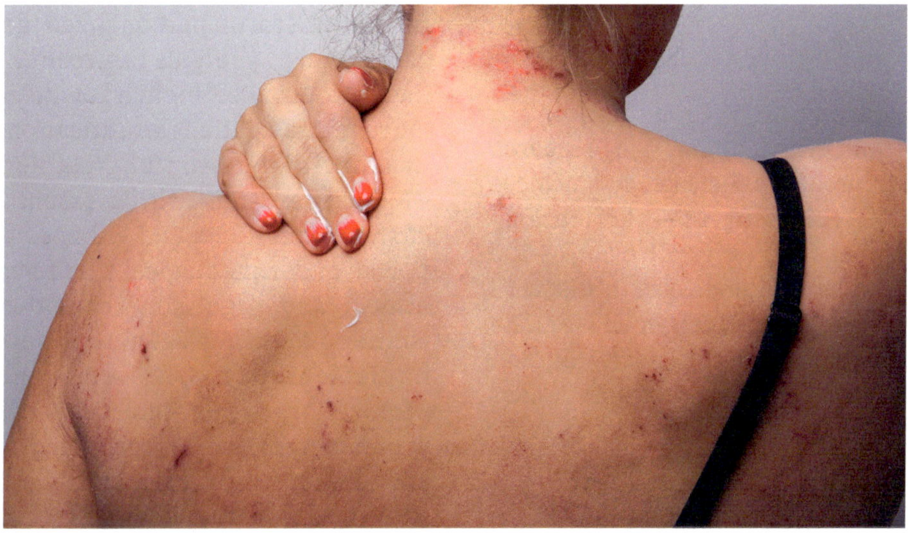

Figure 1.14. Addressing psychological aspects of skin conditions.

Source: https://www.healtheuropa.com/wp-content/uploads/2023/03/1-shutterstockKsenia-Kirillovykh_2078648983.jpg.

Test Your Knowledge

1. Outline the key components of an effective patient management strategy for a chronic dermatological condition such as psoriasis or atopic dermatitis.
2. Discuss the principles of holistic patient management in cases where skin conditions are secondary to systemic diseases (e.g., lupus, diabetes, HIV). How does the internal medicine approach ensure comprehensive care?

1.6. Emerging Research and Future Directions

Learning Outcome

1. Explain the advances in dermatological treatments
2. Discuss the role of technology in dermatology
3. Learn about future trends in internal medicine and dermatology

The field of dermatology is undergoing a transformative shift driven by emerging research and innovative approaches. Specifically, advances in single-cell technologies—particularly single-cell RNA sequencing (scRNA-seq)—are reshaping our understanding of skin diseases at a cellular level. These techniques enable researchers to explore the complexity of skin pathologies by classifying cellular responses and identifying specific disease subtypes. As highlighted by recent studies, integrating scRNA-seq into drug discovery not only improves target identification but also enhances our understanding of therapeutic mechanisms. This foundational research is paving the way for more personalized therapies tailored to individual patient profiles, marking a significant milestone in dermatological care and opening new avenues for disease control (Van et al., 2023). In addition, the integration of AI into dermatology presents a promising frontier for enhancing diagnostic accuracy and treatment effectiveness. A growing body of research highlights AI's potential, showing that machine learning algorithms can diagnose dermatological conditions with remarkable precision. This technology allows clinicians to detect and classify skin diseases more rapidly and accurately. However, the transition from research to clinical application presents several challenges, including the need for standardized datasets and robust ethical frameworks to protect patient privacy. Notably, privacy-preserving technologies such as federated learning are being developed to address these issues, enabling secure data sharing between institutions without compromising confidentiality. Overcoming these barriers is essential for the successful integration of AI in dermatological practice, which has the potential to streamline clinical workflows and improve patient outcomes (Khalid et al., 2023). Looking ahead, the convergence of single-cell analysis and AI is expected to usher in a new era of personalized dermatological care. Future synergies between these fields are likely to advance biomarker discovery, enable more precise patient stratification, and support dynamic monitoring of treatment responses. Ongoing research will be essential to address current limitations and enhance the predictive power of dermatological therapies. Meanwhile, ethical and regulatory considerations must continue to be evaluated to ensure responsible implementation. As such, the future of dermatology within internal medicine appears promising, driven by technological innovation and dedicated to enhancing patient-centered care in an evolving healthcare landscape.

1.6.1. Advances in Dermatological Treatments

In recent years, dermatology practice has seen significant advancements in treatment modalities that have enhanced the management of various skin conditions. Developments in topical therapies, biologic agents, and systemic treatments have broadened the spectrum of options available to clinicians. For example, biologic therapies targeting specific immune pathways have proven effective in managing chronic inflammatory skin disorders such as psoriasis and atopic dermatitis.These medications have transformed the standard of care, offering patients greater efficacy and fewer adverse effects compared to traditional treatments. Additionally, advances in phototherapy—including narrowband UVB (NB-UVB) and excimer laser—have improved the precision and effectiveness of skin disease treatment, resulting in better patient outcomes and highlighting the integration of internal medicine principles into dermatologic care models. Another significant development in dermatology is the growing emphasis on personalized medicine, which tailors treatment plans to each patient's unique characteristics, including genetic profiles and underlying systemic conditions. This is particularly important given the strong connection between cutaneous diseases and systemic metabolic or immune-related disorders. Through genetic screening and biomarker analysis, dermatologists can more accurately predict treatment responses and optimize therapeutic regimens. These approaches help minimize trial-and-error prescribing, improve treatment satisfaction, and enhance patient adherence. According to Bulkley, recognizing the systemic relevance of dermatological conditions is critically important. It compels clinicians to address the multifactorial nature of skin diseases rather than relying solely on localized treatment strategies (N/A, 2022). The emergence of digital health technologies has also revolutionized dermatological care. Teledermatology has become an essential tool, improving access to dermatology specialists, particularly in underserved populations. Additionally, mobile health platforms enable patients to monitor their symptoms, report changes in symptoms, and adhere to treatment plans more effectively. These technologies support improved communication between healthcare providers and patients, ultimately leading to better clinical outcomes. Moreover, as illustrated by the Korean Sepsis Alliance in developing sepsis treatment guidelines, structured clinical protocols can strengthen evidence-based practice and enhance patient safety (Park et al., 2024). The convergence of innovative treatment modalities, personalized medicine, and digital health technologies is poised to reshape dermatological care into a more integrated and universally applicable model that bridges internal medicine and dermatology (Figure 1.15).

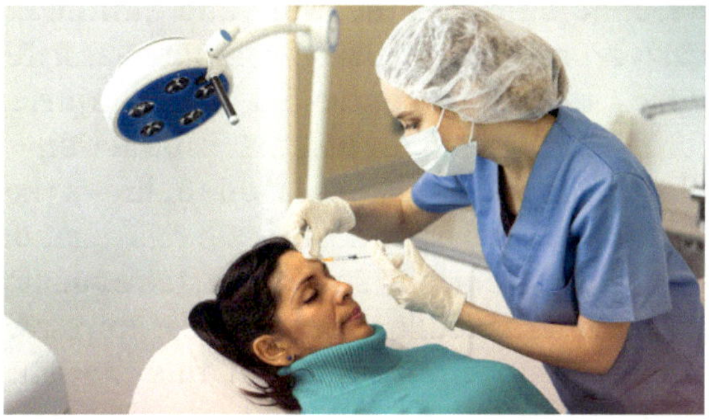

Figure 1.15. The field of dermatology has witnessed significant advances in treatment modalities.

Source: https://www.nanjappahealthcare.com/wp-content/uploads/2024/08/thumbnail-dermatology-768x432.png.

1.6.2 The Role of Technology in Dermatology

The integration of technology in dermatology has revolutionized the management of skin health, offering innovative solutions that enhance clinical practice. Among the most prominent developments is the use of (AI) in diagnostic processes. AI algorithms can analyze dermatological images and identify diseases such as melanoma and other skin pathologies with remarkable precision. This technology not only improves diagnostic accuracy but also enables the early detection of diseases that might otherwise remain undiagnosed during routine clinical examinations. The ongoing development and refinement of AI algorithms underscore the potential of technology to augment human expertise and foster improved patient outcomes. However, as AI becomes more prevalent, dermatologists need to adopt a critical, ethically grounded approach to its implementation. This ensures that the benefits of AI are realized without undermining patient-centered care or the nuanced exercise of clinical judgment (Crowe et al., 2024). Microneedling, a widely employed therapeutic technique in dermatology, exemplifies the convergence of technological innovation and minimally invasive procedures. Using computer-assisted devices to create controlled micro-injuries, microneedling stimulates the production of collagen and elastin, collagen being a key structural protein essential for skin rejuvenation. Recent enhancements, such as radiofrequency-assisted microneedling, have further improved the safety and effectiveness of this modality. These advancements allow dermatologists to treat a wide range of conditions—including wrinkles and acne scarring—with improved outcomes and reduced recovery times. Moreover, the flexibility of microneedling enables its combination with complementary therapies, thereby optimizing both results and patient satisfaction. As technological progress continues, microneedling—for both aesthetic and therapeutic applications—is poised to become a staple in dermatologic practice (Jaiswal et al., 2024). Ethical considerations regarding the adoption of advanced technologies in dermatology remain a top priority. The emergence of generative AI and other sophisticated systems necessitates that practitioners strike a balance between efficiency and the preservation of the empathetic components of patient care. Dermatologists must critically evaluate the scientific validity of new technologies, ensuring their deployment is based on a comprehensive understanding of potential benefits and pitfalls. Healthcare institutions bear responsibility for cultivating environments that support the mindful integration of innovations and foster collaboration between technology experts and clinicians. Ultimately, technology should complement—not supplant—the interpersonal dimension of dermatologic care, serving as a tool that enhances skilled, compassionate practice (Crowe et al., 2024).

1.6.3 Future Trends in Internal Medicine and Dermatology

The convergence of technology and medicine is poised to reshape both internal medicine and dermatology. A key trend is the growing application of AI and machine learning (ML) in diagnostic workflows. These systems can process extensive datasets to deliver accurate, timely diagnoses, especially in complex cases where human judgment may be limited. However, as reliance on AI increases, concerns about the explainability of algorithmic decisions become more urgent. The "black-box" nature of deep learning models—where decision-making processes are not transparent—raises critical issues related to trust, liability, and clinical utility. Consequently, the evolution of eXplainable Machine Learning (XML) has become essential. XML seeks to clarify AI-driven decisions, thereby bolstering clinician and patient confidence and reinforcing evidence-based decision-making (Rasheed et al., 2022). In parallel, nanotechnology represents a cutting-edge frontier in both dermatology and internal medicine. Nanomaterials offer unique physical and chemical characteristics that can significantly enhance drug delivery and therapeutic effectiveness. Nanoparticles can improve the therapeutic index of medications—maintaining effectiveness while reducing systemic side effects—making them particularly suited for localized dermatological interventions. These materials have applications that span therapeutic delivery, bioimaging, tissue regeneration, and antimicrobial treatments, underscoring their clinical versatility. Nevertheless, introducing nanomaterials into practice demands rigorous toxicological evaluation and robust regulatory mechanisms to ensure patient safety. Establishing safe dosage parameters and defining optimal anatomical and morphological specifications will be vital to their successful adoption (Harish et al., 2022). Looking forward, the future of internal medicine and dermatology lies in integrated, interdisciplinary models of care. This approach recognizes the close interplay between systemic diseases and dermatologic manifestations. Increasingly, internal medicine specialists and dermatologists will collaborate to manage conditions such as lupus and diabetes, which often present with significant skin involvement. Coordinated specialty care enables more comprehensive management and streamlined patient pathways, ultimately enhancing health outcomes. Telemedicine further facilitates this model by allowing remote consultation, expanding access to expert care. As these collaborative frameworks proliferate, they will enable tailored, patient-centered treatment strategies, fostering a holistic approach to complex health challenges across both internal medicine and dermatology.

Test Your Knowledge

1. What are some recent advances in biologic therapies for chronic inflammatory skin diseases like psoriasis and atopic dermatitis?
2. What role does AI play in the early detection and diagnosis of skin cancers?
3. What is the significance of pharmacogenomics in guiding systemic therapy for dermatological patients?

SUMMARY

The integration of internal medicine within dermatologic care represents a transformative shift toward holistic patient management. Recognizing the interconnections between skin and systemic conditions enables health professionals to craft treatment plans targeting both dermatologic needs and overall health. For instance, managing psoriasis effectively requires an emphasis on cardiovascular risk assessment, improving quality of life, and reducing long-term complications. This interdisciplinary paradigm underscores the importance of bridging gaps between dermatology and internal medicine to optimize patient outcomes. Emerging research supports evidence-based integration—such as combining opioid analgesics with antipsychotics to enhance pain control in complex dermatological scenarios—thereby advancing internal medicine practices. Synergistic innovations across both disciplines facilitate prompt intervention and sustained management of dermatologic conditions. With vigilant surveillance and adaptive treatment protocols, clinicians can significantly reduce complications originating from skin disease and concurrent systemic processes. Interprofessional collaboration—spanning internal medicine, dermatology, and radiology—bolsters diagnostic and therapeutic efficacy. Evidence points to enhanced disease detection and improved patient outcomes within multidisciplinary care models (Borja et al., 2025). Moreover, encouraging active engagement in clinical discourse improves patient satisfaction and promotes a clearer understanding of care plans (Flavio et al., 2025). Effective care is rooted in robust communication, regular interdisciplinary meetings, and technology-facilitated collaboration. Aligned with internal medicine's comprehensive ethos, this integrated framework elevates dermatologic care and fosters continuous professional development across specialties, ensuring optimal patient-centered outcomes in an evolving healthcare landscape.

KEY TERMS FROM THIS CHAPTER

- Pruritus
- Urticaria
- Anemia
- Autoimmune Disease
- Psoriatic Arthritis
- Malabsorption
- Erythema
- Vasculitis
- Diabetes Mellitus
- Systemic Lupus Erythematosus
- Metabolic Syndrome
- Nutritional Deficiency

CRITICAL THINKING QUESTIONS

1. Which systemic disease is most commonly associated with acanthosis nigricans?

a. Diabetes mellitus

b. Hyperthyroidism

c. Addison's disease

d. Systemic lupus erythematosus

2. Livedo reticularis is typically seen in which of the following conditions?

a. Polyarteritis nodosa

b. Psoriasis

c. Systemic sclerosis

d. Lichen planus

3. Which dermatological manifestation is classically associated with dermatomyositis?

a. Gottron's papules

b. Erythema multiforme

c. Koebner phenomenon

d. Erythroderma

4. A malar rash is most characteristic of which systemic condition?

a. Dermatomyositis

b. Systemic lupus erythematosus

c. Systemic sclerosis

d. Sjögren's syndrome

5. Which of the following is a cutaneous marker of internal malignancy?

a. Erythema nodosum

b. Erythema multiforme

c. Acanthosis nigricans

d. Urticaria

Short Answer Questions

1. What is the significance of acanthosis nigricans in internal medicine?
2. List three systemic diseases associated with livedo reticularis.
3. Describe the cutaneous manifestations of systemic lupus erythematosus (SLE).
4. Explain the significance of heliotrope rash.
5. Describe the skin manifestations of sarcoidosis.

Answers to Critical Thinking Questions

1. (a); 2. (a); 3. (a); 4. (b); 5. (c)

REFERENCES

1. Aggarwal, R., Sounderajah, V., Martin, G., Ting, D. S. W., Karthikesalingam, A., King, D., Ashrafian, H., & Darzi, A. (2021). Diagnostic accuracy of deep learning in medical imaging: a systematic review and meta-analysis. *Npj Digital Medicine*, *4*(1), 65. https://doi.org/10.1038/s41746-021-00438-zAjani, J. A., D'Amico, T. A., Bentrem, D. J., Chao, J., Cooke, D. T., Corvera, C. U., Das, P., et al. (2022). Gastric cancer, Version 2.2022, NCCN clinical practice guidelines in oncology. *Journal of the National Comprehensive Cancer Network*, *20*, 167–192. https://doi.org/10.6004/jnccn.2022.0008 (accessed on 17th July 2025).
2. Awad, Z., Ali–Eldin, A., Allam, M., & Mahmoud, M. I. (2024). Diagnostic role of non-invasive risk scores in prediction of simple steatosis versus non-alcoholic steatohepatitis. *QJM: An International Journal of Medicine*. https://www.semanticscholar.org/paper/09ad3c67b8b04c6bb2c58f2d60ab25b82835a3e5 (accessed on 17th July 2025).
3. Bahr, R., Clarsen, B., Derman, W., Dvořák, J., Emery, C. A., Finch, C. F., Hägglund, M., et al. (2020). International Olympic Committee consensus statement: Methods for recording and reporting of epidemiological data on injury and illness in sports 2020 (Including the STROBE extension for sports injury and illness surveillance (STROBE-SIIS)). *Orthopedic Journal of Sports Medicine*, *8*. https://doi.org/10.1177/2325967120902908 (accessed on 17th July 2025).
4. Bekbolatova, M., Mayer, J., Ong, C. W., & Toma, M. (2024). Transformative potential of AI in healthcare: Definitions, applications, and navigating the ethical landscape and public perspectives. *Healthcare*, *12*, 125–125. https://doi.org/10.3390/healthcare12020125 (accessed on 17th July 2025).
5. Bologna, D., Birra, M., Lugará, A., De Sena, A., Oliva, G., Tirelli, P., Madonna, P., et al. (2024). Skin lesions and the role of the internist: A series of clinical cases. *Italian Journal of Medicine*. https://www.semanticscholar.org/paper/bff968f043e3a442e762c4670991a2d5462d062b (accessed on 17th July 2025).
6. Campbell, C., & Kahwash, R. (2020). Will complement inhibition be the new target in treating COVID-19–related systemic thrombosis? *Circulation*, *141*, 1739–1741. https://doi.org/10.1161/circulationaha.120.047419 (accessed on 17th July 2025).
7. Chan, A. W., Tetzlaff, J., Gøtzsche, P. C., Altman, D. G., Mann, H., Berlin, J. A., Dickersin, K., et al. (2013). SPIRIT 2013 explanation and elaboration: Guidance for protocols of clinical trials. *BMJ*, *346*, e7586–e7586. https://doi.org/10.1136/bmj.e7586 (accessed on 17th July 2025).
8. Chehelgerdi, M., Chehelgerdi, M., Allela, O. Q. B., Pecho, R. D. C., Narayanan, J., Rao, D. P., Thamaraikani, T., et al. (2023). Progressing nanotechnology to improve targeted cancer treatment: Overcoming hurdles in its clinical implementation. *Molecular Cancer*, *22*. https://doi.org/10.1186/s12943-023-01865-0 (accessed on 17th July 2025).
9. Crowe, B., Shah, S. J., Teng, D., Ma, S. P., DeCamp, M., Rosenberg, E. I., Rodriguez, J. A., et al. (2024). Recommendations for clinicians, technologists, and healthcare organizations on the use of generative artificial intelligence in medicine: A position statement from the Society of General Internal Medicine. *Journal of General Internal Medicine*, *40*, 694–702. https://www.semanticscholar.org/paper/70da57c34ea19fe121a8251cae539515105518cb (accessed on 17th July 2025).

10. Esteva, A., Chou, K., Yeung, S., Naik, N., Madani, A., Mottaghi, A., Liu, Y., et al. (2021). Deep learning-enabled medical computer vision. *npj Digital Medicine, 4.* https://doi.org/10.1038/s41746-020-00376-2 (accessed on 17th July 2025).

11. García-Malinis, J., Pérez-Gilaberte, B., Gracia-Cazaña, T., González García, M. P., Planas Linares, D., & Gilaberte, Y. (2024). The impact of shared assistance between dermatology and internal medicine on patients with psoriasis. *Journal of Clinical Medicine, 13.* https://www.semanticscholar.org/paper/2742c85bedf3883ad3756356ab9bb4ba5ca32713 (accessed on 17th July 2025).

12. Gössi, F., Arpagaus, A., Becker, C., Gross, S., Bassetti, S., & Hunziker, S. (2025). Patient perspective of ward rounds in Swiss internal medicine departments: A mixed-methods study. *Swiss Medical Weekly.* https://www.semanticscholar.org/paper/787c79416ac9b0ff1760520aa0c235ca1c1511ed (accessed on 17th July 2025).

13. Grignoli, N., Livoti, S., Greco, A., Pironi, M., Noseda, R., Ceschi, A., Garo, M. L., et al. (2025). The impact of opioid analgesics with concomitant antipsychotic use on pain modulation and management in internal medicine: A cross-sequential study protocol. *Frontiers in Pain Research, 6.* https://www.semanticscholar.org/paper/34ef5021aa7a6d74a9b9a37b7cbb82e08d2ea583 (accessed on 17th July 2025).

14. Hansen, M. S., Klefter, O., Julian, H. O., Lynge, A. M., Pedersen, —, & Heegaard, S. (2017). Management of patients with ocular manifestations in vesiculobullous disorders affecting the mouth. *Oral Diseases, 23*(7), 849–853. https://www.semanticscholar.org/paper/4a3368e15fbe936b18310e34b54ce114c01fea36 (accessed on 17th July 2025).

15. Hashiguchi, T. C. O. (2020). Bringing health care to the patient. *OECD Health Working Papers.* https://doi.org/10.1787/8e56ede7-en (accessed on 17th July 2025).

16. Höhfeld, J., Benzing, T., Bloch, W., Fürst, D. O., Gehlert, S., Hesse, M., Hoffmann, B., et al. (2021). Maintaining proteostasis under mechanical stress. *EMBO Reports, 22.* https://doi.org/10.15252/embr.202152507 (accessed on 17th July 2025).

17. Ikram, M. A., Brusselle, G., Ghanbari, M., Goedegebure, A., Ikram, M., Kavousi, M., Kieboom, B. C. T., et al. (2020). Objectives, design and main findings until 2020 from the Rotterdam Study. *European Journal of Epidemiology, 35,* 483–517. https://doi.org/10.1007/s10654-020-00640-5 (accessed on 17th July 2025).

18. Jaiswal, S., & Jawade, S. A. (2024). Microneedling in dermatology: A comprehensive review of applications, techniques, and outcomes. *Cureus, 16.* https://www.semanticscholar.org/paper/3e0a39a0461a2d4e9fdd9b249f0581ae5fc34aa0 (accessed on 17th July 2025).

19. Ker, J., Wang, L., Rao, J. P., & Lim, C. C. T. (2017). Deep learning applications in medical image analysis. *IEEE Access, 6,* 9375–9389. https://doi.org/10.1109/access.2017.2788044 (accessed on 17th July 2025).

20. Khalid, N., Qayyum, A., Bilal, M., Al-Fuqaha, A., & Qadir, J. (2023). Privacy-preserving artificial intelligence in healthcare: Techniques and applications. *Computers in Biology and Medicine, 158,* 106848–106848. https://doi.org/10.1016/j.compbiomed.2023.106848 (accessed on 17th July 2025).

21. Khanna, G., de Wildt, L. A. M. de S. D. F., Bajaj, M., Lai, J., Gardiner, E., Fonseca, A. M. F. de A., et al. (2020). Improving treatment outcomes for leprosy in Pernambuco, Brazil: A qualitative study exploring the experiences and perceptions of retreatment patients and their careers.

BMC Infectious Diseases, 21. https://www.semanticscholar.org/paper/3f6179b6111fa5441b2a0fbdf073dbcbd4b92eb1 (accessed on 17th July 2025).

22. Kung, T. H., Cheatham, M., Medenilla, A., Sillos, C., De Leon, L., Elepaño, C., Madriaga, M., et al. (2023). Performance of ChatGPT on USMLE: Potential for AI-assisted medical education using large language models. *PLOS Digital Health, 2*, e0000198–e0000198. https://doi.org/10.1371/journal.pdig.0000198 (accessed on 17th July 2025).
23. Mergen, M., Graf, N., & Meyerheim, M. (2024). Reviewing the current state of virtual reality integration in medical education–A scoping review. *BMC Medical Education, 24*. https://doi.org/10.1186/s12909-024-05777-5 (accessed on 17th July 2025).
24. Mulla, S. (2021). Efficacy of Bastikarma in vitiligo. *International Journal of Cosmetics and Dermatology*. https://www.semanticscholar.org/paper/9fcfec6103b5cd13d43bf7fe75263dd0a7bc93fd (accessed on 17th July 2025).
25. Murugaiyan, J., Kumar, P. A., Rao, G. S., Iskandar, K., Hawser, S., Hays, J. P., Mohsen, Y., et al. (2022). Progress in alternative strategies to combat antimicrobial resistance: Focus on antibiotics. *Antibiotics, 11*, 200–200. https://doi.org/10.3390/antibiotics11020200 (accessed on 17th July 2025).
26. Nehme, M., Arsever, S., Tahar, A., Lidsky, D., Chevallier Lugon, C., Braillard, O., Grira, M., et al. (2024). [New developments and perspectives in outpatient general internal medicine]. *Revue Médicale Suisse, 20*(859), 200–206. https://www.semanticscholar.org/paper/09b400d96a9af115f676e7c67cb4f929007c1be9 (accessed on 17th July 2025).
27. Neira Borja, J. E., Plaza Alcívar, A. R., Estay Peralta, K. N., Calero Zea, M. A., & Vaca Rojas, M. de F. (2025). The diagnostic triad: Enhancing patient care through internal medicine, dermatology, and radiology collaboration–A narrative review. *Salud, Ciencia y Technology*. https://www.semanticscholar.org/paper/0c409457510a99449ef2dc3b153da2618b42716a (accessed on 17th July 2025).
28. Park, C., Ku, N. S., Park, D. W., Park, J. H., Ha, T. S., Kim, D. W., Park, S. Y., et al. (2024). Early management of adult sepsis and septic shock: Korean clinical practice guidelines. *Acute and Critical Care, 39*, 445–472. https://www.semanticscholar.org/paper/eb4a787f700a904a1a0b83093d1c4c2186483cca (accessed on 17th July 2025).
29. Qayyum, A., Qadir, J., Bilal, M., & Al-Fuqaha, A. (2020). Secure and robust machine learning for healthcare: A survey. *IEEE Reviews in Biomedical Engineering, 14*, 156–180. https://doi.org/10.1109/rbme.2020.3013489 (accessed on 17th July 2025).
30. Rasheed, K., Qayyum, A., Ghaly, M., Al-Fuqaha, A., Razi, A., & Qadir, J. (2022). Explainable, trustworthy, and ethical machine learning for healthcare: A survey. *Computers in Biology and Medicine, 149*, 106043–106043. https://doi.org/10.1016/j.compbiomed.2022.106043 (accessed on 17th July 2025).
31. Renert-Yuval, Y., Thyssen, J. P., Bissonnette, R., Bieber, T., Kabashima, K., Hijnen, D., & Guttman-Yassky, E. (2021). Biomarkers in atopic dermatitis—A review on behalf of the International Eczema Council. *Journal of Allergy and Clinical Immunology, 147*, 1174–1190.e1. https://doi.org/10.1016/j.jaci.2021.01.013 (accessed on 17th July 2025).
32. Sadeghi, H. M., Adeli, I., Călina, D., Docea, A. O., Mousavi, T., Daniali, M., Nikfar, S., et al. (2022). Polycystic ovary syndrome: A comprehensive review of pathogenesis, management,

and drug repurposing. *International Journal of Molecular Sciences, 23*, 583–583. https://doi.org/10.3390/ijms23020583 (accessed on 17th July 2025).

33. Shaigany, S., Gnirke, M., Guttmann, A., Chong, H. L., Meehan, S., Raabe, V., Louie, E., et al. (2020). An adult with Kawasaki-like multisystem inflammatory syndrome associated with COVID-19. *The Lancet, 396*, e8–e10. https://doi.org/10.1016/s0140-6736(20)31526-9 (accessed on 17th July 2025).

34. Steffel, J., Verhamme, P., Potpara, T., Albaladejo, P., Antz, M., Desteghe, L., Hæusler, K. G., et al. (2018). The 2018 European Heart Rhythm Association practical guide on the use of non-vitamin K antagonist oral anticoagulants in patients with atrial fibrillation. *European Heart Journal, 39*, 1330–1393. https://doi.org/10.1093/eurheartj/ehy136 (accessed on 17th July 2025).

35. Thomas, C. M., Kumar, K. G. S., Ekkalayil, D., Kumar, S. K., & Sithara, K. B. (2023). A case of blue rubber bleb nevus syndrome. *PARIPEX Indian Journal of Research*. https://www.semanticscholar.org/paper/44733fca2235387b16aacf79c16fc45d5c11fb0f (accessed on 17th July 2025).

36. Van de Sande, B., Lee, J. S., Mutasa-Gottgens, E., Naughton, B. J., Bacon, W., Manning, J., Wang, Y., et al. (2023). Applications of single-cell RNA sequencing in drug discovery and development. *Nature Reviews Drug Discovery, 22*, 496–520. https://doi.org/10.1038/s41573-023-00688-4 (accessed on 17th July 2025).

37. Vancha, H., Tewari, D., Gaur, M., Yadav, A. B., Swaroop, S., Bechelany, M., & Barhoum, A. (2022). Review on nanoparticles and nanostructured materials: Bioimaging, biosensing, drug delivery, tissue engineering, antimicrobial, and agro-food applications. *Nanomaterials, 12*, 457–457. https://doi.org/10.3390/nano12030457 (accessed on 17th July 2025).

38. Zhong, F., He, K., Ji, M., Chen, J., Gao, T., Li, S., Zhang, J., et al. (2024). Optimizing vitiligo diagnosis with ResNet and Swin transformer deep learning models: A study on performance and interpretability. *Scientific Reports, 14*. https://doi.org/10.1038/s41598-024-59436-2 (accessed on 17th July 2025).

39. Zhou, Y., Chia, M. A., Wagner, S. K., Ayhan, M. S., Williamson, D. J., Struyven, R., Liu, T., et al. (2023). A foundation model for generalizable disease detection from retinal images. *Nature, 622*, 156–163. https://doi.org/10.1038/s41586-023-06555-x (accessed on 17th July 2025).

40. Zuberbier, T., Abdul Latiff, A. H., Abuzakouk, M., Aquilina, S., Asero, R., Baker, D. R., Ballmer-Weber, B., et al. (2021). The international EAACI/GA^{2}LEN/EuroGuiDerm/APAAACI guideline for the definition, classification, diagnosis, and management of urticaria. *Allergy, 77*, 734–766. https://doi.org/10.1111/all.15090 (accessed on 17th July 2025).

PSYCHIATRY AND BEHAVIORAL MEDICINE

2

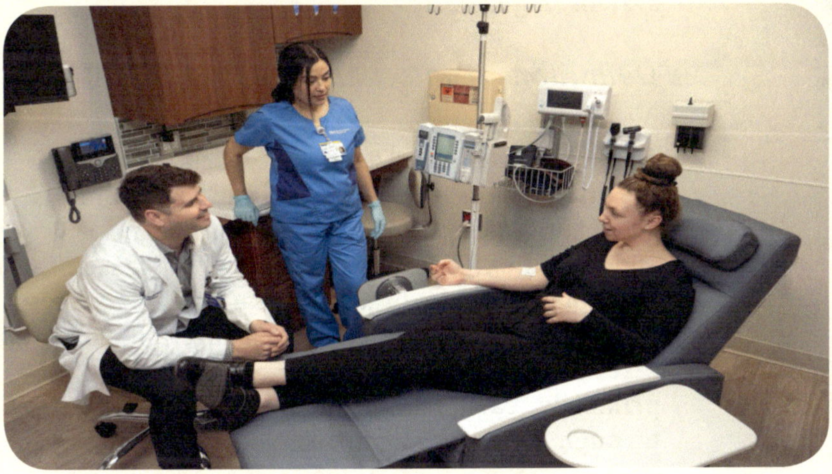

LEARNING OBJECTIVES

After studying this chapter, you will be able to:

1. Discuss the historical context of psychiatry
2. Explain the role of general practitioners in mental health
3. Describe common mental health disorders in internal medicine
4. Discuss diagnostic tools and techniques
5. Focus on treatment approaches in internal medicine
6. Learn about challenges in integrating psychiatry into internal medicine

Introduction

The integration of internal medicine into psychiatry and behavioral medicine is a critical area of research that combines physiological insights with mental health considerations. Such integration recognizes that physical wellness is significantly influenced by psychological factors, emphasizing the need for an interdisciplinary approach to patient care. Discrimination and microaggressions pose serious challenges to both the quality of medical education and the effectiveness of healthcare delivery in modern systems. For instance, while the literature highlights the detrimental effects of bias in healthcare settings—which can undermine trainee development and patient safety—introducing curricula that enhance residents' competencies to address these biases is essential for establishing an inclusive healthcare environment. By prioritizing experiential learning to help residents identify and respond to microaggressions, internal medicine residency programs can foster equity and support across the profession. The significance of addressing mental health is also clearly illustrated in behavioral sleep medicine, an interdisciplinary domain that merges behavioral psychology and sleep science. This field examines how psychological variables affect sleep quality and overall well-being. Referral patterns to behavioral sleep medicine clinics indicate that internal medicine physicians play a key role in connecting patients with appropriate care. However, barriers to initial access—including patient age and insurance status—can hinder effective treatment.

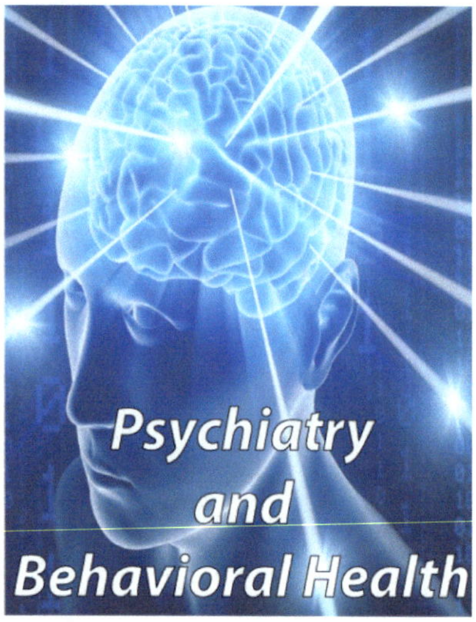

Figure 2.1. The internal medicine within the realms of psychiatry and behavioral medicine.

Source: https://www.sciencexcel.com/images/EdxBR6mNsPQOkteCBinyvEEMRmLvoc2FGMQsZUQk.gif.

Addressing these limitations requires a more integrated, patient-centered model that better supports behavioral health access through primary care pathways. As internal medicine continues to intersect with psychiatry and behavioral science, it becomes increasingly clear that incorporating mental health into general medical care is fundamental for improving patient outcomes. Educating healthcare providers about bias awareness and equipping them to address microaggressions can result in a more culturally competent workforce capable of delivering nuanced care across diverse settings. Additionally, dismantling barriers to behavioral services enhances treatment effectiveness by acknowledging the complex interplay between psychological and physical health. This approach not only improves the educational experience of medical residents but also ensures holistic, responsive patient care. The evolution of internal medicine to include these interdisciplinary elements marks a transformative shift toward a more comprehensive and effective healthcare system (Figure 2.1).

Definition of Internal Medicine

Internal medicine serves as the foundational specialty in integrated healthcare, particularly at the intersection with psychiatry and behavioral medicine. It focuses on the prevention, diagnosis, and treatment of adult non-surgical diseases affecting multiple organ systems. Internists apply specialized knowledge to manage complex cases involving numerous comorbidities. They primarily care for chronically ill patients through a holistic approach that addresses both physiological conditions and psychological factors that influence patient outcomes. The integration of internal medicine with psychiatry is especially crucial in managing chronic illnesses that significantly affect mental health. Conditions such as hypertension, diabetes mellitus, and cardiovascular diseases often lead to psychological consequences, including depression and anxiety. Research indicates that patients with chronic diseases are at an increased risk of developing mental health disorders. Consequently, internists play a vital role not only in managing the physical aspects of these diseases but also in recognizing and addressing their psychological impacts. This comprehensive approach improves overall patient well-being and enhances adherence to treatment regimens, benefiting both psychiatric and physical health outcomes. Modern internal medicine thus adopts a biopsychosocial perspective, recognizing the complex interplay between bodily illness and mental health, and moving toward integrated care models. Behavioral medicine further emphasizes the influence of psychological, behavioral, and cultural factors on physical health and healthcare delivery. Internists who incorporate behavioral assessments into their treatment plans are better equipped to manage medication adherence, lifestyle modifications, and coping strategies among patients. Understanding the interaction between physical and mental health enables internists to tailor interventions that improve patient outcomes, satisfaction, and quality of care. In this evolving landscape, internal medicine transcends traditional boundaries, embracing a broader definition of health that integrates both physical and psychological components.

Overview of Psychiatry and Behavioral Medicine

Psychiatry and behavioral medicine are closely linked disciplines increasingly recognized as essential to holistic patient care. Both fields focus on the impact of psychological and social factors on physical health and overall well-being, and promote integrated treatment strategies. There is growing evidence that mental health substantially influences outcomes in chronic illnesses such as diabetes and cardiovascular disease. Addressing psychiatric and behavioral issues allows healthcare providers to develop personalized interventions that alleviate symptoms and support long-term health maintenance. Psychiatrists specialize in diagnosing and treating mental illnesses, whereas behavioral medicine targets the connection between behavior and health. By employing evidence-based behavioral interventions, behavioral medicine aims to modify maladaptive behaviors and encourage healthier lifestyles. The emphasis on psychosocial factors ensures a comprehensive understanding and management of patient health. The integration of behavioral techniques into psychiatric care enables individualized treatment that addresses each patient's unique needs. This interdisciplinary approach facilitates improved management of coexisting psychiatric and somatic conditions, leading to better prognosis and quality of life. Medical education is evolving to reflect the importance of integrating psychiatry and behavioral medicine into internal medicine. Increasingly, medical curricula include training on the recognition and management of mental health conditions alongside physical illnesses. Exposure to clinical environments where psychiatric and physical care are concurrently provided helps reduce stigma and promotes comprehensive patient care. As psychiatry and behavioral medicine continue to intersect with internal medicine, this collaboration is poised to enhance healthcare delivery significantly, ensuring patients receive holistic and effective treatment (Figure 2.2).

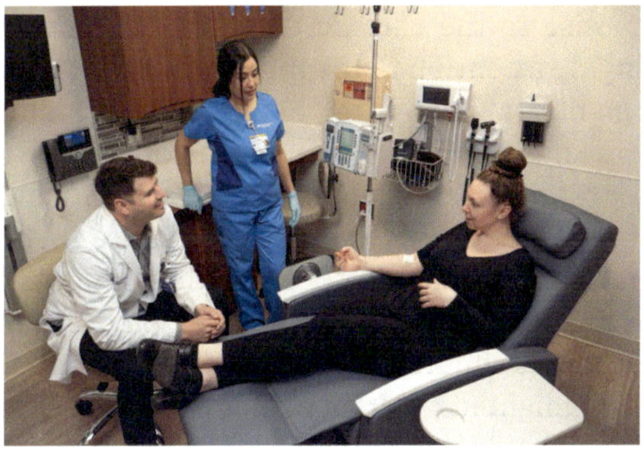

Figure 2.2. The intricate relationship between psychiatry and behavioral medicine.

Source: https://www.nm.org/-/media/northwestern/images/care-areas/behavioral-health/bh-ketamine-infusion.jpg?la=en&h=2800&w=4200&hash=8274435B6A60E89D7C9232270FC3F716.

Importance of Integrating Internal Medicine with Psychiatry

The conjoining of internal medicine and psychiatry is most important in responding to the complexity of patient care, especially with the increasing incidence of comorbid physical and psychiatric illnesses. By joining forces, health professionals are better placed to comprehensively understand and treat patients' health, considering that physical conditions can result from mental illnesses, and mental illnesses can result from physical conditions. For instance, diseases such as depression complicate chronic diseases like diabetes and hypertension to cause poorer health outcomes. With interdisciplinary approaches, practitioners are better positioned to ensure patient compliance with treatment, reduce hospital readmissions, and lower healthcare spending. This process ultimately illustrates a commitment to holistic care, in which every aspect of a patient's physical, psychological, and social health is addressed simultaneously to yield more effective clinical interventions. Moreover, concurrent care programs have grown in popularity as a response to the chronic disease phenomenon, bringing attention to the interconnected nature of mental and physical health. These models are designed to improve health outcomes by integrating professionals from various fields. This synergy has been shown to reduce mental illness stigma, making it easier for patients to feel comfortable accessing help for physical and psychiatric conditions. The COVID-19 pandemic has highlighted the importance of adaptive care models that integrate medical and psychological interventions within healthcare systems. Over this period, telehealth technologies demonstrated how simple such integration can be, bringing essential services to patients from a distance and enabling routine patient follow-up and interaction. The pandemic experience underscores the imperative for present and future integration within the healthcare sector. In behavioral medicine, integrating internal medicine concepts into psychiatric practice provides a treatment algorithm grounded in evidence. By incorporating scientific evidence into mental and physical disease states, clinicians can create individually tailored care plans that meet a patient's needs. This approach allows clinicians to monitor the influence of physical healthcare interventions on mental state and vice versa, enabling a targeted, patient-centered model of care. Research has shown that this integrative method not only enhances patient satisfaction but also delivers superior health outcomes, making it a vital component of modern-day healthcare practice. Through continuous communication and collaboration among healthcare providers, the integration of internal medicine and psychiatry not only optimizes treatment efficacy but also offers opportunities for innovation in medical education and behavioral health training.

2.1. Historical Context of Psychiatry

Learning Outcome

1. Understand the evolution of psychiatric practices
2. Discuss key figures in psychiatry
3. Explain the impact of historical events on psychiatric approaches

The history of psychiatry is therefore associated with the evolution of treatments given by the medical profession and public perception of mental illness. Initially, individuals with symptoms of mental illness were stigmatized and treated harshly, leading to their incarceration in asylums with insensitive care. It was during the Enlightenment era that a shift occurred: influential thinkers began advocating for humane care and the study of mental illnesses. This description not only helped establish institutions to provide care but also encouraged the development of psychiatric theories intended to describe the complexities of the human mind. As a footnote, powerful movements, including the anti-psychiatry movement, strongly rejected conventional medical models, with a focus on the socio-political contexts of mental health care and the priority given to connecting patient experiences and social conditions to psychiatric practice, eventually shaping current psychiatric treatment in internal medicine. In contemporary psychiatry, there is a clear shift toward integrated care models that bring mental health into broader health settings. This change embodies a paradigm shift from ascriptive institutionalization to community-based care that celebrates patient autonomy and social reintegration.

The World Health Organization has also emphasized the need for balanced care systems, with efforts to coordinate across sectors such as education and social services to optimize mental health outcomes. The "balanced care" model offers a compelling prototype for addressing mental health needs in internal medicine because it promotes services closely aligned with patients' milieus. Such integration is critical since mental illness among youth is likely to occur outside of the healthcare system—e.g., school and community settings—posing the challenge for widely based interventions that function outside clinic walls (Annemans et al., 2011). Moreover, the historical trajectory of psychiatry highlights the salience of cultural influences on the construction and regulation of mental health. For instance, the variation in mental health practice between nations, such as Japan and Italy, illustrates how cultural perceptions shape interventions and social representations of mental illness. This variance in understanding highlights the inadequacy of a globalized model of psychiatry, which necessitates understanding local contexts to develop efficient models of mental health care. Empirical research—for instance, observations of modernization's impact during Japan's Edo and Meiji periods—illustrates the influence of cultural models on contemporary psychiatric practice and the emergence of new spaces for social inclusion through community work and art (Bucci et al., 2014). As psychiatry continues to develop, cultural issues such as these remain crucial for establishing integrative treatment models in internal medicine (Figure 2.3).

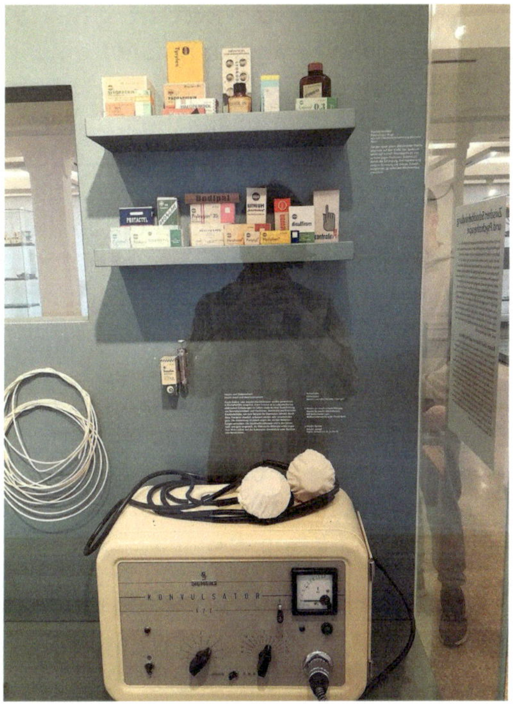

Figure 2.3. The historical context of psychiatry.

Source: https://upload.wikimedia.org/wikipedia/commons/thumb/b/bc/Psychiatric_Items.jpg/800px-Psychiatric_Items.jpg.

2.1.1. Evolution of Psychiatric Practices

The evolution of psychiatric practice has been influenced to a large extent by the transition from institutional to community-based care, most famously observed following the Second World War. The Ministry of Health's decision in 1961 to close down psychiatric hospitals across the UK initiated different trajectories for each region to change its mental health care system. In Scotland, for instance, hospitals did not vanish overnight; instead, they adapted their practices to fit the new mindsets about mental health. This was a process that took place over time, where institutional centers began embracing approaches designed to offer improved care to the patients and thus helped the overall transformation of psychiatric care.

Glasgow psychiatric provision during the 1970s is an example of how a great reliance on under-resourced hospitals co-existed with emerging ideologies of deinstitutionalization, indicating a complex progression rather than a static position of care (Long et al., 2016). Within psychiatric practice, a growing realization of the confluence of art and mental health has also expanded the debate regarding psychiatric care. Performance art, with its often visceral examination of the human condition, poses challenging questions regarding the intersection of physicality, mental illness, and societal responses to notions of sanity. The practices of artists such as Kira O'Reilly demonstrate how institutions are grappling with the implications of showcasing art that overlaps with bodily and psychic experience. In her work 'Wet Cup,' O'Reilly was confronted with institutional issues of health and safety, as well as with ideas of normalcy and sanity. The criticism she was subjected to speaks to a broader societal issue around the portrayal of mental illness in art that is symptomatic of the tension between institutional control and artistic autonomy. These considerations complicate the understanding of psychiatric practice because they are intertwined with mental health and artists' bodily representations of culture (Bartram et al., 2012). The development of psychiatric practice suggests a shift in society at large toward an understanding of mental health from a variety of vantage points, including reform of policy, integration into society, and cultural factors. New practice styles emerged that sought to put patient and community welfare first, ahead of the single task of symptom containment within the walls of an institution. Outpatient programs and community mental health programs were some of the advances that were made to take care beyond the stigma of hospitalization. Psychiatric practice expanded into more integrated practices, so care ideas now include patient autonomy and the maximum use of community resources. The continuous interaction among shifting ideologies, reiterations of policy, and cultural discourse underscores the necessity of an elastic, adaptive psychiatric practice attuned to the subtleties of mental health in contemporary society, thereby fostering wider recognition of human psychological welfare.

2.1.2. Key Figures in Psychiatry

In psychiatry, several prominent individuals have contributed immensely to the evolution and practice of the field, particularly in general settings. Sigmund Freud and other pioneering psychiatrists brought revolutionary ideas of psychoanalysis with far-reaching implications in altering the perception of the human mind and psychosis. Freud's writing focused on unconscious mechanisms and early childhood experiences, offering a theory that has stood the test of time through several modifications within the practice of psychotherapy. His emphasis on talk therapy paved the way for subsequent psychotherapeutic methods, influencing the integration of psychiatric care into internal medicine. These early assumptions have evolved to influence modern methods, enabling clinicians to analyze the subtle manipulations of mental illness through a therapeutic lens. Knowledge of Freud's work thus underscores the value of examining historical patients in psychiatry when assessing modern-day practices in general medicine. There is also Emil Kraepelin, who is universally regarded as the father of contemporary psychiatry due to his extensive studies and classification of mental illness. Kraepelin's methodical approach to psychiatric condition classification based on recognizable symptoms laid the fundamental foundation for the diagnostic procedures employed today. His work not only facilitated a more organized approach to mental illnesses but also paved the way for the development of the Diagnostic and Statistical Manual of Mental Disorders (DSM). This transformation towards evidence-based classification systems demonstrates that Kraepelin's contribution remains relevant to date in guiding general practitioners. With internal medicine increasingly becoming entwined in psychiatric factors, having an understanding of these categories is imperative for accurate diagnosis and treatment so that patients can be provided with appropriate overall care according to their specific mental health needs. Incorporation of evidence-based research into psychiatric care is also emphasized by existing programs, as discussed in psychological therapy services. These services offer a range of empirically grounded therapeutic modalities but encounter implementation challenges in clinical practice, as evidenced in recent evidence-based practice discourse. In seeking the subtlety of collapsing research and day-to-day care, it becomes evident that a comprehensive approach is needed to close the gap between evidence and practice. The intensive review and integration of feedback into such services give clinicians a chance to reflect on their practice while adopting new ways to enhance patient outcomes. Such endeavors resonate with the growing requirement for innovative mental health strategies in internal medicine, stressing the value of ongoing adjustment in the delivery of psychiatric care. With improvements in these services, they not only honor pioneers in psychiatry but also develop alongside contemporary challenges through diligence and research (Iveson et al., 2005; Howardova et al., 2013).

2.1.3. Impact of Historical Events on Psychiatric Approaches

The evolution of psychiatric methods has, in meaningful ways, been directed by historical events that redirected the world's frame of mind and clinical practices. For instance, significant wars have helped shape gains in how psychological trauma is comprehended, so that new psychiatric approaches are developed. World War I and World War II were times when soldiers' mental injuries were brought into the limelight, resulting in the development of psychotherapy and rehabilitation techniques that addressed previously ignored mental disorders. This revolution paved the way for a more compassionate awareness of mental sickness beyond treatments addressing the body. Therefore, integrating psychological dimensions into medical practice was unavoidable, and this was a turning point in reformulating the definition and role of psychiatry within internal medicine. In addition, historical occurrences have also accelerated the transformation of gender perceptions and their effects on mental health. The late 20th-century feminist movements highlighted the unique experiences of women in psychiatric treatment, calling out how gender interactions have a profound influence on psychiatric diagnosis and treatment. Studies show that standard psychiatric procedures previously ignored these gendered problems, creating a vicious cycle of confusion among medical professionals regarding women's mental health issues. For example, the findings of a Q-methodological study helped identify nine distinctive accounts of women's problematic behavior in secure psychiatric settings, pinpointing the moment at which frontline staff too frequently omitted consideration of gender in clinical assessment. This helps to underscore the imperative for feminist concerns to be integrated into psychiatric training and practice, as required by campaigners in the field, thereby informing current models of women's mental health care (Anderson et al., 2003). Moreover, the work of original thinkers in psychiatry has imprinted its own marks on contemporary practices, as seen with the critical considerations of thinkers such as Antoni Kępiński's. His observations about the conjunction of psychiatry and more general philosophical issues set the stage for discussions that continue to hold relevance in today's mental health debates. Comparing Kępiński's work with current paradigms allows tracing the historical development of psychiatric thought according to historical conditions. His emphasis on the psychophysical questions in psychiatry encouraged a more integrated approach to mental illness, accepting the complexity of human existence. Thus, the celebration of the historical roots in psychiatry for strategies is not only an appreciation for the work of earlier thinkers but also an enablement of more profound understanding of their influence on practice today, encouraging developments in the field of psychiatry within internal medicine (Zawiła-Niedźwiecki et al., 2016).

Test Your Knowledge

1. How did the treatment of mental illness evolve from ancient times to the 19th century?
2. were some of the key figures in the development of modern psychiatry, and what were their main contributions?

2.2. Role of General Practitioners in Mental Health

Learning Outcome

1. Understand the first point of contact for patients
2. Deal with the integration of mental health assessments
3. Focus on collaboration with mental health specialists

The role of General Practitioners (GPs) in mental health is increasingly vital, given their frontline role in patient contact. GPs possess a single opportunity to diagnose mental illnesses, depression, or anxiety at the early stages. Their holistic comprehension of patients' illness and social background allows them to see how physical ill-health is entwined with mental health. But this gatekeeping role is flawed when addressing more specific disorders like attention-deficit hyperactivity disorder (ADHD). According to a study, GPs don't always recognize the signs, sometimes due to stigmas regarding mental health diagnosis, or don't want to refer patients to mental health specialists (Ghanizadeh et al., 2016). Therefore, improving knowledge and attitudes among GPs is essential to maximize the diagnosis and treatment of ADHD. GPs play a significant role in offering psychological therapies within the majority of healthcare systems, which is challenging but also very promising for effective mental health management. GPs can play a significant role in providing primary screening and developing treatment plans that strongly impact patient outcomes. However, implementing evidence-based practice in routine clinical environments often encounters setbacks. For instance, the translation of new research into treatment for mental illness can be fraught with difficulties, particularly when evidence may not so easily transfer to everyday practice or the complexities of patients' needs (Iveson et al., 2005). Therefore, GPs must apply their clinical experience to bridge the gap between research evidence and practical implementation, enabling patients to receive care that is both research-informed and tailored to their individual needs. Additionally, integrating mental health into internal medicine has broad implications for healthcare as a whole. Interdisciplinary practice fosters a culture where various health professionals can share opinions and recommendations. GPs can facilitate an integrated view of mental health needs through shared care practice and referral to psychologists and psychiatrists. This collaboration, however, needs continuous training and professional development for GPs to feel assured that they are capable of addressing mental health issues properly. With enhanced skills and learning, GPs are in the best position to handle the subtleties of mental health care, thereby contributing significantly to dismantling access barriers for patients in need. This will decidedly take us in a direction towards a healthcare system that earnestly places mental well-being on par with physical health (Figure 2.4)

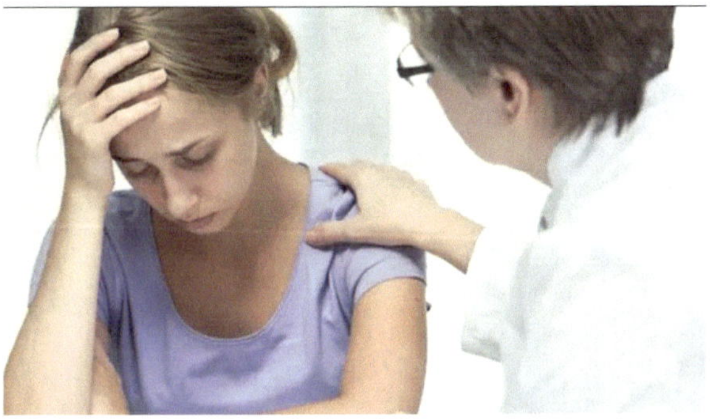

Figure 2.4. A psychiatrist motivating a patient.

Source: https://ichef.bbci.co.uk/ace/ws/640/cpsprodpb/0942/production/_92207320_mentalhealth.jpg.webp.

2.2.1. First Point of Contact for Patients

The position of primary care physicians as the initial point of entry for patients presenting with mental health issues is central in the context of psychiatry in internal medicine. Clinicians most likely see individuals presenting with symptoms of mental illness, but they most commonly feel unprepared to manage such complicated problems. Actually, the majority of general practitioners (GPs) report lacking confidence in recognizing and managing mental illness, which can lead to missed opportunities for earlier intervention. The implications of this deficit are considerable since delayed or poor responses to emotional distress have been found to result in more severe patient conditions and heavy health system burdens. To ensure optimal primary care effectiveness, GP training in evaluating and addressing mental health needs must be increased, enabling improved decision-making and appropriate referrals for additional therapy. The need for smooth communication and interprofessional collaboration between practitioners is also enhanced by the differing needs of mentally ill patients. Since they are the first point of contact, GPs are not only diagnosticians and prescribers of treatment. Still, they must also listen and try to grasp broader social circumstances that affect their patients' health. A qualitative study identifies anger on the part of grieving families, perceiving systemic breakdown when signs of mental illness are overlooked, and the key function that GPs must play in recognizing the warning signs early and responding to them. Furthermore, relatives are worried about over-reliance on drug treatments and prefer a more holistic approach to addressing mental problems with psychosocial interventions. Incorporating patient history, social context, and family contributions into planning will enable GPs to achieve improved mental health outcomes and to assist in building supportive environments for patients who require them. Finally, the first contact in psychiatry is not merely clinical assessment; it is also about building rapport and trust with patients. Mental illness can be highly stigmatizing, and patients may present to their GPs with fear or apprehension of being judged. Therefore, GPs will need to employ methods that create a safe environment for patients to discuss their issues openly. This entails engaging patients directly in discussions about their mental well-being and not belittling their issues or oversimplifying the complexities of their states. Secondly, promoting increased access to mental health care and community resources is vital for directing patients towards integrated care. Such collaborative effort can highlight the critical role played by primary care physicians in preventing mental health crises, as evidenced by the need for proactive outreach and education programs for patients and families to instill awareness of available support systems, culminating in enhanced health outcomes in the area of psychiatric treatment (Thomas et al., 2012; Pearson et al., 2017) (Figure 2.5).

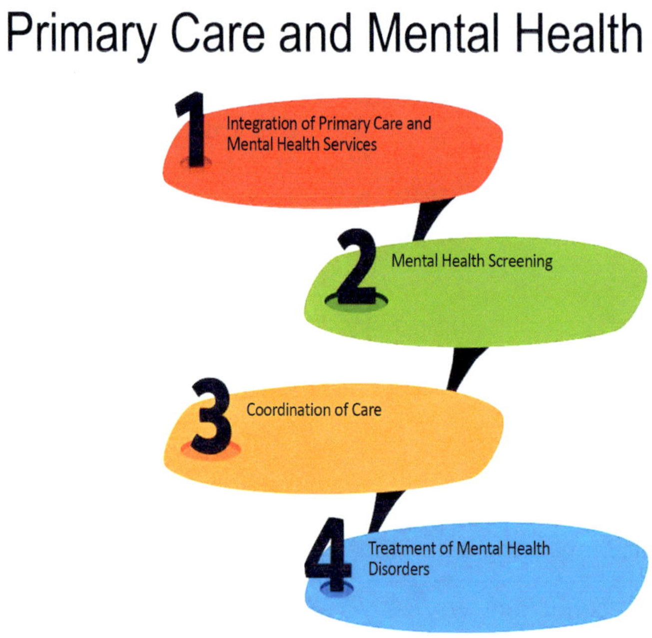

Figure 2.5. Primary care and mental health.

Source: https://fastercapital.co/i/Primary-Care--The-Importance-of-Primary-Care-in-the-Health-Care-Sector--Primary-Care-and-Mental-Health.webp.

2.2.2. Integration of Mental Health Assessments

Integration of mental health screening into internal medicine is imperative to encourage holistic patient care. This enables primary care physicians to identify mental illness that may be masked by the physical presentation of health, thereby promoting a holistic view of patient health. Despite the recognized necessity of mental health screening, most clinicians find it challenging to implement routine assessment. This could result in missing crucial information about a patient's biopsychosocial status, which is essential for case conceptualization and treatment planning. Empirical evidence points to the need for enhanced training and greater accessibility of mental health assessment for general practitioners, so that important information is gathered systematically to guide interventions that advance treatment outcomes (Melchert et al., 2011). Moreover, the meeting of the particular requirements of vulnerable groups, including those suffering from schizophrenia, is necessary in mental health assessments. The emphasis on using physical activity as a helpful intervention here underscores the need for contact-based assessments that consider not only psychological factors but also the patient's physical health. General practitioners must consider barriers to including these groups in physical activity, including the need for mental health assessments that assess psychological well-being alongside physical health metrics. By adding questions on physical activity and its health benefits, practitioners will better understand the issues specific to individuals suffering from mental health disorders. This multidisciplinary approach enables mental health assessment to lead to actionable treatment plans that improve overall quality of life (Connaughton et al., 2016). The success of incorporating mental health assessment into internal medicine depends on developing a multidisciplinary approach. Integration among health practitioners—e.g., psychiatrists, psychologists, and physical therapists—enables the development of comprehensive management plans that address mental and physical well-being. This is significant when managing patients who are likely to have complex health issues. Furthermore, the use of validated questionnaires and tools can facilitate standardized evaluation of mental and physical health complaints, thereby enhancing the efficacy of treatment. Through a systematic approach to mental health assessment, general practitioners can ensure that the patient's overall health is integrated, ultimately leading to improved therapeutic outcomes and increased patient satisfaction in the treatment of psychiatric illness (Melchert et al., 2011; Connaughton et al., 2016) (Figure 2.6).

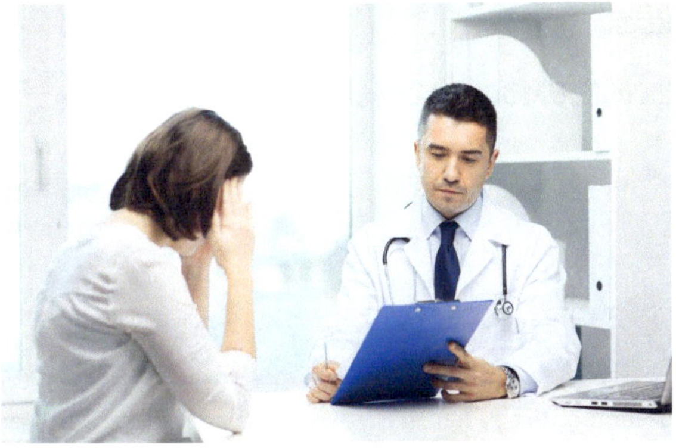

Figure 2.6. The integration of mental health assessments within internal medicine.

Source: https://www.highfocuscenters.com/wp-content/uploads/2017/04/Does-a-Mental-Health-Assessment-Always-Lead-to-Being-Admitted.jpg.

2.2.3. Collaboration with Mental Health Specialists

The integration of mental health specialists into internal medicine is a driving force for optimizing patient outcomes, particularly in child and adolescent psychiatry. GPs might have patients requiring psychiatric treatment and assessment, but do not possess the necessary training in this regard. Through collaboration with mental health specialists, GPs can initiate comprehensive care strategies that address the complex nature of mental illnesses. For instance, research highlighted disparities between admission diagnoses and working diagnoses after joint assessments, underscoring the value of multidisciplinary assessment in streamlining treatment plans and optimizing psychopharmacological interventions. It ensures that GPs are capable of managing psychiatric medication judiciously and provides an environment that facilitates ongoing education and skill development in mental health (Camilleri et al., 2009). The importance of targeted training and ongoing support for GPs cannot be overstated, as they are usually the frontline providers for mentally ill adolescents. In the majority of cases, GPs are expected to manage complex psychiatric disorders that demand expert awareness of emergent treatments and best practice. Collaboration with mental health professionals not only enhances GPs' capacity for accurate diagnosis and handling of such disorders, but also equips them with more straightforward guidelines for when to refer care. The SNAP survey results underscore the need for GPs to be exposed to professional opinion and feedback during consultations, which can significantly enhance the quality of care for young patients with emotional and behavioral issues. Such cooperation ultimately forms a healthier trajectory for young people's mental well-being and health (Barbour et al., 2006). Moreover, having a robust communicative framework between mental health professionals and GPs can be used as a preventive measure against potential misdiagnosis and medication abuse. Data illustrate the need for effective consultation and referral systems, as a large proportion of children previously prescribed antipsychotic medication had their treatment changed following specialist review. This exchange helps cut the risks associated with non-specialist use of psychiatric drugs, resulting in enhanced conformity to evidence-based practice within internal medicine. In addition, frequent interaction among GPs and psychiatrists fosters a culture that makes knowledge sharing part of the fabric and, eventually, shapes the quality of outcomes for adolescents. By giving precedence to such multidisciplinary relations, the field of internal medicine can develop its practice of psychiatry and address the youth mental health crisis more effectively (Camilleri et al., 2009) (Figure 2.7).

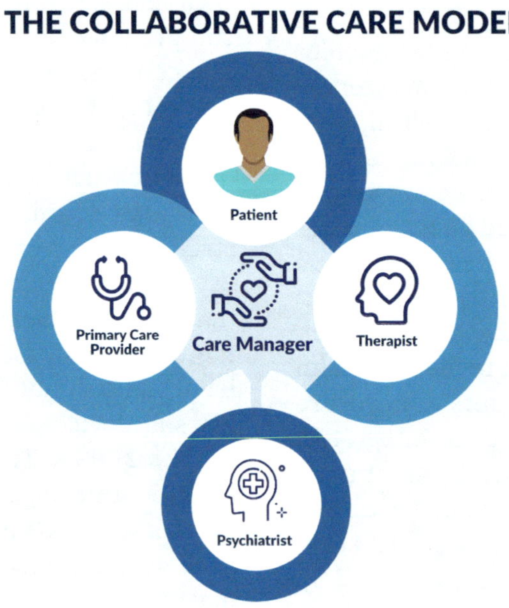

Figure 2.7. Collaboration with mental health specialists.

Source: https://heal.nih.gov/files/Collaborative%20Care%20Model%20%281%29.png.

Test Your Knowledge

1. Why are general practitioners (GPs) often the first point of contact for patients experiencing mental health issues?
2. How do general practitioners collaborate with mental health specialists, such as psychiatrists or psychologists, to provide comprehensive care for patients?

2.3. Common Mental Health Disorders in Internal Medicine

Learning Outcome

1. Understand depression and anxiety disorders;
2. Describe substance use disorders;
3. Explain stress-related disorders.

In the field of internal medicine, psychiatric illnesses are common and include the spectrum of disorders such as depression, anxiety disorders, and bipolar disorder. These conditions have a marked effect on patients' daily functioning and general well-being, which makes it important to identify and treat them in primary care practice. General practitioners are generally the first point of contact for individuals suffering from mental distress, and thus it is important that they are trained to detect and deal with such problems in the most effective manner. Since there are complex interplays between physiological and psychological health, being aware of the nuances of such disorders facilitates better provision of individualized care along with better patient outcomes. Further, early intervention in a familiar healthcare environment is an effective moderator of the impact of these disorders, highlighting the importance of integrating mental health into models of internal medicine.

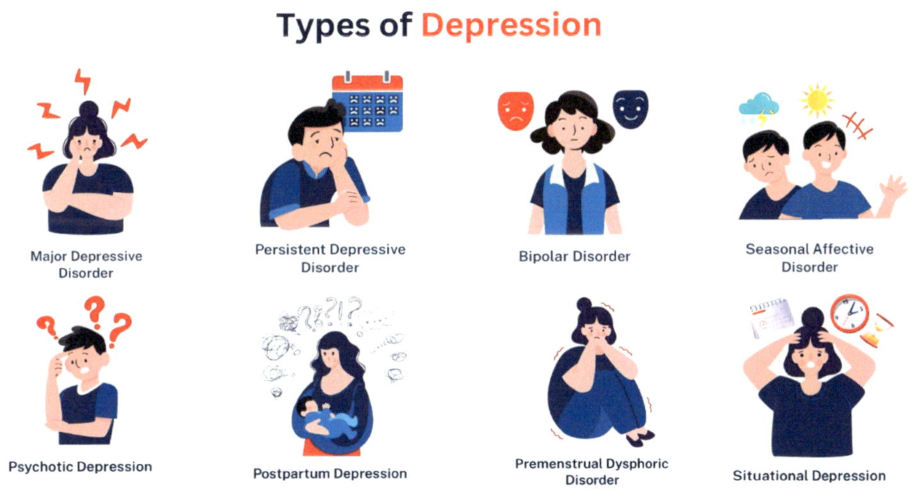

Figure 2.8. Types of depression.

Source: https://relevancerecovery.com/wp-content/uploads/2023/10/httpsrelevancerecovery.comblogwhat-is-grey-area-drinking-2-1024x576.png.

One key factor in addressing mental health conditions in internal medicine is appreciating the role of underlying personality traits, such as neuroticism, which has been linked with numerous psychopathologies. Research now indicates that neuroticism is a general susceptibility that can precipitate the development and perpetuation of common mental disorders, including anxiety disorders and mood disorders (Barlow et al., 2017). These developments give rise to a paradigm shift in treating common mental disorders and promote treatment focusing on modifying stable traits instead of treating the manifestations of specific disorders. By targeting these underlying vulnerabilities, practitioners can enhance the effectiveness and efficacy of psychological treatment, moving toward a more comprehensive understanding of patient health. This approach is conducive to developing models of mental health care that emphasize early intervention and holistic care within internal medicine. An additional complicating factor facing general practitioners in managing mental health is the socio-demographic determinants of parental perception of obesity-related health concerns in children as a reflection of overall psychological concerns. A fascinating study discovered that a significant number of parents did not perceive their overweight child's weight as a health risk, even though the awareness of their child's weight status was important in the understanding of related health problems (Croker et al., 2013). This chasm points to the need for internal medicine practitioners, apart from dealing with diagnosed mental illnesses, to become more aware and to sensitize their patients about the psychological correlates of physical illnesses. By virtue of open discussion of these matters, families can be enabled to identify and treat psychological vulnerabilities at the start, ultimately integrating mental health considerations into patient care plans in the context of internal medicine.

2.3.1. Depression and Anxiety Disorders

Traditional intervention methods have been demonstrated to be lacking in both length and specificity, which tends to limit availability and performance. New developments in psychological science have recently indicated that prevention programs with a cognitive-behavioral orientation, specifically crafted to be transdiagnostic, are promising in averting the onset of anxiety and depression in at-risk groups. The programs target adaptive emotion regulation skills within a brief intervention window, promoting short-term coping skills and long-term resilience. Findings from proof-of-concept experiments demonstrate that participants perceive these interventions not only as acceptable but also as effective in teaching skills necessary for emotional regulation, following a trend toward more inclusive and effective mental health interventions within internal medicine practice (Barlow et al., 2017). The integration of these prevention and intervention models within internal medicine represents an essential opportunity to enhance the quality of mental health care. With the prevalence of depression and anxiety increasing globally, practitioners must adopt a holistic perspective that values the interconnectedness between mind and body. Training general practitioners to identify early signs of mental disorder can lead to early intervention, which eventually benefits patients and healthcare facilities. Furthermore, by embracing evidence-based programs aimed at physical and emotional well-being, healthcare professionals can develop a more comprehensive and balanced approach to patient care. Not only does such innovation produce better outcomes for patients, but it also helps create an improved, more responsive healthcare system capable of addressing the varied needs of its population (N/A, 2011).

2.3.2. Substance Use Disorders

Substance Use Disorders (SUDs) present formidable challenges in the practice of psychiatry in internal medicine, necessitating a sophisticated appreciation of their pathophysiologic mechanisms. The disorders are characterized by compulsive drug use and seeking despite negative consequences resulting from alterations in brain function and structure. Clinicians must realize that SUDs are not merely behavioral disorders but complicated biopsychosocial diseases requiring multifaceted treatment approaches. The translation of neuroscience research into clinical practice is essential but often overlooked. For instance, groups such as the Neuroscience Interest Group of the International Society of Addiction Medicine aim to bridge the divide between addiction neuroscience and clinical application by encouraging the adoption of cognitive assessments and neuroimaging technologies that could enhance the efficacy of treatment strategies for SUDs (Arunogiri et al., 2019). Moreover, translating research evidence into effective clinical practice is critical to improving outcomes in patients with SUDs. Building an RPI model is a collaborative initiative that engages various stakeholders, including researchers, practitioners, and patients, in developing and revising treatment protocols. The model encourages practitioners to apply the latest research findings to inform their clinical interventions and adjust treatment options accordingly. Case studies illustrate the extent to which research findings can directly influence the design of treatment services, particularly in the context of adolescent drug abuse, highlighting the importance of tailoring interventions to patient need and current evidence (Sterling et al., 2006). Research, combined with clinical acumen, is essential to advancing the quality of care for patients with SUDs. Lastly, the management of SUD within internal medicine underscores the need for multimodal treatment approaches integrating pharmacologic and psychosocial interventions. Effective management needs to look not just at the biological dimensions of addiction but also at its psychological, social, and environmental etiologies. Expanding the view in this way can contribute to improved long-term patient outcomes by preventing relapse and promoting better overall health. Application of neuroscience-based interventions, including cognitive training and neuromodulation, in combination with conventional therapies, facilitates a more targeted, likely more effective treatment approach. Encouragement of international collaboration between researchers and clinicians for the advancement of evidence-based practice is important for the future direction of addiction treatment in mainstream psychiatric practice (Arunogiri et al., 2019) (Figure 2.9).

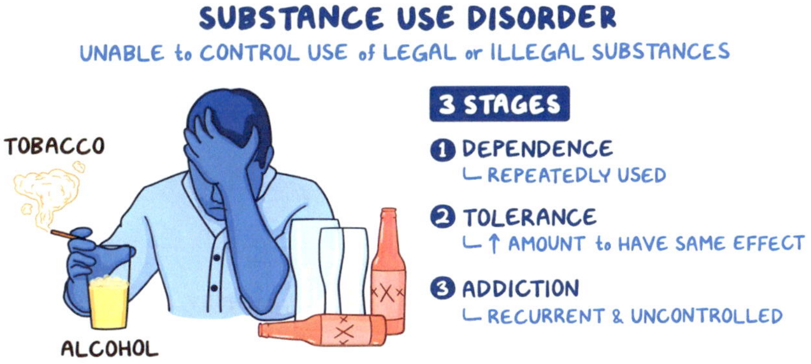

Figure 2.9. Substance use disorders (SUDs) present significant challenges within the realm of psychiatry in internal medicine.

Source: https://www.osmosis.org/_next/image?url=https%3A%2F%2Fd16qt3wv6xm098.cloudfront.net%2FnNkHRDLGSi6CFI-9G-1TKT-0Q4qjL8pU%2F_.jpg&w=3840&q=75.

2.3.3. Stress-Related Disorders

Stress disorders are becoming a major issue in the domain of general psychiatry, reflecting the relationship between mind and body. Disorders like anxiety, depression, and post-traumatic stress disorder (PTSD) usually emerge as a result of chronic stressors and can significantly impede daily functioning. Evidence indicates that patients with both medical and mental conditions experience a higher rate of stress-related disorders, which can lead to increased mortality and a strain on health systems. To effectively treat these conditions, general practitioners must adopt an integrated treatment approach that considers the psychological and physiological aspects of such disorders. This type of approach is in line with evidence that highlights the necessity of integrated care in addressing the complexity posed by stress-related disorders among patients (N/A, 2011). The role of psychoeducational interventions (PIs) cannot be overstated in preventing and managing stress-related disorders, particularly among vulnerable populations such as adolescents. Given the high rates of depression and anxiety among this group, evidence-based psychosocial interventions are paramount. Systematic reviews have shown that PIs are able to offer critical health information, which leads to improved understanding and symptom management. Not only do PIs improve communication and participation, but also enhance mental health outcomes. Family and group interventions, school-based and web-based, have demonstrated efficacy in addressing the subtleties of stress-related disorders and have shown potential to be used as first-line or adjunctive therapy for individuals who suffer from them (Jones et al., 2017). The results of successfully treated stress-related disorders have far-reaching implications beyond individual health, shaping societal-level dynamics. The cost of these disorders often takes the form of a substantial economic burden, resulting from reduced productivity and increased healthcare use. Precise knowledge regarding the causes of stress-related disorders is vital for constructing effective public health strategies of prevention and intervention. Policymakers need to place a high value on evidence-based treatment methods that emphasize self-management support for patients, especially in the internal medicine department. With growing awareness of mental health, integrating stress disorder management into daily medical practice will improve the quality of care and reduce the cost burden on healthcare systems (N/A, 2011).

Test Your Knowledge

1. What are the typical signs and symptoms of depression and anxiety disorders that general practitioners should look for during consultations?
2. What role do general practitioners play in the early identification and management of substance use disorders?
3. How can general practitioners support patients in managing stress-related disorders alongside other physical health conditions?

2.4. Diagnostic Tools and Techniques

Learning Outcome

1. Discuss clinical interviews and assessments
2. Describe standardized screening tools
3. Understand the importance of patient history

The use of diagnostic methods and tools in internal medicine psychiatry is critical to enhanced patient outcomes. Among the many techniques employed, standardized questionnaires and structured interviews have helped quantify a range of psychiatric disorders. The tools enable practitioners to systematically obtain extensive information, thereby enhancing diagnosis. For instance, the use of Autism Diagnostic Observation Schedule (ADOS) has gained recognition for its diagnostic validity in detecting autism spectrum disorders (ASD) in diverse populations. Specifically, research indicates that advances in machine learning are making it increasingly effective to detect ASD, potentially optimizing diagnosis and providing clinicians with better paradigms for differential diagnosis. These developments justify the incorporation of reliable tools to enhance diagnostic accuracy in internal medicine practice, ultimately improving therapeutic interventions. Moreover, the new environment of psychiatric diagnosis necessitates rethinking traditional methodologies in light of contemporary research.

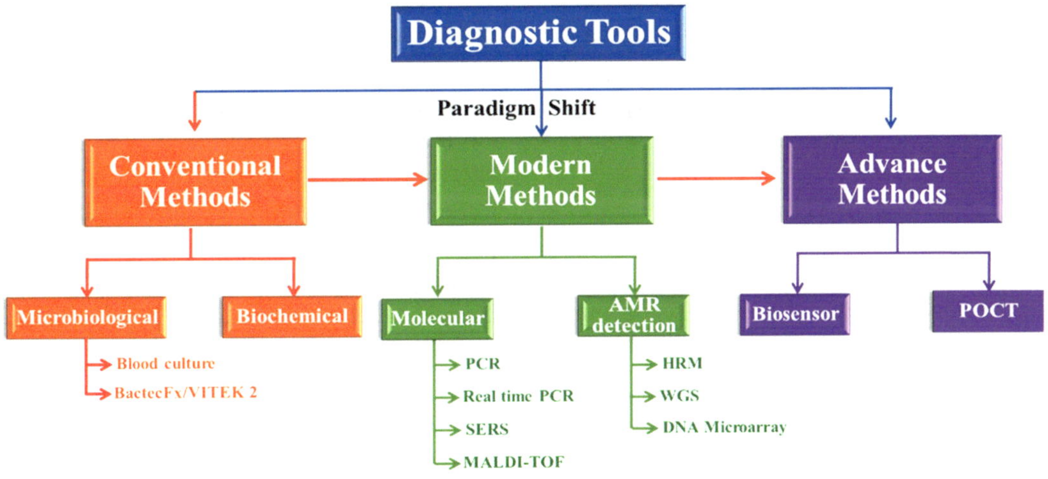

Figure 2.10. The integration of diagnostic tools and techniques.

Source: https://www.mdpi.com/diagnostics/diagnostics-13-00277/article_deploy/html/images/diagnostics-13-00277-g001.png.

The systems of psychiatric diagnosis, traditionally dominated by subjective determination, are increasingly being questioned regarding the extent to which they reflect the range of variability of mental illnesses. Innovative paradigms, such as the National Institute of Mental Health's Research Domain Criteria, promote the complementarity of biological measures and psychological evaluation. This new paradigm highlights the promise of biomarker discovery to sharpen diagnostic criteria and augment treatment options. As clinical professionals adopt these new standards, the intersection of psychological concepts and biomedical approaches is significant for advancing the practice of psychiatry within internal medicine settings, as it redefines the conceptualization of mental health complexities (Aria et al., 2018). Significantly, one must also consider that the use of diagnostic tools in internal medicine psychiatry is not devoid of drawbacks. The appropriate interpretation and use of these tools require clinicians to cultivate an intimate understanding of the psychological constructs that they measure. Despite positive trends within the field, for instance, enhanced ASD diagnostics based on reduced behavioral indicators identified with machine learning, practitioners are still vulnerable to errors that result from poor training or capacity. In addition, the dynamic nature of diagnostic criteria can affect their consistency in clinical practice. Overcoming these problems with continuous education and inter-professional communication is required for optimal utilization of diagnostic tools. In the long term, their use improves patient outcomes and contributes to the knowledge base of complex psychiatric disorders in the general context of internal medicine psychiatry (Hauck et al., 2020) (Figure 2.10).

2.4.1. Clinical Interviews and Assessments

Clinical interviewing and assessment are core aspects of psychiatric care, especially in the internal medicine context, where primary care physicians tend to be the initial contact for patients with mental illness. Clinical interviewing enables clinicians to obtain detailed information about a patient's psychological condition, background, and social environment, which is essential for informing diagnosis and treatment. The complex nature of mental health illnesses necessitates that the clinician is skilled at applying various interviewing techniques that yield credible and meaningful responses. Building rapport in such an interview directly affects the quality of the data gathered, which, in turn, guides clinical decision-making and patient outcomes. Compelling clinical interviews not only foster trust but also allow for an investigation of the patient's symptoms, thoughts, and feelings that may lead to a more precise understanding of their mental health conditions. Furthermore, formal clinical evaluations complement the subjective data gathered through interviews. These evaluations often employ standardized tools that quantify and categorize symptoms, providing a foundation for clinicians to examine mental health disorders systematically. These tools can potentially enhance the validity of diagnoses and guide treatment approaches by highlighting areas of concern. For instance, the use of risk assessment instruments can identify individuals at risk of inflicting self-harm or harm to others, allowing practitioners to adopt the necessary safety protocols. Evidence indicates that veteran clinicians depend on an integration of cues and psychological representations when making educated risk estimates in suicide and self-neglect, which proves the interconnected nature between standardized tests and clinical judgment (Adams et al., 2008). Integration is essential, especially in a primary care environment, where limited resources demand efficient risk assessments to ensure patient safety. Finally, the nuances of capacity assessments in patient care underscore the value of clinicians putting legal and ethical methods into practice in clinical assessment and interviewing. The Mental Capacity Act of 2005 provides a benchmark for determining a patient's ability to make informed decisions, yet, as cited in recent studies, these legal provisions are often inadequately applied in hospitals (Alzheimer's Research Trust et al., 2012). This disparity is the reason why there must be greater awareness and adherence to guidelines by practitioners. With a better understanding of capacity determinations, practitioners can provide patients not only dignified care but also support in making personalized health decisions. This two-pronged approach, combining robust clinical interviews with strict compliance with legal provisions, makes the practice of psychiatry in internal medicine even more effective, ultimately enhancing the provision of care and patient outcomes in mental health care (Figure 2.11).

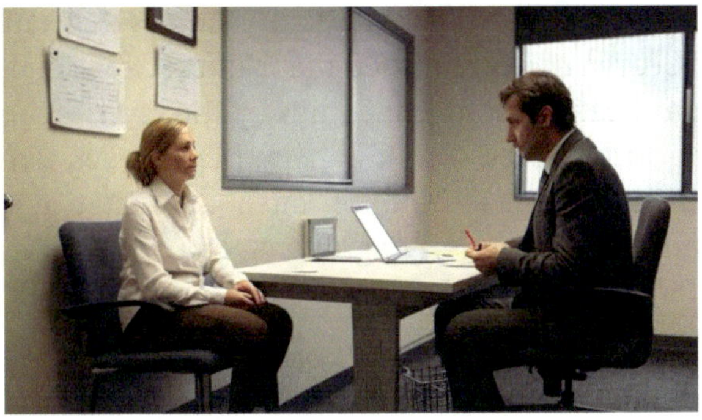

Figure 2.11. Presentation of clinical interview.

Source: https://psychiatristinlahore.com/wp-content/uploads/2024/10/History-Taking.jpg.

2.4.2. Standardized Screening Tools

Implementation of standardized screening tools in internal medicine is essential to enable earlier detection of psychiatric disorders, which would otherwise not be detected until they become full-scale illnesses. Such tools allow primary care providers to perform systematic evaluations, enabling the consistent measurement of similar mental health symptoms across patient populations. Specifically, they provide practitioners with well-tested instruments that can effectively determine psychological disorders, such as depression and anxiety, before their severe disruption of patients' daily living. Furthermore, research indicates that integrating these instruments into routine clinical practice can significantly improve patient care by enabling early interventions and better health outcomes.

By adhering to established guidelines, practitioners can conduct effective, comprehensive health assessments that enhance their proficiency in managing complex mental health cases across diverse practice environments. The incorporation of standard screening instruments into clinical practice requires not only sufficient training for healthcare providers but also ongoing performance monitoring and evaluation. Successful deployment requires insight into patient populations, as these populations may vary in levels of psychological distress; therefore, tailored methods may enhance the specificity of screens. Emerging evidence shows that developmental delays and psychiatric symptoms are common but not adequately detected, particularly in primary care. Equipment designed to test developmental issues, as in recent studies, affirms the necessity of adapting such measures to improve the detection of potential mental health issues among patients, particularly children and the elderly (Sices, 2007). Equipment must be regularly checked and verified to ensure its sensitivity and specificity in detecting subtle presentations of mental health issues. Furthermore, standardized screening instruments can minimize long-term consequences of untreated psychiatric disorders, such as worsening depressive symptoms and excessive utilization of healthcare services. For instance, a study among elderly adults receiving home care documented that nearly 56% exhibited clinically critical depressive symptoms, highlighting the significance of effective screening procedures among this at-risk group (Browne et al., 2014). By employing standardized measures, healthcare professionals can launch evidence-based interventions that reduce depressive symptomatology and improve health-related quality of life. These are particularly vital in enhancing patient outcomes, reducing unnecessary hospitalizations, and eventually decreasing overall healthcare expenses. With the evolving environment of internal medicine, the application of such tools remains a critical component in enabling mental health support so that patients can receive timely and efficient treatment along the continuum of psychiatric services.

2.4.3. Importance of Patient History

Gathering patient history is a fundamental part of psychiatric assessment in internal medicine.

In-depth familiarity with an individual's medical, psychological, and psychosocial background allows clinicians to frame appropriate treatment plans tailored to each patient's needs. The detailed process involves both clinical and contextual factors that influence mental health, ensuring that any underlying issues are identified and addressed beforehand.

For instance, being aware of a patient's history of past experiences with psychiatric treatment, family history of psychosis, or past traumas exposes essential patterns that help in diagnosing current conditions and establishing effective therapeutic interventions. Thus, a deliberate effort to assemble thorough patient histories contributes to better clinical outcomes and to the overall quality of care provided within psychiatric centers. Also, patient background is not the only responsibility of individual assessments; it contributes to suicide risk assessments commonly encountered in emergency departments. Clinicians typically see several barriers and facilitators in suicide risk assessment and emphasize the importance of having a thorough understanding of the patient's background. Multidimensional and collaborative approaches that include patient history enable practitioners to address key topics influencing suicide risk, such as patient engagement and practical communication skills (Berlin et al., 2015).

Establishing rapport via open-ended dialogue about past trauma and mental health issues can lead to enhanced risk assessment and more effective decisions. Hence, obtaining thorough patient histories is critical not only for understanding the patient's current state but also for strategically managing complex clinical issues, where risk management is of utmost importance. Finally, the compilation of findings across different practitioners underscores the significance of advanced knowledge of the determinants of clinicians' decision-making behaviors in risk assessment. Research has established that clinical experience significantly determines how patient histories are interpreted, revealing significant cues that guide risk assessments, such as situational context and underlying reasons (Adams et al., 2008).

Through the integration of these considerations, clinicians can adopt a more informed methodology for determining risk for suicide and self-harm. This enhances clinical judgment and enables identification of evidence-based treatments that consider both actuarial data and patient history. This, accordingly, ensures that the incorporation of history into the patient assessment makes it not only essential to risk evaluations but also highlights the necessity of multidisciplinary care of mental health within internal medicine so that psychiatrists are competent to offer care that is at once effective and empathetic as well as informed (Figure 2.12).

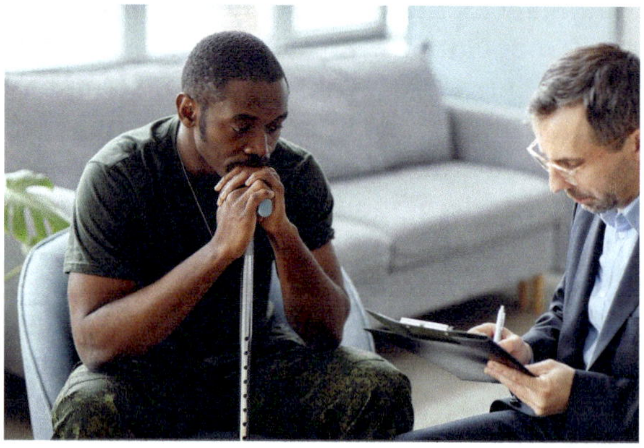

Figure 2.12. Gathering of patient history forms a foundational component of psychiatric assessment.

Source: https://cdn-ikpihob.nitrocdn.com/GJAklxHQfMKMvlVnrUvgDGQlJMJYRDNE/assets/images/optimized/rev-ee31753/therosemarycentre.com.au/wp-content/uploads/2024/11/shutterstock_2150083279-scaled.jpg.

Test Your Knowledge

1. What is the role of clinical interviews in the psychiatric assessment conducted by general practitioners?
2. Which standardized screening tools are commonly used in internal medicine to identify mental health disorders such as depression and anxiety?
3. How does obtaining a comprehensive patient history contribute to accurate diagnosis in psychiatric cases within internal medicine?

2.5. Treatment Approaches in Internal Medicine

Learning Outcome

1. Explain the concept of psychopharmacology
2. Discuss psychotherapy and counseling
3. Focus on lifestyle modifications and support

Internal medicine treatment protocols, particularly in psychiatry, require a combination of evidence-based practice and interprofessional collaboration among medical practitioners. Implementing research findings into clinical practice can help enhance the quality of psychiatric care. Integration of research and practice (RPI) is one model that addresses this, as it emphasizes interprofessional collaboration among the most powerful stakeholders, including clinicians, patients, and researchers. This model has been of great success in alcohol and other drug (AOD) dependence treatment, showing how empirical findings can be translated into practice. Not only does this synergy improve the treatment outcomes, but it also promotes ongoing dialogue that can lead to the formulation of new research questions, hence creating a continuous feedback loop that can enhance clinical practices in psychiatry (Sterling et al., 2006). The other crucial aspect of treatment in internal medicine is treating sensory processing. The way individuals process sensory information can significantly impact their mental well-being, leading to issues such as anxiety, depression, and post-traumatic stress. Using sensory modulation approaches as an intervention can be a helpful treatment for individuals experiencing distress, agitation, or withdrawal. These methods offer a non-coercive alternative to traditional methods such as seclusion and restraint that may cause further psychological harm. Empirical studies have shown that sensory-modulated therapies improve patient engagement and behavioral stabilization, underscoring their flexibility across a wide range of psychiatric conditions. Consequently, their training of healthcare professionals can foster better models of mental health care within internal medicine practice (Hoque et al., 2016). Further, good treatment in internal medicine is not only about clinical interventions but also requires adequate staff education and the redirection of resources. Training programs in the staff during in-service about sensory modulation techniques have shown promise. If the staff understands these methods, they are better placed to develop therapy environments that empower patients and reduce reliance on more coercive interventions. Feedback from training sessions indicates that trainees and employees alike view educational materials as beneficial to their overall practice. This opens a clear avenue for implementing novel treatment approaches into routine practice, ultimately leading to improved patient outcomes and enhanced psychiatric care within internal medicine practices (Sterling et al., 2006; Hoque et al., 2016).

2.5.1. Psychopharmacology

Psychopharmacology is a primary tool in psychiatry for treating and managing mental disease. The establishment of pharmacological treatment as part of internal medicine practice has expanded the scope of care that physicians can provide. While further research in medication therapy continues, practitioners need to remain current in understanding new psychotropic drugs and their efficacy for specific illnesses. The complexity of the treatments necessitates interprofessional collaboration among healthcare workers. Multidisciplinary working enables comprehensive patient care, with therapeutic interventions underpinned by best practice and individualized to patient need. In addition, as more and more general practitioners see patients with psychiatric problems, psychiatric drug management becomes their key skill in optimizing treatment outcomes in a holistic sense. Despite the merits of psychopharmacological therapies, incorporating these practices into general practice remains challenging. Prescription privileges for psychologists raise challenges regarding the controversy surrounding the adequacy of training and safety concerns. Most of the focus has revolved around interprofessional practice, with emphasis on teamwork as a mechanism for enhancing patient care.

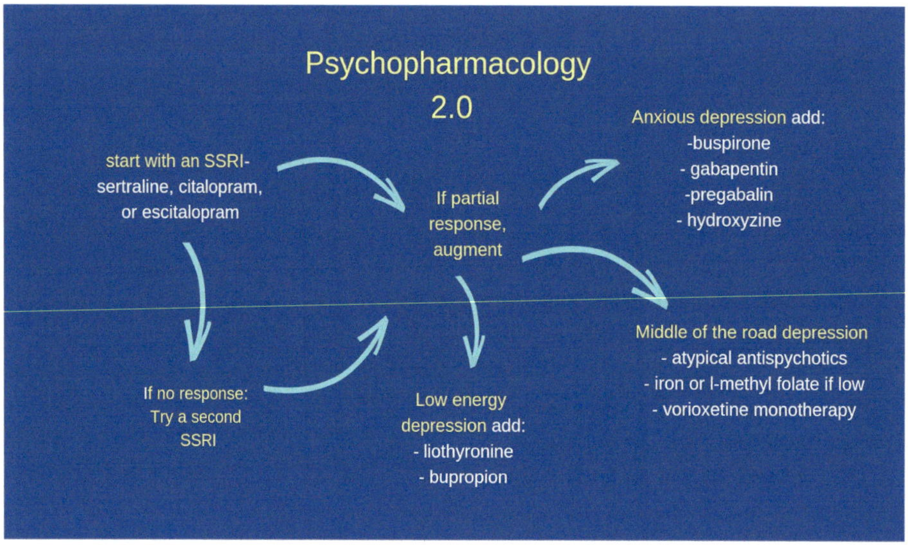

Figure 2.13. The psychopharmacology plays a pivotal role in the treatment and management of mental health disorders.

Source: https://thecurbsiders.com/wp-content/uploads/2019/02/Infographic-The-Curbsiders-140-Psychopharmacology-2.0-antidepressant-algorithm-1024x576.png.

The American Psychological Association's Ad Hoc Task Force recommended a Level of Collaboration consonant with current healthcare reform, emphasizing coordinated models of care over the controversial proposal to grant prescription privileges. Opponents envision inequalities in educational preparation between psychologists and prescribing professionals as creating concerns about the efficacy and safety of patient care. Thus, a shift to collaborative practice can expand access to treatment and minimize the risks associated with psychopharmacological treatment, ultimately putting patient well-being before professional terrain. Additionally, more contemporary approaches such as the Comprehensive Behavioral Intervention for Tics (CBIT) hold promise for evidence-based non-pharmacological interventions, establishing an inclusive model of mental healthcare. Research on CBIT has documented dramatic reductions in tic severity and associated impairment among children with Tourette disorder, suggesting that behavior therapies may complement or, in some cases, displace pharmacologic interventions. Given that neurology and pediatric clinics are often the first sites of encounter for individuals with tics, integrating such therapies into psychiatric care is essential. Positive feedback on satisfaction and therapeutic alliance further underscores the value of an integrated treatment paradigm in which different modalities, such as psychopharmacology, are applied interactively. Therefore, development in the practice of psychiatry by the integration of pharmacological and behavioral interventions improves patient care overall and matches changing healthcare trends (Figure 2.13)

2.5.2. Psychotherapy and Counseling

The integration of psychotherapy and counseling into internal medicine is required to provide holistic mental health care. In current clinical practice, the general practitioner is often presented with patients presenting with psychological distress; hence, mental health is part of primary care. Because practitioners are positioned at the intersection of physical and mental health, they should be well-versed in the fundamentals of various therapeutic modalities, including psychotherapy. This consciousness enables practitioners to recognize the juncture at which patients may benefit from psychotherapeutic intervention, developing a more holistic approach to patient care. In addition, the emphasis on mental health supports long-term treatment strategies, facilitating more effective care for psychological and somatic issues. Psychotherapy is a continually evolving discipline, increasingly employing mindfulness-based therapies that have gained popularity for their positive impact on therapeutic interventions. Research has brought into focus the benefits of mindfulness counseling, demonstrating how it not only reduces stress but also improves emotional regulation and self-awareness for clients. As internal medicine practitioners are often the first line of contact for individuals seeking mental health treatment, they must familiarize themselves with these innovative approaches. The integration of mindfulness as a therapeutic intervention can empower professionals to help their patients better manage their mental health conditions. Mindfulness interventions can also be applied as a preventive measure to promote mental health and resilience, thereby ensuring that the healthcare system is not strained.

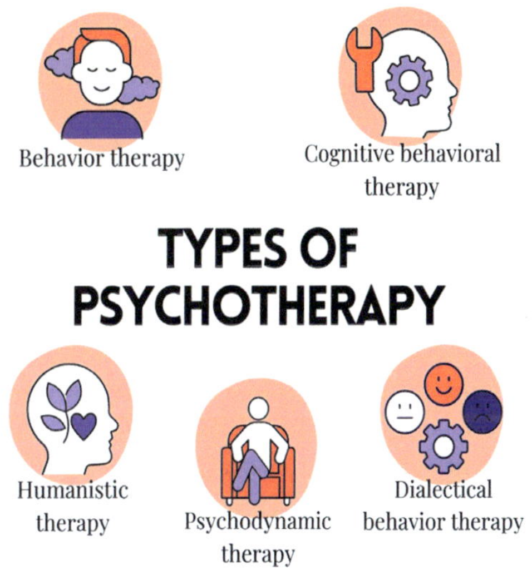

Figure 2.14. Types of psychotherapy.

Source: https://www.simplypsychology.org/wp-content/uploads/Types-of-psychotherapy.jpg.

Furthermore, establishing an integrative platform that combines psychotherapy with spontaneous mechanisms of support is essential to advancing mental health care within internal medicine. The distinction between informal social support and formal psychotherapy can become blurred because both contribute significantly to emotional well-being. Research has shown that integrating these two sources of psychological support can enhance the overall effectiveness of mental health care. By acknowledging the value of social support alongside psychotherapeutic treatments, general practitioners can develop a more comprehensive understanding of their patients' mental health needs. This paradigm shift fosters the development of interprofessional models of care in which healthcare workers collaborate to provide holistic care, enhancing the therapeutic experience for patients and strengthening community resilience (Figure 2.14).

2.5.3. Lifestyle Modifications and Support

Lifestyle modifications play a crucial role in the management of mental health conditions in internal medicine, demonstrating body-mind interdependence. Lifestyle modifications may involve dietary changes, physical exercise, sleep patterns, and social engagement, all of which can significantly influence emotional states and cognitive functions. As an example, habitual exercise has been associated with decreases in symptoms of depression and anxiety, and proper nutrition can improve mood as well as global mental health. The combination of lifestyle changes is particularly relevant when taking into account the high rate of patients with comorbid medical and mental illnesses, which also evokes concerns for mortality rates as well as quality of care. As noted, implementing support strategies to enable patient self-management can help them take an active role in their care, become resilient, and improve the effectiveness of treatment (N/A, 2011). Additionally, formal and informal support systems facilitate effective lifestyle change. Mental health professionals in internal medicine can help patients develop organized plans for implementing change by providing encouragement and motivation. Peer support groups and community programs can further enhance the effectiveness of lifestyle interventions by fostering a sense of accountability and belonging among people with similar issues. Involvement in multidisciplinary teams can also improve care by offering alternative perspectives on behavioral interventions. The recognition of the social determinants of health functions highlights the need to overcome lifestyle change barriers, including socioeconomic status, to enable individuals to enact and sustain changes that promote mental well-being (N/A, 2011). Personalized care strategies, including personalized medicine applications, offer promising avenues for integrating lifestyle modifications into psychiatric interventions. The evolving nature of technology and genomic testing enables tailored interventions that correlate lifestyle changes with an individual's health profile. Individualized care can facilitate streamlined treatment planning by considering genetic risks, lifestyle decisions, and psychosocial factors that affect patient participation and compliance with prescribed changes. As healthcare moves towards a systems medicine and biology-based paradigm, it is increasingly critical to recognize how patient-specific characteristics affect mental health interventions. These advances allow clinicians to offer personalized care, which optimizes the efficacy of lifestyle change and patient care experience alike in individuals affected by mental illness.

Test Your Knowledge

1. What are the common psychopharmacological treatments initiated by general practitioners for conditions like depression and anxiety?
2. How can general practitioners decide when to refer patients for specialized psychotherapy or counseling services?

2.6. Challenges in Integrating Psychiatry into Internal Medicine

Learning Outcome

1. Discuss the stigma surrounding mental health
2. Describe time constraints in internal medicine
3. Focus on limited resources and training challenges

The integration of psychiatry into internal medicine is gravely threatened by resource utilization and the health system's readiness. In the majority of LMICs, the absence of rudimentary infrastructure significantly limits the delivery of mental health care. For instance, the PRIME study identifies critical shortages of trained mental health staff and core medicines across health systems in Ethiopia, India, Nepal, South Africa, and Uganda. These gaps pose a significant obstacle to providing quality mental health services in general practice, as primary care practitioners too frequently lack the assistance required to manage psychiatric disorders adequately. Apart from that, the lack of quality information on available treatment coverage exacerbates difficulties in implementing scalable mental health integration programs and underscores the need for inclusive district plans that align mental health resources with broader general health services (Alem et al., 2014). Most importantly, however, the treatment gap in mental health programs is not only available in LMICs but also exists in more developed nations. Research in the European context identifies significant barriers to the delivery of mental health services due to structural deficits and non-continuous care structures. Health care professionals, e.g., general practitioners, report access and availability limitations in mental health services that hamper the formation of an uninterrupted chain of care. The subtleties of bridging gaps in treatment and facilitating effective referral further complicate the integration process, rendering it difficult for general practitioners to practice integrated care of psychiatric patients. Such fragmentation of the system points to the need for models of cooperation that facilitate the shift in care levels while keeping mental health as part of the overall agenda of internal medicine (Axelsson et al., 2020). Furthermore, the evolution of mental health care in internal medicine must overcome the prevailing attitudes and the stigma that presently prevail regarding psychiatric issues. The majority of patients, particularly from less educated communities, may be reluctant to receive assistance for mental health because prevailing societal attitudes attribute mental illness to a lack of strength or failure. Stigma can lead to treatment avoidance, further exacerbating the already prevalent mhcGAP that has been documented in studies across various countries. To address this, general practitioners must be equipped not only with clinical skills but with the means to foster mental health literacy among patients and families. Through collaboration with resources, including e-mental health technology and community programs, practitioners can provide more accessible pathways for patients' engagement in mental health services, ultimately contributing to greater incorporation of psychiatry into internal medicine and a more comprehensive approach to health care (Axelsson et al., 2020).

2.6.1. Stigma Surrounding Mental Health

The stigma of mental illness is a common obstacle that significantly affects those who need help in the field of internal medicine psychiatry. The stigma can exist in the form of negative stereotypes and social discrimination, which together cause significant issues in coping with the prevailing situation. Fear of judgment or rejection in most people can quell their urge to seek the right treatments or report issues about their conditions. Thus, such hesitancy not only makes their mental disease problems worse but also limits opportunities for healing and help. Unless these long-term stigmas are resolved, the place of psychiatry in internal medicine can be undermined severely, since patient mistrust incapacitates practitioners' ability to provide quality mental health care. In addition, evidence indicates that the effects of stigma extend beyond personal issues; they are a robust factor in public health outcomes as well. Evidence demonstrates that stigma prevents individuals from accessing crucial services such as housing, jobs, and even health benefits since it traps them in a vicious cycle of disadvantage and exclusion. The paper emphasizes that stigma is one of the most significant barriers to recovery. It states that the elimination of such stigmas is necessary for returning individuals with mental illness as an equal member of society.

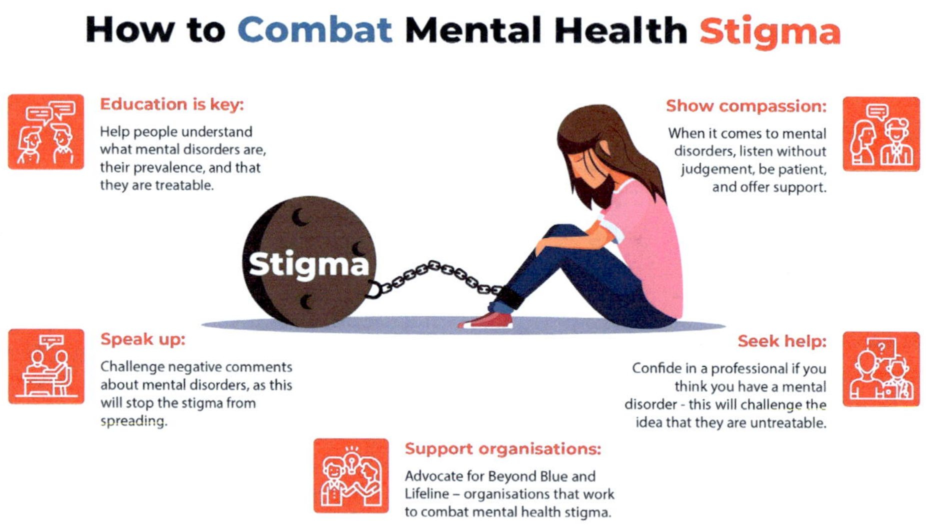

Figure 2.15. Stigma surrounding mental health in internal medicine.

Source: https://www.australiawidefirstaid.com.au/media-library/infographic-on-how-to-beat-stigma-surrounding-mental-health-923w.webp.

Locally and internationally, too, stigma reduction programs have a key role to play in establishing a culture where an individual can seek mental health care without shame or fear (Hocking B). Hence, general practitioners must be equipped with skills and knowledge to combat stigma beforehand as part of routine practice. In addition, the interplay between mental illness stigma and chronic diseases places an additional layer of challenge on treatment methods in the domain of internal medicine. Conditions such as anorexia nervosa, which reveal a distressing prevalence in some patient groups, highlight the intertwinement of physical health and mental health (Chelvanayagam et al., 2012). It is significant for general practitioners to know about the psychological aspects of diseases like anorexia, particularly in the context of social pressure and stigma. It calls for a more holistic approach that not only addresses the physical manifestations of an illness but also the psychological concerns behind a disorder that patients become stigmatized around. By placing a high value on a stigma-free, empathetic approach to addressing mental health issues, practitioners can increase patient engagement and create a better healthcare environment supportive of overall recovery (Figure 2.15).

2.6.2. Time Constraints in Internal Medicine

In the contemporary setting of the healthcare industry, time pressures in internal medicine have posed a significant concern, particularly in managing psychiatric disorders. General practitioners (GPs) tend to work under pressure in managing large volumes of patients in short consultation windows. This tends to erode their ability to conduct thorough examinations needed to diagnose and determine mental illnesses. It is aggravated when it involves complicated disorders like attention deficit hyperactivity disorder (ADHD), which may require more intensive investigation to prevent misdiagnosis and, consequently, appropriate intervention. GPs as gatekeepers to specialist services may be hesitant to refer patients due to constraints of time and a lack of sufficient confidence in identifying ADHD symptoms, leading to underdiagnosis and ineffective treatment (Ghanizadeh et al., 2016). Moreover, GPs' resistance to policy shared care, particularly for mental health, indicates another dimension of the time constraint problem. According to a systematic review, it appears that some GPs are skeptical regarding ADHD because they lack training and counseling on managing psychiatric disorders (Ghanizadeh et al., 2016). This vagueness is particularly problematic in the narrow time frames of internal medicine, where GPs will prioritize physical health issues viewed as more urgent or concrete. As a result, the critical role of mental health screening takes a back seat, contributing to the stigma of mental health illness and perpetuating a cycle of suboptimal care for patients. Overcoming these constraints requires a paradigm shift in training and resource allocation in internal medicine to enhance the provision of psychiatric care (Ghanizadeh et al., 2016). Incorporating screening and brief interventions (SBI) into internal medicine can improve mental health outcomes, even under time pressure. Training in SBI skills has been reported to improve health professionals' readiness to discuss mental health with patients. While implementing such measures may appear time-consuming in the short run, the long-term benefits could easily outweigh the time spent upfront. By giving GPs access to the tools and frameworks they need to handle mental health issues in their practice efficiently, health systems can create an environment where psychiatric matters are more routinely treated and acknowledged. In the end, by keeping training paramount and developing support systems that build on GPs' abilities, better patient outcomes in psychiatric care will result, preventing the negative impacts of time pressures in internal medicine.

2.6.3. Limited Resources and Training

Good psychiatry in internal medicine is significantly threatened by resource and training limitations. General practitioners are not typically well-trained in psychiatry, posing a challenge in diagnosing and managing mental illness. Although there exist evidence-based guidelines for the identification and treatment of psychiatric disorders, their application is frequently eroded by insufficient training in psychiatry and deficient supportive clinical infrastructures. General practitioners may have diverse psychiatric presentations in their patient populations; however, their potential to intervene appropriately may be hampered by minimal levels of exposure to mental health education during medical school. The gap underscores the imperative for more intensive mental health education as part of primary care training curricula. Moreover, integrating psychiatric genetics into internal medicine adds another dimension of limited resources and training. The International Society of Psychiatric Genetics has underscored the importance of incorporating genetic information into psychiatric training programs. Although progress in the elucidation of the genetic determinants of psychiatric disorders is on the horizon, their integration in the clinic is still sporadic. The challenges of genetic testing, such as its relative underutilization in diagnosing conditions like autism and intellectual disability, constitute a core shortcoming in the skillset of general practitioners. There is a clear need for systematic educational frameworks that equip practitioners to interpret and apply genetic information in clinical decision-making (Austin et al., 2018). Moreover, the overall mental health workforce shortage makes the issue of poor resources and training within psychiatry even more complicated. Congressional action has recognized the interconnectedness of quality, access, and cost of mental health care, and how competent providers influence such determinants. The lack of adequately trained mental health professionals directly impacts the quality of care that internal medicine can provide. Furthermore, as mental health needs grow, the gap between the number of trained professionals and the increasing patient demand is a serious issue for policymakers to address (Bagalman et al., 2013). Accordingly, building an appropriately trained mental health workforce through improved training and resource management is instrumental in improving psychiatric care in internal medicine practice.

Test Your Knowledge

1. What are the main challenges in integrating psychiatry into internal medicine practice?
2. Why is it difficult to diagnose psychiatric disorders in patients with medical illnesses?

SUMMARY

The evolution of psychiatry illustrates both progress and pervasive challenges within the discipline. Modern psychiatry has successfully transitioned from rudimentary diagnostic frameworks, such as those embodied in the DSM-III, to a more elaborate system designed to encapsulate the complexities of mental illness. Nevertheless, the ongoing crisis of diagnostic inflation raises concerns about the reliability of psychiatric diagnoses and the appropriateness of interventions. As highlighted, the uncritical acceptance of expanded diagnostic criteria in the DSM-5 has arguably muddied the waters of clinical practice, necessitating a reevaluation of how psychiatric conditions are understood, diagnosed, and treated. Ultimately, the field must navigate the delicate balance between advancing knowledge and maintaining robust, clinically useful frameworks for diagnosis and treatment (Frances A, 2013). Furthermore, the intricate interplay between mental and physical health underscores the critical importance of an integrative approach to patient care. The assertion that there is no health without mental health encapsulates the profound impact that mental disorders have on overall health outcomes and functional capacity at both individual and societal levels. Recognizing the multifaceted nature of mental health, evidenced by the high prevalence of co-morbid conditions and the significant burden of neuropsychiatric disorders globally, necessitates a comprehensive model of care that holistically addresses these interdependencies. It becomes imperative for medical practitioners to adopt a bio-psycho-social framework, as encapsulated in modern psychiatric paradigms, to optimize treatment efficacy and patient well-being (Kallivayalil RA, 2012). Lastly, the continued development of psychiatry as a medical specialty relies on accessible education, effective communication, and the integration of innovative practices within existing healthcare frameworks. The necessity for thorough training in psychiatry for all medical students cannot be overstated, as it equips future healthcare providers with the skills required to regard psychological factors within their practice. Enhanced collaboration across disciplines and within healthcare systems can foster a more nuanced understanding of mental health issues, ultimately improving patient care outcomes. Addressing the systemic barriers to mental healthcare, including those related to stigma and accessibility, remains paramount for the evolution of psychiatry. Thus, the journey toward a more informed, compassionate approach in mental health care is not merely an academic goal; it is essential for the holistic advancement of medicine as a whole (Frances A, 2013).

The integration of internal medicine within psychiatry and behavioral medicine is pivotal for advancing a holistic approach to patient care. A major focus within this interdisciplinary practice is addressing the barriers faced by small primary care practices as they adapt to healthcare reforms. The challenges of transforming these practices are multi-faceted; however, specific options for Medicaid have the potential to catalyze significant improvements. These options include facilitating practice supports that help implement and sustain innovative care models. As noted, the mechanisms that drive change in small practices are essential for ensuring that both physical and mental health care are cohesively managed, which can ultimately enhance patient outcomes and streamline health care delivery. Cognitive health in geriatric patients represents another key area of focus within internal medicine and behavioral medicine. A recent summit conducted by the National Academy of Neuropsychology highlighted the necessity of addressing cognitive impairment in older adults, especially when they present with acute illnesses. The implications of cognitive decline for managing coexisting diseases can complicate treatment strategies; hence, establishing clear guidelines for cognitive screening in medical settings is vital. Participants in the summit underscored the importance of educational initiatives aimed at both providers and patients regarding the value of cognitive assessments. Identifying who should be screened and developing standardized approaches to screening are crucial steps for informing effective and comprehensive care for this vulnerable population. Moreover, the interaction between physical and mental health is evidenced through the recognition of cognitive impairment as a risk factor for dementia and other chronic conditions. The need for validated screening tools that are sensitive to various cultural, linguistic, and educational factors cannot be overstated, as these considerations directly impact the accuracy of cognitive assessments. Electronic health records (EHRs) are emerging as a valuable resource in this area, capable of enhancing cognitive screening procedures and facilitating ongoing tracking of cognitive health over time. This technological integration not only allows for more precise monitoring but also fosters an environment where healthcare providers can respond proactively to the evolving needs of older patients. As such, these developments within psychiatry and behavioral medicine are essential for creating a more interconnected health care system that prioritizes cognitive wellness alongside physical health.

KEY TERMS FROM THIS CHAPTER

- Mental Status Examination
- Depression
- Bipolar Disorder
- Delusion
- Obsessive-Compulsive Disorder
- Substance Use Disorder
- Cognitive Behavioral Therapy
- Neurotransmitter
- Anxiety Disorder
- Schizophrenia
- Hallucination
- Post-Traumatic Stress Disorder
- Psychosis
- Psychopharmacology

CRITICAL THINKING QUESTIONS

1. Which of the following is a positive symptom of schizophrenia?

a. Anhedonia

b. Alogia

c. Hallucinations

d. Avolition

2. Selective Serotonin Reuptake Inhibitors (SSRIs) are most commonly used in the treatment of:

a. Schizophrenia

b. Bipolar disorder

c. Generalized anxiety disorder

d. Obsessive-compulsive disorder

3. Which of the following is NOT part of the mental status examination (MSE)?

a. Thought content

b. Mood and affect

c. Blood pressure

d. Insight and judgment

4. A 25-year-old man believes the government is monitoring his thoughts through his television. This is an example of:

a. Somatic delusion

b. Referential delusion

c. Nihilistic delusion

d. Delusion of control

5. Lithium is most effective in the treatment of:

a. Generalized anxiety disorder

b. Bipolar affective disorder

c. Major depressive disorder

d. Schizoaffective disorder

Short Answer Questions

1. Discuss the etiology, clinical features, diagnostic criteria, and management of Major Depressive Disorder.
2. Explain the pathophysiology, clinical presentation, and management of Schizophrenia.
3. Discuss the role of neurotransmitters in psychiatric disorders.
4. Focus on dopamine, serotonin, and norepinephrine in relation to mood disorders and psychosis.
5. Elaborate on the diagnosis and management of Generalized Anxiety Disorder.

Answers to Critical Thinking Questions

1. (c); 2. (d); 3. (c); 4. (d); 5. (b)

REFERENCES

1. Buckingham, C. D., Adams, A., & Mace, C. (2008). Cues and knowledge structures used by mental-health professionals when making risk assessments. *Journal of Mental Health, 17*(3), 299–314. https://doi.org/10.1080/09638230701498374Alem, A., Bhana, A., Cohen, A., Rahman, A., Fekadu, A., Bradley, E. H., Thornicroft, G., et al. (2014). Challenges and opportunities for implementing integrated mental health care: A district level situation analysis from five low- and middle-income countries. https://core.ac.uk/download/19747695.pdf (accessed on 17th July 2025).

2. Allery, L. A., Bullock, A., MacDonald, J., & Muddiman, D. (2016). 'Black sheep in the herd'? The role, status and identity of generalist doctors in secondary care. https://core.ac.uk/download/74223766.pdf (accessed on 17th July 2025).

3. Alzheimer's Research Trust, Appelbaum, P. S., Bebbington, P., British Medical Association, The Law Society, Brazier, M., et al. (2012). Homeward bound or bound for a home? Assessing the capacity of dementia patients to make decisions about hospital discharge: Comparing practice with legal standards. https://core.ac.uk/download/9990190.pdf (accessed on 17th July 2025).

4. Anderson, J., Bennett, A. J. W., Clayton, P., McKeown, M., et al. (2003). Gender politics and secure services for women: Reflections on a study of staff understandings of challenging behavior. https://core.ac.uk/download/338689.pdf (accessed on 17th July 2025).

5. Annemans, L., Eyssen, M., Mommerency, G., & Schoentjes, E. (2011). *Organisatie Van Geestelijke Gezondheidszorg Voor Kinderen En Jongeren: Literatuurstudie En Internationaal Overzicht.* https://core.ac.uk/download/55771707.pdf (accessed on 17th July 2025).

6. Aria, M., Asperger, H., Bonacich, P., Callon, M., Chuang, K. Y., Cosgrove, L., Cosgrove, R., et al. (2018). Autism research: An objective quantitative review of progress and focus between 1994 and 2015. https://core.ac.uk/download/287581051.pdf (accessed on 17th July 2025).

7. Arunogiri, S., Baldacchino, A., Bates, M. E., Bowden-Jones, H., Lubman, D. I., Lees, R., et al. (2019). A roadmap for integrating neuroscience into addiction treatment: A consensus of the Neuroscience Interest Group of the International Society of Addiction Medicine. https://core.ac.uk/download/286356092.pdf (accessed on 17th July 2025).

8. Austin, J. C., Berrettini, W. H., Besterman, A. D., DeLisi, L. E., et al. (2018). What should a psychiatrist know about genetics? Review and recommendations from the Residency Education Committee of the International Society of Psychiatric Genetics. https://core.ac.uk/download/227054247.pdf (accessed on 17th July 2025).

9. Axelsson, M., Bockting, C., Buysse, A., Desmet, M., van den Broek, A., Podlipny, J., et al. (2020). Healthcare professionals' perspectives on mental health service provision: A pilot focus group study in six European countries. https://core.ac.uk/download/288817269.pdf (accessed on 17th July 2025).

10. Bagalman, E., & Heisler, E. J. (2013). *The Mental Health Workforce: A Primer.* https://core.ac.uk/download/18615793.pdf (accessed on 17th July 2025).

11. Barbour, R. S., Bryce, G., Connelly, G., & Furnivall, J. (2006). *Only Connect: Addressing The Emotional Needs of Scotland's Children and Young People.* https://core.ac.uk/download/9016267.pdf (accessed on 17th July 2025).

12. Barker, C., & Pistrang, N. (2002). Psychotherapy and social support–Integrating research on psychological helping. https://core.ac.uk/download/1670904.pdf (accessed on 17th July 2025).

13. Barlow, D. H., Bentley, K. H., Boettcher, H., & Bullis, J. R. (2017). Development of a single-session, transdiagnostic preventive intervention for young adults at risk for emotional disorders. https://open.bu.edu/bitstream/2144/39785/1/Bentley%20et%20al%202017_UP%20prevention.pdf (accessed on 17th July 2025).

14. Barlow, D. H., Sauer-Zavala, S., & Wilner, J. G. (2017). Addressing neuroticism in psychological treatment. https://open.bu.edu/bitstream/2144/40060/4/Addressing%20Neuroticism%20in%20Psychological%20Treatment%20FINAL-1.pdf (accessed on 17th July 2025).

15. Bartram, A. (2012). The performance of pain: The consequences for the performing body and its portrayal of mental health. https://core.ac.uk/download/17352854.pdf (accessed on 17th July 2025).

16. Begley, M., Condon, M., Garavan, K. C., Holland, W., et al. (1999). Asylum in Ireland–A public health perspective. https://core.ac.uk/download/11309246.pdf (accessed on 17th July 2025).

17. Berlin, J. S., Gutierrez, P. M., Petrik, M. L., & Saunders, S. M. (2015). Barriers and facilitators of suicide risk assessment in emergency departments: A qualitative study of provider perspectives. https://core.ac.uk/download/213077361.pdf (accessed on 17th July 2025).

18. Bevan Jones, R., Jones, I., Simpson, S., & Smith, D. J. (2017). Psychoeducational interventions in adolescent depression: A systematic review. https://core.ac.uk/download/132211505.pdf (accessed on 17th July 2025).

19. Borro, M., Di Sanzo, M., Fineschi, V., Frati, P., et al. (2017). Clinical applications of personalized medicine: A new paradigm and challenge. https://core.ac.uk/download/80315182.pdf (accessed on 17th July 2025).

20. Brabeck, K. M., Holtzman, E. G., & Kene, P. (2018). Integrating mindfulness into the training of helping professionals. https://core.ac.uk/download/215489761.pdf (accessed on 17th July 2025).

21. Browne, G., Busing, B., Forbes, D., Gibson, M., et al. (2014). An interprofessional nurse-led mental health promotion intervention for older home care clients with depressive symptoms. https://core.ac.uk/download/323070460.pdf (accessed on 17th July 2025).

22. Bucci, F. (2014). Cultural representations of mental illness in contemporary Japan. https://core.ac.uk/download/74711749.pdf (accessed on 17th July 2025).

23. Camilleri, N., Cassar Parnis, A., & Cassar, J. R. (2009). Problems associated with the diagnosis and the prescribing of anti-psychotic medication in children and adolescents for psychiatric conditions, by non-psychiatric specialists. https://core.ac.uk/download/46602212.pdf (accessed on 17th July 2025).

24. Chang, P., Cosley, D., Frank, E., Gay, G., et al. (2016). Self-monitoring practices, attitudes, and needs of individuals with bipolar disorder: Implications for the design of technologies to manage mental health. https://core.ac.uk/download/213087764.pdf (accessed on 17th July 2025).

25. Chelvanayagam, S., Collins, B., Duncan, J., O'Brien, K., et al. (2012). Uncovering anorexia nervosa in a biofeedback clinic for bowel dysfunction. https://core.ac.uk/download/20321227.pdf (accessed on 17th July 2025).

26. Connaughton, J., du Plessis, C., Probst, M., & Rosenbaum, S. (2016). What are the top 10 physical activity research questions in schizophrenia? https://core.ac.uk/download/61305032.pdf (accessed on 17th July 2025).

27. Coogle, C. L., & Owens, M. G. (2015). Screening and brief intervention for alcohol misuse in older adults: Training outcomes among physicians and other healthcare practitioners in community-based settings. https://core.ac.uk/download/215483536.pdf (accessed on 17th July 2025).

28. Croker, H., Falconer, C. L., Kessel, A. S., Kinra, S., et al. (2013). Perceptions of health risk among parents of overweight children: A cross-sectional study within a cohort. https://core.ac.uk/download/13117165.pdf (accessed on 17th July 2025).

29. Ely, L. J., Gilbert, D. L., Lipps, T. D., Mink, J. W., et al. (2015). Pilot testing behavior therapy for chronic tic disorders in neurology and developmental pediatrics clinics. https://core.ac.uk/download/213085584.pdf (accessed on 17th July 2025).

30. Fochtmann, L. J., Kunkle, R., Nininger, J. E., Plovnick, R. M., et al. (2014). Who's your expert? Use of an expert opinion survey to inform development of American Psychiatric Association practice guidelines. https://core.ac.uk/download/213444916.pdf (accessed on 17th July 2025).

31. Frances, A. (2013). The past, present and future of psychiatric diagnosis. *World Psychiatry, 12*, 111–112. https://doi.org/10.1002/wps.20027 (accessed on 17th July 2025).

32. Ghanizadeh, A., Heikkinen, A., Rafalovitch, A., Mueller, A. K., Olson, A. L., Miller, A. R., Gavin, B., et al. (2016). What do general practitioners know about ADHD? Attitudes and knowledge among first-contact gatekeepers: Systematic narrative review. https://core.ac.uk/download/159108013.pdf (accessed on 17th July 2025).

33. Grey, B. J. (2015). The future of emotional harm. https://core.ac.uk/download/144230394.pdf (accessed on 17th July 2025).

34. Griffiths, M. D., Shonin, E., & Van Gordon, W. (2015). Mindfulness in mental health: A critical reflection. https://core.ac.uk/download/30649717.pdf (accessed on 17th July 2025).

35. Groom, G., Holmwood, C., & Nicholson, S. A. (2008). *Mental Health Shared Care in Australia 2001: Report for the Commonwealth Department of Health and Aged Care*. https://core.ac.uk/download/14931392.pdf (accessed on 17th July 2025).

36. Hauck, F., Kamp-Becker, I., Kliewer, N., Küpper, C., et al. (2020). Identifying predictive features of autism spectrum disorders in a clinical sample of adolescents and adults using machine learning. https://core.ac.uk/download/288845804.pdf (accessed on 17th July 2025).

37. Hocking, B. (2025). A life without stigma. https://core.ac.uk/download/pdf/30676353.pdf (accessed on 17th July 2025).

38. Hoque, S. (2016). Care team education on the use of sensory resources in inpatient psychiatry. https://core.ac.uk/download/79664899.pdf (accessed on 17th July 2025).

39. Howardova, A., Kallert, T. W., Kiejna, A., Nawka, P., et al. (2013). To what extent could acute general psychiatric day care reduce inpatient admissions? https://core.ac.uk/download/30698054.pdf (accessed on 17th July 2025).

40. Iveson, S., Leach, C., & Lucock, M. (2005). Using evidence to improve psychological therapies services. https://core.ac.uk/download/57835.pdf (accessed on 17th July 2025).

41. Kallivayalil, R. A. (2012). The importance of psychiatry in undergraduate medical education in

India. *Indian Journal of Psychiatry, 54*, 208–208. https://doi.org/10.4103/0019-5545.102336 (accessed on 17th July 2025).

42. Long, V. (2016). 'Heading up a blind alley'? Scottish psychiatric hospitals in the era of deinstitutionalization. https://core.ac.uk/download/293881690.pdf (accessed on 17th July 2025).
43. Melchert, T. P., & Meyer, L. (2011). Examining the content of mental health intake assessments from a biopsychosocial perspective. https://core.ac.uk/download/213064254.pdf (accessed on 17th July 2025).
44. Pearson, A., Glaser, B., Ahmedani, B. K., Pope, C., O'Connor, E., Leavey, G., & McDaid, D. (2017). The failure of suicide prevention in primary care: Family and GP perspectives–A qualitative study. https://core.ac.uk/download/151170770.pdf (accessed on 17th July 2025).
45. Robiner, W. N., Tompkins, T., & Tumlin, T. R. (2013). Psychologists and medications in the era of interprofessional care: Collaboration is less problematic and costly than prescribing. https://core.ac.uk/download/143958393.pdf (accessed on 17th July 2025).
46. Sices, L. (2007). *Developmental Screening in Primary Care: The Effectiveness of Current Practice and Recommendations for Improvement.* https://core.ac.uk/download/71350769.pdf (accessed on 17th July 2025).
47. Sterling, S., & Weisner, C. (2006). Translating research findings into practice: Example of treatment services for adolescents in managed care. https://core.ac.uk/download/323072702.pdf (accessed on 17th July 2025).
48. Thomas, A., Burns, A., Bains, P., Beecham, J., Fox, C., Lawton, C., Ballard, C., et al. (2012). Cost-effectiveness analyses for mirtazapine and sertraline in dementia: Randomized controlled trial. https://core.ac.uk/download/9838269.pdf (accessed on 17th July 2025).
49. Thornton, T. (2011). Recent developments for naturalizing the mind. https://core.ac.uk/download/341071.pdf (accessed on 17th July 2025).
50. Zawiła-Niedźwiecki, J. (2016). Antoni Kępiński's philosophy of medicine–An alternative reading. https://core.ac.uk/download/83117222.pdf (accessed on 17th July 2025).

GERIATRIC MEDICINE

3

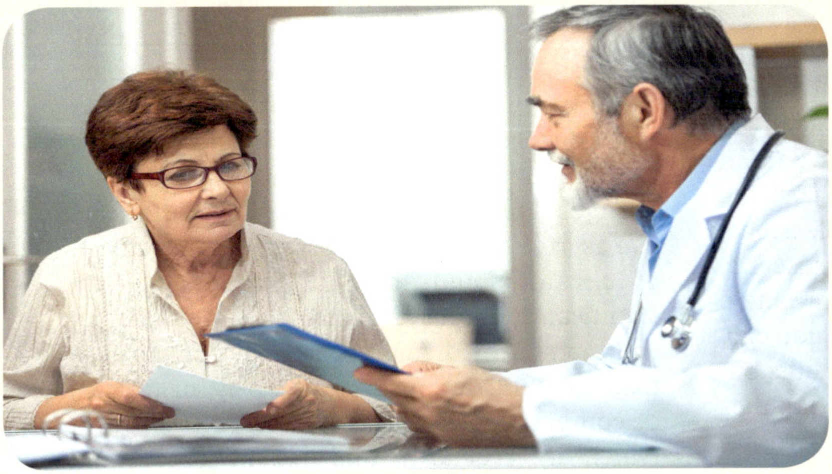

LEARNING OBJECTIVES

After studying this chapter, you will be able to:

1. Understand common health issues in the elderly
2. Discuss geriatric assessment
3. Describe pharmacological considerations
4. Focus on non-pharmacological interventions in geriatric medicine
5. Explain palliative and end-of-life care
6. Deal with challenges in geriatric medicine

Introduction

Geriatric medicine is increasingly recognized as an essential specialty in addressing the unique healthcare needs of the elderly. With aging, the patient typically harbors a mix of complex health conditions resulting from interactions among chronic diseases, functional impairment, and the multifactorial nature of aging itself. This necessitates an encyclopedic system of care that transcends traditional internal medicine. Geriatric internal medicine is concerned not only with the medical management of illness but also with comprehensive care that includes social, emotional, and economic factors. Familiarity with this multifaceted approach is essential for practitioners who want to optimize care for elderly patients. It is at the practice center of internal medicine for the geriatric population that the impact of age-related risks on healthcare quality and cost is recognized. According to existing research, geriatric and aged patients often present with complex healthcare needs that strain the healthcare system. Reducing these effectively has been shown to improve care quality while simultaneously reducing costs. Geriatric care management approaches to older patients can enhance their health outcomes by strengthening the coordination of healthcare professionals. In doing this, the challenge is to implement the strategies uniformly across various healthcare centers, ensuring equal access to quality care. The quest for the effectiveness of care management for older people remains at the core of advancing geriatric medicine and producing sufficient evidence to inform policy translation. Also, geriatric healthcare policy is informed by a strong evidence base for practice-sensitive to older adults' specific needs. The Stern Center's reports identify areas where the research evidence is strong yet remains unrealized in practice, including palliative care and patient self-management. These results underscore the importance of developing an interprofessional practice that incorporates geriatric expertise into broader health systems. By prioritizing prevention and care coordination, the profession not only strives to enhance the health of older adults but also seeks to empower patients and families through informed involvement in care decisions. The future development of geriatric medicine will undoubtedly be based on translating research into policies to address both short- and long-term healthcare challenges in the elderly (Berry-Millett et al., 2009; Morton et al., 2015) (Figure 3.1).

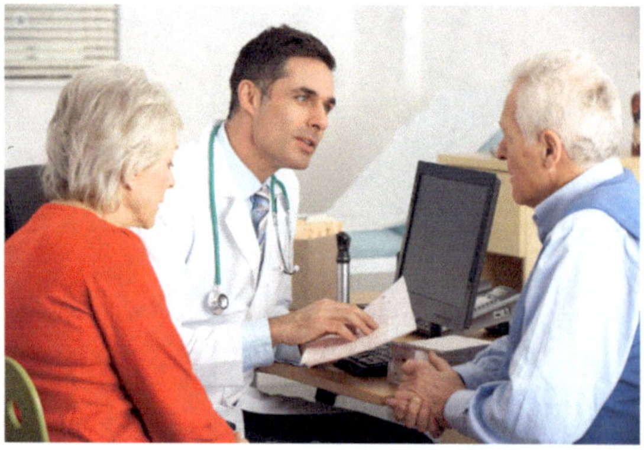

Figure 3.1. The field of geriatric medicine.

Source: https://staticnew-prod.topdoctors.co.uk/files/Image/large/5bd9bdd8-dbf8-41a5-a429-248025bbab96.png.

Definition and Scope of Geriatric Medicine

The three-dimensional definition of internal medicine, particularly in geriatrics, reflects the diversity of health care in elderly groups. Internal medicine, in general, is focused on the diagnosis, treatment, and prevention of a wide variety of illnesses in adults, with special emphasis on comprehensive patient care. This is a specialty especially applicable to geriatric patients, who often present with many comorbid conditions and need a thorough understanding of how these conditions interact. The internal medicine physician must not only possess extensive medical knowledge but also grasp the unique physiological and psychosocial changes that occur in geriatric patients. Its use is relevant because proper management of chronic conditions in the elderly can significantly improve outcomes and quality of life. Internal medicine's role is not only disease management; it is also guided by principles of comprehensive geriatric assessment (CGA), which are crucial in this patient population. CGA involves a multidimensional evaluation that assists in screening for several geriatric syndromes—e.g., frailty, falls, and cognitive impairment—that commonly accompany chronic diseases. For instance, recent studies have found that certain sets of geriatric syndromes are strongly correlated with some of the health hazards and are influenced by conditions like psychosocial factors and fluid imbalance. Thus, prompt and accurate assessment can lead to more accurate prognostic estimates, enabling clinicians to individualize interventions based on specific patient needs appropriately. Targeted intervention is required to improve health outcomes and reduce hospitalization risk among elderly patients. Internal medicine also plays a significant role in the detection and care of prevalent geriatric illnesses, e.g., anemia. Studies have established that anemia is likely to be underdiagnosed among the elderly, even though it has significant correlations with unfavorable health consequences, including mortality and functional loss. Effective treatment of anemia in elderly patients requires active intervention by practitioners in internal medicine, who must make a correct diagnosis and select appropriate treatment approaches. This includes prompt identification of anemia causes, together with attention to the multifaceted nature of health in the elderly. The challenges posed by this population reflect the central role internal medicine plays in maximizing care and the necessity of improved awareness and training in geriatrics among healthcare providers. By bringing together an expansive knowledge base of medical and functional aspects of care, internal medicine can help provide greater assurance about the overall quality of life of older adults (Figure 3.2).

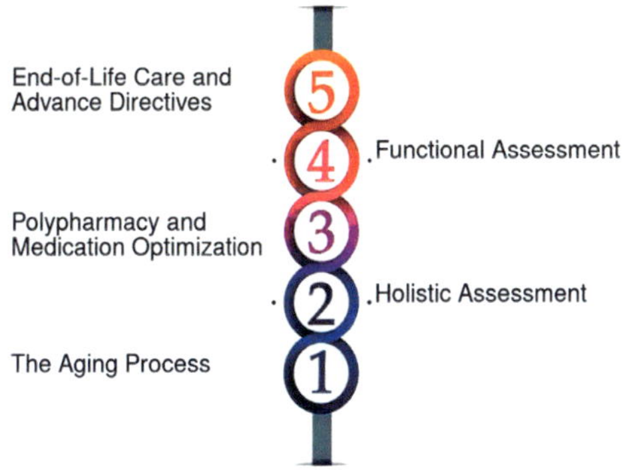

Figure 3.2. Definition of internal medicine is multifaceted.

Source: https://fastercapital.co/i/Geriatric-medicine--The-Specialty-that-Addresses-the-Health-and-Aging-of-Older-Adults--Introduction-to-Geriatric-Medicine.webp.

Importance of Geriatric Medicine

The importance of geriatric medicine cannot be overstated, particularly given the unique health concerns of the aging population. Aging is often accompanied by multiple chronic conditions, which typically complicate disease treatment and call for expert care strategies. Trends in geriatric medicine underscore the need for an integrative viewpoint with physical, mental, and social well-being. As older adults are likely to present with abnormal symptoms, geriatricians play a crucial role in diagnosing and managing conditions that would otherwise remain undetected. Not only does this integral approach improve the quality of life in elderly patients, but it also significantly reduces the healthcare burden and expenses associated with uncontrolled chronic illness. Such effective management can ultimately lead to better health outcomes, underscoring the pivotal importance of geriatric medicine in modern healthcare. In addition, the population's aging trend underscores the growing importance of geriatric medicine in the practice of internal medicine. As life expectancy rises, the healthcare system must adapt itself to meet the complex requirements of the elderly, who are constantly confronted with multiple, interlinked health issues. For instance, conditions like heart disease, diabetes, and cognitive impairment tend to come in clusters and require concerted, multidisciplinary management. Geriatric medicine reorients attention toward imparting knowledge and skills to health professionals so they may better communicate and collaborate to address complex health cases. Furthermore, recognizing the value of standardized care frameworks, such as individualized medication management and advance directives, strengthens the bond between the physician and patient, establishing the trust needed when caring for the sensitive health needs of the elderly. This shift in mindset ultimately translates into improved care and better outcomes for this vulnerable segment of the population. Moreover, geriatric medicine has a key role to play in the management of some geriatric syndromes, such as delirium and frailty, that significantly impact morbidity and mortality in older persons. The nuances of such syndromes allow practitioners to individualize care plans that treat not only symptoms but also prevent complications. As an example, management of postoperative delirium is augmented by guideline-recommended measures that take a proactive approach to preoperative identification of high-risk patients. In addition to maximizing surgical outcomes, this preventive strategy aligns with the overall goals of geriatric medicine, which aim to optimize function and independence in older adults. Thus, the commitment to geriatric medicine, as evidenced in an integrated care model that addresses the specific needs of this age group, is priceless in helping to establish a healthier, more robust society in its elder years.

Overview of the Aging Population and Its Implications

Population aging is a major demographic shift that will affect much of society, particularly the healthcare system. While medical science and technology have extended life expectancy, more individuals are living into old age, thereby increasing the proportion of older individuals in the population. By 2030, individuals aged 65 and older will represent an increasingly larger share of society, raising fundamental questions about whether current healthcare systems can meet their unique health needs. The population change extends beyond numbers; it represents a need for healthcare workers to adapt their services to treat a population with increasing health issues. These include chronic illnesses and cognitive impairments. Therefore, geriatric medicine will be a required science and a challenging field for medical practitioners in addressing the multifaceted issues of elderly patients. Also, the effects of an aging population extend beyond healthcare to include economic and policy implications. An aged population means high medical treatment demands, which may strain existing healthcare resources and infrastructure. Additionally, the rising costs of elderly care require careful policymaking. Studies have brought into sharp focus the value of instituting evidence-based policies that emphasize prevention and care coordination for health outcomes among the elderly. For example, patient self-management and palliative care programs need to be strengthened to reduce the burden on healthcare systems while improving the quality of life for the elderly. The imperative for strategic action that mandates interdisciplinary collaboration is of prime importance to the ongoing viability and effectiveness of geriatric medicine within an evolving health system context, as noted in recent literature. To respond to the distinctive needs of older people, it is necessary to understand and implement CGAs in clinical practice fully. These assessments provide crucial insights about the unique health profiles of geriatric patients, with superior predictive value for morbidity and mortality compared to other tools. Tests identify domains such as social support, frailty, and nutritional status as predictors of meaningful health outcomes.

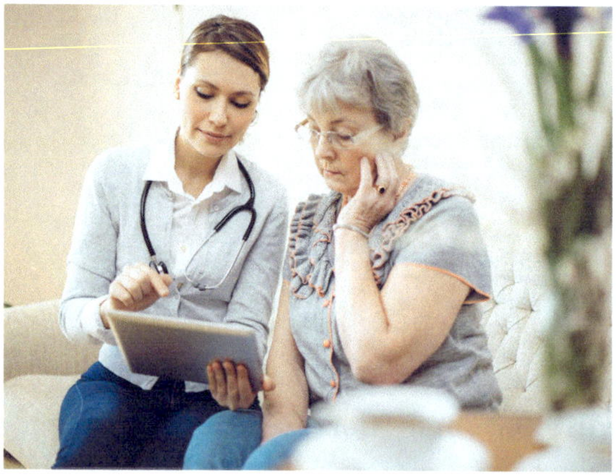

Figure 3.3. The aging population represents a significant demographic shift poised to reverberate through various facets of society.

Source: https://assets.contenthub.wolterskluwer.com/api/public/content/a6b90f9f101541f9a485f307f6e5eeca?v=12f18c4c.

Although their effectiveness has been proven, this essential assessment is performed for only a minority of oncogeriatric patients before surgical treatment. To fill the gap, medical student educational programs are crucial, equipping them to deliver high-quality evaluations in clinical practice settings. Building a solid foundation of geriatric education among future physicians will ultimately improve the delivery of care, as this group continues to grow and requires specialized care and resources, as noted by Lampugnani et al. (2017) and Morton et al. (2015) (Figure 3.3).

3.1. Common Health Issues in the Elderly

Learning Outcome

1. Discuss chronic diseases prevalent in older adults;
2. Focus on mental health challenges, including dementia and depression;
3. Explain mobility and physical health concerns.

Because the aging population continues to grow, it is essential to recognize and address common health issues. The increasing prevalence of chronic diseases such as hypertension, diabetes, and arthritis is a cause for concern. Not only do these diseases diminish the quality of life in the elderly, but they also enhance the demand for healthcare. In particular, hypertension is typically silent but can result in severe complications, such as heart disease and stroke. Management of such chronic conditions thus entails careful consideration of the unique physiological changes with aging. Consequently, health professionals must adopt multidimensional interventions that include drug management, lifestyle modification, and regular monitoring to optimize health outcomes among older patients.

The complexity of treating such conditions underscores the need for specialist education and training for healthcare professionals specializing in geriatric medicine, focusing on care plans tailored to each individual. Cognitive impairment is also a significant health issue for elderly populations, and dementia and Alzheimer's disease are increasingly prevalent conditions. These cognitive impairments not only affect the patients but also cause a severe physical and emotional strain on family members and caregivers. Early identification and treatment are essential to achieve an optimal level of remaining cognitive function and slow the course of the disease. Geriatric assessments play a significant role in diagnosing age-related cognitive disturbances; however, the application of comprehensive assessments is hampered by time constraints for healthcare providers. As quoted, the application of geriatric assessments targeting relevant cognitive areas allows for the recognition of risks and the appropriate conceptualization of interventions to enhance the quality of life in elderly patients with cognitive impairment (Lampugnane et al., 2017). Mental illness issues, particularly depression and anxiety, are prevalent in older people and tend to be exacerbated by loneliness, chronic pain, and loss. They tend to go undiagnosed and untreated, but have the potential to reduce quality of life and lead to significant adverse outcomes. Geriatric medicine practitioners must be especially vigilant in screening for mental illness since it manifests differently in older patients, sometimes mimicking physical illnesses or manifesting as chronic somatic complaints. Mental health treatment is not just pharmacological interventions but also psychosocial measures to promote social interaction and emotional support. Greater sensitivity to the mental health needs of older adults highlights the benefits of having an integrated plan of care that includes mental well-being within overall health planning (Fiorini et al., 2003). Through the encouragement of an open culture in which to discuss mental health, healthcare providers can better address the emotional and psychological needs of the older adult (Figure 3.4).

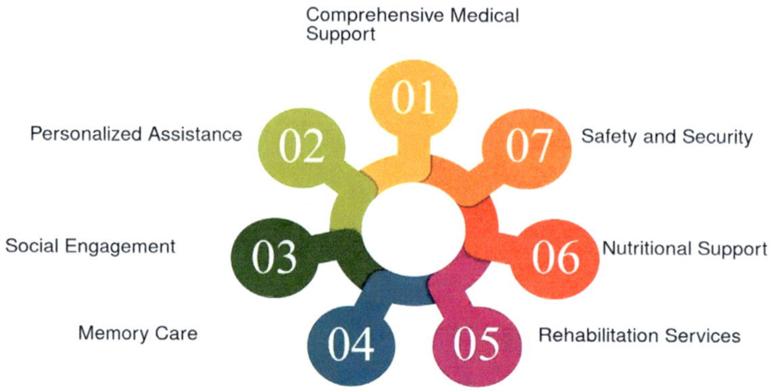

Figure 3.4. Common health issues in the elderly.

Source: https://fastercapital.co/i/Geriatric-Care-Center--Importance-of-Specialized-Care-for-the-Elderly.webp.

3.1.1. Chronic Diseases Prevalent in Older Adults

Chronic diseases are an important area in the practice of geriatric medicine, particularly as the aging population is rising; as a result, chronic conditions such as hypertension, diabetes, and arthritis have become increasingly prevalent . These diseases have an adverse effect on quality of life, leading to functional disability and increased healthcare burdens. Hypertension, for instance, tends to be diagnosed frequently among older adults, often with concomitant chronic disease. Hypertension management is also made more challenging with the occurrence of comorbid conditions, requiring careful medications management to prevent polypharmacy—a prevailing problem in this group of patients. A review highlights that there are many reasons for polypharmacy in elderly cancer patients, including managing adverse drug reactions and comorbidities (Khanal et al., 2019). It also highlights the need for an integrated approach to handle the complex interplay between chronic disease plus polypharmacy in older persons. Diabetes mellitus is also a chronic disorder quite prevalent in elderly populations, which significantly affects their overall health and quality of life. Numerous complications, including cardiovascular disease, neuropathy, and retinopathy, accompany this condition. Diabetes, comorbid with other chronic illnesses, aggravates the older person's health condition, resulting in deteriorating health. In addition, older persons typically require customized management programs that address their own drug physiological response and dietary requirements. Research confirms differences in the management of hypertension, namely that African American older adults have higher levels of hypertension and may be treated with additional anti-hypertensive medication without achieving optimal blood pressure control (Allman et al., 2015). These findings demonstrate that race-specific, gender-specific, and comorbidity-specific healthcare practices are necessary for managing diabetes and its complications among older adults. Arthritis, another prevalent chronic illness in the elderly, poses challenging conditions that compromise mobility and autonomy. Osteoarthritis and rheumatoid diseases produce chronic pain and stiffness that lead to limited physical activity and secondary illnesses such as obesity and depression. The linkage of arthritis to comorbidities is an adverse healthcare environment in geriatric medicine that necessitates multimodal strategies that address pain management and enhance physical function. Effective management strategies are essential for maintaining mobility and quality of life among the elderly with arthritis. Healthcare providers should also take into consideration the risk of polypharmacy among patients and ensure that patients receive no unnecessary medication that worsens underlying health conditions. In conclusion, the management of chronic disease among the elderly must be comprehensive and individualized to achieve maximum health benefits.

3.1.2. Mental Health Challenges, Including Dementia and Depression

As age increases, an individual suffers from a lot of mental illness conditions, such as dementia and depression, which are the most prominent challenges in geriatric practice. Dementia, or a progressive decline in cognitive function, is a high-stakes problem not only for the patient but also for caregivers. Caregiving burden can result in heightened stress, emotional distress, and even mental deterioration among carers, which is why it is essential to address the needs of both patients and those who care for them. Research shows that older carers, who are frequently still underrepresented in research and policymaking agendas, face special sources of stress that overwhelm their own mental health issues. The identification of these dynamics underpins the development of more effective interventions that benefit both the demented elderly and their caregivers, highlighting the need for resilience-building and coping strategies in this group (Henwood et al., 2017). Depression, another common problem with the elderly, is also found to co-occur with chronic physical illness and cognitive impairment, thus complicating clinical assessment and treatment. Depression and dementia interact particularly adversely, with depressive symptoms catalyzing further loss in cognitive ability, creating a self-reinforcing downward spiral for mental and physical health. The issue is one of accurately screening for depressive disorder in the elderly population, especially in those with cognitive impairment. The National Academy of Neuropsychology has emphasized the importance of routine cognitive screening and early detection of mental health disorders among geriatrics, specifically in the case of comorbid conditions (Adler et al., 2018). The multidimensional approach not only improves the quality of care but also enhances overall health outcomes, underscoring the need for tailored screening tools that address the cognitive and emotional complexities of aging populations. Also, it is essential to provide an environment that fosters the mental health of the elderly and emphasizes more preventive care in geriatrics. Inclusion of mental health interventions such as group therapy or social interaction programs can play a significant role in alleviating loneliness and anxiety among elderly individuals.

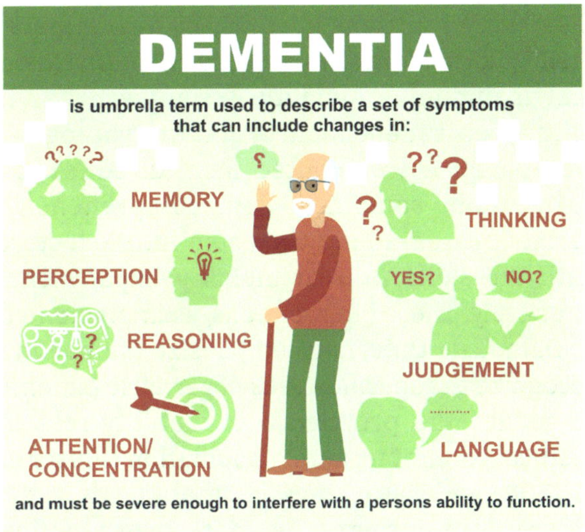

Figure 3.5. Mental health challenges, including dementia and depression.

Source: https://www.careinsurance.com/upload_master/media/dementia-symptoms.webp.

Further, both patients and healthcare providers can be educated on the significance of mental health in the elderly to improve detection and care of disorders like dementia and depression. Healthcare systems should adopt comprehensive models of care that address the physical and mental health needs of older adults, ensuring they receive well-rounded, individualized care. It not only alleviates the short-term symptoms of dementia and depression but also encourages long-term mental and emotional well-being, ultimately enhancing the quality of life for aging populations (Figure 3.5).

3.1.3. Mobility and Physical Health Concerns

With the expanding scope of Geriatric Medicine, mobility and physical functioning problems remain central to the management of the elderly. Older patients are often plagued by a range of mobility issues brought about by musculoskeletal disorders, neurological illnesses, and frailty. These conditions can severely curtail their daily functioning, which in turn impacts their quality of life. Research has demonstrated that maintaining mobility is significant, as it influences independence and psychological well-being. A well-crafted medical education curriculum, combined with comprehensive geriatric care training, can equip future doctors with the skills to treat mobility impairments effectively. These interventions, as implemented at Dalhousie University, emphasize the need to recognize the specific needs of geriatric patients to reduce the prevalence of mobility-related medical conditions in this population (Freter et al., 2003). Physical assessment of health in the elderly also encompasses more than mobility issues; it involves quantifying multimorbidity, support networks, and nutritional status. Comprehensive geriatric assessments are key to understanding the intricate interaction between these variables. Research emphasizes the need to integrate geriatric evaluations, especially in the management of conditions such as cancer, which specifically target older persons. Although their value is acknowledged, most healthcare providers find it challenging to apply these assessments due to time constraints and workload demands. Thus, training programs focused on geriatric assessments can provide a greater understanding of how to optimize physical health, enabling older patients to receive interventions tailored to their specific needs and mobility requirements. Lastly, improving mobility in elderly patients is not merely about medical interventions but also about community-based interventions that support mobility in daily activities. Exercise protocols that include physical activity, balance exercises, and social engagement are extremely valuable when implemented concurrently with geriatric educational programs. One example is encouraging collaboration between geriatricians, physical therapists, and occupational therapists to establish a multidisciplinary support network for geriatric patients. Interdisciplinary treatment can improve mobility outcomes through targeted therapies that enhance musculoskeletal strength and overall physical functioning. With frailty and mobility impairment still spreading in the elderly, concerted efforts in healthcare education and mobilization of social resources will be essential to overcome these pressing issues in Geriatric Medicine (Freter et al., 2003; Lampugnale et al., 2017).

Test Your Knowledge

1. What are the most common chronic diseases affecting older adults?
2. How can early detection of dementia and other cognitive disorders improve the management and care of elderly individual?
3. What are the primary risk factors for depression in older adults?

3.2 Geriatric Assessment Learning Outcomes:

Learning Outcome

1. Understand the comprehensive geriatric assessment process
2. Describe tools and methods used in assessment
3. Explain the importance of individualized care plans

With the aging population, geriatric assessment becomes increasingly important in the practice of geriatric medicine. This comprehensive evaluation is required to establish the multifaceted health care needs of older adults, who have many comorbidities and complex care needs. The assessment typically is a thorough medical history, physical examination, and functional ability, cognitive, and psychosocial assessments. Using a systematic approach, subtle differences in well-being and health can be identified, enabling interventions to be undertaken at the right time to enhance the quality of life of geriatric patients. Furthermore, geriatric assessment supports the guidance of the treatment decision, such as medication management, which is significant given older adults' heightened susceptibility to drug-related side effects and interactions and therefore eradication of the risk of inappropriately prescribing that will lead to further complications, as reported by Corsonello et al. (2016). By using tools and techniques specifically designed for geriatric assessment, patient outcomes can be significantly improved. Medication assessment tools, for instance, are essential for mitigating the polypharmacy hazards commonly faced by older individuals. Inadmissible prescribing implicit and explicit standards help clinicians navigate the complexity of treatment individualization in accordance with appropriate dosing, patient compliance, and potential drug-drug interactions. Interdisciplinary teamwork between health care practitioners is also crucial to ensuring the success of these methods. With the multidisciplinary expertise of pharmacists, physicians, and nurses, geriatric assessment can be conducted with greater detail and rigor. Not only does this team approach effectively streamline pharmaceutical care, but it also aligns with the broader principles of geriatric medicine, which call for multidimensional care to address the unique needs of older patients, as explored by Corsonello et al. (2016). Furthermore, policy concerns regarding geriatric assessment are imperative for improving the care of the elderly. The outcomes of studies reveal a pressing need for evidence-based policies to intensify prevention and coordination of care, as reported in.

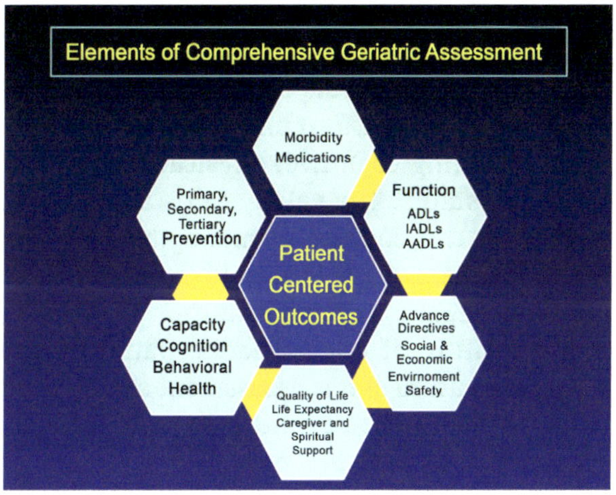

Figure 3.6. The importance of geriatric assessment.

Source: https://media.springernature.com/lw685/springer-static/image/chp%3A10.1007%2F978-3-319-90761-1_8-1/MediaObjects/191085_0_En_8-1_Fig2_HTML.png.

While some topics, including patient self-management and palliative care, have strong evidence supporting their importance, they also reveal a broad policy gap. Resolving these inconsistencies is a high priority, with geriatric evaluation and resulting care interventions made routine and universally available to all older individuals. These evaluations must be integrated into future health care systems from the beginning, bypassing present shortcomings while prioritizing the crucial roles of family caregivers and members of the health care workforce in delivering quality care. By employing information from geriatric assessments, geriatric medicine can enable health improvement in ageing populations (Figure 3.6).

3.2.1. Comprehensive Geriatric Assessment Process

Comprehensive geriatric assessment is a multidimensional, interdisciplinary diagnostic process for determining the medical, psychological, and functional capabilities of older individuals. CGA is broader than a typical medical assessment, as it encompasses multiple areas, including cognitive, physical, social, and emotional status. The value of this assessment is clear in the context of managing complex health needs, where multiple comorbidities often accompany a single condition. Especially in the context of oncogeriatric patients, the integrated nature of this assessment can be used to tailor treatment regimens to both cancer-related issues and the overall well-being of the ageing patient (Lampugnale et al., 2017). By rigorous risk identification and enhanced coordination among healthcare professionals, CGA enables more effective clinical decision-making, ensuring that elderly patients' changing needs are adequately met. Despite the clear benefits of CGA, it still has not been adopted on a broad scale owing to persisting challenges. Time constraints in the clinical environment are the most general barrier, with clinicians often struggling to incorporate detailed assessments into the frenetic workflow. Indeed, evidence suggests that many oncogeriatric individuals receive incomplete assessments, even though their benefits are known to clinicians (Lampugnane et al., 2017). Additionally, staff orientation and training on the topics encompassed by assessments can contribute to the challenge of successful implementation. To correct these conditions, interventions to practicing clinicians and medical students are called for. These interventions would then be formulated based on the most predictive areas for measuring postoperative risk, equipping future clinicians with the skills to perform effective geriatric assessment and enhancing patient outcomes. Data acquired through the CGA process can be a determining factor in individual patient management and in the establishment of healthcare policy for elderly people. All studies have reaffirmed the need for preventive and coordinated care, particularly amid the looming demographic shift in the elderly population.

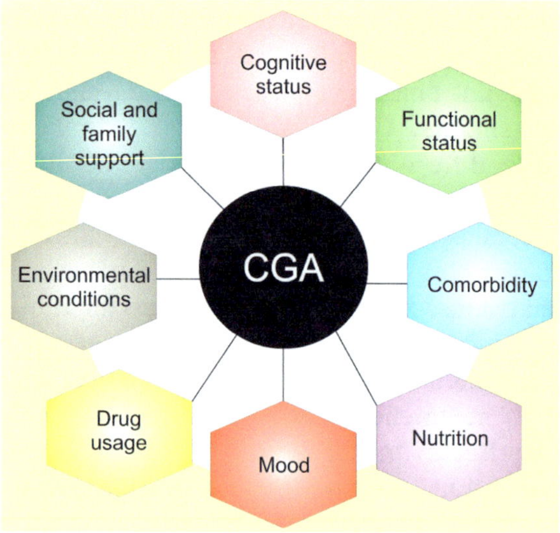

Figure 3.7. Comprehensive geriatric assessment (CGA): An organized evaluation method to provide a multidisciplinary assessment of and care for the elderly.

Source: https://www.researchgate.net/publication/346542805/figure/fig2/AS:11431281211610800@1702468437731/Comprehensive-geriatric-assessment-CGA-is-an-organized-evaluation-method-to-provide-a.tif.

By intentionally connecting assessment findings to evidence-based policy, healthcare systems can refine their plans to improve the health of older adults. Facilitating an interprofessional collaborative culture that includes family caregivers and focuses on patient self-management will ensure that CGA has meaningful impacts beyond clinic environments. As populations grow older, the health sector must recognize the importance of comprehensive assessment to inform policy, enhance service provision, and ultimately improve the quality of care for our aging population (Figure 3.7).

3.2.2. Tools and Methods Used in Assessment

Assessing geriatric patients requires specialized tools and methods tailored to the complexities of aging. The cornerstone of this testing lies in the comprehensive geriatric assessment (CGA), which encompasses physical health, cognitive function, social environment, and functional status. Not only does this more integrated approach enable individualized patient management, but it also enhances the validity of treatment plans through thorough analysis of each patient's particular context. For instance, oncogeriatrics requires a thorough pre-surgical geriatric assessment to arrange surgical procedures that meet the special needs and wishes of older patients. These assessments identify essential predictors of surgical outcomes after operation, thus allowing clinicians to optimize care pathways and mitigate risks of surgical treatment. It is important for healthcare professionals to become sensitized to their use in patient management plans (Lampugnani et al., 2017). In addition, cognitive screening instruments have become more prominent in geriatric medicine, especially in the emergency department, where rapid screening is critical. The Ottawa 3DY (O3DY) and the Short Blessed Test (SBT) have both proven helpful in identifying cognitive impairment among older adults presenting to the emergency department. Empirical research confirms that these tools exhibit moderate sensitivity and specificity, thereby facilitating early identification of cognitive impairments that can significantly impact patient management and outcomes. By using standardized measurement methods, healthcare providers can better prioritize interventions for the geriatric patient population, thereby improving the quality of care. Furthermore, understanding the inter-rater reliability of such assessments is essential to ensure consistent, reproducible results in geriatric cognitive screening among healthcare providers who routinely use them (Barbic et al., 2018).

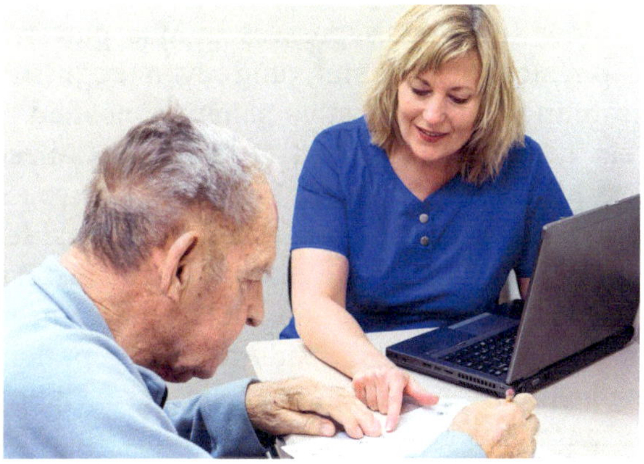

Figure 3.8. Cognitive-assessment for senior.

Source: https://floridaseniorconsulting.com/wp-content/uploads/2024/10/cognitive-assessment-for-seniors-1.jpg.

In addition to complete and cognitive assessments, various other methods are used to screen geriatric patients effectively. These include functional assessments, which examine older adults' ability to perform daily activities, and tests such as the Frailty Index or the Geriatric Depression Scale, which are specifically designed to quantify physiological and psychological parameters relevant to elderly care. The use of these varied assessment tools addresses the multifactorial nature of aging, enabling clinicians to provide patient-centered, holistic care. It can be observed that the use of these different assessment methods enhances understanding of each geriatric patient's needs, enabling more informed clinical decision-making. Ultimately, the successful application of assessment tools in geriatrics improves health outcomes and quality of life among elderly individuals while assisting them with the challenges of aging (Lampugnani et al., 2017) (Figure 3.8).

3.2.3. Importance of Individualized Care Plans

In geriatric medicine, the importance of individualized care plans cannot be overstated. As older individuals possess unique patterns of physical, emotional, and even cognitive disabilities, the respective plans are needed to treat their individualized needs. Personalized care plans encourage an integrated approach in which medical professionals consider factors such as the patient's medical history, personal preferences, and social circumstances. This tailored strategy leads to higher patient engagement and satisfaction because elderly patients feel dignified and at home in their care environment.

It also enables more effective collaboration among interdisciplinary teams, ultimately leading to improved health outcomes and quality of life for seniors. Individualized care plans are also a key pathway to resident-focused care in institutional settings. In nursing homes, for instance, the application of individualized methods can go a long way toward enhancing the quality of interaction dynamics and care interventions among residents. According to the findings of an interdisciplinary panel in 2008, the majority of barriers to effective individualized care stem from poor nurse participation in culture change and inadequate training in resident-focused care (Kantor et al., 2009). Putting individualized plans at the forefront of agendas can structurally address these shortcomings in healthcare facilities, empowering nurses and caregivers to foster a more elderly-resident-friendly environment. All such attempts not only betoken best practices in the care of the elderly but are also central to cultural transformation that honors the unique needs of each individual resident. The implications of individualized care plans are evident at the facilities themselves, as pilot programs to support resident-centered care are increasingly undertaken during regulatory inspections. They illustrate the theoretical benefits of aligning care practices with regulatory expectations, enhancing both the quality of care delivered and residents' overall experience (David et al., 2010). Such initiatives encourage proactive, rather than compliance-based, approaches, emphasizing learning and responding to individualized needs rather than adhering to rigid protocols. By highlighting the usefulness of care tailored to a person within the continuum of care, geriatric medicine can usher in a more compassionate model that honors the singularity of aging individuals while also improving overall health practices (Figure 3.9).

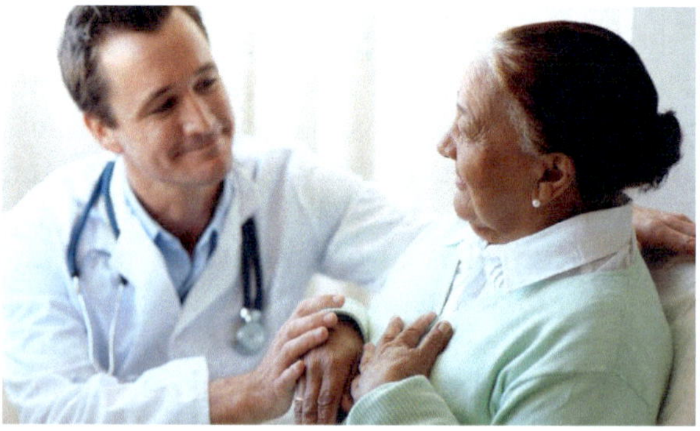

Figure 3.9. Older adults receive tailored healthcare.

Source: https://www.rand.org/content/rand/pubs/commentary/2012/08/addressing-the-geriatrician-shortage-may-help-reduce/_jcr_content/par/blogpost.crop.888x522.cm.jpeg/1720736825659.jpeg.

Test Your Knowledge

1. What is the role of a comprehensive geriatric assessment (CGA) in evaluating the overall health of older adults?
2. Why is it critical to develop individualized care plans based on the results of a geriatric assessment?

3.3. Pharmacological Considerations

Learning Outcome

1. Discuss the phenomenon of polypharmacy in the realm of geriatric medicine
2. Understand age-related changes in drug metabolism
3. Focus on strategies for safe medication management

In geriatric medicine, pharmacological considerations are most crucial given the complex interactions among aging, comorbidity, and polypharmacy. Older patients have characteristic pharmacokinetic and pharmacodynamic changes that can alter the efficacy and safety profile of medications. Such changes may include decreased renal and hepatic function, alterations in body composition, and modifications in receptor sensitivity, which can increase susceptibility to ADRs (Onder et al., 2012). Thus, doctors must be more careful when dealing with drugs, such that the dosing regimens are personalized according to the individual profile of elderly patients. The application of clinical aids, such as the Beers Criteria and STOPP/START criteria, can help practitioners detect potentially inappropriate medications and optimize therapeutic regimens to enhance patient safety and quality of care. The prevalence of ADRs in older patients underscores the need for close monitoring and assessment of drug regimens. One of the key strategies for minimizing ADRs is the use of the GerontoNet ADR Risk Score, which helps identify patients at increased risk of adverse reactions (Onder et al., 2012). This identification of patients at increased risk allows providers to implement targeted interventions that reduce medication-related harm. Such preventive measures can include thorough medication reviews, adjustments in prescribed therapy, and increased patient education on the importance of compliance and the identification of ADRs. Furthermore, interdisciplinary consultation, especially with clinical pharmacists, is a critical element in medication safety because they bring specialized expertise to the review and management of pharmacological treatment for geriatric patients. In addition to individual-level interventions, systemic models of prescribing practice also help decrease harm effects in the elderly. Healthcare systems have an obligation to establish efficient channels of communication between specialists and primary care clinicians to ensure care continuity and, as appropriate, medication adjustments when patients transfer between care settings. Interventions such as geriatric assessment can provide a snapshot of an elderly patient's health profile, revealing subtleties that warrant cautious drug management (Onder et al., 2012). Apart from that, electronic prescribing systems can introduce safety by alerting in real time regarding possible drug interactions and contraindications. Promoting a safety and vigilance culture in prescribing not only improves the quality of medicines prescribed but also significantly improves health outcomes among older individuals in community and clinical settings.

3.3.1. Polypharmacy and Its Risks

The practice of polypharmacy, or concomitant use of multiple drugs, is a significant challenge in the field of geriatric medicine. Amongst the elderly, especially those with comorbid diseases, polypharmacy is prevalent and always because of the complexity in managing many diseases. The implications of polypharmacy, however, are drastic and pervasive. These older patients also tend to develop drug side effects, interactions, and hospitalization, which only adds to their state of morbidity. Complications also lower the quality of life, creating a cycle of medical intervention that exacerbates their conditions further. Thus, these healthcare providers must continue to be mindful of the effects of polypharmacy and seek avenues for preventing them since these are also crucial in maximizing therapeutic outcomes for elderly patients. Further, existing evidence has revealed the intricate association between polypharmacy and geriatric oncology, and results have shown that patients who are older and have cancer are at a higher risk of having suboptimal drug effects. Polypharmacy in such patients generally develops through the combination of necessary therapies for cancer, comorbid disease treatment, and chemotherapy side effects. While clinical pharmacists play a rudimentary role in addressing such concerns in traditionally advanced healthcare systems, their services are insufficient in the majority of resource-limited environments. A well-coordinated approach through the expertise of pharmacists can be the turning point for the detection and management of polypharmacy risk in elderly cancer patients. Such intervention is particularly relevant given that the majority of recent research fails to account for polypharmacy as a predictor of adverse outcomes in geriatric oncology and points to an insufficiency in the existing clinical paradigm (Khanal et al., 2019). The need for universally accepted methods of assessment and treatment of polypharmacy is increasingly evident in geriatric practice. Effective medication review processes are necessary because variations in definitions and measurement techniques can lead to unequal evaluations of polypharmacy's impact. At the core of such an issue is the deprescribing process that aims to minimize medications that cause more harm than benefit. Despite various methods for identifying candidates for deprescribing, their evaluation in the geriatric oncology population remains insufficient. By establishing rigid guidelines for medication assessments, clinicians can address polypharmacy problems more effectively while also promoting enhanced health outcomes in older individuals. In the long term, the integration of standardized interventions will be essential to addressing polypharmacy, along with the delivery of optimal, safest treatment regimens to elderly patients (Aparicio et al., 2016) (Figure 3.10).

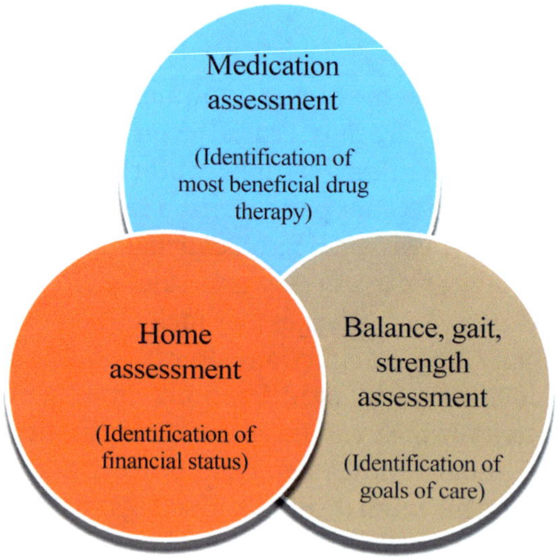

Figure 3.10. Management plans for polypharmacy.

Source: https://www.mdpi.com/geriatrics/geriatrics-07-00097/article_deploy/html/images/geriatrics-07-00097-g003.png.

3.3.2. Age-Related Changes in Drug Metabolism

With aging, numerous physiological alterations significantly affect drug metabolism, posing special challenges in geriatrics. The drug pharmacokinetics of absorption, distribution, metabolism, and excretion are often altered in the elderly due to decreased liver and renal function, changes in body composition, and variability in enzymatic activity. This diminished organ function leads to reduced rates of drug elimination, culminating in drugs that have lasting effects and an increased risk for ADRs. Of particular note is the fact that older individuals are usually on several drugs at once, particularly for managing long-term illness, thereby elevating drug-drug interaction risk and complicating therapy. An understanding of these metabolic changes with increasing age is crucial for individualizing drug therapy to mitigate risks with optimally improved therapeutic benefits in this vulnerable population. Polypharmacy, or the concurrent use of multiple drugs, accentuates drug metabolism issues in elderly patients. This is particularly in patient populations with complex chronic diseases, such as cancer and comorbidities. In such a situation, polypharmacy can be a consequence of additive therapy of cancer, drug toxicity to anti-neoplastic drugs, and drugs for disease states that are associated with cancer. The interdependent nature of these therapies necessitates close monitoring to prevent undesirable drug interactions that could further complicate the case. A big issue is when caregivers do not take into consideration the importance of polypharmacy among the elderly, which tends to lead to inappropriate management of drug regimens. Khanal et al. (2019) emphasize the critical role of clinical pharmacists in addressing polypharmacy problems through medication reviews and appropriate recommendations tailored to individual patients' needs. Reducing the risk brought by impaired drug metabolism among the elderly would necessitate that health systems take issues with comprehensive geriatric assessments (CGAs) seriously. Comprehensive geriatric assessments enable a thorough evaluation of the clinical state of an elderly patient, establishing accurate pharmacological needs, taking into account respective physiological changes. This combined strategy can foster better medication management by drug therapy optimization and ADR prevention. Moreover, greater education and training in geriatric pharmacology among physicians and other healthcare professionals can promote greater awareness of the complexity of drug metabolism in elderly patients. Successful interventions, such as the use of electronic health records that trigger potential pharmacological conflicts and encouraging teamwork among multidisciplinary teams, can lead to safer prescribing practices and lower rates of ADRs. As Onder et al. (2012) argue, these interventions are essential to provide older people with safe, effective, and tailored pharmacotherapy tailored to their evolving state of health.

3.3.3. Strategies for Safe Medication Management

Appropriate medication management in geriatric medicine is crucial, as elderly patients have complex pharmacological needs. In the process of aging, patients are susceptible to polypharmacy, a state that increases the risk of side effects and drug interactions. One recommended strategy is the use of comprehensive medication reviews, in which prescribers review all prescriptions to assess their appropriateness and potential redundancies. These reviews can identify duplicate drugs, enabling practitioners to simplify regimens and customize individualized care plans based on patient requirements. Additionally, facilitating open dialogue between healthcare teams, including physicians, pharmacists, and nurses, can enable an integrated approach to medication management. When there is a common understanding of patients' medication regimens, the likelihood of error decreases, leading to improved overall patient care, particularly for individuals with compromised health and a higher risk of medication-related complications. Aside from careful medication reviews, educational interventions can also significantly contribute to safe medication management in older adults. For example, patient and family education regarding each medication's purpose, possible side effects, and indications of adverse reactions can empower them to assume a more active role in their care. This education can help to allay anxiety over taking medications and prompt early reporting of any concerning symptoms. Moreover, integrating pharmacists into the education process can be highly beneficial, as they are more likely to possess specialized knowledge of drug interactions and patient-specific considerations, especially with complex medication regimens. By including pharmacists in the multidisciplinary team, healthcare professionals can leverage their expertise to create more effective and safer medication regimens for elderly patients, thereby overcoming the issues posed by polypharmacy and improving overall healthcare quality (Khanal et al., 2019). Another key method to ensure safe medication management is the application of practices that provide continuous monitoring of medication safety and efficacy. These practices can include periodic follow-up, the use of electronic health records, and prescription tracking. For instance, the creation of geriatric fracture programs has seen positive outcomes in treating pain from fragility fractures, showing how protocol-based interventions improve pain management and limit opioid addiction. In this case, a team-based intervention that includes diverse forms of pain management—such as acetaminophen and fascia iliaca compartment blocks—can be beneficial in enhancing patient comfort while minimizing the use of opioids. With such precise models, healthcare practitioners can scrutinize and systematically adjust medication regimens, reducing side effects while actively addressing the unique medical needs of the elderly population (Casey et al., 2017) (Figure 3.11).

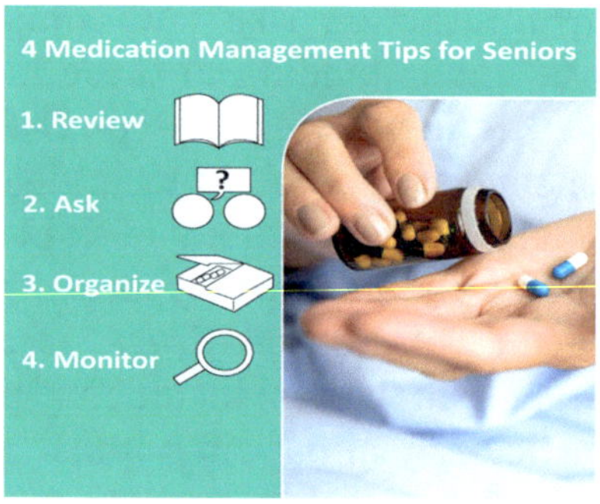

Figure 3.11. Medication management tips for seniors.

Source: https://littlenursinghome.com/wp-content/uploads/2021/03/may-blog.jpg.

Test Your Knowledge

1. What are the primary risks associated with polypharmacy in older adults?
2. How do age-related physiological changes (e.g., alterations in liver and kidney function) affect the pharmacokinetics of medications in elderly individuals?
3. What are some best practices for ensuring safe medication management in geriatric patients?

3.4. Non-Pharmacological Interventions

Learning Outcome

1. Explain the role of physical therapy and rehabilitation in geriatric medicine
2. Understand the importance of nutrition and dietary management
3. Discuss how engagement in social activities influences the mental health of older adults

The increasing focus on non-pharmacological interventions in geriatric practice underscores their importance in maximizing care for older adults. Conventional dependency on pharmacological interventions underestimates the effectiveness of other approaches that can actually meet the necessary complex needs of this group. Non-pharmacological interventions include a range of strategies, including cognitive-behavioral therapy, complementary therapies, and educational interventions, to improve patient outcomes. A systematic review has revealed that such interventions work well in managing chronic pain among the elderly, giving them skills that reduce their reliance on drugs, which are addictive or have adverse effects. The analysis of existing literature shows that, while pharmacological interventions are the most common, there is sufficient evidence to suggest that these alternative approaches are worth exploring and integrating into routine clinical practice (Reid et al., 2006). Non-pharmacological intervention has also proven helpful in individuals with dementia, mainly behavioral and psychological symptoms. A systematic review of randomized controlled trials indicates that family carer training and psychological therapy as individualized interventions significantly improve the lives of community-dwelling individuals with dementia. The interventions not only enhance caregivers' caregiving ability but also improve the quality of life for older individuals with symptomatic distress. The success of such non-pharmacological interventions underscores the importance of healthcare workers working together to devise strategies that address the individual stimuli underlying symptoms and establish a supportive environment. Interventions integrated not only maximize care plans but also de-stress families and healthcare systems, and emphasize their vital contribution in geriatric medicine (Ashaye et al., 2018). Also, the utilization of non-pharmacological interventions necessitates a shift in professional culture for treating the elderly. Traditionally, clinical education for healthcare professionals focuses on pharmacological therapy, often bypassing exploration of alternative measures. However, the evidence supporting non-pharmacological interventions necessitates a genuine reassessment of clinical education and interprofessional collaboration. For instance, nurses and occupational therapists may play significant roles in implementing these interventions, but there is no consensus on the specifics of behavioral and psychological symptoms among workers. To bridge the gap, further research will need to identify the most effective components of complex non-pharmacological interventions so that medical personnel are provided with the information and resources necessary to implement these techniques effectively (Reid et al., 2006; Ashaye et al., 2018).

3.4.1. Role of Physical Therapy and Rehabilitation

The use of physical therapy and rehabilitation in geriatrics is complex and critical to enhancing the quality of life of elderly individuals. As age progresses, the patient loses physical function, limiting the performance of activities of daily living. Physical therapy not only assists in the recovery of mobility but also in building strength, improving balance, and restoring general physical function. This model of active rehabilitation helps prevent comorbid conditions common in older adults. By treating physical impairments and fostering resilience, rehabilitation programs can significantly improve patients' physical and psychological well-being and enable them to regain control of their lives. This requires addressing the central role that physical therapists play in the interprofessional team that ensures the health of older patients. Despite the recognized benefits of rehabilitation, there remain challenges to successful physical therapy for older individuals. Communication between patients and professionals has been identified as a determining factor in one study of older individuals' experiences, with time pressures routinely preventing meaningful interaction between older individuals and professionals (Society et al., 2007). This disruption in communication can lead to unmet rehabilitation needs and unfamiliarity with the roles of the allied health providers providing their care. As healthcare trends shift towards more patient-centered practices, closing such gaps is necessary by ensuring that older patients receive information about the rehabilitation process. Through encouraging open communication, health professionals can better tailor interventions to meet the specific needs of their elderly patients and enhance overall efficiency in rehabilitation services. Besides, the integration of rehabilitation services into geriatric medicine must be underscored to prevent lapsing into indiscriminate residual care, as decried in previous nursing practice (Nolan et al., 1997). As research on the past shows, nursing and rehabilitation activities must not be limited to in-hospital care but must be sustained in home care for elderly individuals after recovery. A greater appreciation of physical therapy in long-term care facilities can help address patients' and caregivers' experiences of powerlessness. Continuing education and training for medical professionals, together with furthering interdisciplinary collaboration, can ensure that rehabilitation services remain a vital component of geriatric care. With such identification of the potential of physical therapy to transform the lives of older adults through a synergistic, coordinated approach, we can foster an atmosphere supportive not only of healing but also of dignity and purposeful aging (Figure 3.12).

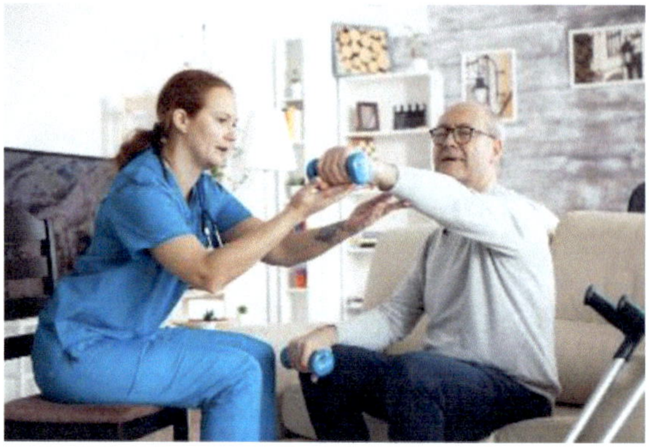

Figure 3.12. Physiotherapist for elderly care.

Source: https://fastrelief.zandupainrelief.com/wp-content/uploads/2023/02/Role-of-Physiotherapy-in-Geriatrics-1.jpg.

3.4.2. Importance of Nutrition and Dietary Management

The role of nutrition in geriatric medicine cannot be overstated, since the quality of life and overall health of older persons primarily rely on eating patterns. As aging advances, physiological alterations necessitate reevaluation of nutritional needs, particularly macronutrient and micronutrient intake. For instance, older individuals are likely to experience reduced appetite and altered metabolism, which can lead to malnutrition and resultant health issues. Thus, personalized dietary management is essential to achieve optimal health status and prevent chronic diseases. Given the relationship between nutrition and health, healthcare policy increasingly emphasizes incorporating evidence-based nutritional advice into the system of geriatric care (Morton et al., 2015). Successful dietary management is thus a vital component of the holistic approach of geriatric medicine. Besides ensuring adequate nutrient intake, nutrition management in geriatrics also entails preventing diseases of aging. Evidence highlights the role of specific nutrients, such as omega-3 fatty acids, vitamins, and minerals, in controlling the effects of diseases like osteoporosis and dementia. By promoting diets high in fruits, vegetables, and whole grains, healthcare providers can promote not only physical but also mental well-being among the elderly. Furthermore, community-level nutrition interventions, such as meal programs and nutrition education, are effective at targeting older adults who may be disproportionately disadvantaged in their efforts to consume nutritiously. The emergence of these community initiatives indicates greater recognition of the central role of nutrition in geriatric health care (Alarcão et al., 2016). In addition, food management goes beyond what the elderly eat and includes understanding personal values and preferences. Effective geriatric care employs tailored nutrition programs that honor cultural identities and individual preferences to improve adherence to diet advice. This person-centered approach encourages motivation among geriatric populations to adopt healthy diets. In addition, family caregiver participation in nutrition therapy has led to favorable outcomes in facilitating dietary modifications. The literature indicates that policies that support caregivers can also strengthen the role of nutrition in promoting geriatric health (Morton et al., 2015). In summary, appreciation of the complex interplay between nutrition and health is critical to the optimal care of elderly populations, underscoring the importance of thorough diet management within geriatric practice.

3.4.3. Social Engagement and Mental Stimulation

Involvement in social activities has a significant impact on the mental health of older individuals, especially those with declining cognition. With advancing age, social interaction may decrease for various reasons, such as health issues, reduced mobility, and the loss of peers. This decline in interpersonal relationships would result in enhanced feelings of loneliness and depression, ultimately leading to the overall well-being being undermined. Research indicates that maintaining close social relationships and participating in group activities can enhance both emotional strength and cognitive ability. For example, intervention programs that include community activity are likely to be effective among older people through fostering companionship and developing care in the environment. Social engagement's multifaceted nature involves both cognitive stimulation and emotional support, which are central to maintaining the quality of life among the aging population. Besides, mental stimulation via structured activities is a component of cognitive functioning in older adults. Engaging in intellectually challenging activities, such as jigsaw puzzles, reading, or joining discussion groups, can help maintain cognitive function and slow the progression of dementia symptoms. Specifically, cognitive stimulation has been shown to yield long-term psychological benefits, particularly when combined with supportive caregiver training. Johnston et al. (2005) illustrate how interventions such as cognitive stimulation and behavioral management both enhance direct cognitive engagement and provide greater knowledge and mastery of neuropsychiatric symptoms among patients with dementia. These stimulation activities provide a channel for older adults to exercise their cognitive function while additionally reinforcing social interaction. Thus, they constitute an essential element of integral care in geriatric medicine. Besides, the physical environment in which social engagement occurs is also key to the effectiveness of mental stimulation in older adults. Novel models such as green care farms highlight the importance of integrating nature into social participation. They provide opportunities for engagement in various physical and cognitive activities and facilitate social relationship-building among participants. Research indicates that dementia patients in these dynamic environments have higher physical activity levels and improved nutritional intake compared to more traditional day care. Bruin et al. (2009) suggest that the variety of program arrangements available in these kinds of facilities can provide for long-term maintenance of cognitive and emotional well-being and enhance quality of life. By facilitating social interaction in lively environments, geriatric medicine can develop holistic approaches that balance the physical and psychological needs of older adults, thereby addressing the complex needs of this group (Figure 3.13).

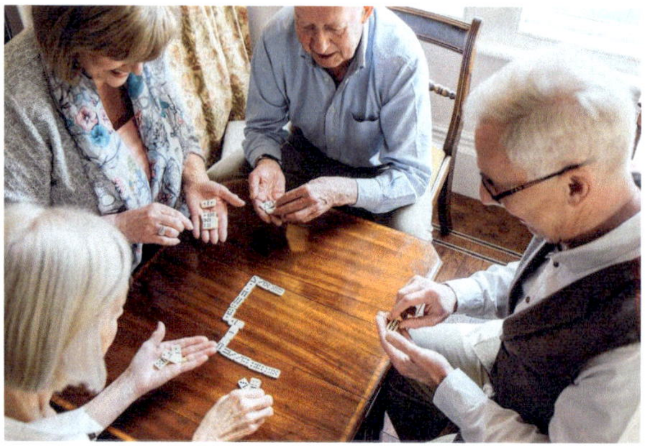

Figure 3.13. Addressing the social needs of older adults.

Source: https://www.mcmasteroptimalaging.org/images/default-source/blog-post-images/unspecified-9.tmb-blogpost.jpeg?Culture=en&sfvrsn=d9ec07d6_8.

Test Your Knowledge

1. What is the role of physical therapy in improving mobility, strength, and balance in older adults?
2. How does proper nutrition impact the health and well-being of older adults?
3. How do social engagement and mental stimulation contribute to the cognitive health and emotional well-being of elderly individuals?

3.5. Palliative and End-of-Life Care

Learning Outcome

1. Explain the principles of palliative care in geriatrics
2. Focus on advanced care planning and decision-making
3. Understand support for families and caregivers in geriatric care

The integration of end-of-life and palliative care into geriatrics is essential to treating the complex needs of an aging population. As people age, they develop conditions that significantly affect the quality of their lives. Palliative care addresses the whole process that, apart from pain, involves psychological and social interventions. It has been designed to improve the well-being of patients and families, enabling high-quality treatment-preference and goal-of-care conversations. Most importantly, evidence indicates that it can provide a more compassionate care experience for older people experiencing serious illness. This is corroborated by evidence showing that palliative care is highly relevant when excellent care preference communication correlates strongly with patient satisfaction, suggesting that palliative care can be a priority in geriatric health care (Morton et al., 2015). Furthermore, the specific challenges faced by aging patients in long-term care facilities underscore the need to integrate palliative care into existing models. Most older adults live in nursing homes or assisted living facilities, settings where they may suffer a loss of both physical and mental function. The quality of life within these settings is often low because there is insufficient personalized care planning that incorporates residents' emotional and psychological demands into the care strategy. Studies have indicated a glaring lack of literature on palliative care in residential settings, particularly given the growing need for sophisticated care among geriatric patients (Clay et al., 2025). Through a quality-improvement approach to palliative care, the physical comfort and emotional well-being of the elderly can be improved, leading to a dignified death process. The evolution toward effective palliative care involves training and reinforcing caregivers treating geriatric patients. Successful provision of palliative and end-of-life care depends on providers having a comprehensive understanding of the complex dimensions of caring for the elderly. In addition, interprofessional collaboration between physicians, nurses, social workers, and therapists is necessary. By using the team-based model, health care professionals can effectively address their patients' multifaceted needs through a single model that optimizes comfort and dignity. Striving to enhance this team-based model will most assuredly improve care coordination and eventually lead to better outcomes for older adults with serious illness. Since policymakers and scholars alike continue to urge growth in this field, it is clear that a robust palliative care infrastructure must be established to meet the evolving needs of an aging population (Morton et al., 2015).

3.5.1. Principles of Palliative Care in Geriatrics

Palliative care principles are essential to the practice of geriatrics because they focus on relieving pain and distress that can accompany serious illness in the elderly. There is a need for an integrated approach that not only addresses physical comfort but also psychological, social, and spiritual concerns. The multidisciplinary paradigm guarantees elderly patients receive coordinated care tailored to their needs. By prioritizing quality of life, palliative care allows for a dignified existence regardless of advanced age or terminal illness. As the population ages, these principles become increasingly essential to integrate into geriatric medicine, balancing medical treatment with what matters most to patients. Disincentives for interprofessional practice continue to exist, however, even as benefits are clear. The majority of health professionals have limited knowledge of other fields, thereby creating care gaps for patients. There is also the absence of shared practice and poor communication across fields, which further strangle effective collaboration. These issues can only be resolved through continuous training and development robust collaborative frameworks. Across multiple-country studies, interdisciplinary collaboration and conversation have been shown to enhance patient outcomes among this group significantly. Thus, improving these communications and shared experiences is equally essential for breaking the barriers that affect the quality of palliative care provided to the elderly, thereby increasing the well-being and health of the vulnerable population (Albers et al., 2016). Aside from this, advocacy for the integration of palliative care ideas into geriatrics training programs is necessary for future healthcare professionals. Establishing academic chairs in palliative care as a subspecialty within geriatrics would support research and education at this interface. Training geriatricians in essential palliative care competencies will better serve to address complex symptoms and improve patient and family communication. Moreover, understanding the ethical problems that most often arise in end-of-life care is necessary to provide compassionate and effective care. By incorporating such principles into the foundation of geriatric education, the healthcare field will be well-positioned to help older individuals better navigate life-altering disease, resulting in improved healthcare experiences and outcomes for an increasingly aging nation (Figure 3.14).

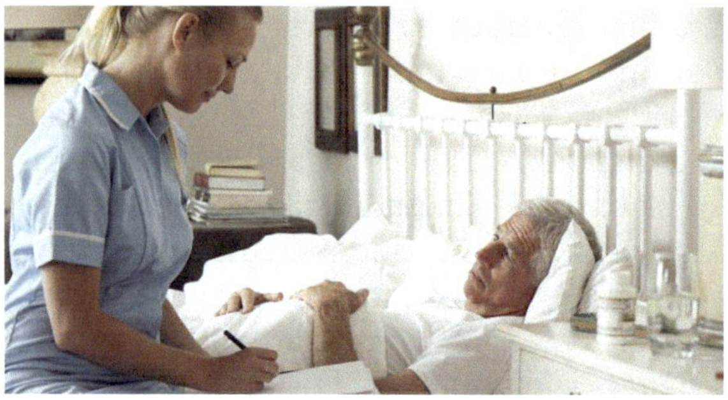

Figure 3.14. Palliative care.

Source: https://papayacare.com/wp-content/uploads/2023/09/Palliative-Care-for-Seniors-papaya-care.jpg.

3.5.2. Advanced Care Planning and Decision-Making

Effective advanced care planning and decision-making are essential components of geriatric medicine, particularly because older patients often present with complex and chronic medical issues. Advanced care planning involves discussion between the patients and their families about the patients' values, goals, and wishes regarding future medical treatment. It equips healthcare providers with the correct information so they can tailor treatment plans to honor patients' decisions. Particularly in the case of progressive diseases, such as dementia, there is an opportunity that an explicit plan will lead to more rational end-of-life care, which is essential to maintaining the dignity and comfort of patients at the end of their lives. To the frustration of clinicians, patients typically do not follow through on advanced care planning; as a result, their wishes are unfulfilled or uncovered, underscoring the importance of preventive actions in geriatric care. Advanced care planning is even more crucial in dementia because cognitive decline will hinder a patient from being able to convey their wishes as the condition progresses. One of the most significant problems with dementia care is being able to accurately predict the patient's needs along the trajectory of the disease's course, particularly at the terminal stage. Research identifies significant barriers to adequate palliative care for individuals with dementia, with the most critical challenges centered on prognostication and communication (Birch et al., 2008). Lack of access to specialist palliative care services is also a significant challenge that leads to enhanced suffering and a reduction in quality of life. Therefore, healthcare professionals should not only engage in discussions about advance directives but also ensure that mechanisms are in place to provide the best possible use of these plans as the disease progresses. Finally, a systematic mapping of research evidence on health policy shows a growing emphasis on advanced care planning in geriatric medicine. Despite the clear benefits of forward thinking—e.g., improved patient self-management and care coordination—the application of research to policy has been inconsistent (Morton et al., 2015). For instance, aligning health systems with the principles of palliative care, such as necessary resources and training, could improve end-of-life care for older adults quite significantly. Accompanying concerted action that benefits both the patient and the family through education and resource leveraging can foster a more compassionate healthcare setting. In this way, complexity in advanced care planning can be effectively addressed, thereby improving the overall quality of care for the elderly.

3.5.3. Support for Families and Caregivers

Support for caregivers and families is highly significant in geriatric medicine, given the growing number of older adults. Families become the caregivers and chief decision-makers of their older relatives, and this can lead to variable degrees of burden and stress. Assisting these caregivers with education, resources, and emotional support is essential to the maintenance of both caregivers' and their loved ones' physical and mental health. Without assistance, caregivers will experience burnout and eventually be disabled from caregiving and supporting. Enforcing systematic interventions that educate families on effective caregiving strategies and on the services provided can address these issues, further enhancing the overall quality of life for both caregivers and the elderly. In addition, comprehensive assessments can significantly help in caring for caregivers and families. Geriatric assessments, although underutilized, have been proven to identify the unique needs of the elderly, which is vital for developing personalized care plans. These assessments, along with social support, mental health, and physical condition assessments, are valuable for identifying target areas where caregivers may need support or guidance. Proactive geriatric assessment has been shown to stratify risk and improve outcomes. By educating caregivers about the complexities of their family members' conditions, health workers empower them to better handle the challenges they face in an environment where caregivers and older patients can live together (Lampugnani et al., 2017). Healthcare institutions and policy decision-makers must also emphasize helping families and caregivers through evidence-based interventions. Recommendations for optimizing this support are enhanced access to palliative care and prevention and care-coordination programs. Of special note, studies highlight the applicability of patient self-management, through which older patients and caregivers assume responsibility for controlling their health problems. At the same time, foster frequent interactions between caregivers and medical practitioners to enable the exchange of critical information and resources for practical caregiver support. With the advancement of geriatric medicine, placing a premium on these policies not only strengthens the healthcare system but also acknowledges the critical role of caregivers in the holistic care of older patients and, hence, in better health outcomes (Morton et al., 2015) (Figure 3.15).

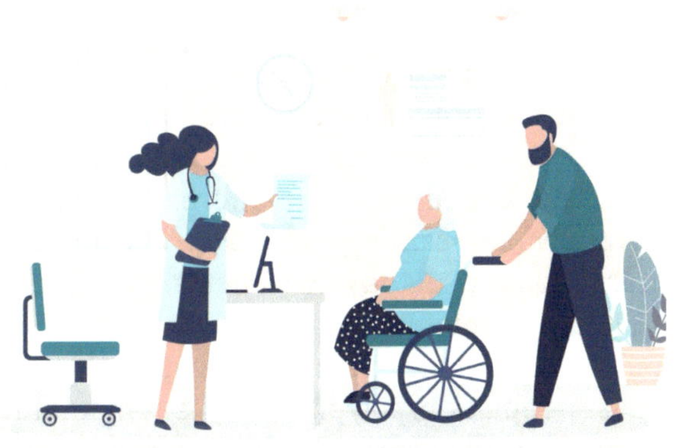

Figure 3.15. The support provided to families and caregivers plays a crucial role in the realm of geriatric medicine.

Source: https://media.capc.org/images/iStock-1263370024.original.jpg.

Test Your Knowledge

1. What are the core principles of palliative care in geriatric medicine?
2. How can healthcare providers facilitate advanced care planning for elderly patients?

3.6. Challenges in Geriatric Medicine

Learning Outcome

1. Discuss the barriers to accessing healthcare for older adults
2. Explain the importance of training and education for healthcare providers for geriatric medicine
3. Focus on ethical considerations in geriatric care

The rising frequency of polypharmacy in the elderly population is a significant challenge in geriatric practice. As elderly patients have multiple chronic diseases, they tend to use various drugs, and therefore complex drug regimens are used. This increased risk of polypharmacy can lead to inappropriate drug interactions, drug adverse effects, and overall medication misuse, especially in developing countries. Evidence points out that, in the aged cancer population, polypharmacy is compounded by the therapy given for both comorbidities and the cancer itself, which creates a critical need for intervention. The role of clinical pharmacists in the treatment of such cases has been found necessary, as they can evaluate drug regimens and recommend alternatives that mitigate risks associated with polypharmacy. The root problems in drug management highlight the imperatives of an interdisciplinary care approach in elderly care, specifically focusing on the complexities of medication management among elderly patients (Khanal et al., 2019). Besides drug management, the occurrence of geriatric injuries raises additional challenges for medical practitioners. The peculiarities of geriatric trauma, involving greater vulnerability to injury, necessitate additional attention to nuance in treatment guidelines. Statistics point to a high percentage of older patients suffering from diverse mechanisms of injury, mainly within the home. High rates of trauma, such as falls and accidents, coupled with the patients' underlying health issues, complicate their entire care and condition. The rates of complications are considerably high, based on the combination of physical debility and potential cognitive dysfunction in this patient population, and can significantly influence recovery while elevating mortality rates. The solution to these issues requires a multidimensional approach that prioritizes prevention and emphasizes the significance of early intervention and integrative trauma care in geriatric practice (Chalya et al., 2012). In addition, incorporating comprehensive geriatrics education into medical training is essential to improve the management of issues in geriatric practice. While elderly patients are increasingly seen, particularly in developing countries, in medical school curricula, the complexities of elderly care are generally neglected, and new clinicians may be inadequately trained. There should be special training on individual geriatric syndromes like dementia and frailty, and also on the care of polypharmacy and geriatric trauma. Vocationally extending training programs to include these aspects could instill a better appreciation for the complexities involved in the management of older people. As the population ages, preparing future medical professionals with the right skills and knowledge will be essential to overcoming geriatric medicine challenges, ultimately leading to improved health outcomes for this vulnerable group.

3.6.1. Barriers to Accessing Healthcare for Older Adults

The ability of elderly individuals to access healthcare services is significantly compromised by a series of barriers, which can severely hamper their overall health. Among these barriers, socioeconomic factors such as limited financial resources and poor insurance coverage often become significant issues. The majority of elderly individuals possess fixed incomes, which impairs their ability to pay for not only standard medical care but also necessary treatments and medication. Furthermore, health-related myths can discourage older people from receiving timely treatment. For instance, older adults may believe that certain diseases are natural consequences of aging and may resist seeking medical attention, thereby exacerbating their health conditions. These challenges must be overcome and require an overarching view of the uniqueness of this age segment's challenges and their need for focused intervention to enhance access to geriatric-focused medical attention. Another significant barrier to healthcare access among older adults is a lack of adequate specialized geriatric care and professional support. Routine healthcare systems typically do not address the specific needs of older patients, exacerbating health inequities. For instance, the lack of integrated oral health assessments in general health check-ups not only affects physical health but also the quality of life, as poor oral health is actually known to be a causative factor for severe systemic diseases. The literature reports that frail older adults frequently do not receive routine dental care due to a multitude of barriers, such as insufficient training among healthcare providers in geriatric oral health (Hajto-Bryk et al., 2017). This knowledge gap underscores the critical imperative for education strategies that equip healthcare professionals with geriatric care competence, thereby optimizing older adult health outcomes. Systematic issues in healthcare policy are equally pivotal drivers of the persistence of access barriers among older adults. Many policies currently in place do not support preventive or coordinated care well, and older adults must contend with broken services that do not meet their needs. Research has shown that evidence-based policies supporting preventative care and effective self-management are implemented poorly, despite being very promising to improving health outcomes (Morton et al., 2015). In addition, the roles of family caregivers are also frequently overlooked despite their central role in the healthcare experience of older adults. More robust policymaking that incorporates caregivers' concerns, fosters citizen engagement, and addresses the specific issues faced by aging populations will be crucial to eliminating these barriers and facilitating health care for older adults (Figure 3.16).

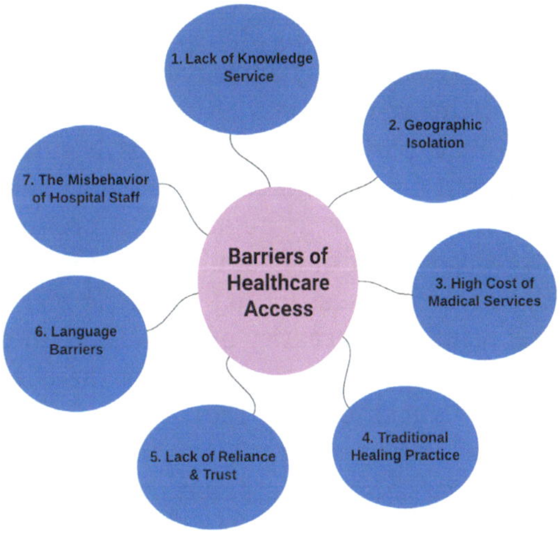

Figure 3.16. Barriers to accessing healthcare for older adults.

Source: https://www.researchgate.net/profile/Md-Sohel-8/publication/373192804/figure/fig1/AS:11431281182216482@1692329024069/Barriers-to-healthcare-access.png.

3.6.2. Training and Education for Healthcare Providers

In the rapidly evolving field of geriatric medicine, it is necessary to prioritize specialized training and education for healthcare professionals. In an aging population, the intricacies of caring for geriatric patients call for providers not only to possess basic medical training but also to understand the special physiological and psychosocial needs of elderly patients. Evidence-based interventions incorporated into innovative training programs are essential for equipping healthcare professionals with the preparation needed to address such problems. An ordered system for mapping research findings to policy guidance can inform curriculum development, thereby boosting training programs aimed at improving health among the elderly. Importantly, the programs are supposed to focus on prevention and care coordination, as current research offers promising, evidence-based policies to target these areas. Thus, early and continuous training specifically in geriatric care can dramatically improve the quality of care for the at-risk population (Morton et al., 2015). Incorporating comprehensive geriatric assessment into healthcare education is also an essential factor in augmenting providers' skills in caring for older adults. Although there is broad consensus among geriatricians and surgeons on the necessity of such assessments, their use remains remarkably low in clinical settings. Causes of this shortage include the time-consuming testing process, which conflicts with clinics' busy timetables. It is therefore vital that training schools for medical providers, i.e., medical students and physician assistants, stress building effective evaluation techniques. Emerging technologies in educational interventions, including simulation training, have helped effectively transfer essential assessment skills while ensuring trainees gain tangible experience under controlled conditions. By educating healthcare providers on the importance of these assessments, risks can be recognized more effectively and treatment plans tailored to their geriatric patients with conditions such as cancer (Lampugnane et al., 2017). Moreover, interdisciplinary collaboration fosters geriatric education. Other practitioners and geriatricians must work together to devise geriatric-specific education. The high level of clinical complexity in addressing comorbidities and surgical procedures in the elderly patient necessitates a multidisciplinary approach in which knowledge sharing and shared care planning are paramount. Integrating joint training modules that allow different practitioners to engage with geriatric concepts not only brings the learning process to life but also fosters cross-specialty agreement on the unique challenges of geriatric medicine. This sort of collaboration can result in improved coordination of care and strengthen the combined health systems' response to the diverse needs of aging populations. As geriatric medicine continues to progress, embracing this collaborative education model will ultimately lead to enhanced care for elderly patients and a more competent healthcare workforce poised to meet the future.

3.6.3. Ethical Considerations in Geriatric Care

The ethical concerns in the care of the elderly are paramount, particularly as population statistics shift towards an aging population. One of the fundamental ethical dilemmas is balancing autonomy with responding to the needs of older patients who may have compromised capacity. Doctors and other healthcare workers have the challenging task of balancing letting people make their own decisions with intervening when there is incapacity or self-neglect. As the aforementioned complexities of self-neglect indicate, the elderly, though proud of their independence, are hard for professionals to distinguish between inability and unwillingness to care for themselves. Such ambivalence raises ethical issues about protecting vulnerable individuals from injury while respecting their autonomy and right to way of life (Braye et al., 2011). Lastly, geriatric care needs to change to emphasize the dignity and independence of aging patients, creating a setting that balances safety and individual empowerment. A second essential ethical factor is access to the proper health care for older people. In most areas, such as Tanzania, it is systematic disregard of the elderly that leads to poor provision of healthcare services, which in turn creates huge inequalities in accessibility and treatment. Elders not only face physical and psychological challenges but also social suffering because of insufficient resources and respect. The 2003 Tanzania National Ageing Policy recognizes older people's rights to access free social services and treatment, but some do not know these rights, thereby worsening their challenges. This disparity is of moral concern for fairness and equity in medicine, whereby the most vulnerable groups may be denied access to primary services. The recurrence of neglect, alongside social complacency, necessitates the promotion of policies and practices that better reflect the rights of elderly people in geriatric care (Kapesa et al., 2016). Furthermore, the ethical mandate to provide compassionate, culturally sensitive care is central to geriatric medicine. It entails knowing and respecting the unique values, backgrounds, and beliefs of older individuals. Clinicians should be trained to appreciate the social and historical context that shapes their patients' lives, particularly in societies where respect for the elderly is highly regarded. Tailoring care to accommodate cultural nuances not only enhances treatment compliance but also fosters trust between clinicians and their older patients. On the other hand, addressing the issue of elder abuse in the case of caregiving is also necessary. In the wake of increased knowledge about elder abuse, it becomes essential to have in place mechanisms that foster not only the physical well-being of the elderly but also their emotional and psychological well-being so that they are treated with respect and dignity (Kapesa et al., 2016).

Test Your Knowledge

1. What are the most common barriers that older adults face in accessing healthcare services?
2. What are some of the key ethical dilemmas that arise in geriatric care?

SUMMARY

The implication of an investigation into geriatric medicine captures the imperative need for individually oriented healthcare practices among the elderly. As people age, with an increase in multimorbidity and chronic diseases, healthcare professionals must transform their practices to address the specific needs of elderly patients. The integration of comprehensive geriatric assessments, particularly in oncology, reflects a significant shortfall in current medical practice. Though geriatricians and surgeons recognize the importance of assessing factors such as frailty, social support, nutrition, and mental health, these instruments are not widely used due to time constraints in healthcare centers. Therefore, awareness and education in geriatric assessments become essential to enhance the quality of care for the elderly population, enabling them to receive the most appropriate and beneficial treatments available. In addition, the problem of an aging population poses challenges beyond those of clinical assessment alone. Effective care management will be required to balance the subtleties of older patients' healthcare presentations against the cost considerations and requirements for quality care. The burden of chronic disease and functional decline in the elderly can contribute to high healthcare costs; therefore, it is essential to develop new models of care that promote better health outcomes while avoiding unnecessary expenditures. By emphasizing an individualized care practice that considers the patient's values, beliefs, and social circumstances, the providers can significantly enhance the healthcare experience of elderly adults. Such strategies not only increase patient satisfaction but also promote treatment adherence, thereby improving health outcomes in geriatric patients. To conclude, promoting the field of geriatric medicine requires an interdisciplinary approach through education programs that equip future healthcare providers with the intricacies of elder care. Supplementing simulation-based educational interventions would significantly enhance medical students' and healthcare providers' skill sets, enabling them to conduct effective geriatric assessments. As has been mentioned, pre-exposing clinicians to prognostic determinants of surgical outcomes and ongoing care management will ultimately improve the treatment environment for patients undergoing oncogeriatric care. As geriatric oncology continues to evolve, most crucially, it will be necessary to fill these gaps in education and create more efficient care models to facilitate better healthcare delivery and improve the quality of life in older patients, so they receive thoughtful, rational, and compassionate medical care in a more complex system of healthcare.

In geriatric medicine, up-to-date developments and academic partnerships are crucial for enhancing the care of older individuals. The establishment of Leicester Academy for the Study of Ageing (LASA) demonstrates a commitment to interdisciplinary research to improve the well-being of the elderly. This initiative gathers diverse stakeholders, including health service providers, universities, and local government agencies, to create an inclusive policy to improve health outcomes. Through applied and translational research, LASA seeks to resolve issues confronting older adults, including functional capability, cognitive function, and social determinants. These collaborative endeavors demonstrate the power of academic collaborations to drive optimal care strategies for older adults and their caregivers through evidence-based practice recommendations and the delivery of healthcare (Agarwal et al., 2019). Apart from collaborative academic endeavors, geriatric medicine practice has also advanced to address the complexities of aging populations better. The Comprehensive Geriatric Assessment (CGA) model has increasingly become central to managing frail older patients, synthesizing multidisciplinary expertise to ensure holistic care. In Leicester, the inclusion of the CGA in acute and emergency care is a salient development in medical practice. The model facilitates early identification of frailty and coordination of appropriate treatment pathways, enabling patients to be triaged to optimal care settings. Furthermore, specialized facility development, such as frail-friendly emergency departments, helps bring further prominence to the emphasis on improving recovery outcomes and reducing hospital-associated complications among aged patients (Agarwal et al., 2019). Research in geriatric medicine also traces its roots to earlier history and provides valuable insights into the discipline's growth. A study of interview studies of leaders in geriatric care brings professional narratives into focus that provided the discipline's initial shape. By examining these oral histories, scholars can observe the challenges and successes of early geriatricians, particularly their efforts to elevate the profession's academic standing. A consideration of these shows how cultural diversity among practitioners can affect career progression in geriatric medicine. Ultimately, such analysis enriches contemporary understanding of the specialty, informing ongoing practice and policy developments that attempt to present a more respectful and efficient approach to elder care.

KEY TERMS FROM THIS CHAPTER

- Geriatrics
- Polypharmacy
- Delirium
- Osteoporosis
- Incontinence
- Malnutrition
- Mobility Impairment
- Frailty
- Dementia
- Sarcopenia
- Falls
- Pressure Ulcer
- Dysphagia
- Cognitive Impairment

CRITICAL THINKING QUESTIONS

1. **Which of the following is the most common chronic condition in elderly individuals?**
   a. Hypertension
   b. Diabetes
   c. Osteoarthritis
   d. Dementia
2. **Which of the following is a key component of a comprehensive geriatric assessment (CGA)?**
   a. Blood pressure measurement
   b. Cognitive function assessment
   c. Complete blood count (CBC)
   d. Chest X-ray
3. **Which of the following is a common challenge in prescribing medications for elderly patients?**
   a. Higher drug metabolism due to aging liver
   b. Increased renal clearance of drugs
   c. Polypharmacy and drug-drug interactions
   d. Reduced sensitivity to medications
4. **Which of the following is a primary goal of palliative care for elderly patients?**
   a. To cure the underlying disease
   b. To delay the progression of the disease
   c. To improve the quality of life and alleviate suffering
   d. To prolong life at any cost
5. **Which of the following is a significant barrier to providing high-quality care for older adults?**
   a. Reduced healthcare costs
   b. High patient turnover in geriatric clinics
   c. Increased access to specialist care
   d. Age-related physical and cognitive decline

Short Answer Questions

1. What is the definition of frailty in elderly patients?
2. How is depression commonly different in presentation in older adults compared to younger patients?
3. Which vaccines are routinely recommended for older adults?
4. What is sarcopenia, and how does it affect the elderly?
5. Explain the difference between aging and disease.

Answers to Critical Thinking Questions

1. (a); 2. (b); 3. (c); 4. (c); 5. (d)

REFERENCES

1. Perry, W., Lacritz, L., Roebuck-Spencer, T., Silver, C., Denney, R. L., Meyers, J., McConnel, C. E., Pliskin, N., Adler, D., Alban, C., Bondi, M., Braun, M., Cagigas, X., Daven, M., Drozdick, L., Foster, N. L., Hwang, U., Ivey, L., Iverson, G., . . . Golden, T. (2018). Population Health solutions for assessing cognitive impairment in geriatric patients. *The Clinical Neuropsychologist, 32*(7), 1193–1225. https://doi.org/10.1080/13854046.2018.1517503Agarwal, S., Bankart, J., Bannerjee, J., Bell, D., et al. (2019). *East Midlands Research into Ageing Network (EMRAN) Discussion Paper Series.* https://core.ac.uk/download/228199189.pdf (accessed on 17th July 2025).
2. Alarcão, V., Bergland, A., Bye, A., Clara, M. I. E., et al. (2016). National survey of the Portuguese elderly nutritional status: Study protocol. https://core.ac.uk/download/77614551.pdf (accessed on 17th July 2025).
3. Albers, G., Deliens, L., EURO-IMPACT, Froggatt, K., et al. (2016). A qualitative exploration of the collaborative working between palliative care and geriatric medicine: Barriers and facilitators from a European perspective. https://core.ac.uk/download/5h5893704.pdf (accessed on 17th July 2025).
4. Allman, R. M., Clay, O. J., Crowther, M., Ford, C. L., et al. (2015). Race and sex differences in correlates of systolic blood pressure in community-dwelling older adults. https://digitalscholarship.unlv.edu/cgi/viewcontent.cgi?article=1269&context=jhdrp (accessed on 17th July 2025).
5. American Geriatric Society, Armstrong-Esther, C. A., Association of Rehabilitation, Birchall, R., British Geriatric Society, Clissett, P., Cooper, G. H., et al. (2007). Older adults' experiences of rehabilitation in acute health care. https://core.ac.uk/download/334072.pdf (accessed on 17th July 2025).
6. Aparicio, A., Appleton, S., Badgwell, B., Balducci, L., Budnitz, T., Bushardt, R., Caillet, P., et al. (2016). Polypharmacy and potentially inappropriate medication use in geriatric oncology. https://core.ac.uk/download/155271770.pdf (accessed on 17th July 2025).
7. Ashaye, K., Braun, A., Dickinson, A., Gage, H., et al. (2018). Managing behavioral and psychological symptoms in community-dwelling older people with dementia: 1. A systematic review of the effectiveness of interventions. https://core.ac.uk/download/287580879.pdf (accessed on 17th July 2025).
8. Backman, A., Cai, Y., Goodman, C., Ocho, O., et al. (2019). Understanding contextual differences in residential LTC provision for cross-national research: Identifying internationally relevant CDEs. https://core.ac.uk/download/287582002.pdf (accessed on 17th July 2025).
9. Barbic, D., Barbic, S. P., Carpenter, C. R., Kemplin, K., et al. (2018). Diagnostic accuracy of the Ottawa 3DY and Short Blessed Test to detect cognitive dysfunction in geriatric patients presenting to the emergency department. https://core.ac.uk/download/212860802.pdf (accessed on 17th July 2025).
10. Berry-Millett, R., & Bodenheimer, T. (2009). Care management of patients with complex health care needs. https://core.ac.uk/download/71346306.pdf (accessed on 17th July 2025).
11. Birch, D., & Draper, J. (2008). A critical literature review exploring the challenges of delivering effective palliative care to older people with dementia in the acute hospital setting. https://core.ac.uk/download/82906952.pdf (accessed on 17th July 2025).

12. Bornat, J. (2005). Recycling the evidence: Different approaches to the reanalysis of gerontological data. https://core.ac.uk/download/12825.pdf (accessed on 17th July 2025).
13. Braye, S., Orr, D., & Preston-Shoot, M. (2011). Self-neglect and adult safeguarding: Findings from research. https://core.ac.uk/download/2721774.pdf (accessed on 17th July 2025).
14. Cankurtaran, M., & Petrovic, M. (2010). Withdrawal of benzodiazepines in the elderly inpatients: How to do it? https://core.ac.uk/download/55843638.pdf (accessed on 17th July 2025).
15. Casey, S. D., Hirsch, C. H., Mumma, B. E., Slee, A., et al. (2017). Emergency department pain management following implementation of a geriatric hip fracture program. https://core.ac.uk/download/323071629.pdf (accessed on 17th July 2025).
16. Chalya, P. L., Dass, R. M., Gilyoma, J. M., Mabula, J. B., et al. (2012). Geriatric injuries among patients attending a regional hospital in Shinyanga, Tanzania. https://core.ac.uk/download/pdf/18410878.pdf (accessed on 17th July 2025).
17. Clay, D., Hyde, J., Nelson, S., & Szczepura, A. (2025). Models for providing improved care in residential care homes: A thematic literature review. https://core.ac.uk/download/49048.pdf (accessed on 17th July 2025).
18. de Bruin, S. R. (2009). *Sowing in the Autumn Season: Exploring Benefits of Green Care Farms for Dementia Patients*. https://core.ac.uk/download/pdf/29250250.pdf (accessed on 17th July 2025).
19. Eberhardt, B., Fachinger, U., & Henke, K. D. (2025). Better health and ambient assisted living (AAL) from a global, regional and local economic perspective. https://core.ac.uk/download/pdf/6497873.pdf (accessed on 17th July 2025).
20. Fiorini, A., & Mallia, P. (2003). Rethinking care for the sick elderly. https://core.ac.uk/download/46601837.pdf (accessed on 17th July 2025).
21. Freter, S., & Gordon, M., et al. (2003). A 3-week geriatric education program for 4th year medical students at Dalhousie University. https://core.ac.uk/download/pdf/85567.pdf (accessed on 17th July 2025).
22. Hajto-Bryk, J., Kossioni, A. E., Maggi, S., McKenna, G., et al. (2017). An expert opinion from the European College of Gerontology and the European Geriatric Medicine Society: European policy recommendations on oral health in older adults. https://core.ac.uk/download/157575136.pdf (accessed on 17th July 2025).
23. Henwood, M., Larkin, M., & Milne, A. (2017). Seeing the wood for the trees. Carer-related research and knowledge: A scoping review. https://core.ac.uk/download/145186527.pdf (accessed on 17th July 2025).
24. Johnston, K., Katona, C., Livingston, G., Lyketsos, C., et al. (2005). Systematic review of psychological approaches to the management of neuropsychiatric symptoms of dementia. https://core.ac.uk/download/1669062.pdf (accessed on 17th July 2025).
25. Kantor, B., Mueller, C., Beck, C., Algase, D., Mitty, E., Rader, J., Anderson, K., et al. (2009). Nurses' involvement in nursing home culture change: Overcoming barriers, advancing opportunities. https://core.ac.uk/download/71353499.pdf (accessed on 17th July 2025).
26. Kapesa, A., Makerere, D. J., Marwa, K., Ngallaba, S., et al. (2016). Common preventable health and social problems encountered by elderly in Shinyanga region in the northern part of Tanzania. https://core.ac.uk/download/pdf/77102115.pdf (accessed on 17th July 2025).

27. Khanal, S., Shrestha, S., & Shrestha, S. (2019). Polypharmacy in elderly cancer patients: Challenges and the way clinical pharmacists can contribute in resource-limited settings. https://core.ac.uk/download/287605655.pdf (accessed on 17th July 2025).

28. Lampugnale, C. A. (2017). *Surgical Assessment of The Geriatric Oncology Patient* [Master's thesis, Boston University]. https://open.bu.edu/bitstream/2144/26707/5/Lampugnale_bu_0017N_13146.pdf (accessed on 17th July 2025).

29. Morton, S., & Dunn, W. (2015). Addressing the health needs of an aging America: New opportunities for evidence-based policy solutions. https://core.ac.uk/download/75783019.pdf (accessed on 17th July 2025).

30. N/A. (2007). Developing national in-home caregiver training standards. https://core.ac.uk/download/71356225.pdf (accessed on 17th July 2025).

31. Nolan, M. (1997). Gerontological nursing: Professional priority or eternal Cinderella? https://core.ac.uk/download/56526.pdf (accessed on 17th July 2025).

32. Onder, G., Petrovic, M., & van der Cammen, T. (2012). Adverse drug reactions in older people: Detection and prevention. https://core.ac.uk/download/55848564.pdf (accessed on 17th July 2025).

33. Reid, D. M., & Schofield, P. (2006). The assessment and management of pain in older people: A systematic review of the literature. https://core.ac.uk/download/177013.pdf (accessed on 17th July 2025).

34. Stevenson, D. G., & Gifford, D. R. (2010). The impact of a regulatory intervention on resident-centered nursing home care: Rhode Island's individualized care pilot. https://core.ac.uk/download/71352138.pdf (accessed on 17th July 2025).

35. Vaughan-Wrobel, B. C., & White, S. (2008). An educational pathway for geriatric home caregivers. https://core.ac.uk/download/71356265.pdf (accessed on 17th July 2025).

INTERNAL MEDICINE FOR ONCOLOGY AND PALLIATIVE CARE

4

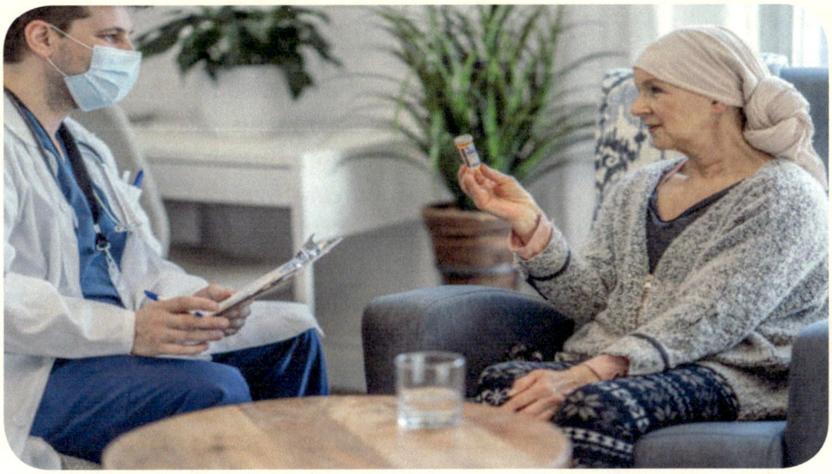

LEARNING OBJECTIVES

After studying this chapter, you will be able to:

1. Discuss the role of internal medicine in oncology;
2. Explain the principles of palliative care;
3. Understand the common oncological conditions;
4. Know challenges in oncology and palliative care;
5. Focus on advances in oncology treatments;
6. Discuss the integration of palliative care in oncology.

Introduction

Integration of internal medicine into oncology and palliative care is a foundational reform in cancer management. As cancer care becomes increasingly complex and grows exponentially, more and more people need to manage it under a multidisciplinary approach. Development of models such as the multidisciplinary palliative tumor board (MPTB) is an indicator of this paradigm shift. The primary aim of the MPTB is to timely refer palliative care to ultimately improve the quality of life in patients with advanced and metastatic cancer. By being patient-focused in its strategy, the MPTB will prevent unnecessary emergency room visits and overdiagnosis, enabling patients to receive appropriate care that aligns with their values and preferences (Mangel et al., 2020). This model emphasizes the value of interprofessional cooperation among various medical professionals and develops a network of care that addresses both the physical and emotional needs of patients. The bi-weekly meetings at the core of the MPTB process serve as valuable forums for case discussion and collaborative decision-making. With their membership including palliative care consultants, medical oncologists, internal medicine physicians, psychologists, psychiatrists, and oncology and palliative medicine nurses, the group meets to examine each patient's unique medical history and current situation. During a given period, the MPTB assessed 93 patients with end-stage disease, allowing thorough examination of 6–10 complex histories per session (László et al., 2020). This collaborative effort not only helps create individualized palliative care plans—whether for outpatient visits, home care, or institutional transfers—but also enables oncologists to shift from a purely curative approach to one that is patient-needs-oriented. The outcomes of applying the MPTB have been promising, especially in reducing unwarranted emergency unit referrals.

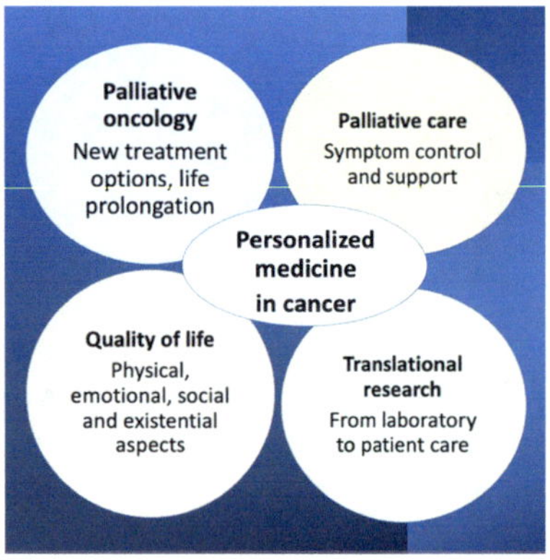

Figure 4.1. The integration of internal medicine into oncology and palliative care.

Source: https://febs.onlinelibrary.wiley.com/cms/asset/95aababf-9373-42d4-8c78-59b80b08874e/mol213278-toc-0001-m.jpg?trick=1750617747314.

The initial stage of emotional intensity in team meetings reflected the overwhelming impact of cancer on patients and also medical experts. The sessions, however, gradually shifted the style of operational and specialist-oriented deliberation. This change indicates the effectiveness of the MPTB model in ensuring the availability of timely, essential palliative care (Mangel et al., 2020). This ripple effect of the model can lead to cultural change in oncology, encouraging healthcare providers to adopt a more sympathetic, non-judgmental attitude. Overall, the MPTB not only improves the quality of patient care but also changes the culture between oncology and palliative services, opening the door to better outcomes for patients and higher-quality care in internal medicine (Figure 4.1).

Definition of Internal Medicine

Internal medicine is a platform for comprehensive care, with an emphasis on the prevention, diagnosis, and treatment of illness in adults. Since it is an inter-medical specialty, internal medicine specialists are uniquely positioned to manage complex cases that commonly involve multiple organ systems. In the areas of oncology and palliative medicine, internal medicine practitioners are central in making the special issues presented by caring for cancer patients manageable. Through intensive training in internal systems, such experts are highly skilled at coordinating between various therapies and balancing both physical and emotional stress patients undergo. Such holistic treatment ensures that all aspects of a patient's health are considered, allowing for treatments to be more effective at addressing patients' needs and preferences, particularly where complex decision-making is involved. In oncology, internal medicine doctors are working with emerging therapies and are often involved in clinical studies to develop new treatment methods. It is their involvement that is critical, as they not only provide frontline patient care but also become integral players in the larger universe of cancer science and evidence-based practice. For example, diagnostic challenges posed by diseases such as adrenocortical carcinoma require a thorough understanding of endocrine function and oncological principles, as emphasized by current clinical guidelines that support extensive assessment and multidisciplinary approaches for the effective management of these rare tumors (Faßnacht et al., 2018). Encouraging the use of evidence-based techniques, internal medicine clinicians can tailor treatments to ensure non-recurrence and improve prognostic outcomes. Moreover, palliative care is a crucial component of internal medicine, particularly for patients with cancer who are facing end-stage cancer. Palliative care values align with the fundamental principles of internal medicine, which focus on the patient's well-being and quality of life. Such care not only entails the management of pain and symptom relief but also psychological support and coping with complex ethical dilemmas of end-of-life care. Internal medicine doctors, with their interdisciplinary perspective, are best positioned to advance such conversations in a way that upholds the patient's values and addresses their needs in their illness. The incorporation of palliative principles in oncology underscores the need for an interdisciplinary healthcare system, underscoring the international nature of internal medicine and its crucial role in advancing patient-centered care across oncology and palliative practice (Alexander et al., 2022).

Overview of Oncology

A critique of oncology presents an elaborate field dedicated to the study, diagnosis, and care of cancer, aiming to provide integrative care that addresses the patient's physical and psychological aspects. Oncology's multidisciplinary nature involves a liaison among several healthcare practitioners, including medical oncologists, radiation oncologists, surgical oncologists, and palliative care specialists. This multidisciplinary sphere ensures that patients receive personalized treatment plans that emphasize not only the elimination of cancer but also symptom management and improved quality of life. Ongoing advancements in research, the addition of novel therapies such as immunotherapy and targeted therapy, reflect the ever-evolving nature of cancer therapy and are necessary for optimizing outcomes in oncologic and palliative care. At the broader oncology level, palliative care is critical in the comprehensive management of cancer patients' varied needs, particularly in the advanced stage of cancer. Palliative care emphasizes symptom control, emotional support, and decision-making assistance, which collectively enhance the patients' and families' quality of life. Evidence indicates that including palliative care in the early stages of oncology can improve psychological outcomes, patient satisfaction, and, in some cases, enhance survival (Morton et al., 2015). By adopting an integrated approach encompassing physical, emotional, and spiritual dimensions, oncology clinics can ensure patients are treated as individuals with unique needs and preferences throughout their healthcare journey.

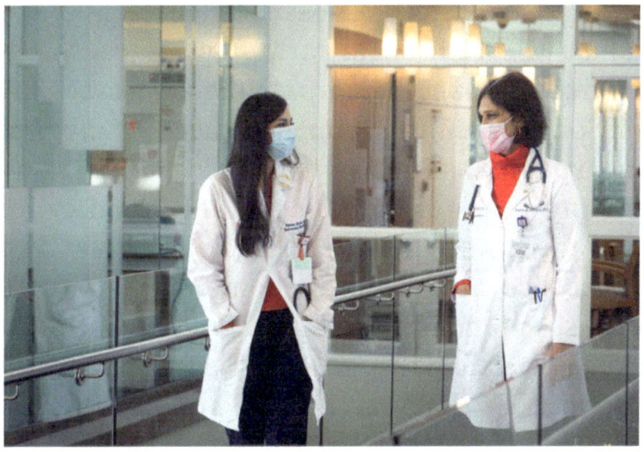

Figure 4.2. An overview of oncology reveals a complex field dedicated to the study.

Source: https://www.southalabama.edu/colleges/com/departments/internalmedicine/images/220208-ozair-sana-2.jpg.

Newly published studies further emphasize the timeliness of integrative approaches to oncology, specifically the use of nature-based therapies. According to studies, exposure to nature has a positive impact on the emotional and psychological condition of cancer patients, suggesting that nature-based therapies could serve as a valuable complement to traditional oncological treatments (Blaschke et al., 2018). Concepts such as meaning-making, distance from distress, and support through nature-based interaction delineate patient needs that extend beyond classic medical interventions. These findings advocate for the incorporation of supportive care interventions into oncology settings to achieve better health outcomes and a more holistic approach to patients' well-being, as part of the general philosophy of palliative care (Figure 4.2).

Importance of Palliative Care in Internal Medicine

Palliative care is an essential part of internal medicine, particularly in oncology, where patients can often face multifaceted symptomatology and complex emotional issues. The integration of palliative care from an early stage of treatment provides a balanced approach that addresses not only physical suffering but also the psychological and spiritual dimensions of the patients. By putting symptom management, quality of life, and communication first, palliative care teams are able to offer some level of care that supplements the treatment of patients. This is particularly crucial for patients with life-limiting illnesses, where the aim of care can shift from curative to comfort-oriented measures. The patient-centered dialogue focus enables alignment between the treatment plan and patients' values, creating a sense of agency and dignity for individuals navigating the complexity of severe illness (Alexander et al., 2022). In addition, the palliative care role in supporting communication among patients, their families, and health care providers cannot be overemphasized. Health care providers, particularly oncologists, are forced to have difficult conversations regarding prognosis, treatment, and end-of-life care. Education on effective communication is a central component of palliative care education, equipping providers with the skills to engage patients in discussions about their health care preferences. Through media such as role-play and case-based learning, as highlighted by current studies, medicine can significantly improve students' confidence in discussing sensitive matters with seriously ill families (Cowfer et al., 2020). Such a capacity for good conversations not only improves patient-centered care but also helps families deal with and come to accept the reality of their condition, fostering a more empathetic healthcare environment. In addition, palliative care has been shown to improve healthcare outcomes, specifically patient satisfaction and resource use. When integrated into regular oncology care, palliative care can reduce hospitalizations and intensive treatments, which are often the sources of patient distress with little impact on quality of life. Palliative care patients demonstrate high levels of satisfaction, owing to better symptom control and emotional support throughout their treatment trajectory. Studies indicate that such patients experience fewer unnecessary interventions and greater insight into their health, reducing their stress and anxiety. As healthcare systems increasingly recognize the value of integrative care approaches, the need to integrate palliative care into internal medicine, particularly oncology, is becoming more pronounced (Alexander et al., 2022).

4.1. Role of Internal Medicine in Oncology

Learning Outcome

1. Discuss the diagnosis and treatment planning;
2. Explain the management of comorbidities;
3. Know coordination of multidisciplinary care.

The internal medicine role in the oncology case is the key to managing the complicated interaction between malignancy and other comorbid conditions. Internists are typically the first point of contact for patients presenting with symptoms suggestive of malignancy. Their intimate knowledge of a patient's medication list, medical history, and overall health allows for accurate diagnosis and referral to an oncologist or other specialist. Besides, internists play an essential role in the coordination of multi-disciplinary care so that cancer therapy does not add to pre-existing disease. This is mainly in the elderly who have co-morbid conditions, making the internist's specialty critical in delivering extensive cancer care. Good communication between internists and oncologists would be far-reaching in enhancing patient outcomes, as shared decision-making aligns patients' treatment plans with their overall health needs and preferences. Additionally, internal medicine's involvement in palliative care is a critical component in addressing the end-of-life process for oncology patients. As patients with late-stage cancer are usually faced with disabling symptoms such as pain, nausea, and fatigue, internists' knowledge of symptom relief and palliative care proves to be highly helpful. Studies have indicated that palliative care programs improve patients' quality of life by reducing somatic and emotional suffering, enhancing clinician-patient relationships, and supporting family caregivers (Elk et al., 2017). Internists are ideally positioned to initiate such palliative interventions early in the course of treatment, which can prevent distress and confusion typically caused by a diagnosis of cancer. By emphasizing patient-centered care, internal medicine specialists ensure that care remains focused on patients' goals, leading to overall satisfaction with the treatment received. Moreover, integrating internal medicine into oncology enhances patient care quality by addressing complex cancer therapies. As cancer treatments become increasingly complex, like personalized therapy and targeted therapy, internists have to keep themselves abreast of the latest developments to manage complications and adverse effects. A survey of treatment practices in pancreatic cancer identified inconsistencies in adherence to established guidelines and suggested improved communication and coordination between medical professions (Boeck et al., 2009). Internists are best positioned to bridge the gap between oncological treatment and overall well-being and to take the necessary preventive measures during the cancer process. By fostering a team environment, internal medicine not only improves treatment compliance but also influences the ultimate prognosis and quality of life of oncology patients (Figure 4.3).

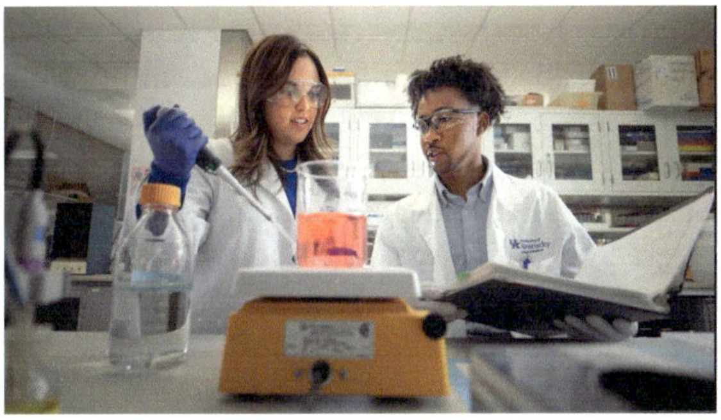

Figure 4.3. The role of internal medicine in oncology.

Source: https://medicine.uky.edu/sites/default/files/styles/split_page_header/public/2022-04/191022MEDICINE368.JPG.webp?itok=cKg82ZfT.

4.1.1. Diagnosis and Treatment Planning

The treatment planning and diagnosis process in internal medicine for oncology and palliative care is intricate and requires a multidisciplinary approach. Correct diagnosis is crucial for preparing patient-specific treatment plans that account for each individual's requirements and context. It involves the integration of multiple diagnostic tests and methods, such as imaging studies, lab tests, and biopsies, all essential for identifying the exact type and extent of cancer. Access to palliative care services is also essential at the right time; early integration can lead to better patient outcomes. Developing a comprehensive treatment plan is not only about treating the cancer itself but also encompasses symptom management, care coordination among many specialists, and end-of-life care decision-making. All this detailed preparation fosters a supportive environment in which patients can become involved in their own care. Palliative care, long considered an afterthought, is now becoming an essential component of oncology treatment planning. The establishment of multidisciplinary palliative tumor boards (MPTB) is a significant step toward early palliative care initiation. Biweekly in nature, these boards analyze high-risk patient histories to facilitate early referral to palliative services, thereby reducing unnecessary emergency visits and enhancing overall care quality. This integrative approach represents a paradigm shift from solely curative intent to a whole-person, caring medical philosophy, so that patient needs in extensive cancer care are addressed comprehensively. This emphasis on multifaceted treatment not only improves symptom management and psychosocial well-being but also aligns treatment goals with patients' values and preferences, underscoring MPTB's role in optimizing cancer care. Moreover, the evolving practice environment of palliative care education increasingly emphasizes training oncologists and clinicians in both oncological principles and palliative care. There has been insufficient emphasis in palliative care training programs on hematological education, despite the high demand for specialty care among the patient population. Because hematological malignancy patients often pose unique challenges to symptom management and have multiple pathways to end-of-life care, including hematology in the palliative care model is essential. As a case point, the absence of proper access to services such as blood transfusions in hospices can serve as a barrier to maximal symptom relief. Resolution of these challenges through the implementation of an efficient training curriculum can enhance healthcare workers' competence to provide comprehensive, equitable palliative care across all cancer types, thereby improving patient outcomes and quality of life (Mangel et al., 2020; Luppi et al., 2023).

4.1.2. Management of Comorbidities

Comanagement of comorbidities is a core component of internal medicine, especially in oncology and end-of-life care settings. Cancer patients often present with multiple diseases that make therapy and prognosis complex. Effective management requires a sophisticated understanding of the manner in which various comorbidities interact with cancer therapy, necessitating meticulous, individualized treatment strategies. For instance, long-term diseases such as diabetes, cardiovascular conditions, and respiratory illnesses can enhance the vulnerability to chemotherapy-induced side effects, leading to increased morbidity and mortality. Additionally, these diseases can influence treatment decisions, as some treatments exacerbate prevalent health issues, necessitating interdisciplinary care to ensure optimal outcomes (Alexander et al., 2022). For hepatobiliary cancers, control of comorbidity is even more crucial due to the delicate balance required between liver function and tumor growth. The National Comprehensive Cancer Network Guidelines emphasize the need for multimodal staging in patients with presentations such as hepatocellular carcinoma (HCC). These recommendations emphasize that, to develop an optimal treatment plan, particularly in liver-impaired patients, a hepatology, oncology, and radiology team is required. The presence of comorbidities may influence therapeutic choices, such as the indication for liver transplantation or the use of novel systemic therapies, such as atezolizumab and bevacizumab, which have shown efficacy in reducing mortality in patients with HCC (Benson et al., 2021). Ultimately, the strategic management of comorbidities in oncology and palliative care impacts not only treatment effectiveness but also the patient's quality of life. Extensive protocol assessments are required to identify and treat comorbid diseases early in the course of treatment. The protocols include regular screening and assessment, as well as patient education about the likely impact of comorbidities on cancer treatment. This proactive approach integrates symptom management, psychosocial treatment, and nutrition interventions to create an overall framework of care. By prioritizing comorbidity management, doctors are improving outcomes, facilitating progress through the various phases of treatment, and enhancing patients' overall well-being over the course of their cancer journey (Figure 4.4).

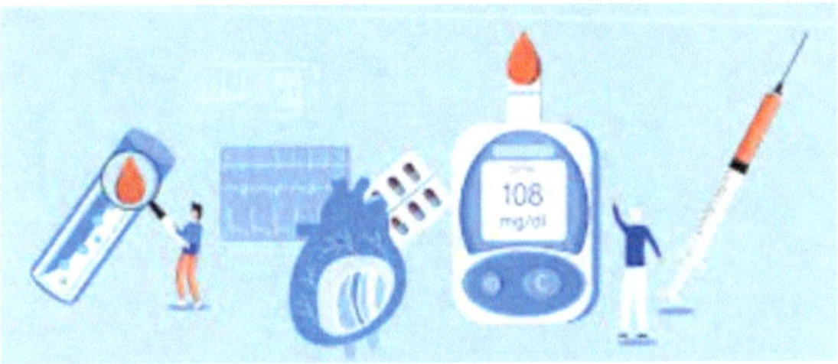

Figure 4.4. Management of comorbidities.

Source: https://encrypted-tbn0.gstatic.com/images?q=tbn:ANd9GcTK0yF42_P6kLM9Fl5hFdv61zpHk8eKa8K_s6QrbVAwyq25Cdo8osh5Y8oWsUlwDkeV3Yo&usqp=CAU.

4.1.3. Coordination of Multidisciplinary Care

Coordination of multidisciplinary care is the bedrock of oncology and palliative care, ensuring that comprehensive treatment plans address patients' various needs. All patients have a combination of issues that require coordinated expertise from multiple specialists, including oncologists, nurses, social workers, and palliative care practitioners. Effective coordination of activities facilitates efficient communication among professionals, which is essential to achieving maximum patient outcomes. By integrating multiple perspectives, healthcare teams can develop personalized treatment plans that not only address disease management but also consider patients' and their families' psychological and emotional well-being. In the case of advanced cancer, the role of multidisciplinary collaboration becomes even more vital, particularly for prognostication and treatment efficacy. Traditional clinician predictions of survival often prove disappointing as new treatments emerge, leading to uncontrolled patient trajectories. For instance, in a recent case of a 53-year-old man with cancer of unknown primary, targeted treatment yielded surprise clinical outcomes, showing that multidisciplinary and flexible designs in oncology are needed. This figure emphasizes the necessity of continuous communication and information exchange among various health professionals to address uncertainty in cancer therapy and palliative care (Torres-Tenor et al., 2025).

This integration, in addition to enhancing clinical decision-making, also enables patient empowerment by aligning treatment plans with individual values and outcomes. The establishment of structured pathways for multidisciplinary treatment also demonstrates the efficiency of this approach in improving patient outcomes. A case in point is the use of a collaborative care pathway for pancreaticobiliary cancer patients, which has proven to be a significant benefit in enabling timely diagnosis and treatment. In this instance, a nurse navigator is an integral person who coordinates necessary referrals and interventions and provides ongoing support to patients. This structured approach minimizes variability in care delivery and optimizes the treatment process, as evidenced by improved timelines for access to care compared with previous cohorts (Sandha et al., 2024). Finally, coordinated multidisciplinary care pathways are a strategic approach aimed at enhancing the quality of care in oncology and palliative settings, enabling patients to receive comprehensive and compassionate care throughout their illness.

Test Your Knowledge

1. What is the role of internal medicine in the supportive care of terminal cancer patients?
2. What are the key components of pre-treatment evaluation in an oncology patient from an internal medicine perspective?

4.2. Principles of Palliative Care

Learning Outcome

1. Definition and goals of palliative care;
2. Focus on the distinction between palliative care and hospice care;
3. Explain the importance of symptom management.

The system of palliative care is based on an integrated design, where the overall health of patients with severe illness takes precedence. The model emphasizes an interdisciplinary team of medical practitioners working together to relieve distress in body, mind, and soul. With cancer prevalence on the rise with the ageing population, the importance of efficient palliative care grows in proportion.

APRNs are increasingly recognized as lead providers of care in this setting, with the capacity to offer the support patients and families need. Educational programs, such as those funded by the National Cancer Institute, are shaping how palliative care is addressed in nursing schools, thereby well equipping future professionals to address the challenging issues in oncology practice (Breakwell et al., 2018). The palliative care guidelines clearly establish clear communication and shared decision-making between healthcare teams and patients. Such a process is necessary not just for symptom control but also for building trust and patient satisfaction with the healthcare process.

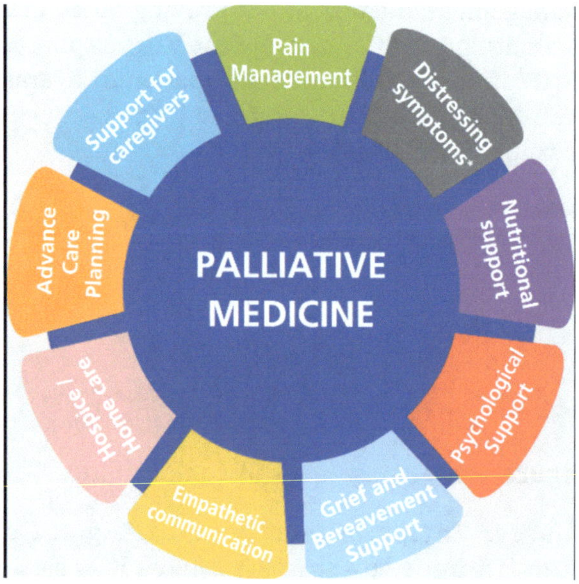

Figure 4.5. The palliative care framework is grounded in its holistic approach.

Source: https://www.fortishealthcare.com/drupal-data/inline-images/Circle%20of%20Care_0.png.

Patients experience unnecessary suffering due to inadequate recognition of their needs across various physical and emotional domains (Elk et al., 2017). Through interdisciplinary methods, palliative care initiatives seek to enhance overall quality of life by addressing unmanaged symptoms that can have a tremendous impact on patient well-being. Expert evaluation by palliative care providers can improve communication, resulting in higher satisfaction among healthcare professionals and families. The implementation of palliative care concepts has also been economically beneficial, as it can lead to more effective use of healthcare resources. Palliative interventions have been associated with reduced costs and lower ICU utilization, indicating a preference for providing care closer to what the patient prefers and values (Elk et al., 2017). These findings highlight the dual benefit of palliative care: improving patients' experiences and also addressing systemic healthcare problems. To the degree that healthcare professionals accept these principles, the focus on patient-centered care and symptom control not only helps people maintain dignity in illness but also aligns with the broader meaning of healthcare provision in cancer treatment and beyond (Breakwell et al., 2018) (Figure 4.5).

4.2.1. Definition and Goals of Palliative Care

Palliative care is a sub-specialty of medical care that focuses not only on relief from suffering for patients but also on their overall well-being during the period of life-threatening illness. It involves a holistic approach to physical, emotional, and spiritual care, with the goal of enhancing the quality of life for both patients and families. Unlike curative treatment, which primarily focuses on curing disease, palliative care aims to optimize comfort and quality of life regardless of the patient's prognosis. Palliative care may be provided alongside curative treatments or as the primary intervention when disease management is no longer possible, underscoring the importance of patient autonomy and informed decision-making throughout treatment. The goals of palliative care extend beyond mere alleviation of physical symptoms; they also encompass a comprehensive system of care that addresses emotional, social, and spiritual issues. Effective palliative care teams work together to assess and respond to the complex needs of patients and families, ensuring open communication about treatment options and goals of care. This multi-disciplinary approach ensures that patients receive care individualized to their unique circumstances and personal beliefs. Secondly, educating patients and families about their condition and what they need to do is crucial in facilitating shared decision-making, thereby allowing them to become actively engaged in their own care pathways. In addition, the importance of good communication skills in palliative care cannot be overstated. The education of healthcare practitioners in these skills is greatly needed to equip them further to feel comfortable and competent when addressing challenging topics such as prognosis, treatment options, and end-of-life therapy. Curricula with communication drills and role-playing exercises have the potential to build medical learners' confidence, as in curricula designed for pediatric palliative care communication (Cowfer et al., 2020). By equipping healthcare workers with these skills, palliative care aims to build better rapport with patients, enabling more effective conversations that address the emotional and ethical needs of patient care. Consequently, palliative care is not only a practice dedicated to the relief of suffering but also a vital part of comprehensive medical practice.

4.2.2. Distinction Between Palliative Care and Hospice Care

The distinction between palliative care and hospice care provides a foundation for understanding the general context of supportive interventions in oncology. Palliative care is a broad model of care designed to alleviate symptoms and enhance the quality of life of any patient at any time during a severe disease process. Importantly, this type of care can be integrated with curative therapies while establishing a patient-medical team alliance. Within such an atmosphere, health practitioners are attentive not only to the physical status but also to the emotional, spiritual, and psychosocial challenges that patients may face while battling their health battle. Such multidimensional care is particularly critical in oncology because patients are likely to suffer intersectoral distress that could disrupt their overall quality of life. On the other hand, hospice care is a specialized form of palliative care, tailored for individuals with terminal illnesses that have a short life expectancy, typically six months or less. The primary objective of hospice is to provide comfort and care, in a manner such that patients can spend the remainder of their time in their preferred environment amidst loving and affectionate care. Compared to palliative care, hospice does not interfere with curative treatment; instead, it shifts the focus to symptom management, pain relief, and emotional support for patients and their families. Thus, hospice care is a service of immense value that adapts to the irrepressible progression of illness, upholding dignity and quality of life during the final stages of life. The integration of hospice and palliative care into oncology practice adds depth to the general model of care for patients with advanced disease. As a recent study confirms, effective palliative care can significantly improve symptoms, quality of life, and patient and caregiver satisfaction (Bickel et al., 2016). Both types of care need to be described to patients and families so they can understand the differences and make informed decisions. Once oncologists properly define palliative care and hospice principles, they help patients make informed decisions about their course of care. In addition, accurate communication about these differences will enable appropriate referrals, allowing patients to easily transition into the supportive care they require at different points in the course of illness (Faßnacht et al., 2018) (Figure 4.6).

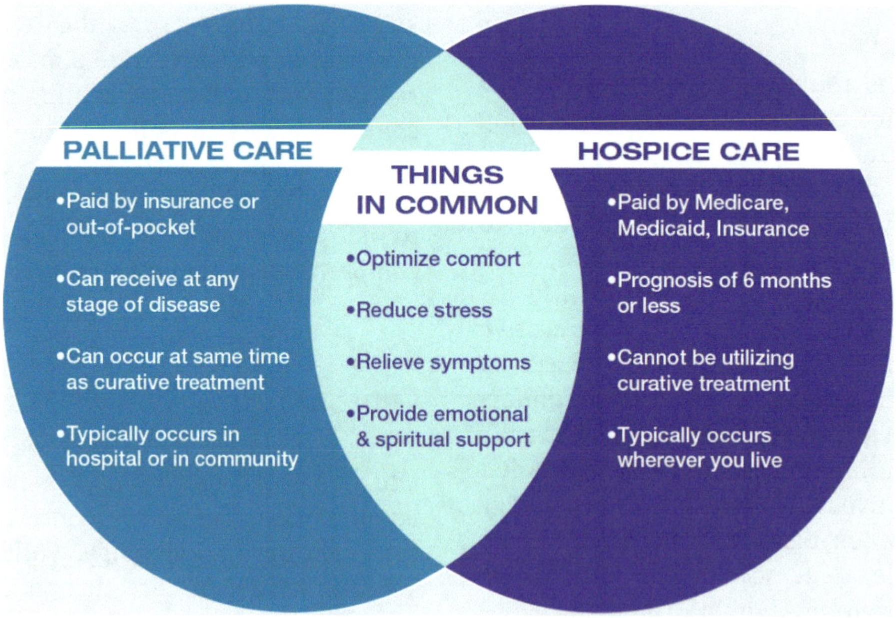

Figure 4.6. The distinction between palliative care and hospice care.

Source: https://lifecare.org/wp-content/uploads/2025/02/Hospice-vs-Palliative-Diagram.webp.

4.2.3. Importance of Symptom Management

Ideal symptom control is the essence of the internal medicine specialty, particularly in oncology and palliative care, as it is an immediate indicator of patient quality of life. Patients with life-limiting illnesses are prone to suffer from unnecessary distress, such as incapacitating pain and psychological distress that not only compromises one's own health but also is a heavy burden on the caregivers (Elk et al., 2017). Through placing symptom control as a priority, healthcare professionals can alleviate this multifaceted distress, allowing patients to experience a better, dignified, and empathetic end-of-life. Research illustrates that interdisciplinary palliative care teams are vital in identifying underrecognized symptoms and unmet needs, thereby enhancing patient–health professional communication—a key determinant of overall satisfaction with care (Elk et al., 2017). Further, effective symptom management measures are particularly required as the demographic composition is changing, with an increase in the proportion of individuals aged 65 years and older. The longer life pattern comes along with a growing number of chronic illnesses necessitating palliative care. Elderly patients have been deprived of adequate palliative care in the past, and this indicates a need for specially tailored systems addressing their distinct concerns. By closing care gaps for older patients, particularly in symptom control for chronic illnesses, health care systems can improve the quality of life for this at-risk population. Facilitating open communication of pain assessment and treatment options empowers older persons to make health care decisions and facilitates a more patient-controlled model of care. The cost implications of effective symptom management in palliative care also support its place. Successfully implemented palliative care interventions have been associated with reduced healthcare costs because they tend to lead to the elimination of preventable hospitalizations and reduced intensive care unit utilization (Elk et al., 2017). By actively managing symptoms, health providers can optimize resource use while improving patient outcomes. This not only boosts the effectiveness of health services but also alleviates the economic and emotional burden on families in difficult times. With mounting population pressures comes the demand for more palliative care, and policy in this area needs to put symptom control first, with patients receiving the tender loving care they so desperately require at the most important part of their life.

Test Your Knowledge

1. What is the primary goal of palliative care in patients with serious illness?
2. How does palliative care differ from hospice care in terms of timing and patient eligibility?
3. Can palliative care be provided alongside curative treatments? Explain briefly.

4.3. Common Oncological Conditions

Learning Outcome

1. Explain the types of cancers treated in internal medicine
2. Discuss epidemiology and risk factors
3. Understand current treatment modalities

Management of recurring oncological illnesses entails a thorough understanding of the illness pathophysiology, as well as psychological and social impacts on patients. Cancers such as breast, lung, and colon cancers are frequent, and therefore, they possess distinctive treatment regimens that match their individual biological behaviors. For instance, the management of breast cancer comprises surgical, chemotherapy, and hormone therapies that are tailored to the characteristics of the tumor. In addition, lung cancer, a highly aggressive and late diagnosis malignancy, tends to require the application of a multidisciplinary team of oncologists, radiologists, and palliative care specialists to address symptom control effectively. This awareness enables healthcare professionals to design patient-centered interventions that not only aim to eliminate the disease but also enhance the quality of life of cancer patients. A critical aspect of the treatment of oncological disorders is the inclusion of psychological well-being in patients. Depression and anxiety among cancer survivors are prevalent but often neglected. The literature favors the assumption that interventions such as cognitive behavioral therapy (CBT) and mindfulness-based stress reduction (MBSR) are effective in reducing symptoms of depression and anxiety among cancer survivors. Specifically, the American Society of Clinical Oncology emphasizes the importance of providing education for mental health issues in addition to traditional cancer treatment to facilitate an evidence-based model of care. In addition, clinicians are encouraged to use a stepped-care model, in which the level of care corresponds to the severity of symptoms, so that every patient receives appropriate care for their mental health issue (Barbara et al., 2023). Also, the importance of continued follow-up and monitoring in oncology cannot be overstressed. When patients transition out of curative treatment into survivorship, there is an immense need to cope with late treatment effects as well as the psychological impact of surviving cancer. Integration of palliative care throughout the spectrum of cancer care is paramount, as it addresses pain management, symptom control, and psychosocial intervention, eventually culminating in patient satisfaction. Significantly, certain oncological conditions, such as chronic myeloid leukemia (CML), necessitate extended monitoring to ensure the efficacy of treatment and the modification of methodologies as needed due to disease progression. Efficient management of common oncological conditions thus necessitates ongoing vigilance over clinical management and general patient care procedures within an established internal medicine practice (Alexander et al., 2022) (Figure 4.7).

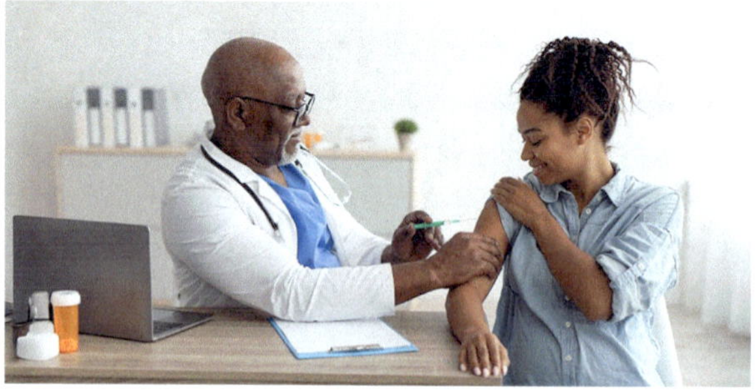

Figure 4.7. The management of common oncological conditions.

Source: https://www.hjhospitals.org/blogimage/zpsVX7KhKI0VQTIElUQw2sueq2tftDPsf17Fe7Cy.jpeg.

4.3.1. Types of Cancers Treated in Internal Medicine

Internal medicine leads the general management of most types of cancer and is typically the first line of treatment for patients. Of neoplasms treated under this specialty, hematologic malignancies such as chronic myeloid leukemia (CML) have become even more prominent. The internist plays an essential role in the management and follow-up of the complexity of these cancers, particularly because they are known to present with systemic symptoms that require proper management. The key focus here is not just the treatment of the tumor but also the control of comorbidities often present in combination with hematological disorders. This management calls for an intimate knowledge of cancer biology and patient-specific factors, the latter of which determine treatment success and quality of life. This multidisciplinary aspect underscores the role of internal medicine in oncology and palliative care and enables patients to receive integrative, personalized treatment plans (Alexander et al., 2022). Solid tumors like head and neck cancers form another significant area where the expertise of internal medicine is highly valuable. Management of these cancers is notoriously difficult due to the intricate anatomy of the head and neck, in which the mode of management hinges on the site, stage, and histopathological characteristics of the tumor. Multidisciplinary management is characterized by the direct involvement of a team of experts, including medical oncologists, radiation oncologists, and surgeons. Internal medicine physicians make valuable contributions to supportive care, such as symptom management and nutritional support, which help maximize patient outcomes. Treatment guidelines may vary based on the latest guidelines from organizations like the National Comprehensive Cancer Network (NCCN), which clearly state that internal medicine physicians must remain up to date with evolving guidelines to maximize the delivery of care. Hence, they stress the need for an integrated management approach in the context of complex malignancies (David et al., 2020). Internal medicine also plays a key role in treating patients with metastatic disease, wherein palliation and quality of life are prioritized. Where malignancies have also extended from their original sites, control of symptoms for pain, fatigue, and psychosocial distress is a key objective. Internal medicine doctors often work in conjunction with palliative care experts to create synchronized treatment plans that address body and mind together. This multidisciplinary teamwork is vital in patients experiencing the compounded effects of cancer and its treatment, optimizing the provision of supportive care against their own unique circumstances. Significantly, physicians should also consider the potential impact of ongoing therapy on patients' general well-being, particularly in managing complications of systemic therapy. The dialogue between oncology and palliative care underscores the crucial role of internal medicine in pushing the boundaries of cancer treatment beyond mere survival, not only guaranteeing survival but also enhancing the quality of life for patients with advanced disease.

4.3.2. Epidemiology and Risk Factors

The discipline of epidemiology is central to the understanding of the incidence, distribution, and determinants of cancer in multicultural populations. By using diverse epidemiological techniques, investigators can identify distinct risk factors for different types of malignancies. For example, environmental exposures, genetic factors, lifestyle, and socio-economic circumstances can all play a significant role in predisposing individuals to develop certain malignancies. This kind of information is imperative to inform public health initiatives and patient-specific care planning in oncology. Furthermore, extensive epidemiological studies provide the foundation for developing preventive interventions that can reduce the cancer burden among high-risk groups, thereby improving overall palliative care effectiveness. The continually evolving nature of such studies, driven by advances in registry science and technology, underscores the need to meticulously prepare these data and interpret them appropriately for patients to inform care processes effectively (N/A, 2020). Modifiable and non-modifiable risk factors of cancer are broadly categorized. Modifiable risk factors include the lifestyle determinants and environmental factors such as smoking, diet, inactivity, and exposure to carcinogens, while non-modifiable risk factors include age, gender, and genetic composition. Understanding these risk factors is important for formulating preventive strategies and customized treatment protocols in oncology. There is evidence to believe that modification of lifestyle can have a significant impact on the development of cancer; e.g., avoidance of smoking and increased physical exercise can lower risks for many cancers. Furthermore, the detection of genetic determinants may lead to screening programs and interventions for individuals at risk, enabling therapeutic intervention at an early stage in palliative care. Thus, a differentiated understanding of these risk factors is enhancing preventive and therapeutic oncology practices, ultimately improving patient outcomes and quality of life (David et al., 2020). In oncology and palliative care, the importance of identifying and addressing epidemiological risk factors extends beyond the treatment of an individual patient. Engaging multidisciplinary teams in the analysis of patient registries and health information can reveal trends that identify key risk factors relevant to specific populations, thereby aiding community-based interventions and care guidelines. For example, integrating findings from registries can inform guidelines for treating cancers of the head and neck, where treatment requires subtle, multidisciplinary approaches (David et al., 2020). Secondarily, the evolving cancer treatment paradigm demands that clinicians stay up to date with emerging epidemiological data to rework patient management strategies longitudinally. Lastly, an aggressive initiative to learn epidemiology and risk factors not only informs clinical practice but also protects health equity by eliminating barriers to vulnerable populations, a fundamental component of both oncology and palliative care models (Figure 4.8).

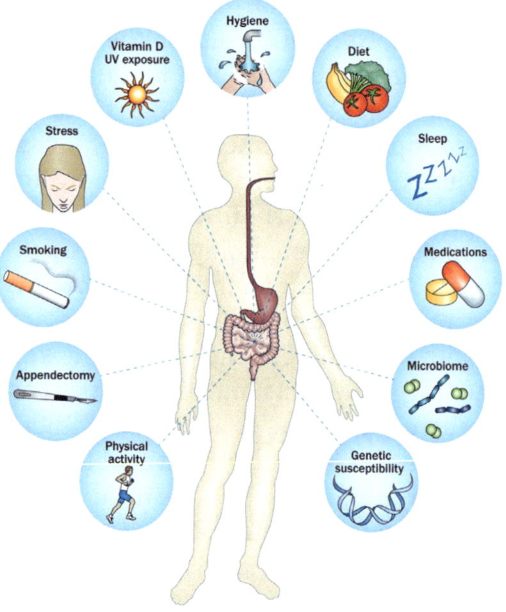

Figure 4.8. The field of epidemiology plays a critical role in understanding the incidence.

Source: https://media.springernature.com/full/springer-static/image/art%3A10.1038%2Fnrgastro.2015.34/MediaObjects/41575_2015_Article_BFnrgastro201534_Fig1_HTML.jpg.

4.3.3. Current Treatment Modalities

The treatment modality landscape in oncology has been revolutionized with the emphasis on personalized therapy optimized to the individual patient profile. The prime driver of this revolution is largely the advancement of genomic medicine, which enables the delineation of tumors at the molecular level and the consequent ability to target aberrations with therapy. For example, the development of targeted therapies has transformed the management of several cancers, such as chronic myeloid leukemia (CML) and hepatocellular carcinoma (HCC). The newer agents are more potent and less toxic than traditional chemotherapy, with promise for a new era of precision oncology. As targeted therapies continue to improve clinical outcomes, the role of the internal medicine specialist is increasingly crucial in managing these complex treatment regimens. Palliative care, a critical part of oncology, focuses on improving the quality of life of patients with serious illnesses, such as those undergoing aggressive treatment modalities. It prioritizes symptom control, psychosocial support, and holistic care, aligning treatment plans with the patient's agenda and desires. Treatment modalities in this situation include not only pharmacologic treatments but also non-pharmacologic treatments, such as counseling and rehabilitation programs. Palliative care upon diagnosis has been shown to enhance patient satisfaction and, in certain groups of cancer patients, even survival. As health care systems recognize the importance of comprehensive care, palliative care is increasingly integrated alongside standard oncology therapy, bridging the gap between curative intent and end-of-life care. Multidisciplinary collaboration is crucial to the successful treatment of complex cancer patients, particularly in the management of hepatocellular carcinoma (HCC). The National Comprehensive Cancer Network (NCCN) emphasizes that optimal treatment benefit can be achieved through an integrated team of specialists, including hepatologists, oncologists, and surgeons. This collaborative approach is invaluable in consideration of the intricacies involved with liver impairment and the multitude of possible treatment modalities such as surgery, transplant, and systemic therapy. Notably, new discoveries have introduced new therapeutic regimens, especially the combination of atezolizumab and bevacizumab, which the FDA has sanctioned as an innovative standard of care for advanced HCC patients, marking a profound turning point in treatment protocols. The mutual synergy of specialists' interactions ensures that patients receive comprehensive care tailored to their unique clinical scenario, ultimately optimizing outcomes and quality of life for those with this challenging disease (Benson et al., 2021; Alexander et al., 2022).

Test Your Knowledge

1. What are two major epidemiological trends observed in global cancer incidence?
2. List three key risk factors associated with the development of colorectal cancer.

4.4. Challenges in Oncology and Palliative Care

Learning Outcome

1. Evaluate communication barriers with patients and families;
2. Know ethical considerations in treatment decisions;
3. Focus on resource allocation and access to care.

Oncology practices are increasingly confronted with a range of problems that directly impact patient survival and care. Rising case complexity is one of the identified challenges, which is worsened by the sheer number of cancer survivors as well as the incorporation of older patients with comorbidities in treatment (Breakwell et al., 2018). A demographic shift such as this necessitates a heightened focus on the education of healthcare providers so that they are adequately trained in oncological and palliative care procedures. Although advanced practice registered nurses have been recognized as significant providers of palliative care, incorporating complementary curricula for such courses into Doctor of Nursing Practice (DNP) education does not typically receive support. These barriers include perceived time limitations, inadequate availability of tenure-line faculty with a focus in palliative care, and inadequate available clinical sites, ultimately limiting the patients' comprehensive care they require along their cancer journeys. Proper communication and interprofessional teamwork are of most significant concern in addressing the challenges of oncology and palliative care. Inpatients with life-threatening ailments usually undergo much suffering, which is brought about by unaddressed physical, psychological, and spiritual issues (Elk et al., 2017).

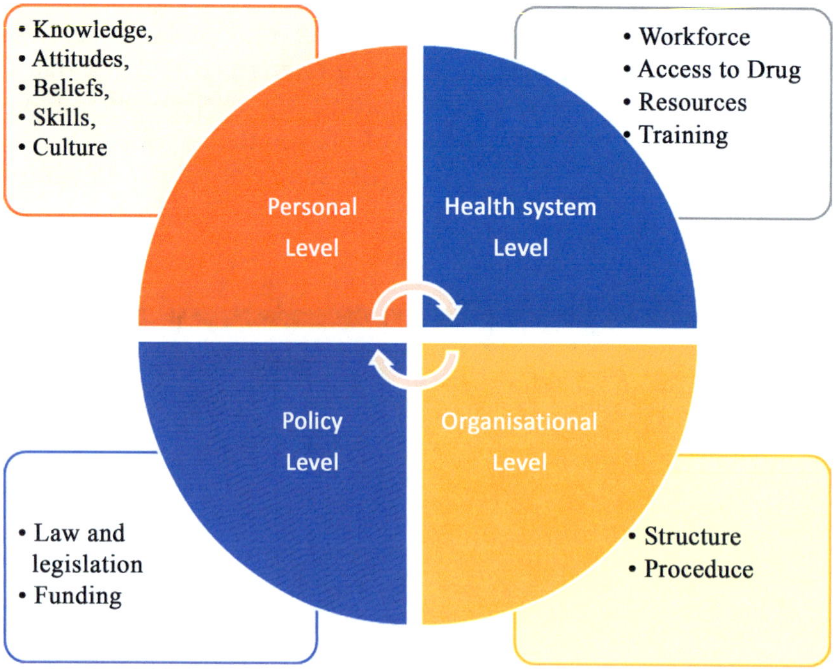

Figure 4.9. Challenges on the provision of palliative care.

Source: https://media.springernature.com/lw685/springer-static/image/art%3A10.1186%2Fs12904-020-00558-5/MediaObjects/12904_2020_558_Fig1_HTML.png.

Miscommunication between patients and health workers can lead to undesirable outcomes, such as excessive pain and distress. Palliative care programs focused on reducing these symptoms play an essential role in improving the overall quality of life of inpatients. These programs promote communication, patient satisfaction with treatment, and family engagement, highlighting the necessity for well-trained health care teams that can recognize and address a range of patient needs. However, implementing these programs within existing health care systems is a challenging endeavor, frequently constrained by systemic barriers and inadequate interdisciplinary education. Additionally, the availability of palliative care services in oncology settings has been associated with improved patient outcomes, yet these services are not uniformly available in healthcare institutions. Research has established that palliative care consultation significantly decreases suffering, enhances satisfaction in care, and lowers hospitalization costs (Elk et al., 2017). However, few hospitals have structured palliative care teams or invest in staff training. This discord poses a significant challenge to the provision of robust oncology care, as without proper integration of palliative care, patients will still experience unmet needs in their physical and emotional well-being. With the ever-evolving field of oncology, overcoming these challenges through better education, interprofessional communication, and structural changes in healthcare delivery will be crucial to improving outcomes for cancer patients and their families (Figure 4.9).

4.4.1. Communication Barriers with Patients and Families

Good communication is essential in internal medicine, especially in oncology and palliative care, where patients and families frequently encounter complicated medical, psychological, and emotional concerns. Communication breakdowns have a wide variety of causes, including cultural, language, and differing health literacy backgrounds. Breakdowns can lead to misunderstandings, mistrust, and increased distress in patients, ultimately impacting their treatment compliance and overall satisfaction with care. The need for healthcare providers to bridge such gaps has become ever more pressing as most discussions migrate to telehealth platforms, which can even exacerbate gaps in certain areas by limiting nonverbal communication and human contact. Bridging such gaps is crucial to ensuring that patients are heard, understood, and empathized with, resulting in better health outcomes and higher patient satisfaction in oncology and palliative care settings. In oncology and palliative care, the emotional effect of an oncological diagnosis is tremendous, and as such, the importance of good communication is paramount. Most patients are disturbed, as defined by the NCCN Guidelines for Distress Management as a multifactorial, unpleasant experience that can interfere with their ability to cope with illness (Michelle et al., 2019). The challenge lies not just in conveying complex medical information simply, but also in providing emotional support. If the healthcare providers are not clear in their communication, then patients become inundated with fear or confusion and end up with their emotional suffering exacerbated. Furthermore, inappropriate communication can retard the appropriate resolution of this distress. It can affect not just the emotional state of the patient but also his or her physical status and outcome of the treatment, particularly in the susceptible setting of cancer treatment. The introduction of telemedicine has also affected communication patterns between healthcare professionals, patients, and their families. While telemedicine enhances the convenience and increased access to medical care, it also presents unique challenges. Lack of personal contact, technical barriers, and the impersonalization of virtual visits can lead to communication failure. The majority of patients and family members are likely to feel isolated or unsupported, hence decreasing their involvement in treatment planning (Rashid et al.,

2020). In order to ensure the successful delivery of oncology and palliative care, healthcare providers must change their communication approaches, leveraging technology to enable more profound understanding and bonding. By deliberately seeking feedback, communicating clearly, and using visuals, providers can better overcome these challenges and establish stronger relationships with their patients and families.

4.4.2. Ethical Considerations in Treatment Decisions

In oncology and palliative care, ethical considerations guide treatment decisions. The complex nature of caring for cancer patients involves a balance among the potential benefits and harms of various therapies. Practitioners are tasked with scrutinizing often gray areas where patient autonomy, informed consent, and the principle of beneficence intersect. For instance, in the management of differentiated thyroid carcinomas with an excellent prognosis, it is crucial to prioritize patients' values and preferences. Patient discussion regarding their treatment goals assists in establishing a shared decision-making environment that respects their autonomy without undermining the reality that they must understand the repercussions of their choice, particularly where surgery or radioactive iodine therapy is advised. This ethical engagement encourages the evolving patient-provider relationship founded upon trust, which ultimately benefits the overall quality of care. Furthermore, ethical issues usually arise when caring for undesirable cancers, such as anaplastic thyroid carcinoma. With the dismal prognosis associated with the tumor, the process of decision-making is made more complicated and replete with ethical considerations. In such a situation, practitioners must weigh the efficacy and side effects of aggressive treatment against the ethical imperative to reduce distress. The application of targeted therapy to patients with recurrent or persistent disease demonstrates the necessity of aligning treatment modalities with ethical principles that accommodate patient comfort and quality of life. Additionally, when discussing available therapies, healthcare professionals are obligated to provide complete information and support so that patients can make informed decisions in accordance with their values and treatment objectives, thereby reasserting the moral imperative of patient-centered care. Aside from this, resource allocation and treatment triage also raise other ethical issues in oncology and palliative care environments.

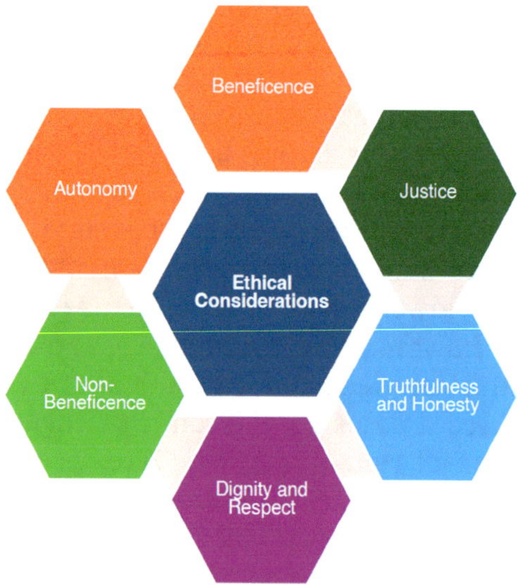

Figure 4.10. Ethical considerations in treatment decisions.

Source: https://www.researchgate.net/profile/I-Made-Dwi-Adnyana/publication/377655909/figure/fig2/AS:11431281219610881@1706107451467/Ethical-considerations.png.

Physicians often face constrained resources and must make decisions that balance individual patient needs with societal interests. The principle of justice enters the picture in determining which treatments to ration based on effectiveness and cost-effectiveness. That is where guidelines developed by organizations such as the National Comprehensive Cancer

Network (NCCN) serve as significant models for ethical decision-making in treatment protocols. For example, recommendations for the surgical management of a series of thyroid cancers offer a systematic approach aimed at optimizing patient outcomes and addressing ethical concerns about resource allocation. In the end, the inclusion of ethical principles in treatment not only enhances patient care but also promotes the moral professionalism of the medical profession through respect, justice, and accountability (Figure 4.10).

4.4.3. Resource Allocation and Access to Care

Health resource planning, particularly in palliative and oncology care, remains a significant hurdle that impedes access to life-prolonging services and medications. Although cancer continues to be one of the leading causes of mortality globally, unequal treatment with proper and timely intervention is appalling. Economic conditions, infrastructure, and health policy may collectively prevent patients from accessing appropriate therapy. For instance, even when essential cancer medicines are on national lists, unaffordability can prevent their use, highlighting the importance of investing in equitable pricing and universal health coverage initiatives to expand access. Correcting for these shortfalls requires a comprehensive understanding of how resources are allocated in healthcare systems to ensure that cancer treatment reaches all stages, from diagnosis through treatment and follow-up, thereby maximizing patient outcomes and survival rates (Cort et al., 2020). The adoption of innovative solutions, such as telemedicine, offers a promising avenue for expanding access to oncology and palliative care, especially for marginalized populations. The increased use of telemedicine within healthcare systems can potentially provide adequate care while reducing the overheads of traditional face-to-face consultations. There is evidence that patients treated via telemedicine achieve outcomes as good, if not superior, to those receiving treatment via conventional services. Nevertheless, there are still hindrances to telemedicine becoming more widely used, including regulatory barriers and differences in health and digital skills among patients. Vulnerable populations, who these services can benefit most, are unable to avail themselves of the benefits that telemedicine offers. Therefore, overcoming these barriers is essential to foster equity and increase overall access to care in oncology settings (Hashiguchi, 2020). With regard to resource spending, expenditure on training health workers and on improved health infrastructure is necessary to increase access to oncology and palliative care. As cancer treatments become increasingly complex, it is vital to equip healthcare professionals with the expertise needed to deliver state-of-the-art treatment modalities. Additionally, improving healthcare delivery through logistics can contribute to optimizing access to drugs and therapies and, ultimately, patient outcomes. Policymakers need to think about integrated strategies that not only allocate funds effectively but also invest in development and training schemes to empower healthcare teams to address evolving oncology and palliative care challenges as needed. This investment will result in a better, more equalized healthcare system with the emphasis on quality cancer care for everyone regardless of their socio-economic status (Cort et al., 2020).

Test Your Knowledge

1. What are two common communication barriers between healthcare providers and patients or families in oncology and palliative care?
2. How can limited healthcare resources impact access to palliative care services in low-resource settings?

4.5. Advances in Oncology Treatments

Learning Outcome

1. Focus on targeted therapies and immunotherapy
2. Discuss the role of clinical trials in treatment options
3. How to impact of technology on patient care

The field of oncology therapy has experienced remarkable advances over the last few decades, revolutionizing cancer treatment and improving patient prognosis. Traditional therapies such as chemotherapy and radiation remain mainstays in the management of cancer; however, the introduction of targeted therapy and immunotherapies has revolutionized therapeutic approaches. Targeted therapy aims to target distinct molecular targets associated with cancer, minimizing toxicities to normal tissues while maximizing effectiveness. Immunotherapies, on the other hand, utilize the body's immune system to target cancer cells. Not only do they provide new avenues of therapy to patients who previously had few alternatives, but they also introduce the possibility of personalized medicine, facilitating more specific therapeutic approaches tailored to patient-specific profiles. Therefore, integrating these advances into oncology is a significant step towards increasing survival rates and improving the quality of life of cancer patients. Despite the promising prospects of newer oncology treatments, challenges with their application and availability persist. Various new therapies require sophisticated assessment protocols, robust healthcare infrastructure, and trained practitioners to ensure optimal delivery of treatment. Additionally, high costs and socioeconomic disparities pose barriers for patients who wish to have access to emerging cancer therapies. Evidence-based policy recommendations are urgently needed to facilitate the integration of oncology treatment innovations into routine clinical practice, particularly in palliative care, research says. As highlighted by current studies, there is a disparity between the known evidence and the policies that actually regulate cancer care, particularly in self-management for patients and palliative care. It is therefore necessary to close these gaps to facilitate equitable access to innovative therapy among all cancer patients (Morton et al., 2015). Further, there is a need to understand problems in controlling cancer pain because therapies in oncology are evolving. With the cancer pain so intricate in its nature, analgesic progress is increasingly becoming relevant. For instance, new techniques such as Transcutaneous Electric Nerve Stimulation (TENS) are promising in symptom relief of cancer pain, potentially supplementing traditional pain management strategies.

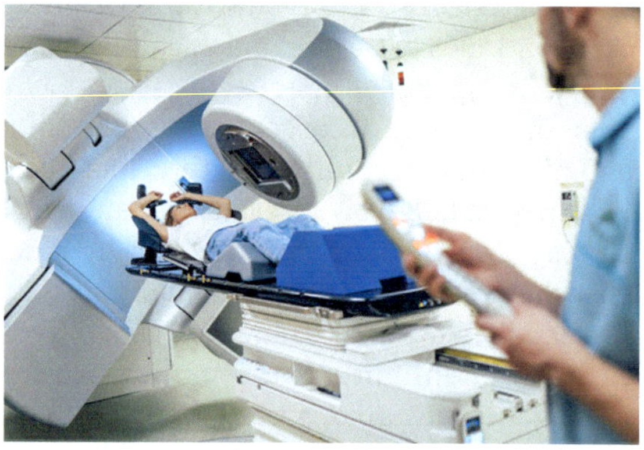

Figure 4.11. The realm of oncology treatments has witnessed remarkable advancements over the last few decades.

Source: https://metrohospitals.com/wp-content/uploads/2025/02/Advanced-Cancer-Treatment-Latest-Innovations-in-Oncology.jpg.

However, systematic reviews have noted the inconclusiveness regarding TENS's effectiveness for this purpose and the need for well-conducted large randomized controlled trials to establish its role in the management of cancer pain (Bennett et al., 2008). In light of the ongoing development of the field, how progress in treatment modalities intersects with integrated pain management strategies will be vital to enhancing overall therapeutic outcomes for patients toward better palliative care (Figure 4.11).

4.5.1. Targeted Therapies and Immunotherapy

With progress in oncology, immunotherapy, and targeted therapies, the industry of cancer treatment has been revolutionized. Targeted therapies aim specifically at molecular targets expressed on cancer cells, providing more targeted treatments with often fewer side effects than traditional chemotherapy. For instance, in metastatic colorectal cancer (mCRC), chemotherapy in combination with targeted therapy, as anti-vascular endothelial growth factor antibodies, has produced remarkable success. In this approach, treatment is targeted to the tumor's individual genetic makeup, optimizing treatment potential with minimal exposure to the broader toxic side effects associated with traditional chemotherapeutic regimens. The strategic use of such treatments underscores the role of genetic profiling in contemporary oncology practice, in which interventions are not one-size-fits-all but are customized to each patient's cancer profile, leading to better patient outcomes. Immunotherapy is yet another oncology revolution, leveraging the body's own immune system to combat cancer. This modality covers a spectrum of approaches, with immune checkpoint inhibitors taking on a more prominent role with their application in the treatment of a variety of malignancies, including melanoma and lung cancer. For mCRC, pembrolizumab is approved for patients who have microsatellite instability-high tumors, demonstrating the personalized approach to this therapy. By engaging with and enhancing the immune response against tumor cells, immunotherapy aims not only to shrink tumors but also to establish long-term immunity, with implications for more prolonged survival and improved quality of life for cancer patients. Immunotherapy is ineffective in some patients, so biomarker understanding is crucial. Therefore, further research is needed to identify which patient populations would benefit most from these new therapies. The integration of targeted therapy and immunotherapy into the mainstream of clinical practice requires an overall, multidisciplinary approach to patient care. Multidisciplinary interaction among oncologists, radiologists, and pathologists enables treatment planning informed by the most up-to-date evidence-based guidelines and genetic data. For example, in pre-treated BRAF V600E–mutant mCRC, combination therapies such as encorafenib and cetuximab are recommended and may offer significant effectiveness. Furthermore, the role of collaborative or shared decision-making between the healthcare provider and the patient cannot be overstated, as it has been proven to strengthen the therapeutic alliance and enhance treatment compliance. Furthermore, as the field of oncology continues to grow, assessing potential risks, side effects, and treatment outcomes is paramount. Keeping up with innovations and ongoing research will remain essential to maximizing care for patients receiving advanced cancer treatments, ultimately changing the face of internal medicine to include oncology and palliative care.

4.5.2. Role of Clinical Trials in Treatment Options

Clinical trials are central to determining treatment options in oncology and palliative care, providing valuable information to support clinical decision-making. Clinical trials allow researchers to systematically compare the effectiveness and tolerability of new therapies, which are essential for keeping pace with the complexity of cancer therapies. As oncology evolves, the increased reliance on clinical trials stems from the need to access evidence-based interventions responsive to patients' unique biological and psychosocial needs. In fact, the heterogeneity of cancer pathology often requires an appreciation of principles beyond standard care, underscoring the significance of trials examining new treatment modalities and innovative therapy combinations. These trials not only increase the likelihood of improved patient outcomes but also enhance our understanding of disease mechanisms, enabling more specific interventions. Additionally, translating trial findings into practice has the potential to close knowledge gaps among health practitioners. A recent study revealed significant gaps in oncology terminology among intensive care and internal medicine physicians, which influence their decision-making in patient management (Gon et al., 2025). It suggests that continuous education, supported by clinical trial outcomes, is pivotal for refining the competence of physicians who care for oncology patients. By standardizing language and streamlining communication in the health system, trials help build a culture that enables physicians to match treatment regimens to evidence-based recommendations more effectively. An educational model grounded on clinical trial results can support the interdisciplinary cooperation necessary for the provision of holistic care to oncology patients. In addition, palliative care's participation in clinical trials exemplifies proactive methods for symptom control and quality-of-life enhancement in patients with palliative illness. Current controversies surrounding psychedelic treatments, in particular psilocybin, reveal a persistent fascination with novel therapies to treat mental health in palliative care (Umbacia et al., 2025). The new methodologies, investigated in clinical trials, could provide critical comfort for palliative patients facing end-of-life challenges. Assessment of these treatments invites further scrutiny of their possible benefits and safety profiles, expanding the arsenal at the disposal of palliative care providers. With further advancement of these trials, they have the potential to transform treatment approaches and open discussions necessary to establish acceptable, patient-centered therapy in oncology and palliative care (Figure 4.12).

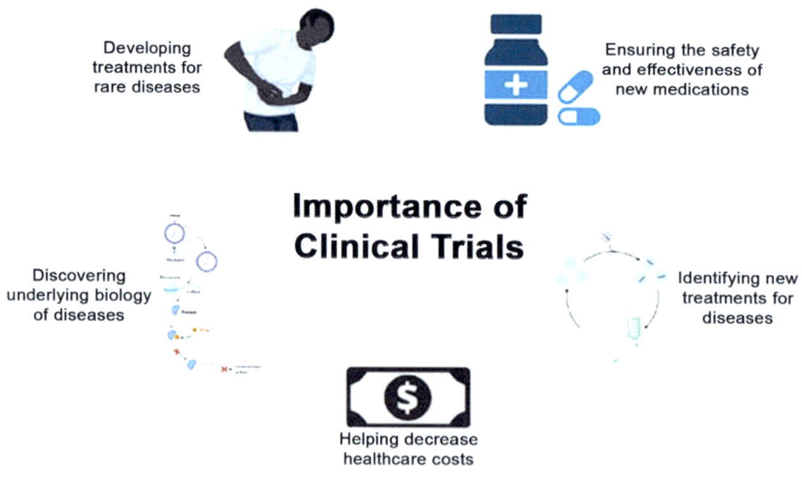

Figure 4.12. Role of clinical trials in treatment options.

Source: https://www.tandfonline.com/cms/asset/a8c64706-d3ac-4e67-b26f-9c8771ac4888/iann_a_2451190_uf0001_c.jpg.

4.5.3. Impact of Technology on Patient Care

The application of technology to patient care has transformed internal medicine as a specialty, with the most obvious being in oncology and hospice care. New diagnostic technologies, such as genomic sequencing and imaging, enhance the accuracy and precision of disease detection and treatment planning. For instance, cardiac magnetic resonance imaging (CMR) has proven helpful in monitoring cardiac disorders secondary to cancer therapies, providing a clear indication of the direct correlation between technological advancement and improved patient outcomes. Moreover, progress in telemedicine has enabled clinicians to maintain ongoing patient interactions and deliver timely interventions that literally alter treatment courses. These innovations not only optimize clinical efficacy but also make individualized medicine a reality, tailoring treatment protocols to each patient's disease pattern and improving the overall quality of life of cancer patients. In oncology, technology is increasingly applied to treatment modalities through electronic systems for precision and efficacy. For example, the application of cardiac implantable electronic devices (CIEDs) has been essential in managing cardiac side effects of cancer therapies. These procedures are a prime example of how technological advancements are required in an effort to attenuate the side effects of aggressive cancer therapies. Such a collaborative relationship between technology and healthcare provision allows multidimensional care strategies that not only cover the primary cancer diagnosis but also the comorbidities that accompany it. The function of an interprofessional team cannot be overstated; the use of various technological solutions ensures that patients receive comprehensive, tailored treatment for their complex health needs. Further, the incorporation of supportive interventions, as described in the NCCN Guidelines for Head and Neck Cancers, demonstrates how technology enables interdisciplinary collaboration among experts, thereby promoting patient safety and the efficacy of treatment regimens. Besides, technology plays a significant role in patient monitoring and data management, which are critical for oncology patient management. With the development of electronic health records (EHRs), it is feasible to have seamless communication among clinicians such that pertinent patient information is accessible and up-to-date at any time. This data streamlining is essential in the effective management of treatment choices, especially in advanced head and neck cancer, where the treatment can be complex and prolonged, like the area of interest for the recent alterations of systemic therapy recommendations in salivary gland tumors. With data analytics, clinicians can more easily track treatment effectiveness and patient response, enabling real-time adjustment of the care plan. Lastly, these innovations not only promote the efficacy of oncology care but also significantly enhance the overall patient experience, affirming the value of embracing innovation in palliative care, as it ultimately results in improved health and patient satisfaction.

Test Your Knowledge

1. What is the key difference between targeted therapy and traditional chemotherapy in cancer treatment?
2. How does immunotherapy help the body fight cancer?
3. Why are clinical trials necessary in advancing oncology treatment options?

4.6. Integration of Palliative Care in Oncology

Learning Outcome

1. Focus on early involvement of palliative care teams;
2. Discuss the benefits of holistic patient management;
3. Identify case studies demonstrating successful integration.

The integration of palliative care into oncology is a revolutionary shift in how cancer treatment is delivered. Oncology has long revolved around a curative purpose and often ignores the psychological and physical suffering experienced by patients. Through a palliative model, healthcare professionals can address complex quality-of-life issues alongside disease treatment. This twinning approach maximizes symptom control while also facilitating emotional and spiritual health, recognizing that cancer affects the whole person, not just the disease itself. Early involvement of palliative care professionals fosters a partnership aimed at achieving a balance between aggressive treatment and the unrelenting need for relief and support. This worldwide perspective rings truer in contemporary oncology practice, calling forth a patient-clinician relationship centered on the goals and priorities of those who live with cancer.

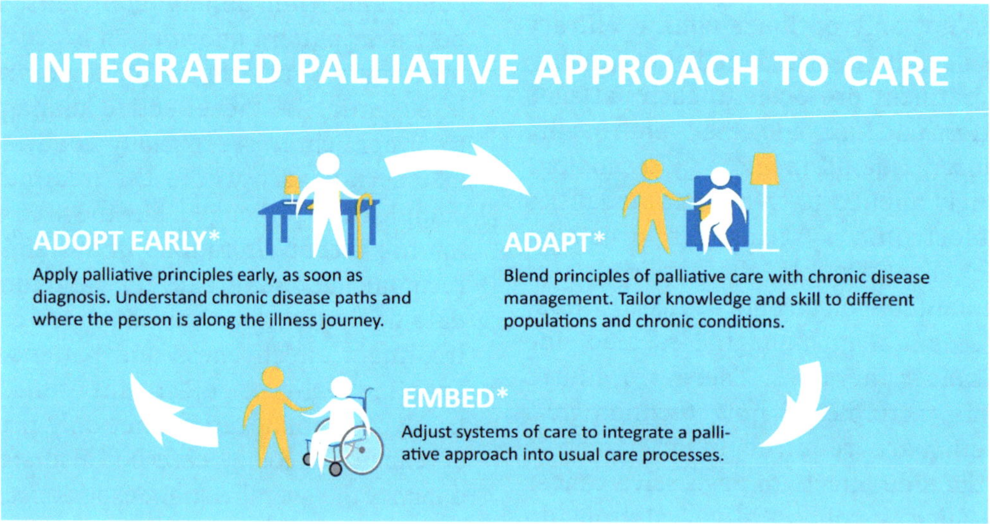

Figure 4.13. The integration of palliative care into oncology.

Source: https://www.cfn-nce.ca/wp-content/uploads/2018/09/CAT2015-32-Stajduhar-Infographic-1024x554.jpg.

The everyday integration of palliative care in oncology settings is not without problems and challenges, however. Clinicians often struggle with practice issues around the implementation of patient-reported outcome measures (PROMs) and patient-reported experience measures (PREMs). These are essential to patient outcomes and need, but are potentially limited by competing priorities within the health system for incorporation into routine care. Among those identified in recent assessments are tensions around standardization, difficulties with measures, and concerns about the scope of practice of clinicians delivering palliative care (Carroll et al., 2018). Navigating these challenges requires responsiveness and sensitivity from health professionals, who must balance competing institutional interests to ensure the quality of cancer care. Optimizing the integration of palliative care in oncology will also involve healthcare policies evolving in support of evidence-based practices. Evidence indicates that enhancing care coordination and preventive strategies has an impressive potential to improve patient outcomes for those with serious diseases (Morton et al., 2015). Areas such as palliative care, however, witness low policy response amid current evidence supporting its efficacy, highlighting a significant disparity in healthcare planning. Continued support for enhancing the health policies that guide palliative care services is critical to disseminating these interventions. By fostering a more caring policy environment, the inclusion of palliative care within oncology can be further established, thereby making cancer treatment a more holistic and human service capable of addressing the needs of patients and families to the utmost (Figure 4.13).

4.6.1. Early Involvement of Palliative Care Teams

The early implementation of palliative care teams in oncology patient treatment has garnered significant recognition in contemporary medical practice. Traditionally viewed as a service applicable only to end-of-life scenarios, palliative care is increasingly being viewed as an intrinsic part of the cancer care continuum. This change in perspective emphasizes the possibility of improving the quality of life and symptom management even during active treatment. Early palliative care integration not only controls the physical symptoms but also addresses psychological, social, and spiritual dimensions of patient wellness. In addition, evidence portrays that patients with earlier palliative interventions have lower hospitalization rates and satisfaction with their care, implicating palliative teams for better-conceived cancer care integration. As oncology environments evolve, the need for multidisciplinary teams is increasingly evident, particularly amid the complexities of cancer symptom management. Palliative care teams may be incorporated to deliver in-depth assessments that inform treatment plans responsive to individual patients' needs. For instance, patients with gastric cancer, characterized by their poor prognosis and distant stage at the time of diagnosis, typically require multidisciplinary management that includes rapid switching of systemic therapy and supportive care measures. The NCCN Guidelines for Gastric Cancer note that initial palliative care involvement is important in patients with unresectable or metastatic disease to assist not only with symptom alleviation but also with informed decision-making about aggressive treatment (Jaffer et al., 2022). By bringing together experts in oncology and palliative care, healthcare systems can marshal a more unified and effective response to the various issues posed by cancer. Combining palliative care teams with the treatment from the beginning also emphasizes the importance of open communication and shared decision-making. As patients move through the often-confusing realm of cancer treatments, frank discussions of prognosis and preferences for care are paramount. Palliative care providers are experienced at broaching these discussions, ensuring that patients' values and needs are prioritized. This model encourages a more patient-focused approach to care, where patients take an active role in decisions about their treatment trajectory. In addition, early palliative care engagement can clarify the purpose of advanced care planning, allowing patients to share their wishes regarding future medical interventions. This proactive strategy not only alleviates stress for patients and families but also ensures care aligned with their wishes, thereby raising overall satisfaction with their cancer care experience, particularly in complex situations such as gastric cancer with systemic complications (Jaffer et al., 2022) (Figure 4.14).

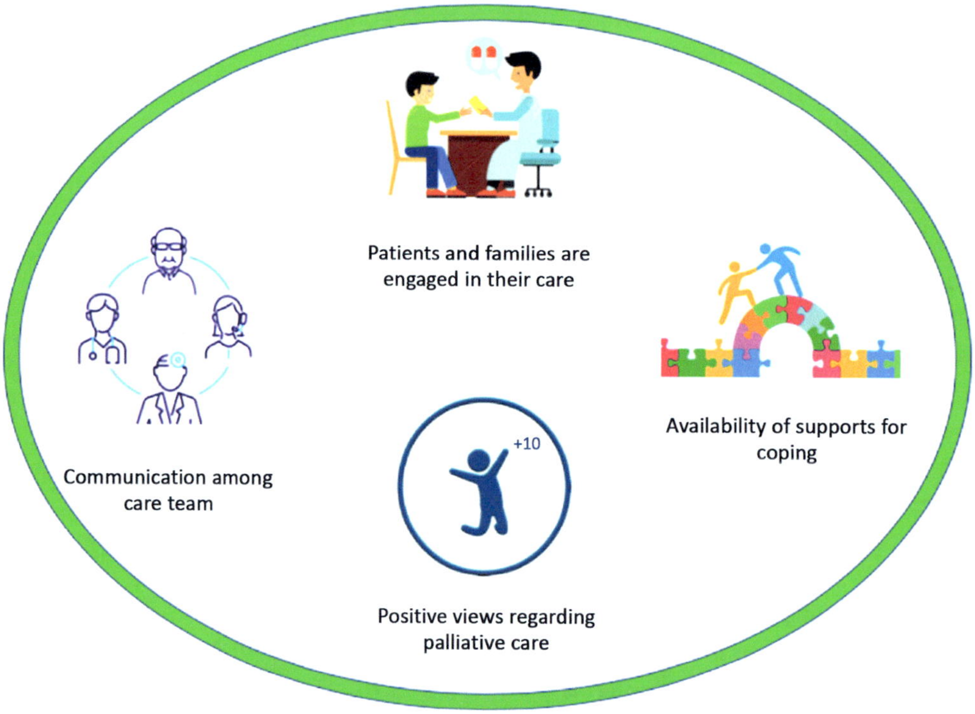

Figure 4.14. Early involvement of palliative care teams.

Source: https://www.researchgate.net/profile/Sadia-Ahmed-17/publication/359077433/figure/fig2/AS:1131764705701890@1646845141853/Patient-and-family-caregiver-experiences-after-early-palliative-care.png.

4.6.2. Benefits of Holistic Patient Management

Integration of holistic patient care into oncology and palliative care has been extremely promising in improving patient outcomes. It is concerned with the understanding of the intricate needs of patients rather than just physiologic factors. By addressing psychological, social, and emotional factors, the health care provider can create a more caring environment for patients undergoing treatment. Evidence supports once again that when health professionals use methods that consider the entire spectrum of patients' experiences—from symptom management to psychological support—patients have higher levels of satisfaction and better quality of life. This type of holistic model closely aligns with current directions in healthcare toward patient-centered care, as seen in changes in standards for cancer treatment delivery. Lastly, holistic management not only empowers patients but also stimulates better therapeutic compliance and health outcomes. Moreover, holistic patient management is central to the creation of successful multidisciplinary teams. Such teams are essential in the oncology and palliative care setting, where the complexities of treatment require collaboration among various specialists. There is an integrative approach in place to ensure that each team member—whether medical oncologists, palliative care providers, social workers, or nutritionists—will work together to understand the patient's needs. They collectively facilitate comprehensive treatment plans receptive to both physical and emotional components of cancer care. The benefit of this interprofessional model resonates through improved communication, as team members are more likely to share information about patients' progress and status. The emphasis on multidisciplinarity, as articulated in technical guidelines, underscores the necessity for integrated care frameworks that are responsive to the individual patient histories (Huang et al., 2020). The economic benefits of holistic patient management must also be considered. By reducing hospital readmissions and treatment-related adverse outcomes through holistic care models, these models can yield significant cost savings for healthcare systems. Prevention of complications of cancer therapy is necessary; therefore, a holistic model makes it possible to provide preventive interventions countering threats. In addition, addressing the patient's psychosocial context can lead to the effective use of resources, ensuring that support services are adequately specialized to meet patient needs. This not only enhances the efficacy of care delivery but also allows patients to be actively engaged in their treatment regimens. Cost-effectiveness with improved patient satisfaction is the icing on the cake in introducing holistic practices into oncology and palliative care, supporting the call that treating diverse patient needs can yield long-term healthcare outcomes (Huang et al., 2020) (Figure 4.15).

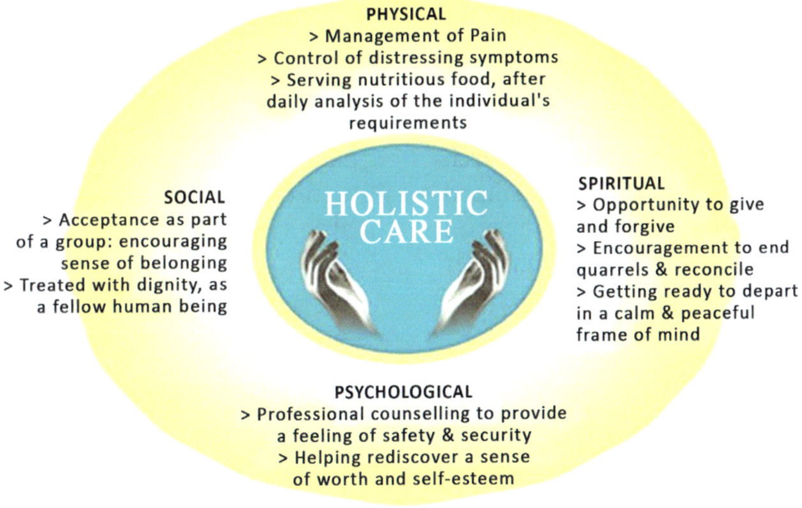

Figure 4.15. Diagrammatic presentation of the components of holistic care.

Source: https://cdnintech.com/media/chapter/72585/1512345123/media/F1.png.

4.6.3. Case Studies Demonstrating Successful Integration

The integration of palliative care into oncology wards is increasingly recognized as central to better patient outcomes and quality of life. A case study of the Charlotte Maxeke Johannesburg Academic Hospital (CMJAH) in South Africa highlights both the challenges and strategies involved in successful implementation in this field. The study highlighted key barriers, such as inadequate budget allocation and lack of support from management, that hinder integration of palliative services into routine oncology care. The study also highlighted enablers, such as increased awareness and a positive attitude among medical professionals, as well as institutionalized training programs that enhance the body of knowledge related to palliative care. These findings emphasize the importance of supportive environments and peer-reviewed models that integrate palliative care into their routine oncology practice, as exemplified by CMJAH's ongoing dedication to advocating patient-centered services within its healthcare model (Pilime et al., 2025). A closer look also reveals that integration challenges are nothing new in South Africa, as a study that evaluated knowledge and communication obstacles between oncology and internal medicine and intensive care physicians concluded that the vast majority of doctors gave their understanding of oncology-related terms a poor rating, and the most frequent confusion was regarding definitional terms like palliative and metastatic. This education gap affects not only clinical decision-making but also underscores the urgent need for standardized educational approaches. Ultimately, addressing these education and communication gaps can lead to more informed patient care practices. Furthermore, the research encourages the development of standardized vocabulary and accessible continuous education for interprofessional collaboration and greater integration of oncology and palliative care (Gon et al., 2025). Successful integration of palliative care into oncology infrastructures requires a multi-faceted approach that both overcomes systemic barriers and enhances training capacity. The implementation of pilot initiatives that engage internal medicine and oncology departments in mutual learning can be a strong model for others to replicate. By enabling interdisciplinary exchange and the development of hybrid protocols, hospitals can effectively break down silos that hinder collaboration across specializations. Furthermore, ongoing monitoring and feedback mechanisms within these integrated programs will ensure that they adapt to the evolving needs of both patients and health professionals. As duly evidenced by successful case studies, such integrative efforts not only improve the quality of care delivery but ultimately improve the patient experience, a paradigm shift in the conceptualization and integration of oncology and palliative care in health systems (Gon et al., 2025; Pilime et al., 2025).

Test Your Knowledge

1. How do palliative care teams contribute to the holistic management of oncology patients?
2. Name two key components of holistic care provided by palliative teams in oncology.

SUMMARY

The study of the role of internal medicines in oncology and palliative care underscores the need for a holistic approach to patient care. Complicated patients, such as those who are battling pancreatic cancer, require more than effective medical treatment; they require extensive emotional and psychological care. The literature indicates that the treatment of pancreatic cancer lacks standardization, with fewer clinicians adhering to available guidelines, reflecting gaps in care provision (Boeck et al., 2009). Such variability creates obstacles to achieving best-case patient outcomes, highlighting the need for standardized protocols to ensure adherence to evidence-based treatment across care settings. Also emphasizing the same, effective communication between healthcare providers and patients plays a significant role in decision-making, leading to more personalized approaches that align with patient preferences and circumstances. Further, transitioning from active treatment to palliative care also needs a careful and individualized approach, especially among culturally diverse patients. It is crucial to recognize the unique issues faced by such patients, like differences in language and cultural attitudes towards disease and death. Such aspects must be identified to enhance the quality of life and ensure a dignified end-of-life process. Emerging themes in qualitative research indicate that trust-building and the inclusion of family dynamics significantly explain patient safety and satisfaction in palliative care (Green et al., 2018). Inclusion of cultural competency in palliative care practice can enable healthcare providers to understand the complexities of patients' backgrounds, ensuring care is respectful and responsive to individualized needs. In conclusion, the approach to addressing the complexities of internal medicine through the umbrella of oncology and palliative care calls for coordinated action by clinicians to improve patient management practices. This not only involves adhering to prescribed treatment protocols but also requires cultural sensitivity and effective communication. The accumulating evidence supporting such practices points to the potential for improved patient outcomes through an integrated and compassionate model of healthcare. By prioritizing these fundamental elements, the healthcare community has a duty to strive for a time when each patient, regardless of background or diagnosis, receives balanced, whole, and tailored care tailored to their specific needs and circumstances. The commitment to continuous evolution in these areas remains at the forefront of enhancing treatment effectiveness and general patient and family satisfaction.

In cancer and palliative care, a general understanding of the modalities of cancer treatment and their influence on patient care is indispensable. The fourth edition of the extensive textbook of cancer treatment rightly lays the foundations of oncology through a comprehensive overview of molecular biology and radiobiology, equipping professionals with a solid scientific background. Chapters detailing various cancer therapies, such as chemotherapy and radiotherapy, provide clinically relevant information and recent trial results to inform treatment planning. The instrument is not merely critical for oncologists but also for clinicians in other branches of medicine, such as palliative care, thereby ensuring interdisciplinarity in the treatment of patients (Gill, 2003). To tackle site-specific cancers, the book provides a critical assessment of malignancies, pathology, staging, and classification systems for diagnosis and management. With a broader spectrum of cancers, starting from hematological malignancies to solid tumors, every chapter explores evidence-based approaches to treatment modalities. With a range of disparate treatment modalities—surgical interventions, chemotherapy regimens, and radiotherapy—happening within its purview, it showcases an extensive cancer management approach. In addition, concise chapters on the management of recurrent and metastatic disease provide practitioners with a comprehensive view of patient care (Glimelius et al., 2001). The final section of the book emphasizes the significance of symptom control and organizational matters of cancer services, with a close association with the evolving situation in palliative care. Principles of communication and the integrative model of oncology are essential in their own right, as they facilitate an integrative model of care that emphasizes the importance of caring for not only physical but also psychological and emotional aspects of cancer care. This paradigm is key to enhancing patients' quality of life, emphasizing that successful palliative care is part of oncology. The systematic review presented in the book is a powerful tool for health workers seeking to match curative treatment with compassionate end-of-life care (Gill, 2003).

KEY TERMS FROM THIS CHAPTER

- Oncology
- Chemotherapy
- Immunotherapy
- Metastasis
- Biopsy
- Cachexia
- Anemia
- Palliative Care
- Radiotherapy
- Targeted Therapy
- Tumor Marker
- Staging
- Neutropenia
- Thrombocytopenia

CRITICAL THINKING QUESTIONS

1. **Tumor lysis syndrome is most commonly associated with:**
   a. Breast cancer
   b. Acute lymphoblastic leukemia
   c. Colon cancer
   d. Renal cell carcinoma
2. **Which electrolyte abnormality is most characteristic of tumor lysis syndrome?**
   a. Hypernatremia
   b. Hypokalemia
   c. Hyperuricemia
   d. Hypophosphatemia
3. **Which of the following is a paraneoplastic syndrome associated with small cell lung carcinoma?**
   a. Hypercalcemia
   b. Cushing's syndrome
   c. Myasthenia gravis
   d. Polycythemia
4. **The most common site of bone metastases in internal malignancies is:**
   a. Skull
   b. Spine
   c. Clavicle
   d. Ribs
5. **Which drug is commonly used for the prevention of chemotherapy-induced nausea and vomiting (CINV)?**
   a. Omeprazole
   b. Ondansetron
   c. Propranolol
   d. Lorazepam

Short Answer Questions

1. What are the common paraneoplastic syndromes associated with lung cancer?
2. Explain the role of internal medicine in the diagnosis and monitoring of hematological malignancies.
3. Describe the role of tumor markers in the diagnosis and follow-up of cancer patients.
4. What is the role of corticosteroids in palliative care?
5. Describe the principles of breaking bad news using the SPIKES protocol.
6. Explain the difference between hospice care and palliative care.

Answers to Critical Thinking Questions

1. (b); 2. (c); 3. (b); 4. (b); 5. (b)

REFERENCES

1. Ajani, J. A., D'Amico, T. A., Bentrem, D. J., Chao, J., Cooke, D., Corvera, C., Das, P., Enzinger, P. C., Enzler, T., Fanta, P., Farjah, F., Gerdes, H., Gibson, M. K., Hochwald, S., Hofstetter, W. L., Ilson, D. H., Keswani, R. N., Kim, S., Kleinberg, L. R., . . . Pluchino, L. A. (2022). Gastric Cancer, Version 2.2022, NCCN Clinical Practice Guidelines in Oncology. *Journal of the National Comprehensive Cancer Network, 20*(2), 167–192. https://doi.org/10.6004/jnccn.2022.0008Andersen, B. L., Lacchetti, C., Ashing, K., Berek, J. S., Berman, B. S., Bolte, S., Dizon, D. S., et al. (2023). Management of anxiety and depression in adult survivors of cancer: ASCO guideline update. *Journal of Clinical Oncology*, *41*, 3426–3453. https://doi.org/10.1200/jco.23.00293 (accessed on 17th July 2025).
2. Bashshur, R. L., Doarn, C. R., Frenk, J., Kvedar, J. C., & Woolliscroft, J. O. (2020). Telemedicine and the COVID-19 pandemic, lessons for the future. *Telemedicine Journal and e-Health*, *26*, 571–573. https://doi.org/10.1089/tmj.2020.29040.rb (accessed on 17th July 2025).
3. Bennett, M. I., Johnson, M. I., Oxberry, S. G., Robb, K., et al. (2008). Transcutaneous electrical nerve stimulation for cancer pain in adults. https://core.ac.uk/download/68503.pdf (accessed on 17th July 2025).
4. Benson, A. B., D'Angelica, M. I., Abbott, D. E., Anaya, D. A., Anders, R. A., Are, C., Bachini, M., et al. (2021). Hepatobiliary cancers, Version 2.2021, NCCN clinical practice guidelines in oncology. *Journal of the National Comprehensive Cancer Network*, *19*, 541–565. https://doi.org/10.6004/jnccn.2021.0022 (accessed on 17th July 2025).
5. Bickel, K., McNiff, K. K., Buss, M. K., Kamal, A. H., Lupu, D., Abernethy, A. P., Broder, M. S., et al. (2016). Defining high-quality palliative care in oncology practice: An American Society of Clinical Oncology/American Academy of Hospice and Palliative Medicine guidance statement. *Journal of Oncology Practice*, *12*, e828–e838. https://doi.org/10.1200/jop.2016.010686 (accessed on 17th July 2025).
6. Biganzoli, L., Cardoso, F., Beishon, M., Cameron, D., Cataliotti, L., Coles, C. E., Delgado Bolton, R. C., et al. (2020). The requirements of a specialist breast center. *The Breast*, *51*, 65–84. https://doi.org/10.1016/j.breast.2020.02.003 (accessed on 17th July 2025).
7. Blaschke, S., O'Callaghan, C., & Schofield, P. (2018). Nature-based supportive care opportunities: A conceptual framework. https://core.ac.uk/download/213607608.pdf (accessed on 17th July 2025).
8. Boeck, S., Bruns, C. J., Heinemann, V., Jauch, K. W., et al. (2009). Current oncological treatment of patients with pancreatic cancer in Germany: Results from a national survey on behalf of the Arbeitsgemeinschaft Internistische Onkologie and the Chirurgische Arbeitsgemeinschaft Onkologie of the Germany Cancer Society. https://core.ac.uk/download/16432402.pdf (accessed on 17th July 2025).
9. Breakwell, S., Fennimore, L., Ferrell, B., Virani, S., et al. (2018). A framework for integrating oncology palliative care in Doctor of Nursing Practice (DNP) education. https://core.ac.uk/download/213089445.pdf (accessed on 17th July 2025).
10. Cohen, R., Krawczyk, M., Laforest, M., Reimer-Kirkham, S., et al. (2018). Micro-meso-macro practice tensions in using patient-reported outcome and experience measures in hospital palliative care. https://core.ac.uk/download/153444956.pdf (accessed on 17th July 2025).

11. Cortés, J., Pérez-García, J. M., Llombart-Cussac, A., Curigliano, G., El Saghir, N. S., Cardoso, F., Barrios, C. H., et al. (2020). Enhancing global access to cancer medicines. *CA: A Cancer Journal for Clinicians, 70*, 105–124. https://doi.org/10.3322/caac.21597 (accessed on 17th July 2025).

12. Cowfer, B., McGrath, C., & Trowbridge, A. (2020). Teaching pediatric palliative care communication skills to fourth-year medical students through role-play. *MedEdPORTAL.* https://doi.org/10.15766/mep_2374-8265.10991 (accessed on 17th July 2025).

13. Elk, R. (2017). The need for culturally-based palliative care programs for African American patients at end-of-life. https://core.ac.uk/download/132289944.pdf (accessed on 17th July 2025).

14. Faßnacht, M., Dekkers, O. M., Else, T., Baudin, E., Berruti, A., de Krijger, R. R., Haak, H. R., et al. (2018). European Society of Endocrinology clinical practice guidelines on the management of adrenocortical carcinoma in adults, in collaboration with the European Network for the Study of Adrenal Tumors. *European Journal of Endocrinology, 179*, G1–G46. https://doi.org/10.1530/eje-18-0608 (accessed on 17th July 2025).

15. Gill, V. (2003). Treatment of cancer (4th edn). *British Journal of Cancer, 88*, 1659–1660. https://www.semanticscholar.org/paper/258afd11fdd977ea4c80e36704762eeb9c09381b (accessed on 17th July 2025).

16. Glimelius, B., Bergh, J., Brandt, L., Brorsson, B., Gunnars, B., Hafström, L., Haglund, U., et al. (2001). The Swedish Council on Technology Assessment in Health Care (SBU) systematic overview of chemotherapy effects in some major tumor types—Summary and conclusions. *Acta Oncological, 40*(2–3), 135–154. https://www.semanticscholar.org/paper/5e19d7cf0273bca39b20ea9bd3427544bc16e934 (accessed on 17th July 2025).

17. Gonçalves, M., Gouveia, R., Barbosa, M., & Meireles, S. (2025). Bridging communication gaps in oncology: Insights from a questionnaire among internal medicine and intensive care physicians. *Cureus, 17.* https://www.semanticscholar.org/paper/dff589856ace862485dd5e96392109af51713e48 (accessed on 17th July 2025).

18. Green, A., Green, M., Jerzmanowska, N., & Lobb, E., et al. (2018). 'Death is difficult in any language': A qualitative study of palliative care professionals' experiences when providing end-of-life care to patients from culturally and linguistically diverse backgrounds. https://core.ac.uk/download/213607752.pdf (accessed on 17th July 2025).

19. Haddad, R. I., Bischoff, L. A., Ball, D. W., Bernet, V., Blomain, E., Busaidy, N. L., Campbell, M. J., et al. (2022). Thyroid carcinoma, Version 2.2022, NCCN clinical practice guidelines in oncology. *Journal of the National Comprehensive Cancer Network, 20*, 925–951. https://doi.org/10.6004/jnccn.2022.0040 (accessed on 17th July 2025).

20. Hashiguchi, T. C. O. (2020). *Bringing Health Care to The Patient.* OECD Health Working Papers. https://doi.org/10.1787/8e56ede7-en (accessed on 17th July 2025).

21. Huang, R., & Zhou, P. K. (2020). DNA damage response signaling pathways and targets for radiotherapy sensitization in cancer. *Signal Transduction and Targeted Therapy, 5.* https://doi.org/10.1038/s41392-020-0150-x (accessed on 17th July 2025).

22. Luppi, M., Bandieri, E., Venditti, A., & Corradini, P. (2023). Hematology and specialist palliative medicine education and training. *BMJ Supportive & Palliative Care, 14.* https://www.semanticscholar.org/paper/6882b27d4a840150bfd71042b83205bb7eb3bcfe (accessed on 17th July 2025).

23. Lyon, A. R., López-Fernández, T., Couch, L. S., Asteggiano, R., Aznar, M. C., Bergler-Klein, J., Boriani, G., et al. (2022). 2022 ESC guidelines on cardio-oncology developed in collaboration with the European Hematology Association (EHA), the European Society for Therapeutic Radiology and Oncology (ESTRO) and the International Cardio-Oncology Society (IC-OS). *European Heart Journal*, *43*, 4229–4361. https://doi.org/10.1093/eurheartj/ehac244 (accessed on 17th July 2025).

24. Mangel, L., Lukács, M., Hajnal, A., Sárkány, H., Forgács-Menyhért, M., Varga, Z., Herendi, E., et al. (2020). The first experiences with the palliative tumor board discussions in the University of Pécs. *Orvosi Hetilap*, *161*(34), 1423–1430. https://www.semanticscholar.org/paper/fceb6dcb27bfb3a61e02a82d99744f9adbf71382 (accessed on 17th July 2025).

25. Morris, V. K., Kennedy, E. B., Baxter, N. N., Benson, A. B., Cercek, A., Cho, M., Ciombor, K. K., et al. (2022). Treatment of metastatic colorectal cancer: ASCO guideline. *Journal of Clinical Oncology*, *41*, 678–700. https://doi.org/10.1200/jco.22.01690 (accessed on 17th July 2025).

26. Morton, S., & Dunn, W. (2015). *Addressing the Health Needs of An Aging America: New Opportunities for Evidence-Based Policy Solutions*. https://core.ac.uk/download/75783019.pdf (accessed on 17th July 2025).

27. N/A. (2004). *Better Palliative Care for Older People*. https://core.ac.uk/download/75777691.pdf (accessed on 17th July 2025).

28. Pfister, D. G., Spencer, S., Adelstein, D. J., Adkins, D. R., Anzai, Y., Brizel, D. M., Bruce, J. Y., et al. (2020). Head and neck cancers, Version 2.2020, NCCN clinical practice guidelines in oncology. *Journal of the National Comprehensive Cancer Network*, *18*, 873–898. https://doi.org/10.6004/jnccn.2020.0031 (accessed on 17th July 2025).

29. Pilime, S., Ratshikana, M., Ojifinni, O., & Ibisomi, L. (2025). Barriers to and enablers of availability and integration of palliative care into routine services at Charlotte Maxeke Johannesburg Academic Hospital, South Africa. *BMC Palliative Care*, *24*. https://www.semanticscholar.org/paper/8ce3d359698896d538ab60ca1472056714555229 (accessed on 17th July 2025).

30. Riba, M. B., Donovan, K. A., Andersen, B. L., Braun, I., Breitbart, W., Brewer, B. W., Buchmann, L., et al. (2019). Distress management, Version 3.2019, NCCN clinical practice guidelines in oncology. *Journal of the National Comprehensive Cancer Network*, *17*, 1229–1249. https://doi.org/10.6004/jnccn.2019.0048 (accessed on 17th July 2025).

31. Sandha, G., Abdulhussain, H., Krahn, T., Timmermans, M., Buchanan, G., Bereznicki, E., Mathura, P., et al. (2024). A112 The Edmonton Pancreaticobiliary Inflammation and Cancer (EPIC) Program–A new multidisciplinary coordination of care initiative. *Journal of the Canadian Association of Gastroenterology*, *7*, 83–85. https://www.semanticscholar.org/paper/900c721d8665e871554161c1e8f4ed1857180a3a (accessed on 17th July 2025).

32. Torres-Tenor, J. L., García-Leal, A., Pérez-Wert, P., Alonso-Babarro, A., & Bruera, E. (2025). Collaboration between palliative care and oncology in the era of personalized medicine. *Journal of Palliative Medicine*. https://www.semanticscholar.org/paper/3389e8d8c03447547829e2656b6a18b05c573f1c (accessed on 17th July 2025).

33. Umbacia, M., Leon, M. X., Quintero, J. M., Castro, L. M., Paez, V., Dodd, S., & Bustos, R. H. (2025). Exploring psilocybin's role in mental health and palliative medicine: A path to improved well-being. *Expert Opinion on Emerging Drugs*, *30*, 99–108. https://www.semanticscholar.org/paper/6cf57d9bfb2164d9f3c053376753cd3a342941c5 (accessed on 17th July 2025).

IMMUNOLOGY AND ALLERGY

5

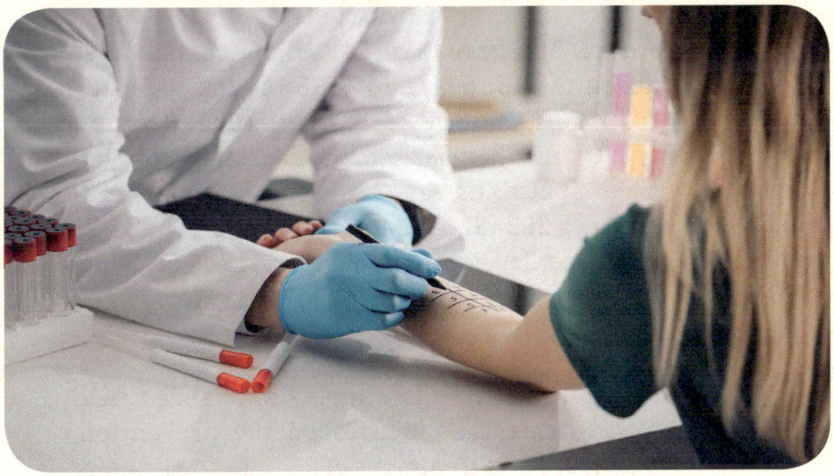

LEARNING OBJECTIVES

After studying this chapter, you will be able to:

1. Explain the types of allergies
2. Understand the mechanisms of allergic reactions
3. Discuss the diagnosis of allergies
4. Describe the treatment options for allergies
5. Define the role of the immune system
6. Focus on current research in allergy and immunology

Introduction

Internal medicine has many subspecialties, of which immunology and allergy are fundamental due to their role in managing complex immune-mediated disorders and allergic conditions. Healthcare workers need to know about these fields, as they can have a profound impact on the quality of life of patients with immunological complications. With improvement in medicine, the demand for well-trained specialists in immunology and allergy, who can interpret the intricate relationship between diseases and the immune system, is growing. The ongoing development of immunodiagnostics supports the demand for this specialty. New technologies developed in immunoassay formats have made diagnostics so effective that the quality of care at clinics has improved. Against this background, internal medicine increasingly integrates understanding from immunology and allergy to the point that it is a central area of study for prospective physicians. The challenge of diagnosing and treating immunological illnesses highlights the need for a firm foundation in internal medicine training. As outlined in comprehensive resources such as First Aid for the Internal Medicine Boards, a firm grounding in knowledge is necessary for internal medicine doctors. Topics of discussion, such as autoimmune and allergic diseases, require an advanced understanding of immune mechanisms to tailor effective treatment algorithms. Not only should internal medicine training encompass such fundamental principles, but it should also be updated on technological advancements in diagnostic equipment. For students preparing for certification examinations, concise note-taking guides and high-yield summaries are invaluable tools for consolidating complex material.

This intersection of intensive training and up-to-date knowledge produces skilled clinicians well-suited to manage the subtle problems encountered in immunology and allergy in the clinic. Immunology and allergy's role in internal medicine extends beyond diagnosis and therapy; it encompasses a significant point of intersection among research, quality improvement, and patient understanding. With immunological disorders and allergies continuously on the rise globally, understanding the epidemiology and management of these conditions is of utmost relevance. The interplay between clinical immunology and other areas of medicine facilitates the development of integrated care plans in multimorbid patients. Further, raising awareness among medical professionals and the public about these conditions could lead to earlier diagnosis and treatment, ultimately improving patient outcomes. Translation of cutting-edge research into practice will pave the way for new treatment approaches, realizing the ultimate goal of enhanced patient care in internal medicine. Immunology and allergy will remain an essential component of modern internal medicine practice and teaching, enabling the healthcare providers to adapt to the evolving needs of the patients (Figure 5.1).

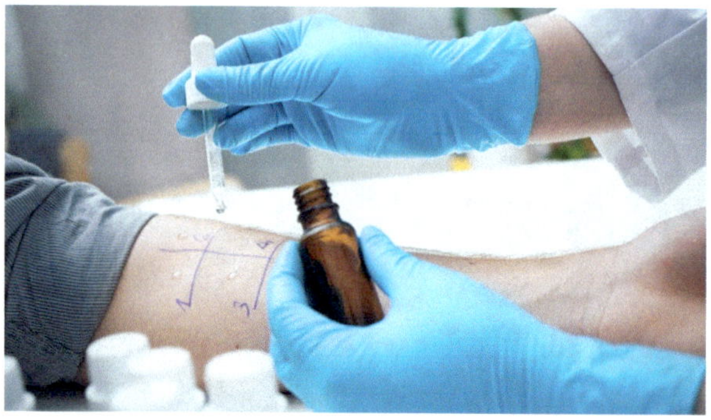

Figure 5.1. Allergy and immunology.

Source: https://cdn.castleconnolly.com/dims4/default/406557f/2147483647/strip/true/crop/1000x563+0+0/resize/840x473!/quality/90/?url=http%3A%2F%2Fcastle-connolly-brightspot.s3.us-east-1.amazonaws.com%2Fdf%2Fa7%2F3432d4134088bf7add8ac125dbc1%2Fpillar-allergy-immunology-49-1200x675.jpg.

Definition of Internal Medicine

Internal medicine is a highly specialized field of medicine that focuses on the prevention, diagnosis, and treatment of a broad spectrum of adult illnesses. It is distinguished by its emphasis on integrative care, particularly in patients with complex diseases that require a highly advanced understanding of multiple organs and their interrelationships. Providers, or internists, are trained to provide overall care, often being a patient's primary care physician while treating acute and chronic illnesses. Such a diversified practice is required in fields like immunology and allergy, where patients may present with complex symptoms that make traditional diagnostic approaches challenging. By merging extensive knowledge of patient pathophysiology and patient history, internists can offer targeted therapies to enhance overall patient outcomes and quality of life. Medicine's ever-changing nature demands that internists stay up to date with the latest studies and guidelines, particularly in the rapidly evolving fields of immunology and allergy management. For instance, contemporary guidelines for urticaria have emerged following global agreement among professional bodies emphasizing evidence-based treatment and diagnostic strategies (Zuberbier et al., 2021). These revisions show commitment to quality patient care through dedication and research, as well as clinical experience. Furthermore, the complexity of managing allergy interventions—including anaphylactic reactions—underscores the critical role of internists as connectors between specialties. They must synthesize recommendations across specialties to ensure safe and effective patient management of intricate immune-related disorders. Besides clinical expertise required, effective communication is also essential in the practice of internal medicine, especially in managing challenging patient cases in immunology and allergy. Internists should communicate risks and benefits of therapy, i.e., vaccines, particularly for potential allergic reactions to products such as polyethylene glycol (Greenhawt et al., 2021). Informed shared decision-making is required because patients want to be more and more involved in their treatment decisions. By fostering a team environment, internists not only enhance patient understanding and compliance but also facilitate individuals' active roles in health care. This interprofessional approach reflects internal medicine's higher goals: providing compassionate, evidence-based treatment while advocating patient independence and thriving amidst increasing health complexities.

Overview of Immunology and Allergy

Immunological mechanisms play a vital role in the practice of medicine, particularly in allergy and clinical immunology. The immune system represents the body's defense against infection, functioning through the intricate interplay of cells, tissues, and organs. It distinguishes between self and non-self and initiates selective responses to eliminate foreign invaders, such as bacteria, viruses, and allergens. The grouping and classification of immune cells, including T cells, B cells, and antigen-presenting cells, highlight their roles in adaptive immunity. Such a response to the immune system can vary in intensity and duration depending on various factors, including the type of pathogen involved and the immune system's prior exposure to it, thereby underscoring the sophistication of the immunological response that can lead to allergic diseases in susceptible subjects. Allergic reactions occur when the immune system overreacts to otherwise harmless substances, called allergens. Some of the most common allergens include pollen, dust mites, mold, pet dander, and food. This overreaction occurs through immunoglobulin E (IgE), an antibody that binds allergens and triggers the release of histamine and other mediators from mast cells and basophils. The induced physiological changes, such as vasodilation and increased blood vessel permeability, can lead to allergy symptoms, including sneezing, itching, and, in extreme cases, anaphylaxis. Understanding the mechanisms behind such allergic reactions is crucial to designing effective remedies. For example, allergy treatment involves pharmacologic therapy, e.g., antihistamines, corticosteroids, and more novel biologic medications that act on specific immune response pathways (John et al., 2022). Current research in immunotherapy has identified promising avenues for treating allergy through patient desensitization to specific allergens. This technique aims to re-educate the immune system over time by gradually exposing patients to allergens, with the long-term goal of reducing the severity of allergic responses. The application of such immunotherapy is most apparent in conditions like allergic rhinitis and food allergy. Meanwhile, ongoing research on vaccines, particularly in response to emerging pathogens such as SARS-CoV-2, underscores the applicability of immunology to both prevention and treatment. The unparalleled speed of vaccine development in the COVID-19 pandemic illustrates the convergence of immunology with ongoing health concerns and emerging pathogens (Connors et al., 2021). Thus, immunology, as a science, continues to expand, advancing vaccine technology and allergy therapy, all in the ultimate pursuit of enhancing patient care in internal medicine clinics (Figure 5.2).

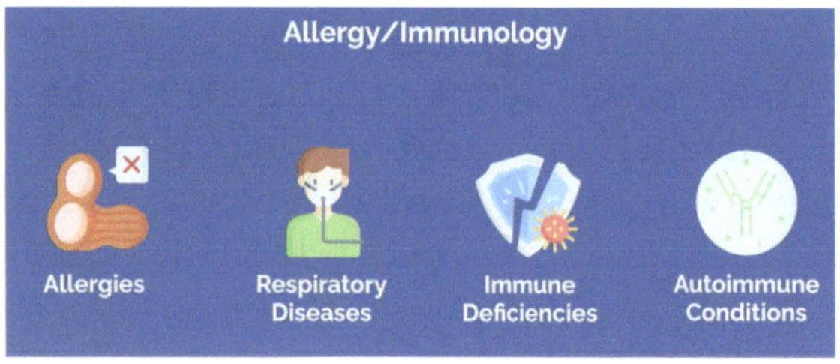

Figure 5.2. An overview of immunology and allergy.

Source: https://medschoolinsiders.com/wp-content/uploads/2023/09/allergy-immunology-examples-graphic-1024x498.png.

Importance of Internal Medicine in Managing Immunological Disorders

Internal medicine plays a pivotal role in treating immunological disorders, serving as the initial point of contact for patients with complex, multifaceted medical issues. Internists can diagnose and treat various diseases stemming from immune dysfunction, such as autoimmune, allergic, and immunodeficiency disorders. This allows them to provide integrative therapy by targeting not only the clinical manifestations but also the intrinsic immunological mechanisms. By combining clinical skill with biopsychosocial principles, internists can develop treatment strategies that are tailored to individual patient considerations, resulting in improved outcomes and quality of life for patients struggling with these challenging disorders.

Chronic inflammatory disorders are a primary focus area in internal medicine and immunology because they often result from abnormal immune mechanisms. Lupus, rheumatoid arthritis, and inflammatory bowel disease are usually challenging for patients and even for healthcare providers. Internists employ varied treatment strategies, such as immunosuppressive medications, biologics, and lifestyle modifications, to dampen inflammation and arrest disease progression. Also, multidisciplinary practice with rheumatologists and allergists allows for more thoughtful treatment planning, considering the whole picture of a patient's health.

This team approach not only ensures optimal quality of care but also helps combat the growing burden of these diseases and makes internal medicine critical to public health. Furthermore, patient education and health awareness regarding immunological disorders are key aspects of internal medicine. General practitioners are generally in a position to advise patients about their conditions, required lifestyle changes, and treatment adherence. They are also involved in screening and early diagnosis, which can significantly contribute to disease prognosis. For example, allergy- or anaphylaxis-risk patients require adequate education on avoidance and appropriate emergency measures, such as the administration of epinephrine auto-injectors. As discussed earlier, underreporting of anaphylaxis is a pointer to the need for well-trained internists in detecting and acting accordingly in emergencies to prevent potentially fatal outcomes (Tanno et al., 2017). In this role, internal medicine improves public health by creating an educated patient base that can effectively manage their conditions preventatively.

5.1. Types of Allergies

Learning Outcome

1. Understand food allergies
- Define environmental allergies
- Describe the prevalence of drug allergies

The classification of allergies is significant in describing their manifestation and management in the field of immunology. There are two broad categories of allergies: IgE-mediated and non-IgE-mediated reactions. IgE-mediated allergies, often characterized by immediate hypersensitivity reactions, are triggered by allergens such as food particles, pollen, and insect stings. These reactions are characterized by the sudden discharge of histamines and other mediators from mast cells when previously familiar allergens are encountered. These reactions have the potential to range from simple rhinitis to fatal anaphylaxis and require prompt medical attention. Delayed reactions are characteristic of non-IgE-mediated allergies, such as contact dermatitis and food protein-induced enterocolitis syndrome. The distinction between them is essential for effective diagnosis and therapeutic control because they rely on different immunological processes and management strategies. Among the IgE-mediated allergies, food allergies are a significant public health problem. Food allergies were a focus in recent studies on rising food allergy rates, particularly in developed countries, leading to evaluations of allergenicity and potential for sensitization. Within the adverse outcome pathway (AOP) framework, researchers have recently begun structuring the molecular and cellular processes underlying IgE-mediated food allergy, thereby expanding understanding of how food proteins can provoke allergic reactions (Benedé et al., 2019). Not only does this framework help scientists reconcile current test methods, but it also informs the development of novel assays to quantify allergen sensitivity. Furthermore, the increasing threat posed by food allergies requires serious risk assessments before new food sources are put on the market, specifically as to their allergenic potential to sensitize vulnerable groups. Not only does allergy control entail avoidance of specific stimuli and control over certain triggers, but also the implementation of preventive methods. Environmental allergies, commonly linked with pollen, dust mites, mold, and pet dander, can lead to chronic ailments such as allergic rhinitis and asthma. In such cases, allergen immunotherapy has emerged as a new ray of hope. This therapy attempts to desensitize an individual to known allergens by exposing them under controlled conditions, thereby reducing the allergic response over time. Apart from this, healthcare professionals have increasingly recognized the importance of personalized treatment plans tailored to a patient's allergy profile. This is further pertinent given research suggests a broad range of impacts from multiple funding approaches in asthma studies, thus informing ongoing efforts to address such complex health issues properly (Watt et al., 2013). It is therefore crucial to learn about the various categories of allergies for clinical practice and ongoing research in allergy and immunology.

5.1.1. Food Allergies

The increased prevalence of food allergy has sparked substantial interest among researchers and clinicians, particularly in defining its pathophysiologic mechanisms. A food allergy occurs when the immune system mistakenly recognizes food proteins as harmful, triggering an abnormal allergic reaction. Immunologic hypersensitivity to food proteins can cause a variety of manifestations ranging from mild illness, such as urticaria and gastrointestinal symptoms, to an anaphylactic reaction that should be aggressively treated (Figure 5.3).

Existing research has indicated that food allergy is not confined to childhood, as prevalence among adults is rising but remains frequently underdiagnosed and undertreated. Findings by studies that have been insufficiently reported have indicated that 5.6% of pregnant women report food allergies. In contrast, the FDA-reported prevalence in the overall adult population is steady, and thus, an ongoing study into adult food allergies is essential (Seita et al., 2013). Awareness of the risk factors that cause food allergies is critical for effective preventive measures and treatment programs. A few factors include genetic susceptibilities, environmental influences, and diet, which all contribute to such hypersensitivities. For instance, babies with parents suffering from allergies are more likely to develop the same sensitivities, indicating that there is a genetic component.

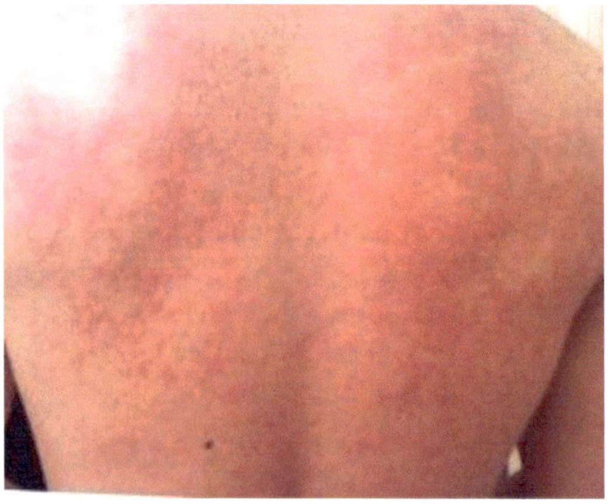

Figure 5.3. Hives on the back are a common allergy symptom.

Source: https://upload.wikimedia.org/wikipedia/commons/b/bb/Hives_on_back.jpg.

Moreover, emphasis has been placed on the importance of the microbiome and early allergen exposure in shaping immune responses. Dysfunctions in early immune tolerance could lead to inappropriate immunity later in life. Investigation into such correlations would go a long way toward broadening our understanding of food allergies to inform the development of targeted interventions that may prevent their establishment (Burns et al., 2019). The impact of food allergies extends beyond the ill individual to public health and safety. With an increasing prevalence of food allergies, their impact on quality of life is a challenge for healthcare providers and food-allergic individuals alike. In pregnant women with food allergies, there is an urgent need to explore maternal health outcomes together with infant development. Recent studies indicate no measurable association between pregnancy food allergies and adverse outcomes, yet the complexities of infancy, pregnancy, and diet demand further research. Furthermore, methods for managing food allergies must be revised to account for both the immediate allergic reaction and the psychological impact of food allergies. Education is at the core of reorienting how food allergies are perceived and managed, thus making room for individuals affected by an increasingly common health condition (Seita et al., 2013) (Figure 5.4).

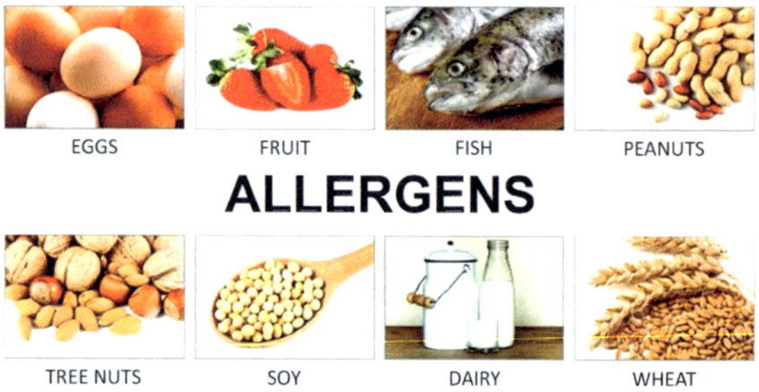

Figure 5.4. Food allergens.

Source: https://www.drbatras.com/sites/default/files/styles/blog/public/2024-04/food-allergies_Header_1.webp?itok=18HBBC8L.

5.1.2. Environmental Allergies

Environmental allergies, also known as allergic responses, are triggered by a variety of agents in our surroundings and constitute a significant portion of allergy and immunology. All such allergies usually arise from exposure to pollen, mold spores, dust mites, and pet dander, ranging from simple nasal congestion to anaphylactic storms. Environmental allergies have increased dramatically over the past decades, a development driven by both genetic predispositions and environmental factors. Several studies suggest that genetic inheritance, genetic mutations, and levels of ecological sensitization influence a person's predisposition to environmental allergens. Establishing these interactions is needed to develop effective preventive measures and therapeutic interventions that minimize the effects of these allergies on affected populations, especially children, who appear more vulnerable to developing hypersensitivity reactions, as indicated by recent observations (Burns et al., 2019). The immune system also plays a key role in the development and manifestation of environmental allergies, mediating subtle, central responses. Upon exposure to allergens, the immune system may respond inappropriately, leading to the overproduction of Immunoglobulin E (IgE), which binds to mast cells and basophils, triggering the release of histamines and other inflammatory mediators. This overreactive response is not only the result of direct contact with allergens but can also be augmented by exposure to different environmental factors, such as pollutants. Recent evidence has explored the intriguing possibility of cross-links between helminth infestations and reduced incidence of allergic sensitization. Research has shown that helminth products may induce regulatory immune responses that downregulate allergic responses, underscoring the complexity of environmental factors in their interactions with the immune response (Mutapi et al., 2012).

Environmental allergy control needs a comprehensive understanding of the epidemiology and treatment protocol that responds to the patient's certain sensitivities. Public health interventions that minimize exposure to common environmental allergens can significantly abate the frequency and intensity of allergic reactions. Of particular importance is improving indoor air quality and promoting hygiene practices, reducing dust and mold burden to relieve the allergic load. Beyond this, increased education and awareness among healthcare providers and patients regarding these ubiquitous allergens can facilitate early recognition and effective management. As the research progresses, namely on mechanisms of pediatric hypersensitivity and on the synergy between environmental exposures and immune mechanisms, the expectation is that more targeted therapies will be developed, ultimately enhancing the quality of life for individuals with environmental allergies (Burns et al., 2019) (Figure 5.5).

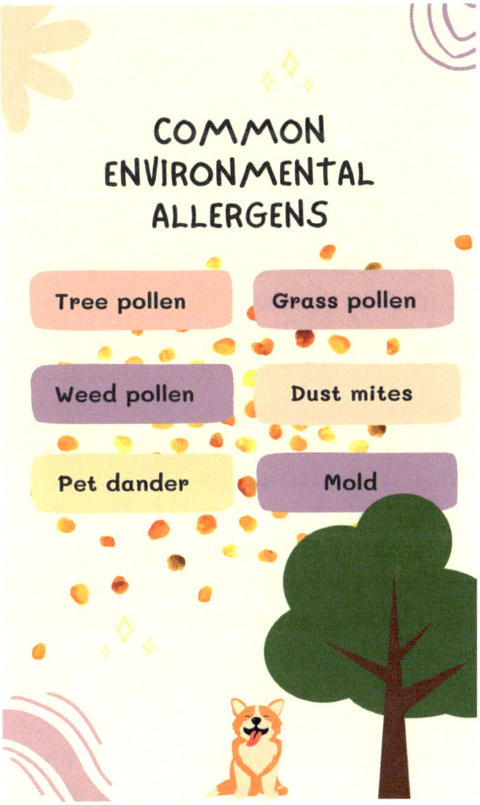

Figure 5.5. Common environmental allergens.

Source: https://foodswithgrace.com/wp-content/uploads/2023/05/Common-environmental-allergens-1-576x1024.png.

5.1.3. Drug Allergies

Drug allergy incidence is a significant public health concern that influences treatment and patient outcomes. Of all the drug allergy subgroups, penicillin allergy is most prominent, attracting attention with its widespread incidence and myth-making surrounding it.

Ironically, while common penicillin allergies are reported, there is a study indicating that only 10% of such patients actually have an allergy, with potential deleterious effects on treatment regimens. This inequality creates more reliance upon other antibiotics, which are either less effective or carry higher side effects. Therefore, understanding the complexity of drug allergies, particularly penicillin, is critical for clinicians to enhance patient care and reduce risks from misdiagnosed allergies, with proper allergy testing in clinical practice being essential. Drug allergies of the mother to even common therapeutic drugs are significant not just for pregnant women but also for fetal health. Research, such as a review of food allergy in pregnant women, underscores the need for a complete understanding of the impacts of allergy on maternal and infant health. Even as the research indicated that food allergies during pregnancy did not correlate with detrimental maternal or infant health outcomes, it emphasizes that pregnant women should be tested for allergies under varying circumstances, including the use of medication. As clinicians deal with the complexity of drug allergy in pregnancy, they must weigh the risks of dealing with allergies against the need for the best treatment for mother and infant so that allergies are correctly read, and drugs utilized are safe for this vulnerable group. Drug allergy diagnosis and treatment in the outpatient setting have taken on ever-greater significance. Pharmacists have now begun playing a critical role in conducting penicillin skin testing (PST), thereby facilitating the re-evaluation of patients with a proven penicillin allergy. This procedure not only de-labels patients but also educates them about their actual allergy risk, thereby allowing them to use beta-lactam antibiotics when necessary. The use of allergy assessment techniques, including PST, highlights the evolving roles between healthcare groups and shows how comprehensive allergy management can enhance therapy effectiveness. With ongoing education and outreach activities solidifying collaboration among allergists, pharmacists, and clinicians, the goal remains to ensure safe and effective care and to minimize the burdens imposed by inappropriately named drug allergies, thereby keeping pace with advances in allergy and immunology treatment (Figure 5.6).

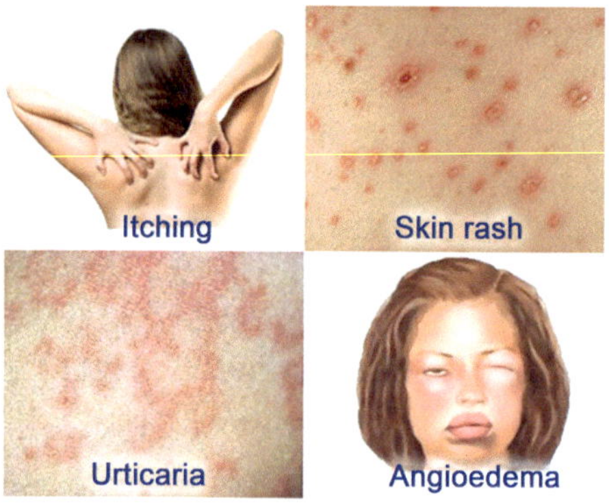

Figure 5.6. Drug allergy.

Source: https://asthmaallergyclinic.in/wp-content/uploads/2023/03/Drug_Allergy_2.png.

Test Your Knowledge

1. What is the primary difference between a food allergy and a food intolerance?
2. Which common environmental allergens are responsible for seasonal allergic rhinitis (hay fever)?
3. What are the typical symptoms of a drug allergy, and how do they differ from common drug side effects?

5.2. Mechanisms of Allergic Reactions

Learning Outcome

1. Explain the role of IgE antibodies
2. Focus on Histamine release and its effects
3. Describe anaphylaxis and severe allergic reactions

An understanding of the physiology of allergic reactions is at the heart of the specialty of Allergy and Immunology. Reactions most commonly occur as a result of an overactive immune response to typically harmless substances, or allergens. After a person encounters an allergen, the immune system mistakenly identifies it as dangerous, triggering a chain of events. The most important players in this process are immunoglobulin E (IgE)- secreting B cells, one of the five antibodies that have a specific function in causing allergic reactions. When an individual is first exposed to an allergen, sensitization occurs, leading to allergen-specific IgE production. This IgE is bound to basophils and mast cells and remains quiescent until the individual is re-exposed to the same allergen. At this point, there is prompt degranulation and release of inflammatory mediators, such as histamine. This mechanism accounts for the fundamental characteristics of allergic reactions and highlights the role of IgE, as enumerated in the results regarding its clinical relevance (Abbas et al., 2011). The phenomenon of allergic reactions has grown dramatically, particularly amid dietary and environmental changes. Notably, food allergy has driven itself to become one of the most common forms of allergic conditions, with a marked increase in incidence among young children. The mechanisms underlying the growing incidence of food allergies remain largely elusive, thereby prompting research into environmental factors, genetic components, and microbiome effects. Recent research has also highlighted the social impact of allergies, showing trends among adult populations previously paid scant attention. Evidence shows that maternal food allergies potentially affect not only their own health but also that of infants as well, and potentially influence pregnancy outcomes. An appreciation of such correlations is essential for both researchers and clinicians and points to the need for greater awareness and research in this dynamic field of Allergy and Immunology (Seita et al., 2013). Such inquiry further reveals profound implications for therapy and management strategies for allergic disease. The salient role of IgE in the initiation of allergic reactions has led to the development of specific therapies, such as monoclonal antibodies, that inhibit IgE binding to its receptors on basophils and mast cells. Additionally, novel desensitization regimens aim to resocialize the immune system to accept specific allergens with reduced sensitivity and diminished reaction intensity. These advances in the management of allergies not only enhance patients' well-being but also advance understanding of immunological tolerance and its mechanisms in the broader field of Allergy and Immunology. As scientific development continues, it becomes critical that a multidisciplinary approach be embraced that integrates clinical insight with the underlying immunology to combat the surging threat of allergies in our contemporary society (Abbas et al., 2011).

5.2.1. Role of IgE Antibodies

The role of Immunoglobulin E (IgE) antibodies is pivotal in allergy and immunology research, particularly in the context of hypersensitivity reactions. IgE is best known for its role in the immune response to allergens, triggering the release of histamine and other mediators from mast cells and basophils. It is this cascade of events that leads to the typical symptoms of an allergic reaction, including itching, swelling, and, in severe cases, anaphylaxis. The synthesis of IgE antibodies is similarly influenced by many other variables, like genetic makeup and environmental exposures. The intricate interactions among these variables have raised fascinating questions about why some individuals develop allergies while others do not. Investigation of such mechanisms remains vital to the discovery of preventive measures and therapeutics that reduce IgE-dependent hypersensitivity. Recent studies have emphasized the complexity of the IgE response, particularly compared with other immune mechanisms, such as helminth infection. Research has reported an inverse relationship between the prevalence of helminth infection and allergic sensitization and suggested that responses to such parasites could modulate IgE production. It has been postulated that helminth antigens can promote regulatory immune responses that suppress IgE-mediated mechanisms typical of allergy. This correlation raises intriguing mechanistic and evolutionary hypotheses about immune adaptation in humans. The ongoing controversy over the clinical significance of such findings underscores the subtle balance between allergic disease development and immune protection. It necessitates further research to fully elucidate the functions of IgE under these conditions, including its relative dynamics with distinct immune responses (Mutapi et al., 2012). Furthermore, increased child allergies have prompted investigation into IgE antibodies, with particular emphasis on identifying the specific risk factors involved in their production among vulnerable children. Genetic predisposition, environmental sensitization, and even nutritional components have all played a part in the increased allergy risk observed in children. Investigations that have examined these risk factors indicate that exposures in early life can have a significant impact on immune function, including the propensity to produce IgE antibodies. By uncovering the mechanisms of hypersensitivity reactions, researchers aim to identify potential interventions that would limit allergic responses in pediatric patients. Detailed knowledge of the risk factors in pediatric hypersensitivity not only enhances our understanding of IgE antibodies but also gives clinician strategies to combat the alarming rise in allergic diseases among children (Burns et al., 2019) (Figure 5.7).

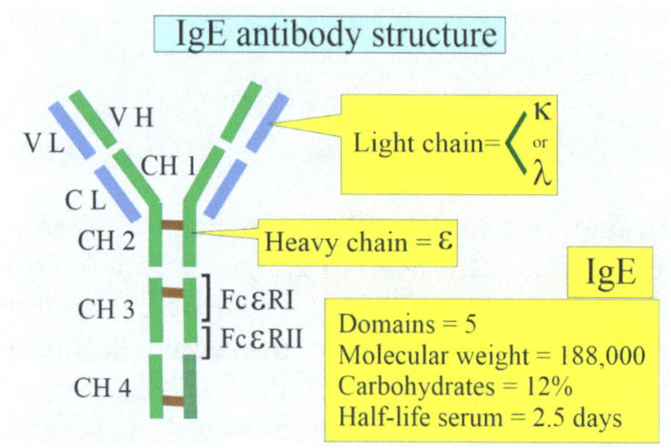

Figure 5.7. The role of immunoglobulin E (IgE) antibodies.

Source: https://labpedia.net/wp-content/uploads/2020/01/IgE-2.jpg.

5.2.2. Histamine Release and Its Effects

Histamine release is a fundamental component of the immune response and triggers allergic reactions. On entry into the body, allergens activate specific IgE antibodies on mast cells and basophils, triggering degranulation. It leads to the release of various mediators, including histamine. Histamine acts on H1 receptors to produce vasodilation, increased vascular permeability, and smooth muscle contraction, all of which together explain the classic features of allergy, such as congestion, swelling, and itching. The complexity of this response makes the relationship between the immune system and the environment clear, indicating room for further research into the mechanisms underlying this relationship to develop practical interventions for patients with hypersensitivity reactions (Burns et al., 2019). Sensitivity to histamine is essential for controlling the environment of allergic disease, particularly as levels of childhood allergy continue to rise. Current studies have focused on identifying risk factors associated with the development of allergy in children, labeling these incidences as both genetically and environmentally related. Pediatric hypersensitivities are linked with significant health consequences, and it is essential to explore mechanisms of histamine release and biological consequences. The relationship between environmental sensitization and allergic reaction underscores the need for multi-pronged strategies to anticipate and potentially avoid the increasing prevalence of such conditions among children (Seita et al., 2013). Also, the role of histamine extends beyond acute allergic responses; it is also involved in chronic diseases such as asthma and atopic dermatitis. These conditions demonstrate how sustained histamine release and receptor stimulation can lead to more severe pathological consequences, triggering a chronic inflammatory response and contributing to tissue remodeling. The convergence of histamine activity and chronic inflammatory diseases necessitates greater familiarity with therapeutic approaches targeting histamine pathways to alleviate symptoms and improve patient quality of life. Studies on the pharmacologic modulation of histamine release and its receptors hold promise for identifying new therapies for allergic and immunologic disorders (Burns et al., 2019).

5.2.3. Anaphylaxis and Severe Allergic Reactions

Anaphylaxis is one of the most severe allergic reactions, with an acute course and the possibility of death if left untreated. Anaphylaxis can be caused by a variety of allergens, including food, drugs, insect bites, and latex. The body's immune system overreacts to the offending agents, leading to the release of mediators such as histamines, which cause excessive vasodilation, bronchoconstriction, and increased blood vessel permeability. As this sequence of events continues, symptoms may be life-threatening in the form of breathlessness, hypotension, and loss of consciousness. Although anaphylaxis is recognized in different age ranges, its prevalence is stated to be rising, particularly with the rise in food allergy among children, something which underscores the necessity for continued research and public awareness (Seita et al., 2013). Treatment of anaphylaxis is outlined according to standard guidelines, with emphasis on early intervention. Intramuscular injection of adrenaline constitutes the backbone of the treatment, followed by adjunct therapies, such as antihistamines and corticosteroids, to alleviate symptoms and downregulate inflammation. Despite global recommendations, there is a significant gap between guidelines and their practical application in clinical practice. A German-Austrian-Swiss survey examining anaphylaxis treatment in allergy consultation clinics discovered complete underreporting of adrenaline injection and adjunctive treatments with acute attacks. Specifically, fewer than a fifth of cases received intramuscular adrenaline, while a notable proportion received inadequate advice on allergen avoidance or on self-administration of epinephrine injectors (Gough et al., 2012). These differences highlight the need for more training and education on managing anaphylaxis among healthcare providers. Additionally, knowledge of anaphylaxis epidemiology is necessary to address the issue on a broader scale. It has been proven that food allergy is one of the leading causes of anaphylaxis, particularly in children and young adults. However, as the number of cases of these allergies increases, there is surprisingly little epidemiological data available concerning adult populations experiencing anaphylaxis. By incorporating diverse demographic characteristics and conducting full-scale data collection, it is possible to fully inform the extent of food allergies' contribution to public health. Furthermore, an ongoing study of the overlap between maternal food allergies and adverse perinatal outcomes is potentially a valuable insight that can be gleaned. As our understanding of these complex interactions becomes more sophisticated, prevention can be individualized, and there is promise for improved management and reduced frequency of severe allergic reactions in diverse populations (Seita et al., 2013) (Figure 5.8).

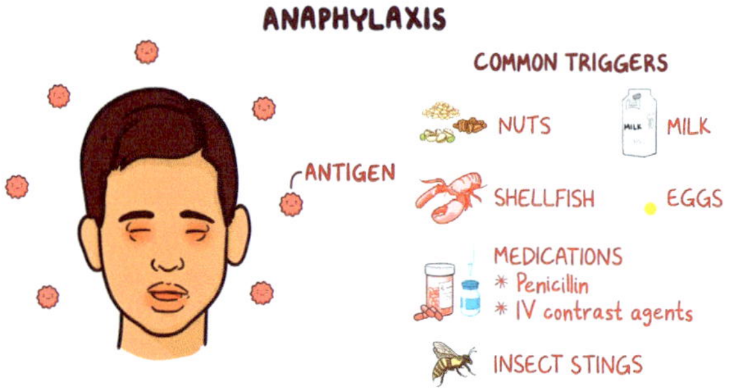

Figure 5.8. Anaphylaxis represents one of the most severe forms of allergic reactions.

Source: https://www.osmosis.org/_next/image?url=https%3A%2F%2Fd16qt3wv6xm098.cloudfront.net%2F8f5BveRWShieZwwPrO8LAhKnSvy0TNy5%2F_.jpg&w=3840&q=75.

Test Your Knowledge

1. What role do IgE antibodies play in allergic reactions, and how are they involved in the immune system's response to allergens?
2. Which cells release histamine during an allergic reaction, and what are the typical effects of histamine on the body?

5.3. Diagnosis of Allergies

Learning Outcome

1. Discuss skin prick tests
2. Explain blood tests for allergens
3. Explain the role of patient history and symptom assessment in the realm of allergy and immunology

The diagnosis of allergies is a critical juncture of clinical experience and patient history in allergy and immunology. Diagnosis must be established by careful evaluation of symptoms and patient history, and often by a series of tests. The assessment starts with clinicians gathering thorough information on patients' medical history, previous allergic reactions, and atopic family history. This core knowledge helps identify probable allergens and individualize the diagnosis process. Based on the presentation, practitioners may use skin prick tests, IgE blood tests, or oral food challenges to diagnose. Each of them has strengths and limitations, involving careful consideration of choice in individual patient cases. Skin prick testing has long been a staple in the identification of allergies because it delivers rapid results and diagnostic outcomes. Skin prick tests, when properly administered, can identify sensitivities to a wide range of allergens, such as pollen, pet hair, and foods. The method is to inject a minimal dose of an allergen into the skin and observe localized reactions showing sensitivity. Even though this process is safe and effective in general, variables such as drug use or cutaneous illness can influence outcomes and produce false positives or negatives. Therefore, to ensure the validity of the allergy diagnosis, practitioners must interpret findings in conjunction with clinical histories and physical examinations. Complete diagnostic planning ultimately facilitates more precise implementation of treatment protocols. Beyond usual practice, advances in allergy diagnosis are also contributing to more subtle, patient-oriented strategies. Techniques like molecular allergology enable a more detailed examination of specific proteins in allergic reactions, thereby enabling more precise diagnostic measures. By identifying the particular molecules that provoke an immune response, doctors can provide patients with more specific guidance on minimizing exposure and managing symptoms more effectively. Additionally, local initiatives to advance standardized measurement activities, as mentioned in relation to monitoring method development, indicate a growing emphasis on quality assurance in allergy diagnosis and treatment. Activities that enhance provider productivity and encourage patients to make informed healthcare decisions are well-suited to contemporary trends in patient-oriented medical homes for allergy and immunology (N/A, 2005; Amaducci et al., 2018).

5.3.1. Skin Prick Tests

Skin prick test (SPT) is a mainstay diagnostic test in allergy and immunology, employed primarily to identify specific allergens responsible for hypersensitivity in patients. SPT is performed by applying tiny amounts of suspected allergens to the skin, usually the forearm or the back. After exposure to the allergen, if the patient is sensitive to the substance, the body's immune system will respond, leading to localized inflammation characterized by redness and swelling. Measurement of the wheal developed after approximately 15–20 minutes yields a clear reading of sensitivity to the allergen. Moreover, skin prick tests are simple to perform, relatively cheap, and capable of yielding prompt results, enabling physicians to make effective decisions regarding further management strategies for allergic disease. A significant advantage of skin prick tests is their versatility, as they can be used against a broad spectrum of allergens, e.g., pollen, cat and dog hair, dust mites, and fungi.

This multidisciplinary application allows clinicians to tailor treatment strategies more effectively to the specific allergens to which a patient is sensitized. SPTs can be used to diagnose conditions such as allergic rhinitis, asthma, and atopic dermatitis, providing greater insight into the underlying immunological processes. Notably, the correlation between allergen characteristics and patient response has been explored in some detail. For instance, plant allergens have been of interest because their protein structures are challenging, and features such as N-glycosylation influence allergenicity (Blanca et al., 2013). In practice, skin prick tests have been described to have pragmatic effects on different populations, including hard-to-reach populations. A pilot cross-sectional study in the Sololá district of Guatemala illustrates this, providing evidence on the prevalence and trends of allergic disease in an indigenous population. The results for the subsample that underwent SPTs were for low rates of common allergen positivity and suggested that allergic symptoms might be relatively rare in this population (Makvandi-Nejad et al., 2023). By demonstrating the feasibility of such testing across various environments, this study underscores the need to adapt allergy testing methods to enhance understanding and control of allergic diseases across different populations. More insight gained by research like this can ultimately guide public health interventions towards better allergy control and education in underserved communities (Figure 5.9).

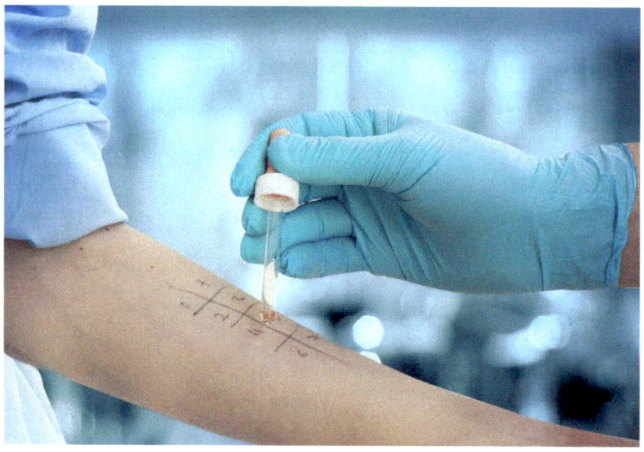

Figure 5.9. Skin prick test.

Source: https://foodallergiesatlanta.com/wp-content/uploads/2022/08/food-allergy-testing.jpeg.

5.3.2. Blood Tests for Allergens

Blood tests are now an integral part of diagnosing allergic disease, offering a valuable adjunct to traditional skin prick testing. This test measures specific IgE antibodies in the blood, produced after exposure to an allergen. In individuals for whom skin testing is unacceptable, such as those with extensive skin disease or those on certain antihistamines, blood testing is an acceptable alternative. In addition, blood testing can provide information on multiple allergens simultaneously, aiding clinicians in assessing patterns of sensitization. Current studies are investigating the correlation between IgE levels and clinical symptoms, driven by increasing knowledge about allergies, which may improve the precision of allergy diagnoses and treatment in allergy and immunology (Seita et al., 2013). The use of blood tests also includes evaluating food allergies, which have increased, particularly among children. Existing studies indicate that maternal food allergies can also have an impact on infant health conditions, suggesting a complex relationship between genetic and environmental factors (Seita et al., 2013). Used to diagnose food allergies, blood tests can help trigger the appropriate dietary changes to reduce exposure. Although blood tests are not definitive, they reduce uncertainty significantly and help patients manage diet and lifestyle for food sensitivities. Moreover, the relationship between established food allergies and actual allergic reactions remains a topic of ongoing research, underscoring the need for further investigation in the field. Although they are helpful, blood tests for allergens are not without their own problems. Interpreting IgE levels can lead to false positives or false negatives, so the accuracy of proper diagnosis is questionable. Furthermore, the cost of such tests could be prohibitive for certain patients. Physicians must interpret blood test results in the context of the patient's clinical history and symptomatology to avoid misdiagnosis. The need for precise diagnostic tools in allergy and immunology has led to ongoing refinement of testing techniques, and the future may see more definitive and accurate assays. For obtaining an overall view of allergy processes, such tests are an essential part of better patient care and management regimens as the technology develops (Figure 5.10).

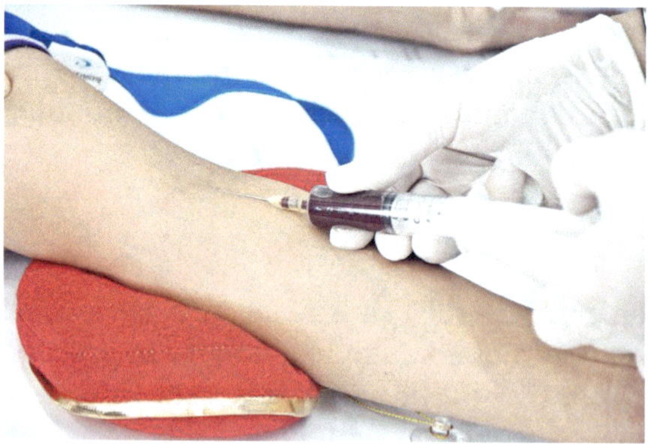

Figure 5.10. Blood tests for allergies.

Source: https://www.allergiesandhealth.com/wp-content/uploads/allergy-blood-testing.jpg.

5.3.3. Patient History and Symptom Assessment

In immunology and allergy, clear and thorough patient history and symptom assessment are foundational aspects to effective diagnosis and care. The patient-practitioner interaction can illuminate the picture of the allergic episode, for example, what triggers it, how frequently it happens, and its severity. An effectively organized patient history should encompass not just information about previous allergic episodes but also any familial predisposition towards allergies or autoimmune diseases. In addition, the history of symptom development—seasonal or precipitated by exposure to specific foods or environments—is helpful. The integration of these data facilitates more tailored interventions in management approaches, including the application of immunotherapy, which has been effective in reducing symptoms of refractory severe allergic rhinitis, as per the literature (Barton et al., 2013). Moreover, symptom assessment is crucial in ascertaining the severity and complicating features of allergies. Symptoms such as respiratory impairment, skin manifestations, or gastrointestinal upset need to be evaluated by medical practitioners with diligence to conceptualize appropriate interventions. For instance, anaphylaxis, an imminent allergic reaction, necessitates urgent intervention and aggressive initial treatment. Recommendations from the World Allergy Organization emphasize the importance of early clinical diagnosis and intervention, with a focus on patient risk factors and a systematic emergency protocol. It is this tactful understanding that enables experts to determine which symptoms are likely indicators of severe allergic reactions and to ensure adequate preventive measures against recurrent episodes, thereby maintaining patient safety and well-being. Finally, thorough patient education becomes a crucial aspect of effective allergy control, heavily reliant on patient history and symptom assessment. More awareness of personal triggers, symptom identification, and steps needed to allow for immediate intervention can help patients act independently. Furthermore, it provides channels for communicating immunomodulation strategies, such as allergy immunotherapy, aimed at maximizing long-term outcomes by modulating allergic responses to specific allergens. Including patients as active partners in their care not only fosters a sense of self-efficacy but also optimizes the effectiveness of treatment regimens based on their individual histories and symptomologies. By emphasizing the integration of exhaustive evaluations with patient education, the healthcare provider can greatly improve the well-being of individuals with allergic disorders.

Test Your Knowledge

1. How does a skin prick test work, and what does a positive result indicate?
2. What information can a blood test provide, and how does it compare to skin testing?
3. Why is a detailed patient history important in diagnosing allergies, even before performing any tests?

5.4. Treatment Options for Allergies

Learning Outcome

1. Understand the role of antihistamines and decongestants for allergies
2. Discuss the concept of Immunotherapy and allergy shots
3. Focus on lifestyle modifications and avoidance strategies

The treatment of allergy is multifactorial, as the presentation and extent of the allergic reaction also differ. Avoidance of recognized allergens is ideal in the initial place; however, this cannot always be offered in everyday life. Relief from symptoms can then be sought with over-the-counter antihistamines, which act quickly on minor allergic processes such as hay fever and contact dermatitis. When cases are more severe, such as with anaphylaxis, urgent medical care is the priority. Current recommendations include intramuscular adrenaline in the case of severe reactions, supplemented by other antihistamines and corticosteroids to alleviate symptoms upon exposure. Unfortunately, evidence indicates a significant disparity between these recommendations and their practice, requiring improved education and training for healthcare professionals to ensure optimal patient outcomes (Gough et al., 2012). For individuals with persistent allergic disease, immunotherapy provides an extended-duration treatment. It is achieved through gradual desensitization of the immune system to the offending allergen and can significantly reduce the severity of allergic reactions.

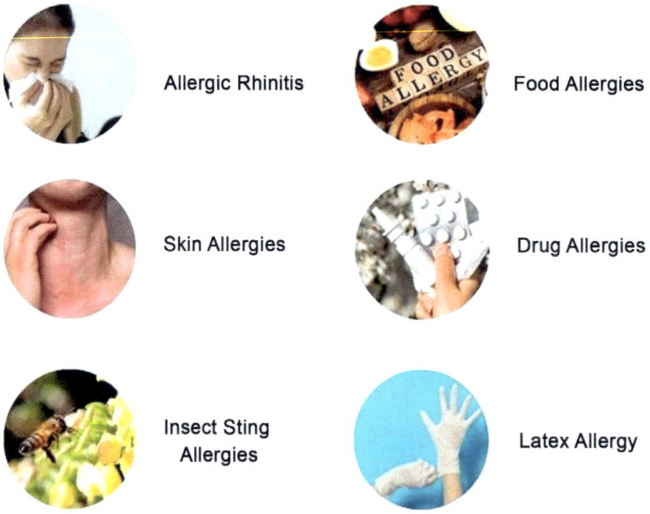

Figure 5.11. The treatment options for allergies are diverse.

Source: https://max-website20-images.s3.ap-south-1.amazonaws.com/Types_of_Allergies_8d3af3219e.jpg.

The most traditional approach is subcutaneous immunotherapy (SCIT), which requires regular injections over a prolonged duration. As an alternative, sublingual immunotherapy (SLIT) has gained popularity due to its ease of administration and acceptable safety profile. Evidence supports greater emphasis on home treatment of acute attacks, particularly in patients with hereditary angioedema due to C1 inhibitor deficiency, highlighting the importance of access to emergency therapeutic modalities and patient education (Ashworth et al., 2015). This changing treatment profile allows for more individualized management strategies to accommodate diverse patient needs. Furthermore, ongoing developments continuously broaden the options in the care of allergies. Individual immune pathway-targeted biologic therapies have shown promise for diseases such as chronic rhinosinusitis with nasal polyps and refractory asthma and have helped patients who have not responded to conventional pharmacotherapy.

These new therapies generally require careful patient selection and follow-up as they represent a radical paradigm shift in the treatment of allergies. The more profound our understanding of the immune system, the greater the chance of new treatments emerging, which will improve the quality of life and clinical outcomes for millions of people with allergies. For this, ongoing research and collaborative efforts among healthcare providers, patients, and researchers will be imperative to advancing care and aligning treatment practices with the latest evidence (Figure 5.11).

5.4.1. Antihistamines and Decongestants

Antihistamines and decongestants play a crucial role in the management of allergic rhinitis and other allergies. Antihistamines inhibit the action of histamine receptors, thereby blocking allergic reactions such as sneezing, itching, and nasal congestion. Antihistamines are classified into first-generation and second-generation antihistamines. While in certain situations effective, the first-generation antihistamines cause sedation due to their ability to cross the blood-brain barrier. Conversely, second-generation antihistamines induce less somnolence and are a better choice for patients who need sustained alertness all day long. As an adjunct to other treatments such as intranasal corticosteroids, the effectiveness of antihistamines can be significantly boosted, thereby improving patient outcomes in the management of allergic reactions and improving quality of life (Al-Samarrae et al., 2011). Decongestants, on the other hand, relieve symptoms by narrowing blood vessels in the nasal passages, reducing swelling and congestion. They are generally used in allergic and non-allergic rhinitis. Decongestants can either be ingested or applied topically, and the latter acts faster. Chronic use of topical decongestants leads to rebound congestion, a condition known as rhinitis medicamentosa. This impact demands caution and careful use of decongestants, as long-term use can lead to persistent nasal obstruction and other issues. They include sinusitis and nasal polyp formation (Kalinowska et al., 2025). As such, medical professionals demand an integrated treatment strategy for decongestants that results in effective symptom relief and reduces the risk of continued use. While drugs such as antihistamines and decongestants are effective, the administration of these medications as a component of an overall management plan for allergic rhinitis is most critical. This could include allergen avoidance strategies and other treatment programs, such as intranasal corticosteroids, which are the cornerstone of treatment for anti-inflammatory management. The combination of these strategies allows simultaneous targeting of multiple allergic inflammatory mechanisms and improved symptom control. Moreover, personalized treatment protocols, possibly involving immunotherapy for permanent relief, are required to address each patient's unique allergic profile. With improvements in allergy and immunology research, ongoing research aims to optimize these pharmacological treatments and their applications, resulting in better patient outcomes and reduced burden of allergy-related diseases (Al-Samarrae et al., 2011).

5.4.2. Immunotherapy and Allergy Shots

Immunotherapy has emerged as an essential treatment modality for a variety of allergies, particularly through allergy shots and oral immunotherapy (OIT). Allergy shots, also called subcutaneous immunotherapy, involve gradually increasing doses of allergens to induce tolerance in the immune system. It has been well researched and proven effective in alleviating the symptoms of seasonal and perennial allergies. By immunizing the immune system against overreacting to specific allergens, patients typically experience a significant reduction in allergy symptoms. The widespread availability of this treatment has made it an orthodoxy in allergy treatment, ensuring long-term relief for many who live with chronic allergic disorders. Over the past decade or so, developments in OIT have introduced a new method in the field of immunotherapy, most notably in the treatment of food allergy. As underscored by recent studies, OIT allows patients to gradually consume allergenic foods under a physician's guidance to develop a desensitized immune response. The treatment method is particularly hopeful for patients with severe food allergies, e.g., peanuts, which pose serious threats, such as anaphylaxis, on exposure (Rauscher et al., 2015). While OIT is not a definitive treatment for food allergy, its use is a giant step in the direction of treating allergies that takes away the chronic anxiety and quality of life issues faced by patients and their families. Research on OIT has led to the establishment of specialized programs at private and academic centers, enhancing appreciation of this treatment's efficacy and safety. With further developments in allergology, the integration of immunotherapy in the form of allergy shots and OIT involves a stringent balancing of efficacy and safety. Ongoing research is necessary to further refine these therapies, particularly as their use increases. For instance, further research is needed better to understand subject response variability to therapy and desensitization risk (Olson et al., 2019). As more clinical trials come in, focus will shift to refining these therapies so they can be used more widely and effectively by more patients. Ideally, the ultimate goal would be to enhance the quality of life for individuals who are afflicted with allergies, reducing the disability caused by such diseases and the pervasive shadow of allergy-related reactions (Figure 5.12).

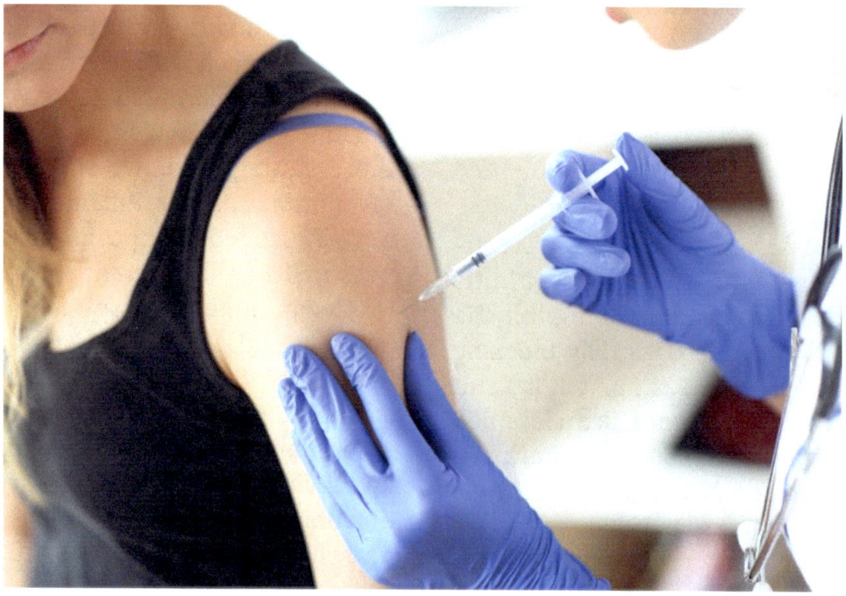

Figure 5.12. Immunotherapy has emerged as a pivotal treatment strategy for managing various allergies.

Source: https://cdn-prod.medicalnewstoday.com/content/images/articles/320/320402/allergy-shot-injection-being-given-to-young-woman.jpg.

5.4.3. Lifestyle Modifications and Avoidance Strategies

In the practice of allergy and immunology, lifestyle modification and avoidance strategies are critical in the management of allergic diseases. Allergy sufferers should adopt strategic approaches to avoid allergens. The methods include meticulous reading of food labels to identify potential culprits, as even tiny remnants may trigger severe reactions. In addition, residents can reduce dust mites and mold by using air purifiers, controlling humidity, and following regular cleaning regimens. All these adjustments provide access to a healthy environment and reduce the risk of allergen exposure, emphasizing preparatory action for one's own health. Equally important is the role of social considerations in lifestyle modifications, as allergic reactions can have drastic effects on daily activities and social engagements. People suffering from food allergies, for instance, are hindered from dining out or joining communal meals. To effectively manage such situations, people need to make their allergies public knowledge among relatives and friends to ensure a supportive base familiar with their dietary limitations. Also, the use of tools such as allergy action plans can assist patients and care providers in responding effectively to allergic episodes, further supporting awareness and preparedness in social settings. With alterations in social strategies, these enhance the quality of life and safety for those with allergies. The rising prevalence of allergic disorders calls for a holistic approach in managing lifestyle, particularly among the elderly. With age, the risk of developing or worsening allergies increases, necessitating lifestyle modifications to support physiological changes and heightened sensitivity. Encouraging regular physical activity is presented as an imperative not only for general well-being but also for combating respiratory allergies such as asthma. In addition, the introduction of allergen immunotherapy (AIT) into treatment can yield long-term benefits for older individuals, significantly improving their quality of life and reducing the impact of allergic disease. These lifestyle changes cultivate a holistic approach towards fighting allergies and highlight the need to gain a better understanding of the impact of aging on immune responses and allergy reactions (Bonini et al., 2017; Olson et al., 2019).

Test Your Knowledge

1. How do antihistamines work to relieve allergy symptoms?
2. What is the role of decongestants in allergy treatment, and why should they be used with caution over long periods?
3. How does allergy immunotherapy help reduce sensitivity to allergens over time?

5.5. The Role of the Immune System

Learning Outcome

1. Differentiate between innate and adaptive immunity
2. Discuss the immune response to allergens
3. Understand tolerance and sensitization

The immune system is responsible for maintaining the body in homeostasis and defending it against pathogenic attack. It is a highly organized collection of tissues, cells, and organs that collaborate to identify and eliminate foreign invaders such as bacteria, viruses, and allergens. At the core of the defense mechanism are two significant responses: the innate and adaptive immune responses. The natural immune response constitutes the initial line of defense, using barriers such as skin and mucous membranes, as well as cell components like macrophages and neutrophils. The adaptive immune system, however, is characterized by its ability to remember specific pathogens through immunological memory, facilitated by T and B lymphocytes. This difference is essential, particularly about allergies, where the immune system falsely recognizes harmless substances as dangerous and deploys inappropriately exaggerated reactions that call for further research and information. The immune system's role in allergic responses defines the precise balance it must maintain. Immunoglobulin E (IgE) is the primary antibody responsible for allergies, regulating them to a large extent. This immune malfunction leads to the stimulation of basophils and mast cells, which, in turn, release inflammatory mediators such as histamine, triggering the symptoms of allergic reactions. Recent advancements in allergy studies have strongly emphasized the need for appropriate risk assessments before introducing new food proteins to the market. In particular, an adverse outcome pathway (AOP) approach has been proposed to elucidate the mechanistic pathways underlying IgE-mediated food allergies. This approach provides a platform for integrating in vitro strategies and for identifying gaps that can hamper the efficient testing of the sensitizing potential of different food proteins, thereby enhancing understanding of immune system interactions with allergens (Benedé et al., 2019). In addition, the immune system is affected by numerous external agents, such as environmental exposures and infections. Epidemiology reveals that people who live in low-infection environments can develop hyperreactive immune responses that might become the cause of allergies and autoimmune diseases. Immune modulation by parasitic infections is an interesting example; helminths, especially, can suppress inflammatory responses and are therefore under investigation for therapeutic use in the treatment of inflammatory diseases. This exchange calls into question the timing and quality of immune conditioning—how early exposures shape immunity versus the influence of later exposures. As greater understanding of the regulatory mechanisms involved is gained, the twofold role of the immune system as a protective mechanism and a potential source of dysregulation becomes increasingly apparent, emphasizing its central role in allergy and immunology (Maizels et al., 2014).

5.5.1. Innate versus Adaptive Immunity

Innate immunity is the body's immediate, non-specific response to pathogens and comprises physical barriers as well as immune responses. It contains several elements, such as epithelial cells, phagocytic cells, and natural killer (NK) cells, that react instantaneously to intruders. Innate immunity is activated within hours of pathogen exposure, and its elements cannot enhance or recall their contact with pathogens. Significantly, innate immune responses can activate adaptive immunity, providing a unifying link between the two. In allergic reactions, innate immune cells such as type II innate lymphoid cells (ILC2) also play a role, as they produce Th2 cytokines that drive allergic inflammation, further complicating the immune response paradigm. It is crucial to understand the role of innate immunity for the development of therapeutic approaches toward allergy diseases (Doherty et al., 2013). Adaptive immunity, however, operates with a delay, taking days to become maximally effective. Such a system is characterized by its antigen-specific response and ability to remember previously encountered pathogens, thanks to specialized cells such as T and B lymphocytes. Adaptive immunity can be further classified into cellular and humoral responses. In contrast, the latter involves the secretion of antibodies by B cells; the former includes the activation of T cells, which can kill infected host cells directly or complement other immune cells. This memory and specificity are the pillars of vaccine efficacy and are employed to develop a long-term immunity against recurring infections. However, when adaptive immune function is dysregulated, it can contribute to pathological responses, such as allergy, in which sensitized B cells produce IgE antibodies inappropriately. The interaction between innate and adaptive mechanisms illustrates the complexity of the immune response and its importance in allergic disease. The intricate interaction between innate and adaptive immunity is best observed in the context of the hygiene hypothesis, where diminished microbial exposure may alter immune responses and predispose to allergic disease. With lifestyle changes in the contemporary world minimizing exposure to diverse microbial environments, the stakes for the maturation of the immune system are high. It is said that low levels of exposure to microbes can limit the growth of regulatory immune cells, which, in turn, can enhance hypersensitivity and allergy formation. This continues even in later life after early childhood, affecting the establishment of the immune system even in fetal life, as maternal microbial interactions decide the developing fetus's immune environment. These observations point to the multifactorial nature of allergic disease, emphasizing the role of early microbial exposure in the context of differential immune trajectories (Apostol et al., 2020) (Figure 5.13).

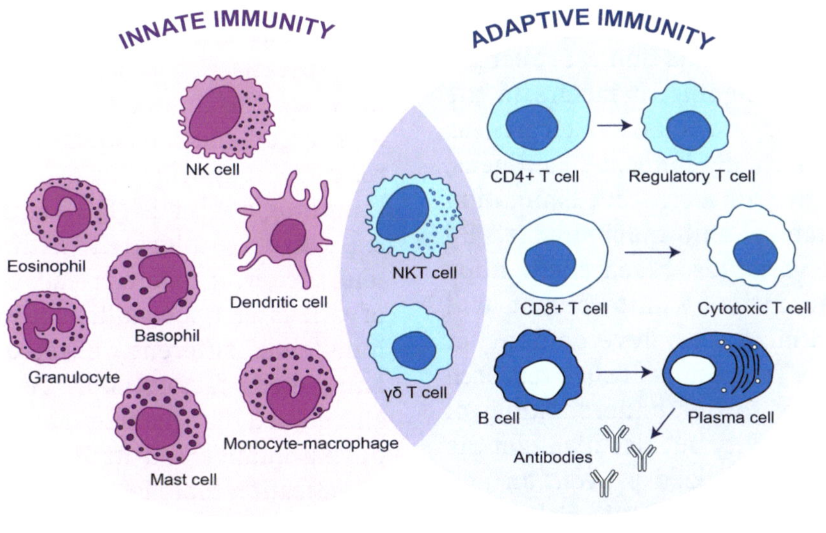

Figure 5.13. Innate immunity versus adaptive immunity.

Source: https://www.researchgate.net/publication/383092819/figure/fig1/AS:11431281271426097@1723615474820/Innate-immunity-vs-adaptive-immunity-The-innate-immunity-is-the-first-line-of-defense.tif.

5.5.2. Immune Response to Allergens

The immune response to allergens is a complex dynamic among the various components of the immune system, dominated by hypersensitivity reactions mediated by Immunoglobulin E (IgE). Upon first contact with an allergen, the immune system misperceives it as harmful, and T and B cells specific for the allergen are activated. This response results in the production of IgE antibodies that sensitize basophils and mast cells. In repeated exposures to the same allergen, these sensitized cells release histamines and other mediators, causing the characteristic symptoms of allergic reactions, including sneezing, itching, and in certain instances, anaphylaxis. Elucidating this initial process of sensitization is critical to the development of therapeutic interventions, as it serves as the foundation for an integrated approach to allergy management and for addressing both clinical and therapeutic interventions in immunology. Scientists have recently become interested in the mechanisms of immune-mediated hypersensitivity reactions, particularly in children. Increasing evidence now suggests that genetic predispositions, environmental influences, and timing of allergen introduction are the significant factors in the development of allergy. Pediatric allergies, as overreactions to normally innocuous antigens, create an imperative for a critical examination of causative factors and mechanisms. By analyzing these variables, researchers hope to identify intervention windows that will prevent or minimize the development of allergy in children. The results of such research not only contribute to our understanding of pediatric hypersensitivity but also highlight the importance of individualized prevention and potential new treatments for this risk group (Burns et al., 2019). Besides environmental and genetic factors, the innate immune system also contributes to the determination of the allergenic response. Recent advances in applying the adverse outcome pathway (AOP) concept provide a systematic approach to understanding the cellular and molecular processes underlying IgE-mediated food allergy. The idea enables discussion of existing in vitro strategies for assessing the sensitizing potency of various food proteins and other allergens. Evaluation of the natural immune response is more likely to yield accessible assays than assessment of the adaptive immune response, owing to the low number of allergen-specific T and B cells. The addition of new ex vivo culture methods can help elucidate mechanisms underlying sensitization, thereby reducing reliance on animal testing and enabling the identification of targeted interventions against allergies (Benedé et al., 2019).

5.5.3. Tolerance and Sensitization

Tolerance and sensitization mechanisms underlie the immune dynamics of allergy in immunology. Tolerance is the capacity of the immune system to recognize and accommodate the presence of specific allergens without reacting with an adverse response. This is crucial in preventing inappropriate reactions to harmless environmental antigens while maintaining homeostasis. Conversely, sensitization is a state in which the immune system gets exposed to an allergen and subsequently has an overactive response, typically through the production of Immunoglobulin E (IgE) antibodies. Chronic exposure to allergens without appropriate tolerance, over time, can lead to the development of various allergic conditions, each of which affects individuals differently based on environmental and genetic factors. More recent research has also guided the schedule of allergen presentation during infancy and its impact on tolerance or sensitization establishment. A systematic review found that delaying the introduction of solid foods containing allergens did not significantly reduce the risk of allergic disease; instead, it was associated with a higher risk of food allergy among high- and low-risk infants (Haglund et al., 2016). This finding underscores the importance of early exposure to food as a trigger to induce immune tolerance. Clinicians are currently advised to suggest introducing foods with common allergens at four to six months of age, which will induce immune tolerance rather than promote sensitization. By understanding these relationships, health professionals can develop better strategies to prevent allergies at the early stages of development. Food allergy and sensitization mechanisms are not specific to children; the trend appears alarming among adults, too, according to the evidence. A study of pregnant women has confirmed that maternal food allergies do affect neonatal health outcomes. Still, a high correlation between maternal allergies and effects on infant health was not established (Seita et al., 2013). This underscores the nuances of immune responses and etiologic agents in the development of allergen responses throughout life. With environmental exposures and genetic susceptibilities caught up in one another, the latest research has sought to decipher the intricate mechanisms of tolerance and sensitization. Elucidating these concepts is paramount for formulating targeted interventions and guidelines to reduce the immunoburden of allergic diseases in populations (Figure 5.14).

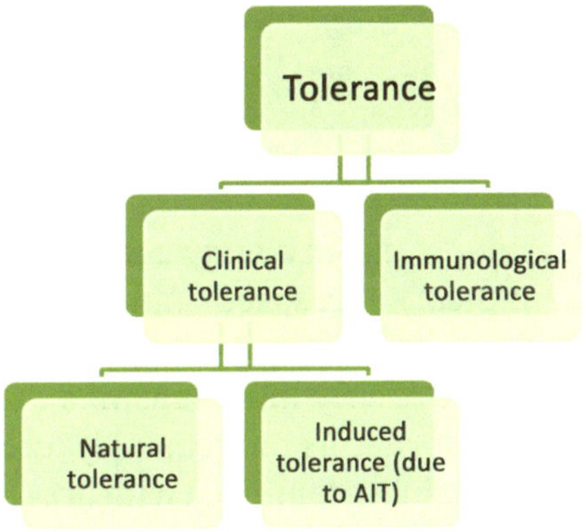

Figure 5.14. The concepts of tolerance and sensitization.

Source: https://clinmedjournals.org/articles/ijam/ijam-2-013-001.gif.

Test Your Knowledge

1. What is the primary difference between the innate and adaptive immune systems?
2. Define immunological tolerance and explain how its failure can lead to allergic reactions.

5.6. Current Research in Allergy and Immunology

Learning Outcome

1. Understand the advances in allergy treatments
2. Discuss genetic factors in allergies
3. The impact of climate change on allergy prevalence

Recent developments in allergy and immunology research indicate increased understanding of the genetic and environmental determinants of asthma, particularly in nations like Pakistan, where the disorder is increasingly common. Genetic susceptibility combined with urban living, environmental pollution, and so on influences nearly 20% of children in the population. Traditionally, environmental influences were considered significant, but recent research emphasizes the role of numerous genes in disease manifestation. Over 100 genes related to asthma have been identified globally, but, unfortunately, studies focusing on Pakistan are not as extensive. Scientists have begun exploring the genetic influence on asthma, recognizing that environmental exposure and genetics interact to significantly impact disease outcomes in local communities, underscoring the need for targeted research to address the unique genetic and demographic nuances of asthma prevention and care planning (Akram et al., 2018). Simultaneously, the identification of therapeutic molecules from natural products is an exciting area of research in allergy and immunology. Plant compounds, such as those found in medicinal plants, have been used in traditional medicine for centuries, and recent scientific studies are now validating their efficacy. Carnosol, a diterpene of *Rosmarinus officinalis*, has recently emerged as of interest due to its therapeutic potential in the management of autoimmune illnesses such as multiple sclerosis. Research indicates that carnosol not only reduces symptoms in animal models of autoimmune encephalomyelitis but also modulates disease-causing inflammatory mechanisms by inhibiting key disease-promoting pathways. By inhibiting Th17 cell differentiation and inflammatory infiltration, carnosol is twice as effective against autoimmune responses. These findings highlight the need to integrate traditional medicinal knowledge with contemporary research methods to develop novel therapeutic modalities in allergy and immunology (Zhang et al., 2018). Overall, the integration of genetics, environment, and nature-derived therapeutic agents represents the frontier of allergy and immunology research. With increasing understanding of the complex interactions underlying allergic disease, there is an urgent need for new approaches that incorporate both genetic studies and natural pharmacological developments. Increased communication among scientists, doctors, and traditional healers can potentially offer combined insights to enhance the prevention, diagnosis, and therapy of allergic diseases. From an integrated point of view, experts can disentangle the intricacies of immunologic and allergic illnesses, paving the way for personalized treatments that reflect patients' unique genetic fingerprints, environmental exposure, and health behaviors, towards a more customized approach to these omnipresent health conditions among heterogeneous populations (Akram et al., 2018; Zhang et al., 2018).

5.6.1. Advances in Allergy Treatments

The discoveries over the past few years in allergy treatments have revolutionized the management of allergic disorders, enhancing patients' quality of life. Among the promising fields of therapeutic research is the use of biologic drugs, including monoclonal antibodies that target immunoglobulin E (IgE) and other mediators of allergic inflammation. These biologics, such as omalizumab, have been truly impressive in reducing the frequency and severity of allergic attacks, particularly in individuals with allergen-evoked mild to severe asthma. This molecular pathway enables more targeted therapeutic strategies, with treatments tailored to individual patient profiles, thereby optimizing treatment concordance and efficacy. Also, technological improvements in sublingual immunotherapy (SLIT) have expanded the scope of allergy treatments, particularly environmental allergens such as pollen and dust mites. SLIT is more convenient and has a favorable safety profile compared to traditional subcutaneous immunotherapy, and thus, it is now accessible to a larger patient population. Recent findings have also demonstrated that SLIT is effective in desensitizing individuals to specific allergens, with long-term tolerance even after treatment discontinuation (Figure 5.15).

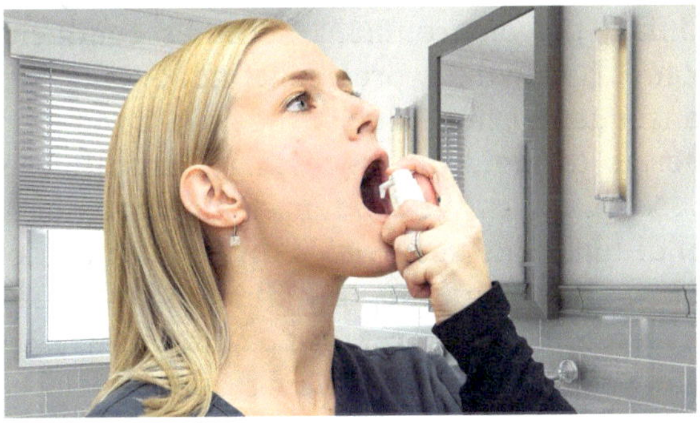

Figure 5.15. Sublingual immunotherapy (SLIT)–allergy relief without injections.

Source: https://www.phillymag.com/wp-content/uploads/sites/3/2016/10/AASpost4.jpg.

By inducing controlled allergen exposure, SLIT not only alleviates symptoms but also acts on the underlying pathophysiological mechanisms of allergic diseases, making it a possible disease-modifying treatment with the potential to transform long-term management strategies in allergy and immunology. An area attracting increasing attention in allergy interventions is the integration of personalized medicine and digital health technologies. This crossing enables clinicians to leverage mobile applications and digital platforms to monitor symptoms and medication adherence, and to adjust treatment plans based on real-time data. Furthermore, digital platforms can enhance patient education on triggers and avoidance strategies, which are critical components of allergy management. These novel approaches align with broader trends in healthcare toward more holistic, patient-centered care. With continued research, there is a need to identify technological advancements and integrate them into existing treatment methods so that patients receive comprehensive and effective care that addresses both their short-term needs and long-term well-being, as supported by ongoing projects referenced by Agache et al. (2016) and Gevaert et al. (2019).

5.6.2. Genetic Factors in Allergies

Genetic contributions to allergy susceptibility have attracted significant attention in the field of immunology. A lot of evidence indicates that an individual can be born with the susceptibility to an allergic disease, with genetic polymorphisms affecting various parts of the immune system. The variations can affect cytokine production, IgE response, and skin barrier integrity. In particular, the pathogenesis of conditions like atopic dermatitis is driven by genetic factors that affect the skin barrier and the immune system. Although the exact genotype correlations with the progression of atopic dermatitis are yet to be researched, current research is beginning to establish key genetic markers. More understanding of these genetic factors is needed to develop personalized therapeutic strategies and prevention protocols for the treatment of allergy, which represents a critical interface between genetics and allergy research (Martyna, 2013). Furthermore, the interaction between genes and environment plays a significant role in determining an individual's response to allergens. For instance, the hygiene hypothesis proposes that reduced exposure to pathogens during childhood may contribute to the development of allergies. This can further be quantified in terms of inherited immune responses. Genetic predisposition may be paired with environmental exposures, such as allergens and helminths, to alter immune system pathways, which might explain why some individuals develop allergies while others do not. Surprisingly, a negative correlation between allergic sensitization and helminth infection has been observed, suggesting that genetic immunomodulation can be multi-factorial and complex. Examining these interactions enhances our understanding of the allergic mechanism and could be pivotal in developing effective interventions (Mutapi et al., 2012). Ultimately, studying genetic factors in allergies involves an in-depth comprehension of both environmental influences and genetic susceptibilities. As one continues to uncover the intricate genetic basis for diseases like atopic dermatitis, genetics' role in determining not only susceptibility but also the overall immune phenotype of those affected becomes increasingly apparent. In addition, uncovering the interplay between genetic and environmental factors, especially infectious threats such as helminths, can uncover new avenues for the prevention and treatment of allergy. With these conditions in mind, further research is needed to fully understand the extent of genetic contribution to allergic diseases, in an effort to develop solid foundations for more personalized and efficient immune treatments in allergy and immunology (Mutapi et al., 2012; Martyna, 2013).

5.6.3. The Impact of Climate Change on Allergy Prevalence

The intricate relationship between global warming and the prevalence of allergies is increasingly recognized as a vital public health issue. With rising global temperatures, the higher concentration of environmental allergens, particularly pollen from trees, grasses, and weeds, poses greater risks for individuals prone to allergic reactions. Rising temperatures advance the growing season of these plants, increasing pollen production and the exposure period for susceptible populations. Moreover, higher carbon dioxide concentrations can enhance plant growth and allergen production, exacerbating symptoms in patients with respiratory allergies. As such, identifying these climate-driven dynamics provides valuable insights into allergy epidemiology and the exacerbation of conditions like asthma, which are directly linked to environmental alterations now further magnified by current climate change. Apart from the direct impact of warmer weather on the quantity of allergens, climate change is broadly to blame for alterations in weather patterns that can further influence allergy prevalence. With increased humidity and rainfall, the environment becomes conducive to mold growth, a prevalent indoor allergen. Consequently, individuals who have never been allergic to mold are becoming susceptible as these fungi thrive under changing climatic conditions. The recurrence and dissemination of these allergens into new areas also stimulate an increase in the incidence of allergic diseases among city residents who are not otherwise exposed to them. As highlighted in emerging research, the broader public health implications of climate change include rethinking existing management strategies for allergens and reaffirming the necessity of anticipatory intervention in allergy prevention. In addition, public health responses will need to be adapted to address the growing threat of climate change in the management and prevention of allergies. As noted in current studies, national and global health agencies must work together to develop comprehensive strategies to address the synergistic effects of climate change and allergic diseases. This also involves not only monitoring variations in allergen levels but also raising public awareness of the potential health impacts of increasing allergens in the environment. For instance, strategies such as improving indoor air quality and ventilation systems can effectively counteract the effects of allergens. However, research has found that such measures can vary in effectiveness in real life (Ahlstedt et al., 2009). Lastly, educated communities with information on how climate change impacts the prevalence of allergies are crucial to optimizing overall public health gain (Petruzelli et al., 2020) (Figure 5.16).

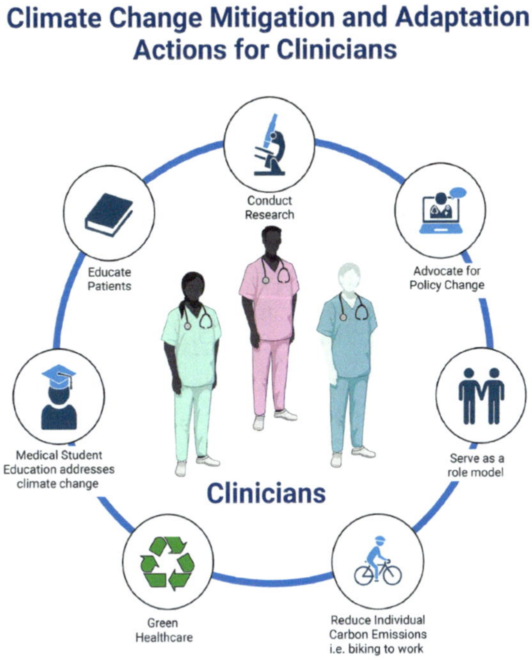

Figure 5.16. The impact of climate change on allergy prevalence.

Source: https://www.annallergy.org/cms/10.1016/j.anai.2023.08.610/asset/d2f8ef46-cf17-4609-9866-50355f1aab93/main.assets/gr2_lrg.jpg.

Test Your Knowledge

1. What are some recent advances in immunotherapy for treating allergies?
2. How do genetic predispositions influence an individual's likelihood of developing allergies?
3. In what ways is climate change believed to affect the prevalence and severity of allergic diseases?

SUMMARY

The conclusion of an essay on Allergy and Immunology not just captures the essence of the significant findings but also reflects on the future research directions and clinical implications of these findings. Weaving together the different strands of discussion, breakthroughs in our knowledge and treatment of allergies reinforce a multi-pronged strategy. For instance, the recent review of management of anaphylaxis has highlighted unsettling discrepancies between contemporary guidelines and their application within clinics. In addition to being a concern for patient safety, this discrepancy also highlights the urgent need for greater medical training and education in the management of severe allergy, as evidenced by the data review of allergy referral centers (Gough et al., 2012). Solutions to these issues will necessitate concerted effort from healthcare providers and policymakers. Education regarding the prevalence and burden of food allergy, especially in high-risk populations such as pregnant women, is essential for the design of effective interventions. Current studies indicate that, while food allergy prevalence among pregnant females is comparable to that of the general adult population, further scrutiny of its actual impact on mothers' and infants' health is still necessary. The retrospective study points out that, despite maternal food allergies falling within the range of predictability, their correlation with poor health outcomes warrants greater attention (Seita et al., 2013). Thus, research in this area may yield significant insights that support better management policies and improved health guidelines, resulting in better maternal and infant care. Lastly, the advancement in the area of Allergy and Immunology rests on bridging the knowledge gaps ascertained through ongoing research and clinical reports. The apparent disparity in the application of anaphylaxis treatment protocols necessitates joint efforts to streamline procedures and enhance public awareness of allergy management. Additionally, with the growing prevalence of food allergies across various populations under closer scrutiny, the importance of sustained research to elucidate the complex etiology of these conditions is greater than ever before. By focusing on interdisciplinary collaboration and integrating new evidence into clinical care, the field can expect to make dramatic strides in patient outcomes and to foster a culture in which allergic disorders are better understood and treated.

Allergy and Immunology is a field with a broad range of health concerns that emphasizes the importance of research expenditures and impact assessment. Asthma UK, one of the major stakeholders here, has been involved in measuring the multidisciplinary implications of its research expenditures. Using the Payback Framework, scientists analyzed the societal and academic paybacks arising from a variety of funded studies. This systematic review concluded that, in spite of the fact that the majority of societal effects were brought about by a minority of projects, there were improvements, such as the development of new asthma treatments. This suggests the vital role of targeted funding strategies in facilitating successful research that can drive clinical guidelines and translate into substantial improvements in patient health outcomes (Watt et al., 2013). A second priority area in Allergy and Immunology is self-management of anaphylaxis, especially for patient self-care. At the same time, it is advised that at-risk individuals carry epinephrine auto-injectors; far too many do not. Research has shown that obstacles such as inconsistent advice from healthcare providers, felt stigma associated with holding the device, and insufficient training significantly hinder successful self-management. In-depth interviews reveal why and how patients consistently fail to carry their auto-injectors with them, due to misconceptions about emergency services or aversion to the device's design. Solutions must be implemented over these variables to enhance patient empowerment in allergy treatment (Barnett et al., 2013). Synthesis of findings from each study, such as asthma research and anaphylaxis treatment, provides a broader lesson in Allergy and Immunology. Enhanced research output and patient engagement intertwine, guiding an exciting imperative for integrated processes that align clinical practices with research progress. Enabling interdisciplinary collaboration between patient groups and healthcare professionals, the goal is to create an environment conducive to improved health outcomes. Attention to patient education, adherence to self-care guidelines, and product redesign is important for achieving these objectives. Ultimately, a comprehensive system that synthesizes research impact assessment and patient empowerment will enhance the practice of Allergy and Immunology and the quality of life of those afflicted (Barnett et al., 2013; Watt et al., 2013).

KEY TERMS FROM THIS CHAPTER

- Immunity
- Antibody
- Adaptive Immunity
- Allergy
- Immunoglobulin E
- Histamine
- T Lymphocyte
- Antigen
- Innate Immunity
- Hypersensitivity
- Anaphylaxis
- Mast Cell
- Cytokine
- B Lymphocyte

CRITICAL THINKING QUESTIONS

1. **Which immunoglobulin is primarily involved in immediate allergic reactions?**
   a. IgA
   b. IgG
   c. IgM
   d. IgE
2. **What is the role of mast cells in allergic reactions?**
   a. They produce antibodies
   b. They destroy infected cells
   c. They release histamine and other mediators
   d. They inhibit inflammation
3. **Which of the following is a common cause of food allergies?**
   a. Gluten
   b. Soy
   c. Shellfish
   d. All of the above
4. **What is the gold standard for diagnosing an IgE-mediated allergy?**
   a. Total IgE level
   b. Skin prick testing
   c. Eosinophil count
   d. Chest X-ray
5. **Which medication is commonly used as first-line treatment for anaphylaxis?**
   a. Diphenhydramine
   b. Hydrocortisone
   c. Epinephrine
   d. Loratadine

Short Answer Questions

1. What are the four main types of hypersensitivity reactions, and which ones are typically involved in allergic responses?
2. Describe the process of sensitization and re-exposure in an IgE-mediated allergic reaction.
3. Name two common diagnostic tests for allergies and describe how they work.
4. List and briefly explain three common treatment strategies for allergic conditions.
5. How do food allergies differ from food intolerances in terms of immune involvement?
6. What is anaphylaxis, and what is the first-line treatment?

Answers to Critical Thinking Questions

1. (d); 2. (c); 3. (d); 4. (b); 5. (c)

REFERENCES

1. Amarasekera, M. (2011). Immunoglobulin E in health and disease. *Asia Pacific Allergy, 1*(1), 12–15. https://doi.org/10.5415/apallergy.2011.1.1.12Agache, I., Bachert, C., Bedbrook, A., Bergmann, K. C., et al. (2016). ARIA 2016: Care pathways implementing emerging technologies for predictive medicine in rhinitis and asthma across the life cycle. https://core.ac.uk/download/77614616.pdf (accessed on 17th July 2025).
2. Ahlstedt, S., Arlian, L. G., Benninger, M., British Thoracic Society, Brooks, C., Brugge, D., et al. (2009). Effect of improved home ventilation on asthma control and house dust mite allergen levels. https://core.ac.uk/download/9025603.pdf (accessed on 17th July 2025).
3. Akram, M., Awan, F. I., Ghani, M. U., Idrees, F., et al. (2018). Awareness of asthma genetics in Pakistan: A review with some recommendations. https://core.ac.uk/download/268082381.pdf (accessed on 17th July 2025).
4. Al-Riyami, L., Harnett, M. M., Harnett, W., Pineda, M. A., et al. (2014). Lessons from helminth infections: ES-62 highlights new interventional approaches in rheumatoid arthritis. https://core.ac.uk/download/42352576.pdf (accessed on 17th July 2025).
5. al-Samarrae, A., Banov, C., Benninger, M., Bernstein, J., Bhargava, S., Blaiss, M., Blom, H. M., et al. (2011). Management of rhinitis: Allergic and non-allergic. https://core.ac.uk/download/pdf/8583828.pdf (accessed on 17th July 2025).
6. Alvarez-Twose, R., Muraro, A., Arga, M., Armstrong, L., Arroabarren, E., Sheikh, A., Barnett, D., et al. (2014). International consensus on (ICON) anaphylaxis. https://core.ac.uk/download/28978204.pdf (accessed on 17th July 2025).
7. Amaducci, S., Bacci, E., Baldacci, S., Bartoli, M., et al. (2018). Inhalation therapy in the next decade: Determinants of adherence to treatment in asthma and COPD. https://core.ac.uk/download/152415584.pdf (accessed on 17th July 2025).
8. Apostol, A. C., Beaudin, A. E., & Jensen, K. D. C. (2020). Training the fetal immune system through maternal inflammation—A layered hygiene hypothesis. https://core.ac.uk/download/288432714.pdf (accessed on 17th July 2025).
9. Ashworth, F., Bethune, C., Cale, C., Dempster, J., et al. (2015). C1 inhibitor deficiency: 2014 United Kingdom consensus document. https://core.ac.uk/download/30611190.pdf (accessed on 17th July 2025).
10. Avery, L. M., Bookstaver, P. B., Justo, J. A., Kufel, W. D., et al. (2019). Penicillin allergy assessment and skin testing in the outpatient setting. https://core.ac.uk/download/231841951.pdf (accessed on 17th July 2025).
11. Barnett, J., Kuljis, J., Lucas, J., Money, A., et al. (2013). Patient perceptions of epinephrine auto-injectors: Exploring barriers to use. https://core.ac.uk/download/29140206.pdf (accessed on 17th July 2025).
12. Barton, P., Dretzke, J., Fry-Smith, A., Huissoon, A., et al. (2013). A systematic review and economic evaluation of subcutaneous and sublingual allergen immunotherapy in adults and children with seasonal allergic rhinitis. https://core.ac.uk/download/18488555.pdf (accessed on 17th July 2025).
13. Benedé, S., Bouchaud, G., Costa, A., Denery-Papini, S., et al. (2019). Applying the adverse

outcome pathway (AOP) for food sensitization to support *in vitro* testing strategies. https://core.ac.uk/download/232112908.pdf (accessed on 17th July 2025).

14. Bieber, T., Bissonette, R., Brown, S. J., Dhar, S., et al. (2018). Human and computational models of atopic dermatitis: A review and perspectives by an expert panel of the International Eczema Council. https://core.ac.uk/download/195291206.pdf (accessed on 17th July 2025).
15. Blanca, M., Blanco, C., Cuesta-Herranz, J., Diaz Perales, A., et al. (2013). Enriched mannose glycosylation contributes to Act d 2 allergenicity. https://oa.upm.es/30046/1/INVE_MEM_2013_164273.pdf (accessed on 17th July 2025).
16. Bonini, M., Canonica, G. W., Del Giacco, S., Gangemi, S., Lombardi, C., Minciullo, P. L., et al. (2017). Allergic diseases in the elderly: Biological characteristics and main immunological and non-immunological mechanisms. https://core.ac.uk/download/80193935.pdf (accessed on 17th July 2025).
17. Burns, H. (2019). The development of hypersensitivity reactions in the pediatric population: A review. https://core.ac.uk/download/213464303.pdf (accessed on 17th July 2025).
18. Doherty, T. A., Lund, S., & Walford, H. H. (2013). Type 2 innate lymphoid cells in allergic disease. https://core.ac.uk/download/323064316.pdf (accessed on 17th July 2025).
19. Else, K. J., Garcia, F. T., McSharry, C., Nakajima, H., Oku, Y., Pawlowski, Z., Petit-Frere, C., et al. (2014). Mucosal immune responses following intestinal nematode infection. https://core.ac.uk/download/29469509.pdf (accessed on 17th July 2025).
20. Evans-Agnew, R. A. (2012). Asthma management: An ecosocial framework for disparity research. https://digitalscholarship.unlv.edu/cgi/viewcontent.cgi?article=1011&context=jhdrp (accessed on 17th July 2025).
21. Gevaert, K., Impens, F., Laval, K., Nauwynck, H., et al. (2019). Pollens destroy respiratory epithelial cell anchors and drive alpha herpesvirus infection. https://core.ac.uk/download/222452376.pdf (accessed on 17th July 2025).
22. Gough, H., Grabenhenrich, L., Hawranek, T., Hompes, S., et al. (2012). Implementation of anaphylaxis management guidelines. https://core.ac.uk/download/12175690.pdf (accessed on 17th July 2025).
23. Haglund, K., Larson, K., McLaughlin, J., Stonehouse, M., et al. (2016). Introducing allergenic food into infants' diets: Systematic review. https://core.ac.uk/download/213072398.pdf (accessed on 17th July 2025).
24. Kalinowska, Z., Krężel, M., Matera, W., Snoch, B., et al. (2025). Drug-induced rhinitis as a complication of using mucosal decongestants. https://core.ac.uk/download/656518361.pdf (accessed on 17th July 2025).
25. Maizels, R. M., McSorley, H. J., & Smyth, D. J. (2014). Helminths in the hygiene hypothesis: Sooner or later? https://core.ac.uk/download/287602009.pdf (accessed on 17th July 2025).
26. Makvandi-Nejad, S. (2023). Prevalence of allergic diseases in Mayan population of Lake Atitlan, Guatemala: A cross-sectional pilot study. https://core.ac.uk/download/580972364.pdf (accessed on 17th July 2025).
27. Mutapi, F., Rujeni, N., & Taylor, D. W. (2012). Human *Schistosome* infection and allergic sensitization. https://core.ac.uk/download/28974396.pdf (accessed on 17th July 2025).

28. N/A (2005). Advancing physician performance measurement: Using administrative data to assess physician quality and efficiency. https://core.ac.uk/download/71349215.pdf (accessed on 17th July 2025).

29. Olson, K. (2019). Pilot study: Program evaluation of peanut oral immunotherapy in a private clinic. https://core.ac.uk/download/223074370.pdf (accessed on 17th July 2025).

30. Petruzelli, N. (2020). The influence of climate change on disease and public health. https://core.ac.uk/download/322826252.pdf (accessed on 17th July 2025).

31. Rauscher, B. (2015). Use of immunotherapy in the treatment of peanut allergies in the pediatric population. https://core.ac.uk/download/58826198.pdf (accessed on 17th July 2025).

32. Seita, H. M. (2013). Food allergies in pregnant women: A study of prevalence in expecting mothers and association with neonatal outcomes. https://open.bu.edu/bitstream/2144/12219/6/Seita_Helene_2013.pdf (accessed on 17th July 2025).

33. Watt, A., Jadad, A. R., British Thoracic Society and Scottish Intercollegiate Guidelines Network, Canadian Academy of Medical Sciences, Brightling, C. E., Cooksey, D., et al. (2013). Conducting retrospective impact analysis to inform a medical research charity's funding strategies: The case of Asthma UK. https://core.ac.uk/download/13641690.pdf (accessed on 17th July 2025).

34. Wesserling, M. (2013). Role of genetic aspect in pathogenesis of atopic dermatitis. https://core.ac.uk/download/71976799.pdf (accessed on 17th July 2025).

35. Zhang, F., Zhang, G. X., Han, J. J., Zhao, L., Zhu, L., Liu, S., Li, X., et al. (2018). Carnosol modulates Th17 cell differentiation and microglial switch in experimental autoimmune encephalomyelitis. https://core.ac.uk/download/213443169.pdf (accessed on 17th July 2025).

TROPICAL AND TRAVEL MEDICINE

6

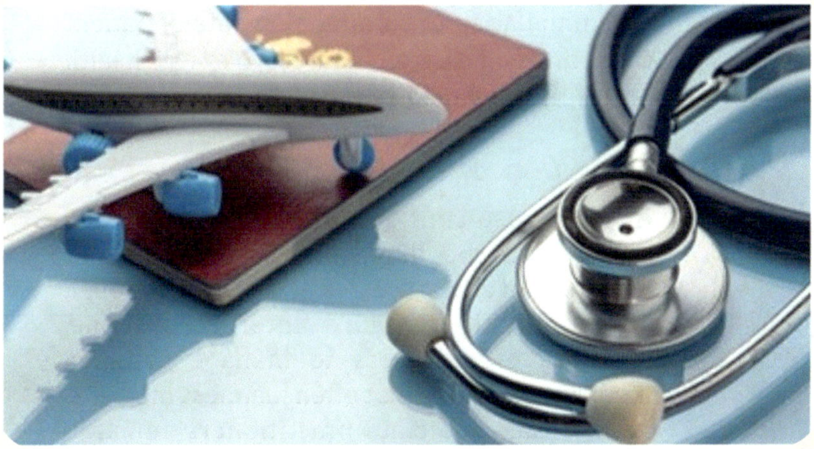

LEARNING OBJECTIVES

After studying this chapter, you will be able to:

1. Discus the historical context
2. Explain the common tropical diseases
3. Focus on preventive measures
4. Understand diagnosis and treatment
5. Discus the role of travel medicine
6. Learn about global health perspectives

Introduction

The development of tropical and travel medicine within internal medicine is crucial for understanding the peculiar health problems of individuals in diverse geographical and environmental settings. With international travel on the rise and exposure to tropical diseases increasingly frequent, doctors must adapt their approach in diagnosing and treating diseases that differ considerably from indigenous diseases. Most experts also agree that timely and accurate diagnosis is crucial for minimizing the impact of such illnesses, especially in low- and middle-income countries with scarce resources (Fleming et al., 2021). An excellent clinical approach, thus, calls for a deep understanding of the epidemiology, pathology, and management of infections and conditions common in such regions. This emphasizes the importance of ongoing training and education in internal medicine, equipping practitioners to address global health issues. Moreover, tropical and travel medicine has a significant overlap with the public health programs aimed at increasing diagnostic capacity and access to health care. A significant issue highlighted is the diagnostic gap across many health facilities, weakening the quality of care for affected groups. The COVID-19 pandemic has further escalated the problem, highlighting the urgent need for increased access to diagnostic equipment and services in both rural and urban health facilities (Fleming et al., 2021). Consequently, internal medicine practitioners must be prepared to utilize innovative solutions, enabled by technological and informatics advancements, to enhance diagnostic capabilities in health systems in low-resource settings.

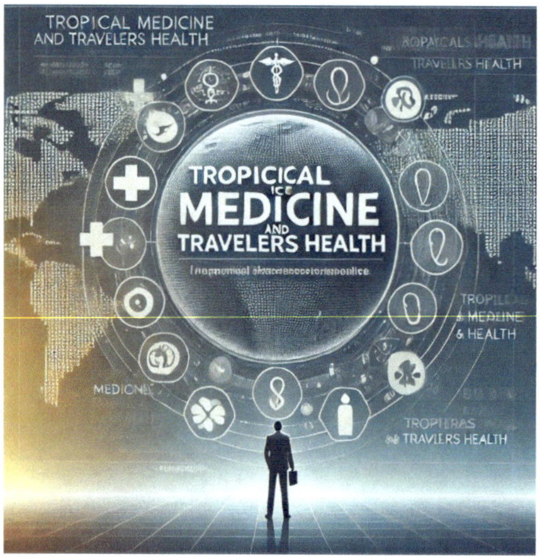

Figure 6.1. The internal medicine for tropical and travel medicine.

Source: https://lwfiles.mycourse.app/66e83b55fe489daea705fb51-public/33456e1d955817619d390f09cdd716af.jpg.

That concordance is not only needed to cure immediate health problems but also to sustain long-term patient outcomes and health equity enhancement. Beyond developments in diagnostics, an appreciation of the role of culturally appropriate care is vital for clinicians in tropical and travel medicine. Many patients who attend to be treated for tropical diseases are likely to be of different ethnic groups and have particular beliefs regarding health, possibly affecting their adherence to traditional medical regimes. By integrating knowledge of cultural influences and potential barriers to healthcare access, internal medicine practitioners will be able to build relationships with patients and increase compliance with treatment regimens. Additionally, the historical use of medicinal plants across cultures, including essential oils with varying biological activities, must be considered. This holistic approach not only solves clinical problems of medicine but is also respectful and accommodating of cultural elements of patient care, finally to better address tropical health issues in the globalized world (Figure 6.1).

Definition of Internal Medicine

Internal medicine is a branch of medicine focused on the diagnosis, prevention, and treatment of adult diseases. It entails a thorough understanding of many internal systems, enabling practitioners to manage complex medical conditions that often manifest in adults. In internal medicine, practitioners function as primary physicians who specialize in the diagnosis and management of chronic diseases, acute diseases, and other complicated health conditions. The knowledge required to excel in this area is immense, as internists must integrate clinical information with an understanding of pathophysiology, pharmacology, and preventive medicine. This underpinning nature sets internal medicine apart from other specialties, highlighting its contribution to ensuring whole-person care and effective management of chronic disease across a multi-ethnic patient population, particularly when dealing with tropical and travel-related health conditions. The particular geography of travel and tropical medicine introduces additional subtleties that internal medicine experts must guide. In disease-endemic areas such as the Zika virus and malaria, internists must use targeted interventions and prevention guidelines through the most recent epidemiological data and clinical practice guidelines. For instance, the

European Network for Tropical Medicine and Travel Health highlights disparate treatment regimens for complex malaria, which requires an immense demand for skilled internists who can adapt to such variations (Antinori et al., 2017). Furthermore, practice of internal medicine in the tropics frequently involves collaboration with the public health agencies in managing significant problems, implementing the need for prevention intervention and health education among travelers and indigenous populations. Disease management in such environments requires an advanced understanding of infectious disease, vaccine policy, and emergency treatment. Internal medicine is also critical in establishing the debate on ethical healthcare practices, particularly regarding disease prevention in the tropics. The Zika virus outbreak exemplifies ethical decision-making, whereby doctors are faced with dilemmas of utilizing contraception and offering reproductive health advice to patients (Clark et al., 2016). The intersection of internal medicine and public health calls on practitioners to be not only well-informed in medicine but also to be skilled in the manipulation of sociocultural contexts and ethical debates. Through education on such distinguished issues, internists enhance their ability to promote patient welfare against regional health challenges. Thus, the scope of internal medicine extends far beyond clinical practice, encompassing an ethos of social responsibility and ethical health care in responding to the challenges of travel and tropical medicine.

Importance of Tropical and Travel Medicine

The relevance of travel and tropical medicine lies not only in the management of disease but also in an overall understanding of environmental exposures and health vulnerabilities. With global mobility on the rise and geographical borders eroding, the potential for infectious diseases rises, underlining the need for expert medical care in this field. Tropical medicine focuses on understanding the epidemiology and vectors of disease transmission in tropical regions, such as malaria and dengue fever. In addition, travelers enter foreign environments to which their bodies are not adapted, encountering pathogens to which they have minimal or no immunity. Thus, practitioners of tropical medicine not only have the duty to provide preventive measures such as vaccinations and prophylactic drugs, but also must inform travelers about the risks posed by some locales to enable informed choices that are crucial to public health. The importance of tropical and travel medicine is then further amplified by the interface between ecological changes and their health implications. Environmental changes, whether driven by climate change or urbanization, affect the spread and vulnerability to disease. For instance, the concept of ecological resilience, meaning a system's ability to endure in the presence of disturbances, is critical when considering the health impacts of altered environments. Increased understanding of ecological resilience can inform public health interventions and build preparedness against new infectious diseases, and thus reduce vulnerability in the targeted populations. The dynamics of infection transmission can change significantly as ecosystems evolve, and a robust scientific investigation of these interconnected dynamics must precede health emergencies. By employing epidemiological techniques to quantify resilience, as discussed in the literature, clinicians can formulate customized interventions that consider the evolving dynamics of tropical and travel health risks (Scheffer et al., 2015). Finally, cultural competence inherent in tropical and travel medicine cannot be overstated. With culturally diverse communities of travelers and residents in impact areas, health professionals are challenged with varying health beliefs, practices, and expectations. Trust and compliance are established through effective communication and empathetic health education, supported by sensitivity to cultural awareness. Additionally, most traditional healing modalities and herbalism are based on specific cultures and, therefore, are deserving of respect and understanding from health professionals. Essential oils, for example, have been traditionally utilized for their biological activities, illustrating a historic relationship between health and culture (Sharifi et al., 2017). Understanding these intricate relationships can make interventions more effective, which, in turn, will lead to enhanced health outcomes. Thus, tropical and travel medicine is not only a field of study but also an essential paradigm to bring to bear upon global health and health inequities in the era of high connectivity (Figure 6.2).

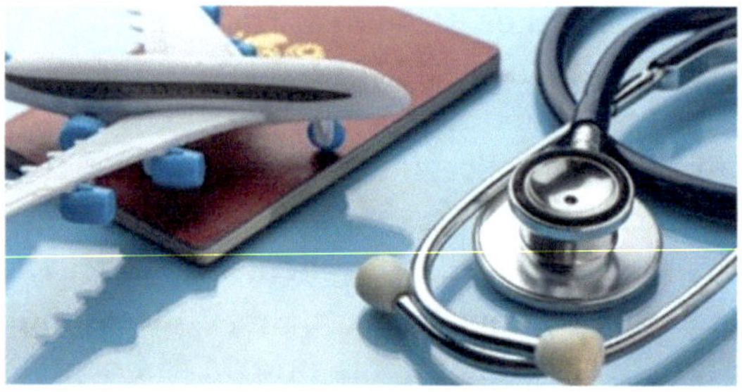

Figure 6.2. The significance of tropical and travel medicine extends beyond the mere treatment of diseases.

Source: https://media.springernature.com/lw725/springer-cms/rest/v1/content/26494678/data/v3.

6.1. Historical Context

Learning Outcome

1. Evolution of internal medicine
2. Development of tropical medicine
3. Impact of travel on disease spread

The historical evolution of travel and tropical medicine is inextricably linked with world exploration, trade routes, and, consequently, disease exchange. When explorers and traders journeyed to distant territories, they were exposed to a broad spectrum of infectious diseases to which they were not previously exposed in their homelands. In the 19th century, the expansion of the British Empire into places like India and Africa triggered extensive documentation of tropical diseases, which bred an interest in learning about and curing such diseases as cholera and malaria. This was the era when the first tropical schools of medicine were opened, whose purpose was to prepare doctors with the expert knowledge necessary to fight these foreign pathogens. These early steps laid the groundwork for subsequent advancements both in internal medicine and in public health, and they emphasize the importance of historical context in shaping contemporary practice in the field. The integration of indigenous medicine with Western medicine has also played an essential role in shaping the institute of internal medicine for tropical and travel medicine. Historical evidence shows the use of traditional treatments and medicinal approaches, a vast majority of which trace their origins to ancient civilizations. Essential oils, for example, have been used for centuries in various healing traditions, which are renowned for their biological activities, e.g., antimicrobial and anti-inflammatory activities (Sharifi et al., 2017). When doctors began investigating these traditional practices, cross-pollination of knowledge widened the scope of internal medicine. This continuous dialogue between these various systems of medicine has not only encouraged a fuller comprehension of tropical diseases but also an appreciation and understanding of the holistic approach to treatment that considers the patient's cultural beliefs and heritage. Today, the historical background of tropical and travel medicine is not only relevant in solving modern problems such as antibiotic resistance and global pandemics. Still, it is an essential component of modern medicine. Lessons from historical experiences with infectious diseases inform present disease prevention and control measures. Public health programs, for instance, base their understanding of disease patterns of spread on history to plan effective vaccination efforts. Moreover, the reality of global travel necessitates consideration of diseases that may occur or recur due to human movement (Slater et al., 2016). An understanding of how earlier responses to tropical diseases have shaped current medical practice yields lessons for managing public health challenges, keeping history's wisdom alive as internal medicine evolves to counter new threats to global health.

6.1.1. Evolution of Internal Medicine

The evolution of internal medicine has been significantly influenced by advances in medical science and technology, as well as the increasing complexity of illnesses encountered across various settings. Having initially focused on the diagnosis and care of disease among the urban populations of industrialized countries, internal medicine has expanded to encompass broader knowledge of health and disease across various settings. This is most relevant in tropical medicine and travel medicine, where clinicians must contend with atypical infectious diseases that do not occur in temperate climates. The historical shift from a symptom-based model to a more sophisticated understanding of disease processes reflects the need for internal medicine practitioners to address complex health issues, with a focus on prevention, treatment, and patient care across diverse geographical settings. Among the significant areas of internal medicine development is the convergence of advanced technologies and techniques of disease diagnosis and treatment. Telemedicine, mobile health technology, and artificial intelligence are some of the innovations that have transformed patient engagement and delivery of care, particularly in resource-limited settings where access to care is limited. These technologies are central to the practice of tropical and travel medicine, where the ability to diagnose quickly can have far-reaching consequences for disease outcomes. Telemedicine has made it possible to provide specialist care to patients in remote locations that would not have been available in the not-so-distant past. The application of these technologies in practice enhances not only the efficiency of care but also the role of internal medicine in bridging health disparities globally, promoting greater access to medical care for disadvantaged populations.

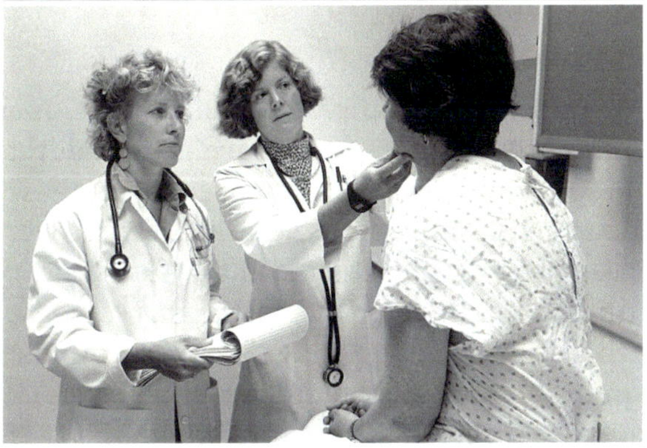

Figure 6.3. Physicians conducting a clinical examination of a patient, demonstrating hands-on diagnostic evaluation.

Source: https://upload.wikimedia.org/wikipedia/commons/thumb/4/45/Seattle_physician_with_patient_1999.jpg/960px-Seattle_physician_with_patient_1999.jpg.

The need for an interdisciplinary system has also characterized the evolution of internal medicine, especially for tropical and travel medicine specialties. With the more mobile world and more connected populations, physicians must possess an advanced understanding of the complex cultural, environmental, and socioeconomic determinants of health. This transition is reflected in greater emphasis on preventive care and health education targeted explicitly to combating the unique demands of traveler and population exposures in endemic areas. This broader context is also supported by growing concerns about antimicrobial resistance and rising incidences of vector-borne infections, as addressed in recent studies on the influence of chronic infections in immunocompromised hosts (Mertes et al., 2023). By adopting an integrative, multidisciplinary approach, internal medicine continues to develop and adapt to the demands of evolving global health, enabling practitioners to effectively address multifaceted health issues (Matthew et al., 2021) (Figure 6.3).

6.1.2. Development of Tropical Medicine

The history of tropical medicine developed as an essential branch of learning to address the specific health issues posed by diseases characteristic of the tropics. Early advances were driven by colonial medicine in the 19th century, with the main focus on managing diseases such as malaria and yellow fever that afflicted expatriates and soldiers. Seeing the endemic nature of diseases among local populations led to a broader, more inclusive policy towards public health. The discovery of pathogens, such as the Plasmodium parasite that causes malaria, underscored the significance of scientific research on tropical diseases. Tropical medicine is now characterized by its multifaceted strategies, including epidemiological studies, environmental management, and health education to tackle health crises in the hot climes around the world. As a result of increased international travel, the interface between tropical medicine and travel medicine is receiving special attention. Travelers are increasingly being exposed to the same tropical infections that attack the local populace, which necessitates a proactive approach in vaccination and prophylaxis. Physicians with training in travel medicine advise against illnesses prevalent in particular regions and use vaccination and preventive medication protocols. This intersection of practice highlights the importance of health awareness and preparedness for both going-out and coming-in travelers. Furthermore, emergent trends in zoonotic disease driven by ecological changes pose new challenges and underscore the need for updated medical curricula that consider both local and global health contexts. Thus, tropical medicine has become priceless in a world where travel and climate change continually shift disease patterns. The application of ecological and socio-economic models has also enhanced its effectiveness. In acknowledging that health is interwoven with societal structures and environmental forces, tropical medicine now adopts multi-pronged methods addressing these fronts. Studies increasingly emphasize the role of ecological degradation in disease spread, such as the increasing caseloads of malaria associated with deforestation and climate change. In view of these challenges, the planetary health concept has emerged, calling for convergence across policy sectors to deliver sustainable health solutions. Advances in technology and interdisciplinarity allow for a detailed understanding of how health consequences are influenced by socio-economic status and cultural traditions in the tropics. So, the persistent development of tropical medicine requires an adaptive model responsive to shifts in the environment and society, while upholding the fundamental values of internal medicine to address issues of global health (Whitmee et al., 2015; Schwellnus et al., 2016).

6.1.3. Impact of Travel on Disease Spread

The increased global connectivity has significantly expanded the role of tourism in the spread of diseases, particularly in travel and tropical medicine. As humans travel across international borders to work, play, or study, they unknowingly transport infectious agents from one continent to another. This was well illustrated by the COVID-19 pandemic, where initial outbreaks were fueled by international travel, showing how quickly pathogens can cross continents. The World Health Organization has noted travel-related illness presents vast challenges, particularly to tourists traveling in tropical regions where vector-borne illnesses such as malaria and dengue are prevalent. Touristic and business travel to these destinations tends to coincide with rising cases of these illnesses, which points to the complex interaction between traveler behavior and public health risks. In addition to spreading infectious diseases, travel has the capability to influence the occurrence and recurrence of disease in a population. When individuals travel to areas with endemic infections or poorly contained disease epidemics, they risk exposure to pathogens that may not be present in their native countries. This makes such areas potential reservoirs for the disease if such travelers return home without receiving preventive education. For instance, the resurgence of such diseases as Zika virus and chikungunya in non-endemic nations can typically be traced to returnees who have visited the infected zones. Although intensified surveillance and public health interventions are needed to contain the risks associated with travel, a strong recommendation is for rigorous pre-travel medical consultations and pre-emptive vaccination. In addition, the contribution of environmental determinants to intensified travel cannot be excluded. Several studies have established that land-use transformation and urbanization, triggered in some cases by tourism and migration, can alter local ecosystems and biodiversity, thereby affecting disease transmission dynamics. For example, as urbanization advances into previously natural or unexplored environments, human-wildlife contact increases, raising the risk of zoonotic disease spillover into human populations. This association underscores the importance of a multisectoral approach that integrates public health, environmental health, and biodiversity conservation, as evidenced by models linking biodiversity to human health presented in several research papers. Neglecting these interrelated problems can worsen global health threats in a more mobile world, thereby necessitating holistic approaches that integrate health and environmental sustainability, as confirmed by Melissa et al. (2021) (Figure 6.4).

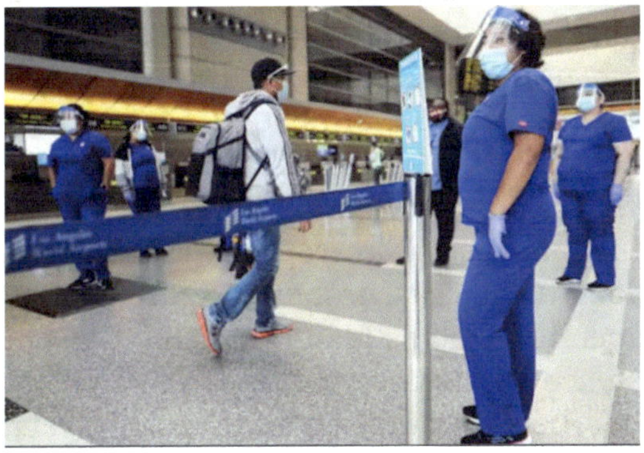

Figure 6.4. The increased global interconnectedness has significantly intensified the impact of travel on the spread of diseases.

Source: https://images.theconversation.com/files/355169/original/file-20200827-18-1fw8hni.jpg?ixlib=rb-4.1.0&rect=14%2C21%2C4723%2C3125&q=20&auto=format&w=320&fit=clip&dpr=2&usm=12&cs=strip.

Test Your Knowledge

1. Why did tropical medicine emerge as a distinct field in the late 19th and early 20th centuries?
2. How has increased global travel contributed to the spread of infectious diseases in modern times?

6.2. Common Tropical Diseases

Learning Outcome

1. Malaria
2. Dengue fever
3. Schistosomiasis

Section 6.2 discusses the prevalence of tropical diseases, which predominantly affect populations in resource-limited settings. The World Health Organization identifies tropical diseases such as malaria, dengue fever, and schistosomiasis as significant public health threats, causing high morbidity and mortality. Such conditions thrive in specific climatic conditions, and most of them are found in tropical and subtropical regions, in which environmental factors such as temperature and humidity are conducive to the existence of disease vectors. Trends over the recent past indicate an increase in travel-related cases, underscoring the importance of knowledge about these diseases within the umbrella of travel medicine. With continued global warming and urbanization, those diseases might spread to non-endemic areas, putting more and more travelers at risk and necessitating early preventive measures and effective management strategies in internal medicine clinics. The presentation and treatment of most tropical diseases can differ significantly from those of non-tropical diseases, and thus medical personnel require specialized knowledge. For instance, malaria is most typically seen with fever, chills, and flu-like symptoms, but if not treated early, it progresses to severe complications and death. Dengue fever also presents with high fever and muscle and joint aching, occasionally leading to life-threatening hemorrhagic presentations. To combat these issues, the medical staff should be proficient in diagnosing such diseases through appropriate laboratory investigations, e.g., rapid diagnostic tests for malaria and serological tests for dengue. Apart from this, clinicians should also be able to manage complications as the patient's outcome efficiently greatly depends upon timely intervention and specific therapeutic measures, and hence education and training in tropical medicine is a continuous requirement for practitioners of internal medicine. Advances in biomedical research have led to the deployment of novel forms of therapy for tropical diseases, such as the manufacture of monoclonal antibodies (mAbs). As of late 2023, an unprecedented increase in approved mAbs underscores their growing importance in the preventive and curative arsenal against infectious diseases. These developments have the potential to advance therapy for tropical diseases, particularly for malaria and rabies, where therapeutics have hitherto been lacking. With the availability of possible prophylactics and therapeutics, mAbs could potentially significantly reduce morbidity and mortality caused by these diseases. Cost, availability, and resistance risk, however, are some of the hurdles that must be surmounted to achieve their optimal application in the clinic. Thus, future research into the application of mAbs will be crucial for their proper incorporation into travel medicine in an effort to better safeguard travelers from these widespread tropical infections (Hanna et al., 2024).

6.2.1. Malaria

Malaria remains a significant problem in internal medicine, particularly in the subtropical and tropical regions where malaria has been endemic. The causative agent, Plasmodium, is transmitted to human beings through the bite of infected Anopheles mosquitoes, and this leads to a variety of clinical presentations ranging from fever and chills to life-threatening anemia and multi-organ failure . Proper management of malaria requires a strong understanding of its pathophysiology, which differs across the five *Plasmodium* species that infect humans. The doctors must be skilled at recognizing the clinical manifestations and possible complications specific to each type and initiating timely treatment. Because malaria is often misdiagnosed due to cross-reactive signs with other fever conditions, microscopy and rapid diagnostic testing remain essential to accurate diagnosis and timely treatment. Community health worker (CHW) programs have emerged as feasible alternatives in the fight against malaria in recent years, particularly in resource-poor settings. Inclusion of CHWs within health systems can facilitate outreach services, enabling early case detection and treatment adherence among high-risk populations. These interventions strengthen communities through active involvement and ownership of malaria control, leading to improved health outcomes. It has been found that aspects such as supportive supervision, continuing education, and logistical support significantly enhance the effects of CHW interventions. It also needs to take into consideration the rights and interests of these workers because it has an impact on their effectiveness in promoting awareness of malaria and prevention. Sustainability for these programs lies in their flexibility at the local level, in responding to local needs and challenges, and in keeping pace with health system objectives (Scott et al., 2018). The ongoing risk of malaria is compounded by the occurrence of drug-resistant strains and also by the socio-ecological factors influencing the dissemination of the disease. Malaria epidemiology has an intimate relationship with environmental components, wherein climate variations influence vector populations and human exposure. Researchers have indicated that the pandemic of zoonotic diseases, strongly associated with environmental changes, underscores the importance of an effective infectious disease control policy. Given that malaria is still an overwhelming public health and economic challenge, the onus of creating new ways to fight this age-old disease becomes increasingly urgent. There has to be a concerted effort toward building surveillance systems, guaranteeing greater access to productive cures, and pursuing overall vaccination policies. Lastly, a multifaceted approach, driven by the vibrant interplay among social, economic, and environmental factors, will be required in the global fight against malaria and other NTDs (Nii-Trebi, 2017) (Figure 6.5).

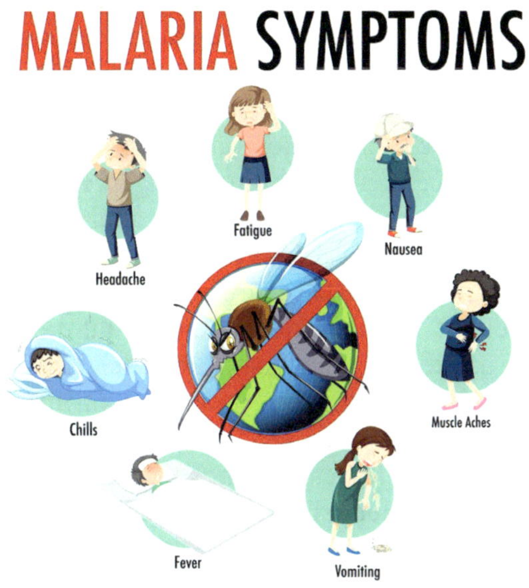

Figure 6.5. Malaria symptoms.

Source: https://max-website20-images.s3.ap-south-1.amazonaws.com/1698649899_21200688_cc6922e92c.jpeg.

6.2.2. Dengue Fever

Dengue fever, a viral infection transmitted primarily by the Aedes aegypti mosquito, is a serious public health threat in tropical and subtropical regions worldwide. The World Health Organization has reported a startling rise in the incidence and geographical extent of dengue, with cases around the world increasing and intensifying, mostly in urban environments. This growth is due to multiple factors, including climate change, urbanization, and increased human mobility, which facilitate the spread of the mosquito vector. Thus, dengue fever is not only a threat to the affected population but also a burden on health systems that must cope with the increased demand for diagnostic, treatment, and preventive interventions. The pathophysiology of dengue and its clinical manifestations are something that internal medicine practitioners who deal with tropical diseases must be aware of to provide timely intervention and improved outcomes for patients. Dengue fever must be managed through an integrated approach that includes early detection and response practices. Symptomatic treatment in the past was the focus of clinical attention, primarily fluid replacement and pain management, since no antiviral drug is currently available. Early detection of warning signs indicative of probable progression towards severe dengue is required to prevent complications. Recent guidelines, such as those discussed in the "Dengue Contingency Planning" manual, emphasize the need to develop local contingency plans to address outbreaks. These plans specify well-defined alert signals that health workers can use to detect outbreaks at the earliest, thereby enabling timely interventions that can significantly reduce morbidity and mortality from severe dengue cases (Runge-Ranzinger et al., 2016). Joint studies by various institutions have elucidated various facts concerning dengue control and prevention measures. One of the major focus areas is educating healthcare workers in affected regions, which has been identified as a priority for improving disease management. Collaborative efforts between indigenous universities and foreign research institutions can help build a highly educated population capable of identifying, diagnosing, and effectively managing dengue fever. Furthermore, the integration of zoonotic disease thinking within training modules can promote understanding of disease transmission dynamics and increase readiness for emerging infectious disease risks (Bourhy et al., 2012). Through resource and expertise sharing, such collaborations aim to respond to the ongoing dengue epidemic and enhance public health resilience overall in tropical settings.

6.2.3. Schistosomiasis

Schistosomiasis, a parasitic disease caused by the *Schistosoma* species, directly affects only tropical and subtropical regions where snail hosts are present and common. Schistosomiasis is not only a significant public health issue but also reflects broader environmental and ecological issues. Schistosomiasis is acquired primarily through contact with contaminated freshwater, placing populations with agricultural or recreational water use at high risk. The clinical syndromes range from acute fever and abdominal pain presentation to long-term liver, intestinal, and urinary tract complications that contribute to significant morbidity. Management and control of schistosomiasis, therefore, require an understanding of its epidemiological patterns that inform interventions such as mass drug administration and vector control. Control of schistosomiasis, therefore, requires a multidisciplinary intervention involving preservation of the environment, health education, and agricultural practices that are sustainable. Association between schistosomiasis prevalence and biodiversity is an indicator of a critical area of disease ecology. Despite providing significant ecological services, biodiversity can reorganize disease dynamics by influencing host and vector populations. For instance, a rich and well-endowed ecosystem may have more host snail diversity, leading to higher transmission rates of schistosomiasis among susceptible human groups. Conversely, biodiversity can enhance natural predation, reduce the number of intermediate hosts, and hence restrict the transmission of the disease. Such knowledge guides public health policy, as it underscores the necessity of preserving biodiversity as a safeguard against diseases such as schistosomiasis. It is important to note that the protection of ecosystems is not only for its own sake but also for sustaining human health through orchestrated public health programs (Melissa et al., 2021). Climate change is a driving force behind the acceleration of schistosomiasis transmission patterns, influencing freshwater availability and shifting habitats. As climate change continues to produce severe weather patterns, the risk of population displacement and eventual migration of individuals into endemic areas of schistosomiasis remains. The migrants, lacking appropriate access to health care, become highly susceptible to infectious diseases, including schistosomiasis. Also, as warmer temperatures spread to previously non-conducive areas, the potential for broader dissemination of Schistosoma species and, potentially, outbreaks in previously non-infected regions increases. This necessitates health systems to reposition through enhanced surveillance and public health interventions grounded in shifting demographic and environmental trends. Preparedness planning must include measures to mitigate the effects of climate change, travel, and migration on schistosomiasis epidemiology to safeguard public health (Jan et al., 2019) (Figure 6.6).

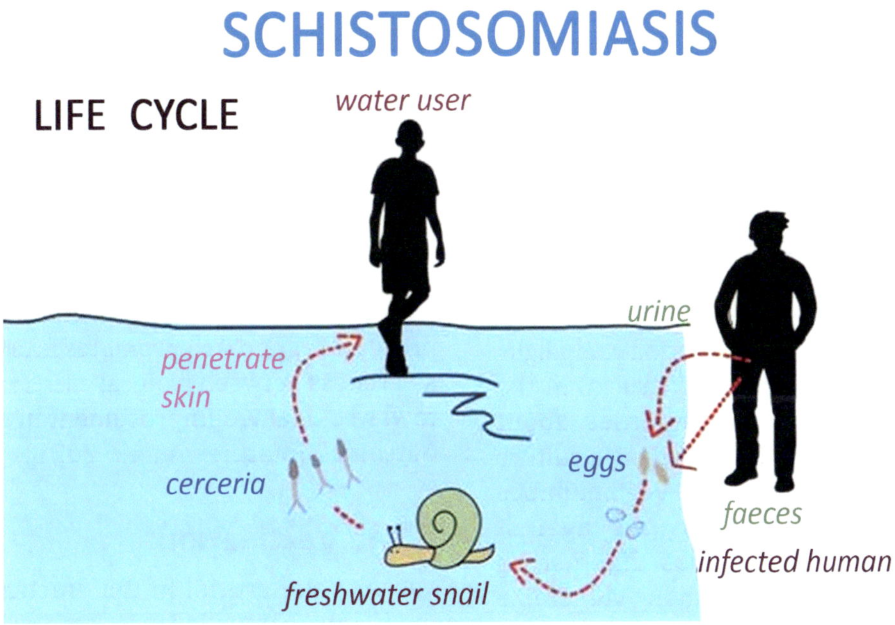

Figure 6.6. Schistosomiasis, a parasitic disease caused by *Schistosoma* species.

Source: https://www.who.int/images/default-source/departments/ntd-library/schistosomiasis/schistosomiasis-(bilharzia)-clip-an-overview.tmb-549v.jpg?Culture=en&sfvrsn=918ebcbf_2.

Test Your Knowledge

1. What is the primary parasite species responsible for the most severe form of malaria, and how is it transmitted?
2. What is a key clinical warning sign of severe dengue, and which vector is responsible for its transmission?
3. Which stage of the Schistosoma parasite penetrates human skin, and what type of water source poses a risk for infection?

6.3. Preventive Measures

Learning Outcome

1. Vaccinations
2. Prophylactic medications
3. Health education and awareness

Preventive measures are essential components of internal medicine, particularly in tropical and travel medicine, where many health hazards are prevalent. Core principles include immunization, preventive medications, and public health education to prevent the spread of infectious diseases. Immunization has proven useful in preventing most tropical illnesses, such as yellow fever and dengue fever, significantly reducing morbidity and mortality. Furthermore, prophylactic medicines such as antimalarials are required for travelers to high-risk destinations, underscoring the importance of pre-travel consultations. Public health education campaigns targeting the masses are equally crucial in the sense that they inform communities about preventive strategies, thereby fostering a culture of health awareness that empowers communities to undertake proactive measures against disease transmission as well as diminishing health inequalities, especially among vulnerable groups (Matthew et al., 2021). In addition to vaccination and prophylaxis, vector control and environmental measures play a key role in preventing disease outbreaks in tropical regions. Proper regulation of water sources to avoid the presence of standing water will successfully reduce mosquito breeding, hence the spread of vector-borne diseases such as malaria and Zika virus. This is important in low-income nations where infrastructure may not be well developed. Involving CHWs in prevention interventions enhances coverage (Scott et al., 2018). CHWs also serve as bridges between healthcare authorities and communities, ensuring that preventive interventions are accessible and culturally appropriate. Inclusion of CHWs not only enhances the program's effectiveness but also builds community confidence. Ongoing training and supportive supervision must be employed to provide ongoing high levels of care and involvement among CHWs and ultimately to enhance local health systems. Finally, a multifaceted intervention for prevention must incorporate research and technological advances aimed at improving health outcomes. For instance, telemedicine innovations have the potential to increase access to health care among marginalized groups by facilitating timely consultations and interventions. Moreover, geographic information systems (GIS) may assist epidemiologists in monitoring epidemics and predicting disease transmission in real time, thereby enabling more effective responses. These are complementary to traditional preventive measures and emphasize the imperative for an adaptive health system employing evidence-based approaches to counter novel travel and tropical disease risks. Ultimately, a holistic preventive approach promotes integrated health awareness between tropical and travel medicine, toward sustained improvement in public health outcomes (Matthew et al., 2021).

6.3.1. Vaccinations

Vaccines are crucial in the practice of internal medicine, particularly in tropical and travel medicine. Not only are these vaccinations a protection against other infectious diseases that are so common in other regions, but they are also a way of reducing the likelihood of outbreaks. For instance, visitors to areas with high disease rates for illnesses such as yellow fever, hepatitis A, and typhoid fever are often mandated or strongly advised to receive vaccinations before traveling. The World Health Organization notes the importance of such vaccinations, particularly because they can prevent incapacitating illnesses that not only affect individual health outcomes but also general public health efforts. In addition, the dynamic nature of international travel increases the need for current vaccination procedures to adapt to shifting epidemiological patterns and emerging pathogens. Aside from keeping individual travelers safe, vaccination helps to establish herd immunity and therefore promotes collective health. Vaccinating a significant percentage of the population against certain diseases changes the dynamics of transmission and makes it less probable for outbreaks to take place. This is especially crucial in low- and middle-income countries, where outbreaks of vaccine-preventable diseases can result in severe health crises, economic instability, and high mortality. Vaccination campaigns supported and funded by global health institutions have been shown to eradicate some diseases, such as smallpox, and bring others, such as polio and measles, to heel. The connection between vaccination programs and the socio-economic determinants of health is critical, as full access to vaccines can reduce inequities and diminish disease burden in at-risk groups. Despite the established benefits of vaccinations, achieving high immunization coverage remains challenging, particularly in low-resource settings. Inadequate healthcare infrastructure, misconceptions regarding vaccine safety, and cultural beliefs could make vaccinating more difficult.

These problems have been evidenced in reports of efforts to increase vaccine coverage in various regions (Mertes et al., 2023). Regular monitoring and research on the efficacy and safety of vaccines are necessary as new vaccines are emerging and being introduced into the arsenal. Introduction of new technology has the potential to improve immunization by enhancing monitoring, delivery, and mobilization at the community level. Lastly, an integrated approach combining education, policymaking, and access to healthcare is essential to improve vaccination rates in tropical and travel medicine and ensure diverse populations are well vaccinated against deadly illnesses (Matthew et al., 2021) (Figure 6.7).

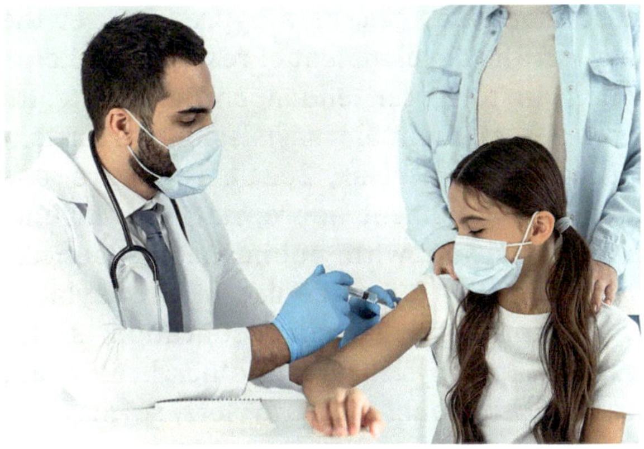

Figure 6.7. Vaccinations play a crucial role in the field of internal med.

Source: https://srhospital.in/wp-content/uploads/2024/05/Vaccinate.jpg.

6.3.2. Prophylactic Medications

In travel and tropical medicine, prophylactic medication is a valuable means of prevention against a variety of infectious illnesses that may be acquired by travelers. The drugs are specifically designed to prevent infection before exposure, particularly in disease-endemic regions such as malaria, typhoid fever, and dengue. The selection of effective prophylactic therapy must consider patient-specific factors, including destination, travel time, and existing health conditions. For instance, some antimalarial drugs, such as atovaquone-proguanil or doxycycline, are prescribed based on the specific malaria transmission risk of the destination country. This pre-emptive action not only protects individual tourists but also contributes to public health by reducing the incidence of such diseases in vulnerable populations. Secondly, prophylactic drug effectiveness is highly dependent on ongoing developments in medical science and understanding of infectious disease dynamics. It is essential information, considering also the phenomenon of antibiotic resistance, in relation to aquaculture practices, as far as the administration of antibiotics with prophylactic intent. The broad application of these medicines can, as a byproduct, set the stage for the development of resistant bacteria, which, in turn, can endanger human health through the potential transmission of resistant pathogens (Pepi et al., 2021). Therefore, one needs to implement appropriate prescribing in combination with public health policies promoting the judicious use of prophylactic drugs. Appropriate medical education is also essential for physicians and other health care practitioners counseling travelers, so they can stay up to date on the latest guidelines and potential hazards associated with prophylactic drugs. Lastly, there is room for alternative preventive interventions, such as the use of essential oils, in tropical and travel medicine. While traditional medications have been effective, the prospect of essential oils, known for their anti-inflammatory and antimicrobial properties, is a fascinating area for investigation (Sharifi et al., 2017). Despite promising results noted in preclinical studies, there remains a wide gap in well-designed clinical trials demonstrating their safety and efficacy in humans. This gap limits the ability to fully endorse essential oils as effective prophylactic agents. Thus, the integration of these adjunct therapies must strike a balance between evidence from clinical research and conventional practice to further augment the roster of preventive methods at travelers' disposal while ensuring their safety and health during foreign travel.

6.3.3. Health Education and Awareness

In travel and tropical medicine, the role of health awareness and education cannot be overemphasized. Travelers go through various geographical landscapes and are subjected to several types of health risks that require multi-dimensional knowledge. Good health education equips travelers with the basic understanding of local diseases, precautions, and good health facilities in the host nations. This data is particularly significant in resource-limited environments, where consistent access to health care is compromised. Identifying gaps in countries like Nigeria, where poverty and wealth coexist, underscores the importance of the transmission of health information that holds the promise of dramatic improvements in population health. As seen, Nigeria's health problems are complex and inequity-based, thus requiring an earnest effort to improve health education for travelers and residents to enhance health literacy and outcomes (Abubakar et al., 2022). Additionally, the COVID-19 pandemic has further underscored the need for robust health education systems. The insights gained during the pandemic hastened the understanding of diagnostic capabilities and public health preparedness worldwide, demonstrating how information sharing can transform health outcomes. Countries with strong health education programs were better equipped to respond to pandemics and disseminate valuable information on health guidelines and vaccine administration. In that regard, this especially fits where technology innovation, from telehealth care to electronic health platforms, can assist in ensuring that vital health information reaches even the most vulnerable populations. Such application of technology to health education is, in itself, a significant channel through which individuals can be empowered, thus democratizing access to vital health information and resources (Fleming et al., 2021). The impact of such health education programs permeates deeply, especially in promoting the prevention of disease and healthy practices among travelers and host populations. Last but not least, the eradication of health inequalities requires a multisectoral approach that engages various stakeholders in tropical and travel medicine. There must be coordination among health educators, government authorities, non-governmental organizations, and host populations when formulating context-specific, culturally tailored integrated health education programs. Such partnerships can facilitate the establishment of focused programs raising awareness of specific diseases prevalent in given regions, encouraging public involvement and preventive interventions. Through local focus and utilizing the community's resources, programs have the potential to enhance health literacy leading to better health outcomes. Appreciation of the fact that health education is not a one-size-fits-all intervention highlights the imperative for locally derived solutions appealing to diverse populations. Lastly, raising awareness through education constructs a more informed populace capable of making healthier decisions and in the process propel the overall goals of internal medicine in tropical and travel settings (Abubakar et al., 2022) (Figure 6.8).

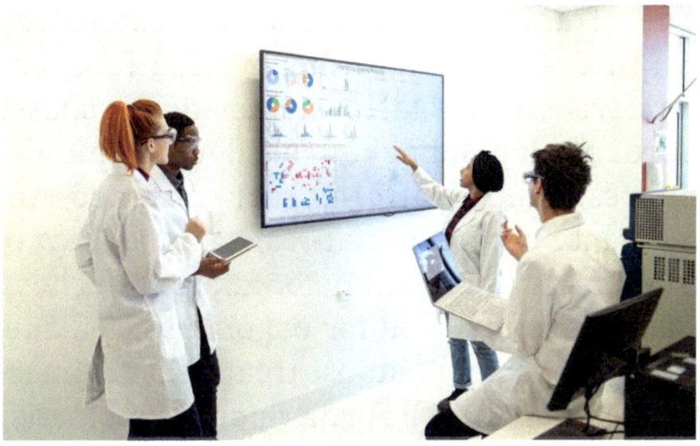

Figure 6.8. Health education and awareness.

Source: https://www.ruseducation.in/wp-content/uploads/2023/11/Addressing-Challenges-in-Medical-Education-for-Sustainable-Development.webp.

Test Your Knowledge

1. Name one commonly used prophylactic medication for malaria prevention and explain when it should be started.
2. Why is health education important in preventing dengue fever in tropical regions?

6.4. Diagnosis and Treatment

Learning Outcome

1. Diagnostic techniques
- Treatment protocols
- Challenges in treatment

Effective diagnosis and treatment of tropical and travel medicine are key to controlling infectious tropical diseases prevalent in specific geographic regions. Many factors contribute to the making of the diagnostic process more complicated, including overlapping presentations of various tropical illnesses and the relative infrequency of quick diagnostic tests. For instance, conditions such as malaria, dengue, and chikungunya can present with superimposable clinical manifestations, necessitating good insight into patient history, exposure, and geography in order to achieve appropriate diagnoses. The use of investigative tools, such as polymerase chain reaction (PCR) analysis, may enhance specificity in the identification of pathogens shared by tropical regions, as demonstrated in research recently carried out. In addition, clinicians must remain vigilant for re-emerging and emerging infections, particularly in immunocompromised patients with atypical presentations. The vigilance is pivotal in providing timely and adequate intervention to avoid morbidity and mortality of such diseases, emphasizing the need for robust diagnostic capabilities in the internal medicine practice of travel and tropical medicine (Mertes et al., 2023). In treatment management, the selection of effective therapeutic regimens is primarily guided by the identified pathogen and host factors such as immunological status and underlying health conditions. The rapidly developing issue of antimicrobial resistance extensively complicates the treatment situation, and therefore it necessitates an individually chosen approach depending on local epidemiology and resistance patterns. For instance, the emergence of tecovirimat-resistant monkeypox virus strains among immunocompromised hosts underscores the need for ongoing surveillance and the capacity to adjust treatment regimens (Mertes et al., 2023). Furthermore, combination therapy or the use of adjunctive drugs may enhance clinical outcomes, particularly in severe cases or resistance to conventional therapy. Clinicians must also stress the role of preventive intervention, such as vaccination and patient education, in order to reduce exposure risks in risk groups going to endemic regions to sustain the success of the treatment strategy. Multidisciplinary intervention is essential to the successful diagnosis and treatment of diseases encountered in tropical and travel medicine. Multidisciplinary intervention among infectious disease specialists, public health experts, and global health professionals ensures inclusive, context-sensitive care delivery. Combinations of clinical and epidemiologic knowledge, for example, may be used to guide interventions in areas of high transmission. Investigation also plays an essential role in the evolution of treatment models, with ongoing research revealing new therapeutics and infection-prevention strategies for tropical world-endemic infections. By fostering a culture of continuous learning and adaptation, health professionals are better equipped to navigate the complexities of diagnosis and treatment in this rapidly evolving field of medicine. Collectively, these initiatives ensure the long-term sustainability of health care systems for managing infectious diseases, underscoring the importance of internal medicine in global health.

6.4.1. Diagnostic Techniques

The function of diagnostic techniques in internal medicine, but particularly in tropical and travel medicine, is vital. They are essential for accurate diagnosis of diseases endemic to some regions but may still be unfamiliar to practitioners outside those localities. These diagnostic techniques can range from standard laboratory tests to advanced imaging modalities. In tropical medicine, where there are many endemic diseases, precise diagnostic skills assist clinicians in distinguishing among overlapping presentations. For instance, dengue fever, malaria, and typhoid fever can share overlapping manifestations, necessitating individual tests to guide appropriate treatment. In the absence of these approaches, misdiagnosis would be followed by increased morbidity, particularly among vulnerable groups who can be denied early intervention by medical practitioners, hence the significance of strict diagnostic procedures in such medical fields. Diagnostic techniques within the realm of travel medicine are key in predisposing travelers to encounter imminent health risks in the countries they visit. Pre-travel counseling, for the most part, emphasizes immunizations and prophylactic medications; nonetheless, the diagnosis of potential travel-acquired disease on return is also critical. Diagnostic methods, including serologic testing or polymerase chain reaction (PCR) assays, enable clinicians to diagnose viral infections such as Zika or West Nile virus in returned travelers from outbreak regions. Moreover, the value of early diagnosis extends beyond immediate patient care because accurate detection of recurrent cases has implications for public health response, informing outbreak surveillance and control activities. Expansion of these diagnostic techniques to primary care thus potentially facilitates better health outcomes and contributes to greater disease awareness among travelers. Besides, as global health concerns continue to evolve, so do the diagnostic techniques employed in travel and tropical medicine. Novel pathogens, such as those responsible for viral hemorrhagic fevers, pose significant diagnostic challenges, typically requiring specialized skills and technology. The application of novel molecular techniques, including next-generation sequencing, enables rapid identification and characterization of novel pathogens, thereby enhancing diagnostic accuracy. In addition, the use of telemedicine as an investigative service, particularly in rural settings, has gained traction, providing timely consultations and enhancing access to diagnostic centers. The application of these new technologies helps not only with clinical decision-making but also fortifies local health systems in low and middle-income countries (LMICs) with the highest rates of endemic diseases. Consequently, interventions to improve diagnostic techniques are essential for promoting equitable health care and aligning with global health programs, as required by Matthew et al. (2021) and Lain et al. (2020) (Figure 6.9).

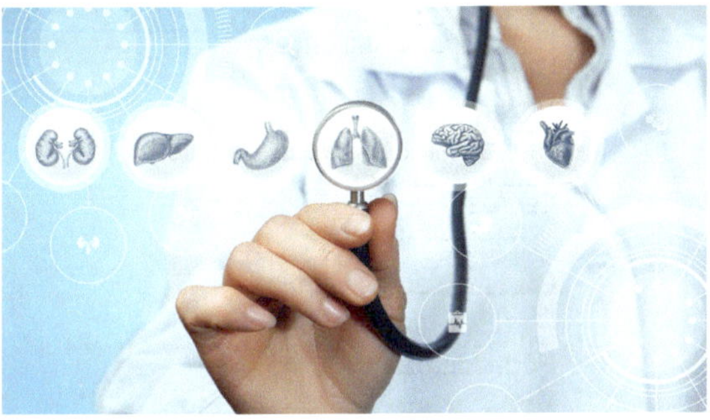

Figure 6.9. The importance of diagnostic techniques in internal medicine.

Source: https://www.bahealthpoint.com/images/content/actual/Internal-Medicine-Bahealthpoint.jpg.

6.4.2. Treatment Protocols

Treatment protocols in travel and tropical medicine form the hub of disease diagnosis and disease control in prevalent diseases in specific geographic areas. The protocols are important not only for the detection and treatment of infections endemic in the tropics, such as malaria, dengue fever, and schistosomiasis, but also for the particular demands of overseas travel. When patients return from endemic regions of these conditions, early detection and treatment in line with evidence-based guidelines can prevent severe health consequences. In addition, standardized treatment protocols provide healthcare professionals with a systematic approach to patient care, which ensures consistency in clinical practice, a quality that, in emergency care, can be a matter of utmost significance since rapid decision-making is of paramount importance. Incorporation of alternative and standard therapies into treatment protocols is critical in tropical and travel medicine. Historically, essential oils and plant extracts have been employed for therapeutic purposes, exhibiting antimicrobial, anti-inflammatory, and antioxidant properties, as outlined in various preclinical studies. While such natural treatments are a component of traditional medical systems around the globe, their incorporation into mainstream treatment regimens is justified, subject to close examination. The potential benefits must be weighed against the vast gaps in clinical trials that define efficacy and safety in man, as outlined in the literature. As the medical community continues to explore these therapeutic compounds, rigorous clinical trials are essential to determine their efficacy and realize their full potential as treatment options for tropical diseases (Sharifi et al., 2017). Besides, the global public health response to infectious disease outbreaks is radically different, tempered by experience gained from past emergencies. The Ebola outbreak underscores the critical need for concerted treatment approaches that integrate prevention, detection, and response mechanisms. The panel's suggestions focus on calling on countries to invest in high-quality healthcare infrastructure that can facilitate rapid intervention upon outbreak occurrence. By offering an early reporting and intensive treatment model for infectious diseases, nations can improve their preparedness for epidemics to come. Regimes that combine treatments should therefore be supported not only by short-term clinical treatment but also by a comprehensive public health response aimed at the socio-political determinants of health, eventually leading to the development of strong health systems that can withstand new health challenges (Moon et al., 2015).

6.4.3. Challenges in Treatment

The complexity of tropical infections and travel-related diseases stems from both biological and logistical limitations. To begin with, tropical infections possess diverse pathophysiological mechanisms; thus, they are complicated to diagnose and treat. Malaria, dengue fever, and schistosomiasis all require tailored treatment based on their etiologies and drug resistance. With more widespread drug-resistant strains, as evidenced by rising counts of resistant malaria cases, practitioners are faced with the continuous challenge of needing to adjust treatment protocols to achieve optimal efficacy and minimize morbidity. In addition, inaccurate diagnostic tests in low-resource countries further complicate treatment delays, limiting patients' access to timely intervention. Therefore, addressing these issues requires an extensive understanding of the epidemiological contexts in which these diseases occur and a commitment to enhancing diagnostic and treatment capabilities (Matthew et al., 2021).

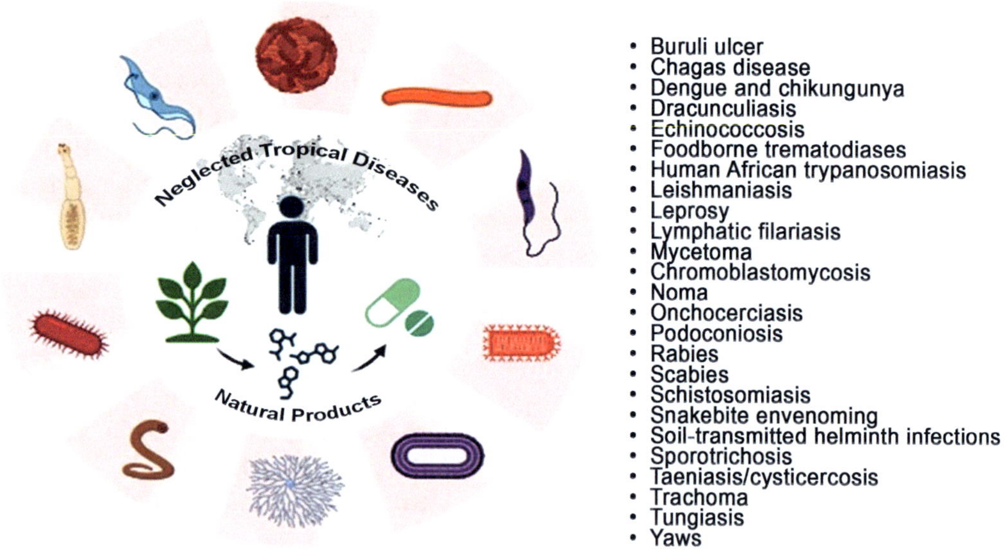

Figure 6.10. The multifaceted challenges in treating tropical and travel-related diseases stem from both biological and logistical barriers.

Source: https://www.mdpi.com/files/special_issues_graphic_abstract/3020/ga_banner_natural_products_against_NTD.png.

Logistical issues also serve as a catalyzing agent in changing treatment options for tropical diseases. Healthcare provision in middle-income and low-income countries (LMICs) is often compromised by inadequate infrastructure, which limits the timely delivery of medicines and healthcare. Political instability and economic constraints also challenge this factor, potentially weakening supply chains and access to the much-needed medication. The over-proportionate morbidity of tropical diseases among children, women, and marginalized groups further complicates the provision of healthcare. These groups usually face barriers to accessing care due to underlying societal inequalities, and hence it is imperative that healthcare providers craft inclusive policies that serve vulnerable groups. Successful treatment of tropical diseases, therefore, requires not only better medical care but also an effective system that addresses the social determinants of health and makes a concerted effort to reduce disparities in access to care (Lain et al., 2020). The interface between climate change and the evolution of emerging pathogens is another challenge for the practice of tropical and travel medicine. As temperatures rise globally, the range of most infectious diseases shifts, with more habitats for vector-borne diseases like Zika and Lyme disease, respectively, through mosquitoes and ticks. This shifting epidemiology continues to challenge clinicians and public health authorities to predict disease epidemics and implement prevention interventions effectively. In addition, as international mobility increases, individuals can unknowingly introduce pathogens into new regions, complicating local healthcare efforts. To counter these emerging challenges, interdisciplinary collaboration, strong surveillance mechanisms, and flexible treatment protocols will be essential. Through an interactive process, the global health community can better adapt to the evolving patterns of tropical diseases to keep therapeutic interventions both effective and available to populations most at risk (Matthew et al., 2021) (Figure 6.10).

Test Your Knowledge

1. What is the gold standard diagnostic method for confirming malaria infection?
2. Which class of drugs is commonly used to treat schistosomiasis, and what is the standard treatment?
3. What is one major challenge in treating dengue fever?

6.5. Role of Travel Medicine

Learning Outcome

1. Pre-travel consultations
2. Risk assessment
3. Post-travel follow-up

Travel medicine is a significant component of internal medicine, particularly in the prevention and treatment of diseases arising from travel to foreign countries. Travel medicine addresses pre-travel planning, identifying potential health hazards for every country, and protective measures such as immunizations and health warnings. By considering a person's past, current health, and planned itinerary, doctors can modify recommendations and interventions to reduce the risk of travel-related illness, particularly endemic tropical diseases. This visionary approach not only protects public health but also allows people to enjoy their travels safely, underscoring the vital role of travel medicine in internal medicine for tropical and travel diseases. Progressive globalization of travel has increased the importance of travel medicine, especially in the management of infectious diseases. They are at risk of exposure to pathogens not typically encountered in their home countries due to varying levels of public health and hygiene. The travel medicine practitioner also has a role in educating travelers on prevention, including safe food handling and the consumption of clean water. Further, these specialists monitor and respond to foreign health threats, such as outbreaks of diseases like Zika or cholera, to support critical responses to new health conditions that may affect returning travelers and communities that harbor them. Through a convergence of individual health and global health forces, travel medicine is then a combination of personal patient care and public health monitoring. With the complexities of travel, the practice of travel medicine is not merely prevention against infectious disease, but instead an expansive umbrella of health concerns, including mental illness and chronic disease management. Pretravel patients with established disease, i.e., diabetes or cardiovascular disease, require careful planning when traveling overseas because stress associated with travel can potentially exacerbate such disease. Travel medicine physicians offer comprehensive assessments and treatment recommendations, suggesting medication needs when traveling and potential changes needed due to variations in time zones or diet. The overall view elevates the role of travel medicine within internal medicine, with its holistic approach to health and well-being—essential to the provision of safe global mobility and to the encouragement of healthy intercultural exchange among travelers.

6.5.1. Pre-Travel Consultations

Pre-travel consultations are an essential component of travel medicine that serves as a pre-emptive measure in equipping travelers with the necessary information and interventions to minimize health risks associated with foreign travel. Personal health needs are assessed, and particular diseases common in the destination nation are considered, which can vary widely depending on geographical and seasonal factors. For example, travelers to the tropics may need to be vaccinated against, for instance, yellow fever or typhoid, and others may need to take antimalarial medication to protect against malaria. Such personalized advice is not just beneficial to one's health but also serves an invaluable role in disease prevention at a collective level, even cutting down on outbreaks back home among populations upon the traveler's return. Through such consultations, travelers are adequately prepared to respond to health risks efficiently, creating an active response to their travel experience. Pre-travel consultations are being compelled by the new health security dynamics of global health threats, as exemplified, particularly in the wake of the COVID-19 pandemic. In deliberations on models of public health, an operational primary health care system is essential for managing endemic and emergent health problems. Travel medicine practitioners must stay abreast of current health advisories, which typically include vaccine recommendations, safety measures, and the likelihood of needing medical equipment during the journey. The dynamic nature of health advisories means that a good understanding of health requirements at home and abroad is required so that travelers are provided with accurate and up-to-date information. To that end, consultation then is not just an opportunity for personal health assessment but also an arena in which travelers are educated about responsible health behavior and compliance with national health guidelines. Further, the role of pre-travel consultation extends beyond explicit health counseling, linking public health and personal healthcare. It provides an opportunity to assess other social determinants of health, including familiarity with the destination country's health systems, presence of medical centers, and availability of emergency services. For tourists from low- and middle-income countries, familiarity with local health care may be beneficial, as health service inequalities will affect their travel schedules and security. As enumerated in ongoing health discourses, addressing these inequalities is essential to guarantee comprehensive care.

Pre-travel consultations are beneficial to the single traveler but also help foster a shared understanding of health risks, enhance universal health coverage, make it more applicable, and underscore the necessity of equal access to the right health resources. Through this awareness, travelers can navigate global environments more securely and confidently, advancing the overall goals of travel medicine (Figure 6.11).

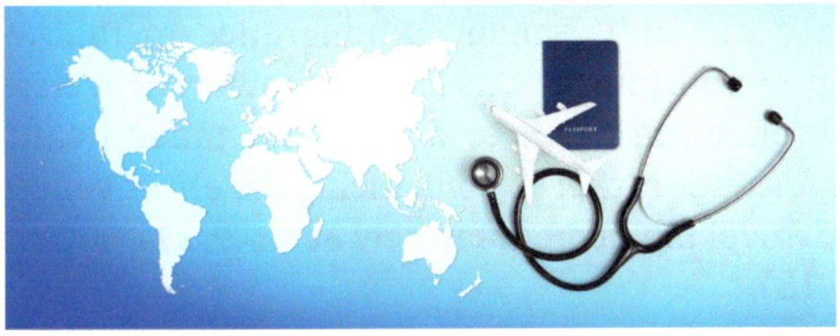

Figure 6.11. Pre-travel consultations are a crucial component of travel medicine.

Source: https://blog.oncallinternational.com/wp-content/uploads/2023/05/iStock-1159847006.jpg.

6.5.2. Risk Assessment

Risk assessment plays a key role in internal medicine for travel and tropical medicine in directing clinical decision-making. Appropriate risk assessment begins with identifying potential health risks to travelers and residents in tropical regions. This might involve evaluating the prevalence of infectious diseases, such as malaria, dengue fever, and the Zika virus, which are known to pose significant health risks in such settings. Sound collection and analysis of data, including that from the WHO, enable the creation of targeted recommendations and interventions. The confluence of epidemiological data and patient history is key to the creation of a general risk profile, which can be used to guide preventive interventions such as vaccination and prophylactic drug administration (Heymann et al., 2020). In addition, the changing nature of infectious disease epidemiology necessitates continued risk assessment throughout the travel experience. As travelers transit from place to place, the risk of exposure to diverse pathogens differs dramatically. For instance, travelers will encounter places where outbreaks of diseases that were formerly under control are occurring. Temporal management of testing is important; policies written in the context of an outbreak must be adaptable as new information is acquired and public health scenarios evolve. This highlights the importance of situational details and effective communication among public health authorities and healthcare providers, so that tourists are informed timely manner on the basis of current data (Slater et al., 2016). Beyond infectious conditions, climate variability is a significant factor in risk assessments in tropical and travel medicine. Climate change can lead to the emergence and re-emergence of various vector-borne infections, thus posing new risks for the healthcare system. Risk assessments must consider not only the current health situation but also future directions based on climatic variations. More international travel creates greater population interconnectedness, raising the demand for more comprehensive risk assessment models that include environmental determinants of health. These have to integrate evidence from epidemiological studies, patient history, and environmental inquiry to maximize preventive care and more efficiently defend public health (Heymann et al., 2020).

6.5.3. Post-Travel Follow-Up

On return from foreign travel, especially to the tropics or an endemic region, there is a need for organized follow-up to diagnose and treat any health issues developed during travel. The follow-up should begin with a proper history of the traveler's medical conditions, including symptoms that could suggest infections or illnesses acquired abroad. These include typical conditions such as malaria, dengue fever, and typhoid, which are significant considerations, particularly in low- and middle-income countries where travelers might be exposed.

As stated, a high proportion of travelers might have related illnesses that remain undetected during initial assessment, thus requiring follow-up visits for early diagnosis and treatment. Educational campaigns should also highlight the necessity of follow-up care and symptom reporting to reduce risks and promote improved health outcomes (Matthew et al., 2021). The use of community-based health workers (CHWs) can enhance the effectiveness of post-travel follow-up, as their well-established connections with communities will lead to stronger compliance with the follow-up protocol. CHWs are responsible for the dissemination of continuing education on returning traveler symptoms and for enabling individuals to seek appropriate medical care. In addition, studies have indicated that CHW programs are more effective in terms of health outcomes when properly integrated into community health systems, providing the logistical support and resources needed for program sustainability (Scott et al., 2018). This approach recognizes that community-level interventions can help fill gaps in healthcare delivery by ensuring that even marginalized groups receive timely, adequate follow-up care. By leveraging CHWs' strengths, health systems can effectively screen travelers for post-travel syndromes and respond more efficiently. Furthermore, technology can significantly improve post-travel follow-up care. Digital health technologies, such as telemedicine and mobile health applications, can empower healthcare workers to maintain contact with travelers, monitor for symptoms, and guide them through recovery phases remotely. This becomes particularly crucial for individuals who may face geographical constraints or find it challenging to access healthcare facilities upon their return. Effective health communication can prompt timely reminders about preventive practices or tests and even deliver essential information about them. The integration of such technological advancements into post-travel care not only enhances adherence to follow-up appointments but also empowers travelers by enabling them to access and tailor health information, thereby enhancing the effectiveness of travel medicine (Matthew et al., 2021) (Figure 6.12).

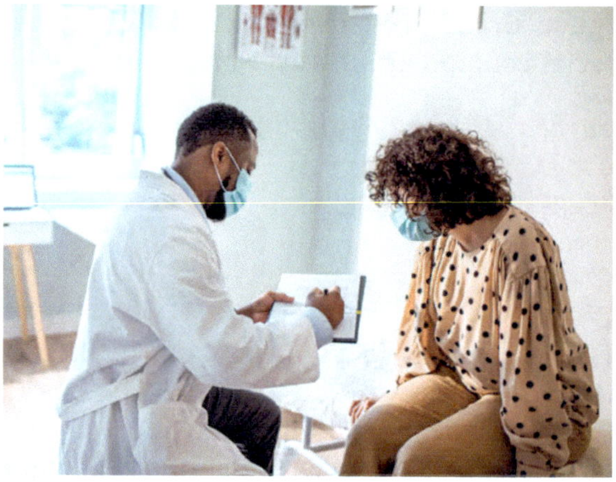

Figure 6.12. Upon returning from international travel.

Source: https://media.post.rvohealth.io/wp-content/uploads/2020/07/doctor-doing-a-medical-exam-732x549-thumbnail.jpg.

Test Your Knowledge

1. What is the primary purpose of a pre-travel medical consultation?
2. Why is post-travel follow-up necessary for travelers returning from tropical regions?

6.6. Global Health Perspectives

Learning Outcome

1. Impact of climate change
2. Socioeconomic factors
3. International collaboration in disease control

The intersection of global health thought and internal medicine, particularly in tropical and travel medicine, is a cross-disciplinary knowledge of health inequalities and structural inequities that define regions of the world. The COVID-19 pandemic brutally exposed disparities, underscoring the need for real-time, accurate diagnostics to ensure optimal healthcare delivery. Consequently, the Lancet Commission on Diagnostics identified the need to enhance diagnostic capacity in low and middle-income countries (LMICs), where access to testing remains largely inadequate. Of most significant concern is the described diagnostic gap, in which a high percentage of the population remains undiagnosed for major conditions and therefore cannot be directed along effective treatment paths (Fleming et al., 2021). In consequence, the implications of poor diagnostic facilities point to a specific area of necessity for practitioners in travel and tropical medicine: the development of robust diagnostic systems to address such persistent shortcomings in international health care systems. Placing a focus on global health in internal medicine goes beyond diagnosis to encompass the broader context of health equity. One of the very crucial components of this is eye health, which has emerged as a key consideration in striving for universal health coverage in an integrated way. Vision impairment disproportionately affects populations in LMICs, where accessible, quality eye care does not exist. With over half a billion people affected by visual impairments, predominantly due to avoidable or treatable conditions, the importance of integrated health interventions becomes clear (Matthew et al., 2021). The effective management of such conditions, in turn, is associated with the implementation of integrative healthcare policies aimed at reducing overall health disparities. It is imperative for internal medicine and travel medicine practitioners to understand how vision health intersects with integrative care plans.

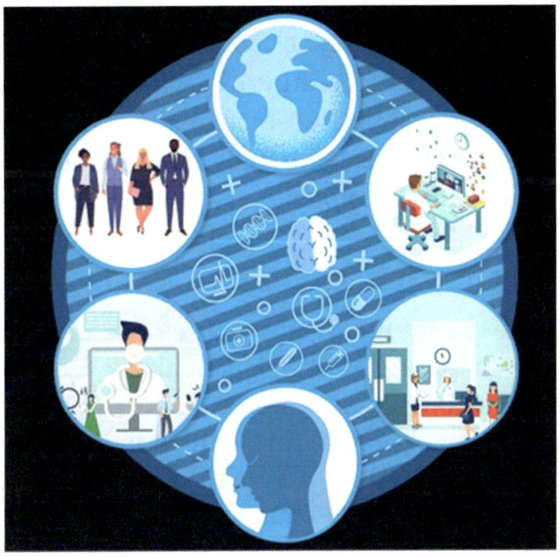

Figure 6.13. The intersection of global health perspectives with internal medicine.

Source: https://media.deloitte.com/is/image/deloitte/gx-lshc-2022-health-care-outlook-banner:Mobile?$Responsive$&fmt=webp&fit=stretch,1&dpr=on,2.625.

Closing these gaps not only maximizes individual results but also enhances community health resilience, leading to a more equitable global model of health. Finally, a critical analysis of innovation's role within global health discourse focuses on the potential of technological innovations to address weaknesses in the healthcare delivery system. In tropical and travel medicine, embracing digital health technologies, telemedicine, and point-of-care testing can radically enhance access to essential healthcare services, particularly in resource-limited settings. The recent rapid progress in innovation has opened new paths in diagnostics and treatment, creating opportunities to democratize healthcare access for marginalized communities. Furthermore, overcoming the challenges to effective utilization of such technologies is essential, as evidenced by the persistence of underfunding and inadequate infrastructure in most regions (Fleming et al., 2021). The path forward entails advocating for profound policy changes that prioritize investment in technology within existing healthcare systems, so that health technology success translates into real improvements in health outcomes globally (Figure 6.13).

6.6.1. Impact of Climate Change

Climate change is also emerging as a determining factor in public health, particularly in travel medicine and tropical medicine. As the climate warms globally, the trends in infectious diseases and disease vectors are rapidly transforming. For instance, climate-change-related alterations in precipitation and humidity patterns create permissive niches for pathogens such as those responsible for dengue fever and malaria, making erstwhile low-risk locales susceptible. Aside from direct health implications, secondary effects such as food insecurity may also result from climate change, adding to the stress on healthcare systems in affected communities. Unhealthy vision has also been linked to climatic factors, with increased exposure to UV light worsening vision problems such as cataracts and macular degeneration, underscoring the need for widespread eye health interventions amid changing environmental conditions (Matthew et al., 2021). Apart from infectious diseases, food-borne disease incidence is also expected to rise due to climate change. The impact of rising temperatures on food safety cannot be underestimated, particularly because they create favorable conditions for the growth of food-borne pathogens. Zoonotic infections, in which pathogens predominantly originate from animal foodstuffs, will likely thrive under such conditions, increasing the risk of human infection through consumption of infected foodstuffs (Abebe et al., 2020). This poses compelling challenges to travel medicine experts. Travelers to the tropics, however, are also at risk of these conditions and therefore need to have good pre-travel health counseling that includes dietary precautions to avoid potential food-related health risks. Climate change also exacerbates existing health inequalities, particularly in low- and middle-income countries (LMICs), whose healthcare systems are less likely to cope with upcoming challenges. Susceptible populations such as women and children are disproportionately affected, with greater exposure to climate change health impacts and limited accessibility to healthcare resources. The intersection between the healthcare sector and climate change in such populations requires a more comprehensive approach to tropical and travel medicine. Eye care and vision-related problems, as well as general health issues, need to be addressed to improve overall health in the affected population. It involves investing in health facilities and adopting green practices to mitigate the negative impacts while optimizing public health outcomes (Matthew et al., 2021).

6.6.2. Socioeconomic Factors

The influence of socioeconomic determinants on health outcomes, in general and particularly in tropical and travel medicine, is far-reaching and profound. Poverty, a ubiquitous feature across most of the globe, aggravates the vulnerability of populations to most diseases, including the neglected tropical diseases such as Human African Trypanosomiasis (HAT). The compromised level of access to healthcare resources by lower socioeconomic status impedes timely diagnoses and treatments, allowing diseases to propagate unchecked. The current disease detection and control systems do not reach poor communities, underscoring the need for integrated health interventions that prioritize economic accessibility. The strategies must incorporate improving participation and infrastructure with a direct impact on accessibility to healthcare, ultimately pursuing the elimination of diseases that arise from socioeconomic disparities, such as in the instances of HAT, where effective control measures remain insufficient (Chappuis et al., 2011). Besides poverty, education has a very significant effect on health literacy and, consequently, on health outcomes in the tropics. Poor education is characterized by limited knowledge of disease prevention and control, including endemic diseases such as anemia in children. A study in Tanzania, for example, revealed very high rates of child anemia under five years and socioeconomic status as the primary determinant factor of underlying risk determinants. For instance, the deficit of anemia treatments and non-awareness of its importance can lead to severe effects on health, as most of the cases remain undetected until they reach critical stages (Schellenberg et al., 2003). Therefore, investing in health literacy schemes that educate individuals can help them understand health problems and advocate for themselves, improving public health. Besides, the interplay between socioeconomic determinants and environmental conditions cannot be overstated in tropical medicine. Where sanitation and access to clean water are poor, susceptibility to infectious disease increases significantly. Populations plagued by poverty usually live in settings that are conducive to vector transmission, such as tsetse flies that cause HAT. This overlap between socioeconomic distress and environmental degradation calls for a multilayered public health response. Interventions must target improvements in living standards alongside access to healthcare, reflecting an integrated understanding of how socioeconomic determinants shape health. In responding to these underlying factors, public health interventions can yield more effective interventions that diminish the impact of tropical diseases and advance international health equity (Chappuis et al., 2011) (Figure 6.14).

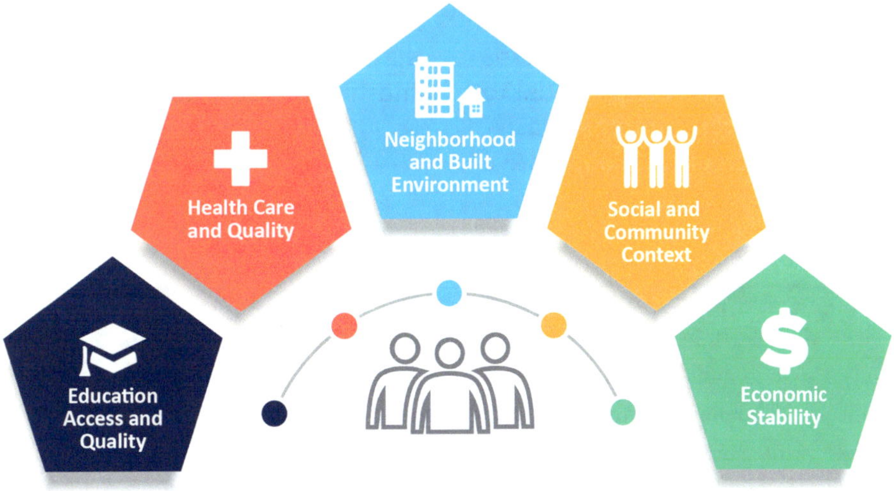

Figure 6.14. The influence of socioeconomic factors on health outcomes.

Source: https://www.cdc.gov/public-health-gateway/media/images/images/sdoh/SDOH-icons.png.

6.6.3. International Collaboration in Disease Control

Increased global interconnectedness has emphasized the necessity of global collaboration in disease control, particularly in tropical and travel medicine. As international travel continues to increase, infectious diseases cross borders, posing a significant threat to health systems worldwide. The COVID-19 outbreak highlighted the sheer necessity of early and accurate diagnostics, exposing stark disparities in diagnostic capacity across regions. These disparities are most dramatic among low- and middle-income nations, where almost 47% of the population lacks adequate access to essential diagnostics. Without convergent diagnostic capacity, outbreak control is severely compromised, underpinning the need for a joint global response enabled by global funds, international know-how, and innovation (Fleming et al., 2021). Furthermore, the presence of tropical diseases is of immense utility in contextualizing solutions to the attendant complex problems they pose, which disproportionately affect high-risk groups in resource-limited settings. Multi-sectoral control of disease should incorporate research, surveillance, and the implementation of interventions consistent with local health priorities. Involvement of various stakeholders, including governments, non-governmental organizations, and private sector partners, facilitates knowledge sharing and the attainment of innovative solutions tailored to unique epidemiological contexts. For instance, the integration of the use of telecommunications and mobile health projects has the potential to enhance the tracking and responding capacity of diseases in hard-to-reach areas. Cooperative structures should also pledge to invest in the health workforce's capacity, ensuring that health workers are equipped with the skills and tools necessary to combat infectious diseases (Matthew et al., 2021). Ultimately, the future of disease control depends on ongoing international collaboration, particularly in addressing emerging health threats. The interconnected environment of the current globalized world requires the establishment of coalitions that transcend geographical boundaries and enable the exchange of information, technologies, and best practices. Mobilization of resources and capacities for the building of integrated health strategies as a vehicle for enhancing preparedness and response to infectious disease outbreaks becomes a necessity. Against this backdrop, the encouragement of a culture of interdisciplinarity, sectoral cooperation, and global collaboration seems a pillar towards improved global health outcomes. As the COVID-19 pandemic has shown, collaboration is crucial towards building strong health systems that can withstand future adversity in tropical and travel medicine (Fleming et al., 2021).

Test Your Knowledge

1. How does climate change influence the spread of tropical diseases like malaria and dengue?
2. Why are low-income communities more vulnerable to tropical diseases?
3. Give one example of international collaboration in controlling tropical diseases.

SUMMARY

An internal medicine review for travel and tropical medicine; it is also critical to be sensitive to the myriad challenges posed by endemic diseases, as well as the impact of globalization on health. With increasing ease of travel, exposure to multiple endemic infections poses a growing risk, necessitating a sophisticated understanding of infectious diseases among health practitioners. Effective management of such conditions also relies heavily on continuous education, targeted preventive care, and an emphasis on high-burden areas, primarily in the developing world. Complications arising from susceptibility to zoonotic diseases make it all the more challenging, as food-borne transmission of bacterial pathogens, a foremost contributor to global morbidity, underscores safe food handling in conjunction with effective healthcare strategies (Abebe et al., 2020). Thus, an integrated strategy must account for the interlinkages among public health, behavior, and travel. In addition, the use of community-based health worker (CHW) programs offers a pragmatic solution to bridging gaps in healthcare delivery for tropical and travel medicine. Evidence shows that successful CHW programs are characterized by integration within the community, support, and adequate logistical capacity, making them more efficient (Scott et al., 2018). These kinds of programs are significant avenues for the transmission of health information, the articulation of preventive regimens, and the care of urgent health issues among travelers and inhabitants of endemic areas, in like manner. Besides, community participation in the operation of the programs increases a sense of belongingness and accountability, which are essential for the long-term sustainability of health programs. With education and resource empowerment of the local population, CHWs can reduce infectious disease transmission and improve overall health outcomes in the target communities. Finally, the convergence of educational initiatives, effective surveillance systems, and the empowerment of community health assets is a key part of addressing the complexities of internal medicine and its linkages to tropical and travel medicine. The advent of multidrug-resistant zoonotic pathogens necessitates an organized response towards monitoring and surveillance, especially in resource-poor environments where healthcare infrastructure may be poor (Abebe et al., 2020). Secondly, scale-up of interventions through CHW programs with local contextual adaptations can enhance their sustainability and impact (Scott et al., 2018). A commitment, therefore, to interdisciplinarity and policy adaptability emerges as key to strengthening global public health endeavors in the wake of an increasingly developing international world. The merging of successful practice with innovative community engagement is sure to chart the course of internal medicine, particularly in tropical and travel medicine paradigms.

The internal medicine specialty is relevant to the practice of tropical and travel medicine because its practitioners must have a firm understanding of the unique health conditions arising from international travel and tropical diseases. As globalization increases, medical professionals must contend with infectious diseases one can contract while traveling overseas. Key considerations include preventive measures, such as vaccinations and prophylactic medications, to avoid the dangers posed by diseases such as malaria, dengue fever, and typhoid. Internal medicine also highlights the importance of pre-travel consultation, during which medical personnel can assess personal risk and provide individualized guidance. Pre-trip review of entry requirements, regional health alerts, and endemic diseases not only informs travelers with data but also helps avoid theoretical public health risks, illustrating the central role of internal medicine in the safety of travelers and indigenous populations. Concurrent with preventive therapy, internal medicine of tropical and travel medicine emphasizes the necessity of proper diagnosis and management of tropical diseases upon patients' return to their home countries. The range of possible infections can vary from well-known diseases such as schistosomiasis and leishmaniasis to more emergent situations caused by newly discovered pathogens, as seen in recent outbreaks. It is crucial to understand the epidemiology, modes of transmission, and clinical features of these diseases to effectively treat and control them. The professionals here must also remain alert to complications resulting from misdiagnosis or delayed treatment, which can drastically alter patients' outcomes. Research indicates that early interventions significantly affect morbidity and mortality rates for infections treated early compared with untreated infections, further confirming the critical role internal medicine professionals play in acute clinical presentations (Xifaras et al., 2022). In addition to individual patient practice, practice in internal medicine of tropical and travel medicine involves a more population health approach, at least in terms of the implications of genetic testing and advances in diagnostic technology. Genetic considerations come into play, in particular in the at-risk populations for hereditary disease and infectious disease with genetic susceptibilities, such as certain forms of malaria. Diagnostic approaches, facilitated by next-generation sequencing, provide data that can inform family and individual health plans. However, there are still challenges, including a need for greater genetic literacy among clinicians and enhanced insurance coverage for genetic testing. These challenges highlight the importance of integrating genetic counseling into standard care pathways. According to modern literature, the evolving landscape of genetic testing holds the potential to improve patient diagnoses and inform preventive measures, thereby forming a more streamlined path for internal medicine in the evolving interplay between personalized healthcare and public health (Kiryluk et al., 2019).

KEY TERMS FROM THIS CHAPTER

- Beyond developments
- Clinical practice guidelines
- Diagnostic capabilities
- Disease transmission
- ecological changes
- Foreign pathogens
- Health challenges
- Clinical information
- Contemporary
- Diagnostic equipment
- Distant territories
- Ecological resilience
- Global pandemics
- Health professionals

CRITICAL THINKING QUESTIONS

1. **Which organism causes malaria?**
   a. *Aedes aegypti*
   b. *Trypanosoma cruzi*
   c. *Plasmodium* spp.
   d. *Leishmania donovani*
2. **What is the primary vector for Dengue Fever?**
   a. Anopheles mosquito
   b. Aedes aegypti mosquito
   c. Culex mosquito
   d. Tsetse fly
3. **Which disease is prevented by the yellow fever vaccine?**
   a. Zika virus
   b. Malaria
   c. Yellow fever
   d. Typhoid
4. **Which medication is commonly used for malaria prophylaxis?**
   a. Azithromycin
   b. Doxycycline
   c. Amoxicillin
   d. Metronidazole
5. **Schistosomiasis is acquired through exposure to:**
   a. Infected blood
   b. Contaminated food
   c. Freshwater containing cercariae
   d. Insect bites

Short Answer Questions

1. What are the most common tropical diseases transmitted by mosquitoes?
2. Which vaccine is recommended for travelers going to sub-Saharan Africa to prevent yellow fever?
3. What is the first-line treatment for uncomplicated malaria?
4. Which parasite causes schistosomiasis?
5. What are the typical symptoms of dengue fever?

Answers to Critical Thinking Questions

1. (c); 2. (b); 3. (c); 4. (b); 5. (c)

REFERENCES

1. Abebe, E., Gugsa, G., & Ahmed, M. (2020). Review on Major Food-Borne Zoonotic Bacterial Pathogens. *Journal of Tropical Medicine, 2020*, 1–19. https://doi.org/10.1155/2020/4674235 Abubakar, I., Dalglish, S. L., Angell, B., Sanuade, O. A., Abímbọ́lá, Ṣ., Adamu, A. L., Adetifa, I., et al. (2022). The Lancet Nigeria Commission: Investing in health and the future of the nation. *The Lancet, 399*, 1155–1200. https://doi.org/10.1016/s0140-6736(21)02488-0 (accessed on 17th July 2025).
2. Antinori, S., Clerinx, J., Develoux, M., Gjorup, K., et al. (2017). An 8-year multi-center observational study. https://core.ac.uk/download/199420704.pdf (accessed on 17th July 2025).
3. Armstrong Schellenberg, J. R. M., Mbuya, C., Mgalula, L., Mushi, A., et al. (2003). The silent burden of anemia in Tanzania children: A community-based study. https://core.ac.uk/download/pdf/11307081.pdf (accessed on 17th July 2025).
4. Bourhy, H., Gaidet, N., & Molia, S. (2012). Mission to Indonesia to participate to the 1st Indonesia-France Seminar in Medicine & Public Health and investigate potential collaborations on animal health: 2nd–9th of November 2012. http://agritrop.cirad.fr/567354/1/document_567354.pdf (accessed on 17th July 2025).
5. Burton, M. J., Ramke, J., Marques, A. P., Bourne, R., Congdon, N., Jones, I., Ah Tong, B. A. M., et al. (2021). The Lancet Global Health Commission on global eye health: Vision beyond 2020. *The Lancet Global Health, 9*, e489–e551. https://doi.org/10.1016/s2214-109x(20)30488-5 (accessed on 17th July 2025).
6. Chappuis, F., & Malvy, D. (2011). Sleeping sickness. https://core.ac.uk/download/pdf/10674293.pdf (accessed on 17th July 2025).
7. Clark, P. A., Edara, R. S., Lee, M. J. H., Myers, A., et al. (2016). Zika virus: Can artificial contraception be condoned? https://core.ac.uk/download/131207271.pdf (accessed on 17th July 2025).
8. de Jong, H. K., & Grobusch, M. (2024). Monoclonal antibody applications in travel medicine. *Tropical Diseases, Travel Medicine and Vaccines, 10*. https://www.semanticscholar.org/paper/117073b00913d7d2caf86cdd75b231fc1352042d (accessed on 17th July 2025).
9. Fleming, K. A., Horton, S., Wilson, M. L., Atun, R., DeStigter, K., Flanigan, J., Sayed, S., et al. (2021). The Lancet Commission on diagnostics: Transforming access to diagnostics. *The Lancet, 398*, 1997–2050. https://doi.org/10.1016/s0140-6736(21)00673-5 (accessed on 17th July 2025).
10. Grandmaison, G., Grobéty, T., Vaucher, J., Hayoz, D., & Suter, P. (2024). Prevalence of critical errors and insufficient peak inspiratory flow in patients hospitalized with COPD in a department of general internal medicine: A cross-sectional study. *Chronic Obstructive Pulmonary Diseases*. https://www.semanticscholar.org/paper/779fce36de569bcf34cb7440d377344e1c132a23 (accessed on 17th July 2025).
11. Hanson, K., Brikci, N., Erlangga, D., Abebe, A., De Allegri, M., Balabanova, D., Blecher, M., et al. (2022). The Lancet Global Health Commission on financing primary health care: Putting people at the centre. *The Lancet Global Health, 10*, e715–e772. https://doi.org/10.1016/s2214-109x(22)00005-5 (accessed on 17th July 2025).

12. Heymann, D., & Shindo, N. (2020). COVID-19: What is next for public health? *The Lancet, 395*, 542–545. https://doi.org/10.1016/s0140-6736(20)30374-3 (accessed on 17th July 2025).

13. Kiryluk, K., Goldstein, D., Rowe, J., Gharavi, A., Wapner, R., & Chung, W. (2019). Precision medicine in internal medicine. *Annals of Internal Medicine, 170*, 635–642. https://www.semanticscholar.org/paper/c7199e8a5226f8d9d55777da0e15e91797bb459a (accessed on 17th July 2025).

14. Lainé, C., Cotton, D., & Moyer, D. V. (2020). COVID-19 vaccine: Promoting vaccine acceptance. *Annals of Internal Medicine, 174*, 252–253. https://doi.org/10.7326/m20-8008 (accessed on 17th July 2025).

15. Marselle, M. R., Hartig, T., Cox, D. T. C., de Bell, S., Knapp, S., Lindley, S., Triguero-Mas, M., et al. (2021). Pathways linking biodiversity to human health: A conceptual framework. *Environment International, 150*, 106420–106420. https://doi.org/10.1016/j.envint.2021.106420 (accessed on 17th July 2025).

16. Mertes, H., Rezende, A. M., Brosius, I., Naesens, R., Míchiels, J., de Block, T., Coppens, J., et al. (2023). Tecovirimat resistance in an immunocompromised patient with Mpox and prolonged viral shedding. *Annals of Internal Medicine, 176*, 1141–1143. https://doi.org/10.7326/l23-0131 (accessed on 17th July 2025).

17. Moon, S., Sridhar, D., Pate, M. A., Jha, A. K., Clinton, C., Delaunay, S., Edwin, V., et al. (2015). Will Ebola change the game? Ten essential reforms before the next pandemic. The report of the Harvard-LSHTM Independent Panel on the Global Response to Ebola. *The Lancet, 386*, 2204–2221. https://doi.org/10.1016/s0140-6736(15)00946-0 (accessed on 17th July 2025).

18. Nii-Trebi, N. I. (2017). Emerging and neglected infectious diseases: Insights, advances, and challenges. *BioMed Research International, 2017*, 1–15. https://doi.org/10.1155/2017/5245021 (accessed on 17th July 2025).

19. Pepi, M., & Focardi, S. (2021). Antibiotic-resistant bacteria in aquaculture and climate change: A challenge for health in the Mediterranean area. *International Journal of Environmental Research and Public Health, 18*, 5723–5723. https://doi.org/10.3390/ijerph18115723 (accessed on 17th July 2025).

20. Runge-Ranzinger, S., TDR, & WHO. (2016). *Technical Handbook for Dengue Surveillance, Dengue Outbreak Prediction/Detection and Outbreak Response (Model Contingency Plan).* https://core.ac.uk/download/74363862.pdf (accessed on 17th July 2025).

21. Scheffer, M., Carpenter, S. R., Dakos, V., & van Nes, E. H. (2015). Generic indicators of ecological resilience: Inferring the chance of a critical transition. *Annual Review of Ecology, Evolution, and Systematics, 46*, 145–167. https://doi.org/10.1146/annurev-ecolsys-112414-054242 (accessed on 17th July 2025).

22. Schwellnus, M., Soligard, T., Alonso, J. M., Bahr, R., Clarsen, B., Dijkstra, H. P., Gabbett, T. J., et al. (2016). How much is too much? (Part 2) International Olympic Committee consensus statement on load in sport and risk of illness. *British Journal of Sports Medicine, 50*, 1043–1052. https://doi.org/10.1136/bjsports-2016-096572 (accessed on 17th July 2025).

23. Scott, K., Beckham, S. W., Gross, M., Pariyo, G., Rao, K. D., Cometto, G., & Perry, H. B. (2018). What do we know about community-based health worker programs? A systematic review of existing reviews on community health workers. *Human Resources for Health, 16*. https://doi.org/10.1186/s12960-018-0304-x (accessed on 17th July 2025).

24. Semenza, J. C., & Ebi, K. L. (2019). Climate change impact on migration, travel, travel destinations and the tourism industry. *Journal of Travel Medicine, 26.* https://doi.org/10.1093/jtm/taz026 (accessed on 17th July 2025).

25. Sharifi-Rad, J., Sureda, A., Tenore, G. C., Daglia, M., Sharifi-Rad, M., Valussi, M., Tundis, R., et al. (2017). Biological activities of essential oils: From plant chemo ecology to traditional healing systems. *Molecules, 22*, 70–70. https://doi.org/10.3390/molecules22010070 (accessed on 17th July 2025).

26. Slater, M., & Sánchez-Vives, M. V. (2016). Enhancing our lives with immersive virtual reality. *Frontiers in Robotics and AI, 3.* https://doi.org/10.3389/frobt.2016.00074 (accessed on 17th July 2025).

27. Whitmee, S., Haines, A., Beyrer, C., Boltz, F., Capon, A., de Souza Dias, B. F., Ezeh, A., et al. (2015). Safeguarding human health in the Anthropocene epoch: Report of The Rockefeller Foundation–Lancet Commission on planetary health. *The Lancet, 386*, 1973–2028. https://doi.org/10.1016/s0140-6736(15)60901-1 (accessed on 17th July 2025).

28. Xifaras, N., Roubou, E., & Altsitzioglou, P. (2022). Analyzing hospital travel times in central Athens using Google Maps services. *The European Journal of Public Health, 32.* https://www.semanticscholar.org/paper/81edc33bc8b1bc6fdee156999b90a24a5f137438 (accessed on 17th July 2025).

GENETICS AND GENOMIC MEDICINE

7

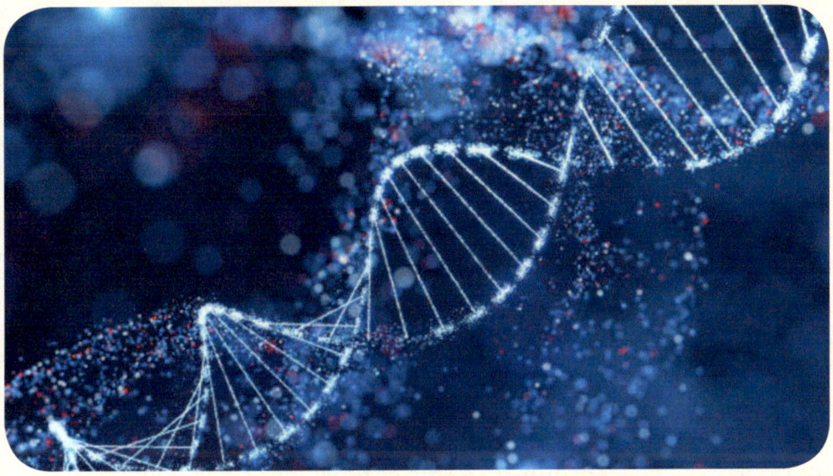

LEARNING OBJECTIVES

After studying this chapter, you will be able to:

1. Discuss the historical background of genetics
2. Explain basic concepts of genetics
3. Focus on advances in genomic medicine
4. Understand applications of genomic medicine
5. Know ethical considerations in genetics
6. Learn about future directions in genetics and genomic medicine

Introduction

The genetic and genomic medicine research is a paradigm shift in the healthcare sector, with the potential to transform prevention, diagnosis, and treatment of diseases. As more is learned about how genes affect health outcomes, future trends in precision medicine are being unraveled day by day. The ability to measure an individual's genomic data enables genetically informed, individually tailored interventions, thereby optimizing treatment efficiency. As such, this new science not only provokes rejection of traditional medical models but also poses ethical issues concerning privacy, consent, and accessibility of genetic information. Positioning the debate within the context of genomic medicine, we are witnessing a fundamental shift towards more personalized care that addresses each patient's specific biological picture. At the center of building genomic medicine is the addition of advanced technologies such as whole genome sequencing (WGS). WGS enables one to examine in very fine detail a person's entire genetic code, facilitating the detection of genetic variants of a wide variety of diseases. WGS is highly useful in rare diseases, where conventional diagnostic methods are generally inadequate. Diagnostic letters based on WGS results demonstrate the complexity and uncertainty of the interpretation of genome data. As quoted in recent reviews, the presentation of such findings to families highlights the challenge practitioners face in presenting often complex and nuanced information. This interaction between technology and patient communication highlights the necessity for clear guidelines and best practices appropriate to genetic testing contexts to enable patients to be adequately prepared to understand their findings and the implications thereof on health management (Ellard et al., 2024). Also, the educational setting in genetics and genomic medicine plays a critical role in cultivating advanced levels of comprehension among practitioners and patients. As recognized in scholarly discourse, integrating genomic concepts into the biology curriculum not only enriches education but also, more significantly, strengthens the connection between molecular biology and clinical applications (Babian et al., 2024). By emphasizing actual contexts, for instance, the case of cystic fibrosis, educators can effectively close the gap between theory and practice. This pedagogical exercise prepares future healthcare professionals to navigate the complexities of genomic medicine by appropriateness, enabling them to promote patient-centered practice. As genomic science continues to advance, a balanced education becomes increasingly important to equip future generations with the tools to advance the science while addressing the ethical and practical challenges.

Definition of Genetics and Genomic Medicine

The field of genetics encompasses the study of heredity and variation of hereditary characteristics in living organisms. It studies how genes and chromosomes pass on traits and diseases from one generation to the next through DNA processes. Being the science of heredity, genetics studies the various genetic diseases, their molecular causes, and genetic mutations that lead to their manifestation. Geneticists employ methods such as gene mapping and sequencing to elucidate intricate associations between genotype and phenotype, an advancement that has led to advances in personalized medicine. This basic understanding is critical in genomic medicine, where the emphasis shifts from single-gene work to whole-genome analysis, enabling one to appreciate the full extent of disease susceptibility and the effectiveness of treatment. Genomic medicine is a revolutionary innovation in health care that integrates genetic knowledge with genomic information to tailor medical therapy. The integration of genomic information makes the strategy more targeted for diagnosing and treating disease, and hence moves beyond traditional methods based solely on clinical presentation. This paradigm also reflects the importance of genetic heterogeneity, which is considered central to understanding individuals' responses to medicines and disease susceptibility. In this context, genomic medicine leverages advanced technologies, such as next-generation sequencing and bioinformatics, to generate vast volumes of genomic data. This data is applied to tailor treatment regimens such that healthcare professionals have data to aid them in making decisions and improving patient outcomes in numerous medical conditions. Furthermore, integration of artificial intelligence (AI) and the Internet of Medical Things (IoMT) into genomic medicine significantly enhances its functionality. By applying AI algorithms, physicians can more effectively and efficiently process rich genomic data, diagnose diseases earlier, and develop novel therapies. This integration bypasses the interpretive challenges posed by big data generated by genomic sequencing and enhances the performance of point-of-care devices, which are currently used extensively in precision medicine. These advancements foster a broader understanding of health ailments, ultimately leading to more personalized and successful treatment regimens. The convergence of genomic medicine, AI, and IoMT not only holds the potential to revolutionize patient care but also to reverse the existing public health challenges of complex diseases and antimicrobial resistance, which characterizes the dynamic, interconnected, and symbiotic nature of modern medical practices (Miethke et al., 2021; Manickam et al., 2022) (Figure 7.1).

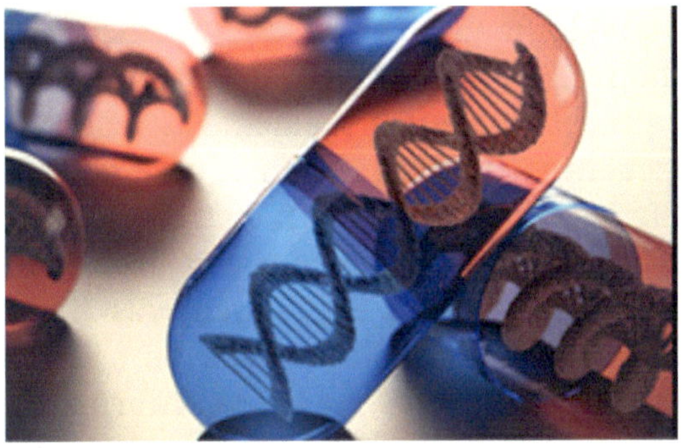

Figure 7.1. Definition of genetics and genomic medicine.

Source: https://www.thelancet.com/do/10.1016/series-do.2019.07.26.107972/full_with_header/genomicmedicine_hubimage.jpeg.

Importance of Genetics in Modern Healthcare

Genetics has become an integral part of contemporary medicine, transforming diagnostic and therapeutic approaches and enabling insights into individual patient care like never before. With improved genome sequencing technologies, clinicians can obtain highly specific genetic profiles at a fraction of the cost of previous decades. This ability enables individualizing treatment regimens based on each patient's unique genetic profile, a fundamental principle of personalized medicine. For instance, genetic predispositions can enable proactive disease prevention and lead to better results in the treatment of long-term conditions. But with the promise of these advances come tremendous implications regarding data privacy, particularly given that genome information tends to be linked to sensitive personal information. These problems reflect the necessity of establishing robust regulatory frameworks to protect individual privacy while harnessing the potential value of genetic information in healthcare (Ayday et al., 2015). Furthermore, genomic medicine has a key role in advancing pharmacogenomics, which investigates how genetic variations affect patients' responses to medications. This field, where clinical pharmacology converges with genetics, enables physicians to prescribe more precisely based on an individual's genetic profile. By identifying genetic markers associated with drug metabolism and efficacy, clinicians can minimize drug side effects and improve therapeutic efficacy. As an example, people who carry specific genetic variants may react very well to certain drugs and be severely injured by others. Thus, this implicit interpretation offers an opportunity to propose a more rational and even more secure policy for drug therapy, significantly enhancing the quality of healthcare provision (Terzic et al., 2017). The use of genetic information in everyday clinical practice is a hallmark of the shift towards evidence-based medicine, charting a new course toward integrated patient management. In modern healthcare, the relevance of genetics extends beyond certain treatment models to encompass greater public health issues as well. The ability to analyze population genetic trends can lead to more effective public health programs and interventions. For instance, the determination of genetic predisposition to specific diseases can inform screening programs and preventive interventions for at-risk groups, ultimately resulting in better health outcomes at the community level. Further, as the accumulation of genomic data assumes greater prominence, ethical dimensions of data use and privacy become critical. Maintenance of the highest possible standards in managing data, ensuring they are handled with respect and in accordance with ethical standards, is critical to establishing public trust in genomic medicine. By resolving such intricacies, genetics can not only enhance patient care at the individual level but also inform better-informed health policy and equitable access to medical resources, shaping the future of modern medicine (Ayday et al., 2015).

7.1. Historical Background of Genetics

Learning Outcome

1. Key discoveries in genetics
2. The human genome project
3. Evolution of genetic testing

The origins of genetics lie in Gregor Mendel's early experiments in the mid-19th century. Mendel's work on pea plants formed the basis of what is now known as genetics. By carefully observing the patterns of inheritance of characters such as flower color and seed shape, he developed the laws of segregation and independent assortment. Although Mendel's studies were largely ignored during his lifetime, they gained recognition in the first half of the 20th century when scientists such as Hugo de Vries and Carl Correns rediscovered his laws independently. The rediscovery changed the course of history and led to the acknowledgement of genetics as a renowned scientific discipline. The early 1900s also saw the formulation of the chromosome theory of inheritance, which provided a physical basis for Mendelian laws, thereby connecting the abstract heredity hypotheses with tangible biological processes. As genetics evolved further, it began to blur into other sciences, most notably in the early 20th century, when scientists began using fruit flies to study genetic linkage and gene mapping by scientists such as Thomas Hunt Morgan. Morgan's work demonstrated that the genes are on chromosomes and that the genes can play a huge role in patterns of inheritance. This period gave a greater understanding of genetic processes, which was further supplemented by the discovery of the structure of DNA by James Watson and Frances Crick in 1953. Describing the double helix provided a molecular framework for heredity, validating the importance of genetics as a significant part of biochemistry. Thus, the second half of the 20th century witnessed the advent of molecular genetics, putting the topic at the centre stage of biological science and heralding the development of genomic medicine. The relationship between earlier progress in genetics and modern genomic medicine is fascinating, particularly with the emergence of personalised medicine, which aims to tailor treatment to an individual's genetic makeup. Projects like the Human Genome Project, which was finished in the early 2000s, have given us a detailed map of human genes, hence transforming our healthcare strategy. The use of genetic data in practice has led to treatments targeting specific genetic mutations, as illustrated by Ivacaftor for cystic fibrosis.

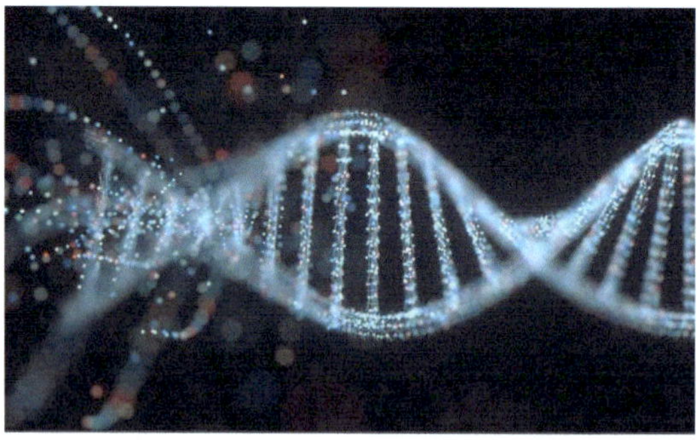

Figure 7.2. Historical background of genetics.

Source: https://media.healthecareers.com/wp-content/uploads/2022/02/11200209/geneticsinternal.jpg.webp.

This drug is a classic example of the trend of treating the cause of disease, offering a clear example of how historical genetic research influences today's medical protocols. With the continued development of genomic medicine, it has intricate interactions with its genetic heritage, affirming the importance of understanding the background to appreciate the promise and dangers of ongoing progress in medicine (Aultman et al., 2006; Cabré et al., 2017) (Figure 7.2).

7.1.1. Key Discoveries in Genetics

Genetics has seen profound advances, particularly in the genetic etiology of congenital heart defects (CHDs), which occur in approximately 1% of all live births. Defects are an intimidating problem in paediatrics, with a variety of phenotypic expressions that render diagnosis and management challenging. Recent research underscores the importance of identifying the genetic and environmental etiologies of CHDs, a challenge that remains in delineating the underlying genetic variants. To rectify this, a systematic multilevel approach is proposed linking phenotypic characterisation to high-throughput sequencing. This model is designed to refine individual treatment protocols and ultimately refine diagnostic precision, thus improving the quality of life for the affected population. Each of these findings more accurately delineates the intricate relationship between genomic profiles and clinical outcomes, a milestone towards personal medicine in pediatric cardiology (Reemtsen et al., 2017). In the broader context of genetics and genomic medicine, the rapid growth of genetic data has created unparalleled opportunities for innovation and discovery. The time in which we are living is characterized by abundant genetic information for research and the clinic, propelling advances in understanding the molecular basis of human disease. But with this deluge of data come challenges, the most significant of which is the ethical management of genetic privacy. As they become increasingly reliant on shared datasets to make advances, ensuring the confidentiality of data originators is paramount. Privacy-protecting strategies for the release of genetic data, which are being contemplated, will weigh risks against the necessity of advancing our understanding of genetic disease to move unimpeded. Thus, it is essential to find a balance between data use and privacy for the creation of an ethical setting in genomics research (Acquisti et al., 2013). Additionally, the translation of genetic findings into clinical care is transforming diagnostic and treatment paradigms in different areas of medicine. The potential to associate specific genetic mutations with illnesses or health conditions could change how care is delivered to patients through personalized medicine. Using knowledge gained from genetic research, physicians can deliver personalized treatments based on patients' genetic profiles, leading to improved drug response. Therefore, the role of genetics in medicine is not merely a matter of knowledge, but also an unprecedented ability to enhance therapeutic control, minimize side effects, and optimize total patient care. The sustained collaboration between genetic research and clinical practice underscores the necessity of ongoing discovery in its role as a cornerstone within the evolving landscape of genomic medicine (Reemtsen et al., 2017).

7.1.2. The Human Genome Project

The Human Genome Project (HGP), initiated in 1990 and completed in 2003, was a colossal feat of the practice of genetics and genomic medicine. This grand international initiative attempted to map and detail all the genes of the human species, from approximately 20,000 to 25,000 genes in the 3 billion base pairs of human chromosomes' DNA. By providing a longer reference sequence, the HGP has profoundly influenced genetic knowledge of differences and their implications for disease and health. This research, which paved the way for novel therapeutic and diagnostic innovations, not only facilitated advances in genetic research but also brought about the age of personalized medicine. The Human Genome Project has significant implications beyond academia and impacts the ethical dimensions of genetic testing and privacy, particularly for children. Genetic testing is very informative about genetic diseases; however, it also raises extremely significant questions about the right not to know, particularly in the case of children. Protecting this right is of utmost significance and entails careful consideration of when and how genetic information is disclosed to children, as presented in recent discussions. For instance, early genetic testing undermines the autonomy of the person by removing the choice of not knowing one's genetic predispositions.

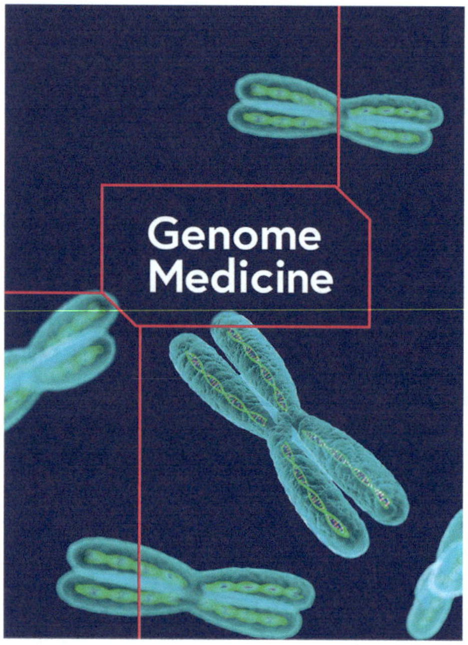

Figure 7.3. The human genome project (HGP).

Source: https://media.springernature.com/full/springer-static/cover-hires/journal/13073.

These ethical concerns have emerged as direct-to-consumer genetic testing kits proliferate, demanding an elegant response to safeguard the interests of susceptible populations while continuing with genetic research (Borry et al., 2014). Moreover, the advancement of genomic technologies, stimulated by the HGP, has profound effects on other species and areas of research, demonstrating the broader importance of the project. As an example, advances in equine genomics have shown that an improved-quality reference genome is linked to improved health and performance in horses. These developments reveal not only the technical achievements enabled by the HGP but also the enduring value of reference genomes for investigations of genetic diversity and evolution within a species. With progressively sophisticated genomic tools, it is promised to characterize the molecular basis of Mendelian and complex traits and further complete the loop between genomics and real-world application in medicine and elsewhere (Bellone et al., 2019) (Figure 7.3).

7.1.3. Evolution of Genetic Testing

The evolution of genetic testing has transformed the art of medicine by integrating technological advances with the basic principles of genetics. Emerging from the discovery of single-gene diseases, genetic testing has expanded to encompass a broad array of applications, from carrier screening to whole genome sequencing. The Human Genome Project timeline ushered in a new era, with scientists and physicians able to push beyond standard practices to more sophisticated ones. Sensitive technologies, including next-generation sequencing (NGS), have not only increased the capacity to manage large genomic datasets but also improved understanding of genetic diversity within populations. As a result, genetic testing is increasingly being embraced as an integral part of preventive and personalized medicine, guiding treatment decisions based on a patient's genetic profile. This trend underscores the need for continued research and the ethical aspects of the practice. Within the broad ambit of genomic medicine, the rapid pace of evolution in genetic testing has brought to the fore the interface between technology and clinical practice. Most likely among these is pharmacogenetics, the science of how genes affect responses to medicines. Although pharmacogenetic testing has the potential to guide effective drug therapy, it is not yet used in everyday clinical practice. Reliability of results between various genetic variations, as well as the absence of standard guidelines, are some of the reasons for this delay. However, as highlighted by recent developments in NGS technology, such hurdles are being met through collaborative efforts to establish homogeneous protocols. Enhanced reproducible datasets and evidence-based guideline emphasis portend a future in which pharmacogenetics could revolutionize therapeutic approaches, thereby optimizing treatment outcomes for patients through personalized interventions. The paradigm shift in thinking about genetics, particularly given the Human Microbiome Project, also underscores the complexity underlying the development of genetic testing. Rather than viewing genes in isolation, this project brings to the forefront the interrelatedness of human genomes and microbial genomes. It proposes that we are actually superorganisms within a web of symbiotic interactions. This shift in perspective calls for greater philosophical respect for genetic information and its health and disease implications. As clinicians and investigators encounter such findings, ethical aspects of interpreting genetic data and incorporating this information into practice must be considered. Understanding the intricate interactions of our biological systems heightens the controversy over genetic testing, forcing us to reconsider how we practice genomic medicine and how it shapes the course of health in diverse populations.

Test Your Knowledge

1. What was Gregor Mendel's key contribution to the field of genetics?
2. What was the primary goal of the Human Genome Project, and when was it completed?
3. How has genetic testing evolved from traditional karyotyping to modern-day molecular diagnostics?

7.2. Basic Concepts of Genetics

Learning Outcome

1. DNA structure and function
2. Genes and alleles
3. Genetic variation and inheritance patterns

The fundamental concepts of genetics provide a foundation for investigating inherited traits and the molecular machinery of life. At the core of these concepts is the gene, the hereditary building block, composed of DNA sequences that instruct biological processes and traits. The mechanisms of inheritance were elegantly explained by Gregor Mendel in the 19th century, leading to the formulation of fundamental principles, such as the law of segregation and the law of independent assortment. These laws explain how alleles, or different versions of a gene, influence the phenotypic expression of offspring. The blending of Mendelian genetics and contemporary genomic knowledge has profoundly impacted our understanding of the intricate patterns of inheritance and the multi-factorial basis of most diseases, thus providing the foundation for progress in genetic testing and targeted medicine. Aside from the initial theories developed by Mendelian genetics, the genomic explosion has necessitated the development of new conceptual frameworks in evolutionary biology. As researchers unravel the complexities of genomes, phenotypes, and biological interactions, they are faced with issues that require a reinterpretation of existing paradigms.

The technological breakthrough offered by next-generation sequencing provides unparalleled insights into the genetic basis of traits and diseases and suggest that an integrated approach is required for an exhaustive exploration of evolutionary processes. This integration of large genomic datasets with evolutionary theory, as highlighted in the call for new paradigms, positions genetics as a static science of heredity rather than as a dynamic discipline integrated with evolutionary medicine and biology (Arnold et al., 2013). Even as the evolution of genomic technologies holds a lot of promise for improved healthcare, it also raises ethical concerns that must be critically examined. Epistemic injustice theory, specifically in the context of genetic and genomic sequencing technologies (GSTs), reveals healthcare system issues that affect patients as knowers of their own health. Epistemic capture and value partitioning are channels through which biomedical technologies may unwittingly perpetuate disparities, rendering patients disempowered.

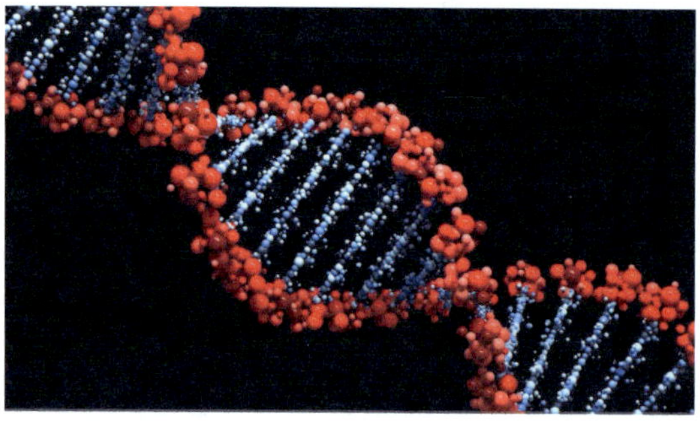

Figure 7.4. The principles of genetics.

Source: https://online.stanford.edu/sites/default/files/styles/widescreen_tiny/public/2018-03/geneticsandgenomics_main.jpg?itok=TYAX14UU.

This critical vision enables us to appreciate the broader ethical implications of genomic medicine, highlighting the need for fair provision of healthcare that values patients as individuals, not just of genomic data but also as co-authors of their health journeys (Michelle et al., 2020). Mitigating these challenges enables the progress of genetics and genomic medicine to be both scientifically credible and socially responsible (Figure 7.4).

7.2.1. DNA Structure and Function

The double helix structure of DNA, as described by Watson and Crick, is the basis for genetic information storage and transmission. Comprised of nucleotides containing a phosphate group, a deoxyribose sugar, and one of four nitrogenous bases (adenine, thymine, cytosine, and guanine), the structure of DNA allows for the specific base pairing: adenine-thymine and cytosine-guanine. This pairing mechanism not only enables accurate duplication of DNA but also facilitates transcription, in which genetic information is passed from DNA to RNA. This kind of intricate architecture is essential for fidelity of inheritance, and any irregularity in this architecture may lead to mutations, which can be manifest in several genetic diseases. An appreciation of this intricate architecture paves the way for breakthroughs in genomic medicine because the detection of these mutations is critical for diagnosis and therapy. Concurrent with structural elucidation, the functional character of DNA is bound up with its sequence, which contains the information necessary for protein assembly. Genes, as the functional units of transmission, define the primary structure of proteins that ultimately give cells their function. In recent years, the use of genomic medicine has highlighted the disease susceptibility and treatment response predictive potential of personal genetic profiles. The developments in the methodology of molecular analysis enable more research of not only protein-coding genes but also non-coding regions of the genome involved in gene regulation and the overall genome structure. Those discoveries are central to the development of targeted therapies because understanding how genes regulate gene expression can lead to novel treatments tailored to an individual's genetic makeup. The evolution of predictive medicine reflects these advances, enabling doctors to deliver more precise and personalized treatment.

Moreover, advances in genomic technologies also shed light on complex genetic diseases, such as infertility with respect to assisted reproductive technology (ART). In recent research, genetic mutations were identified in individuals who have repeated ART failures, furnishing critical information regarding associated genetic disorders.

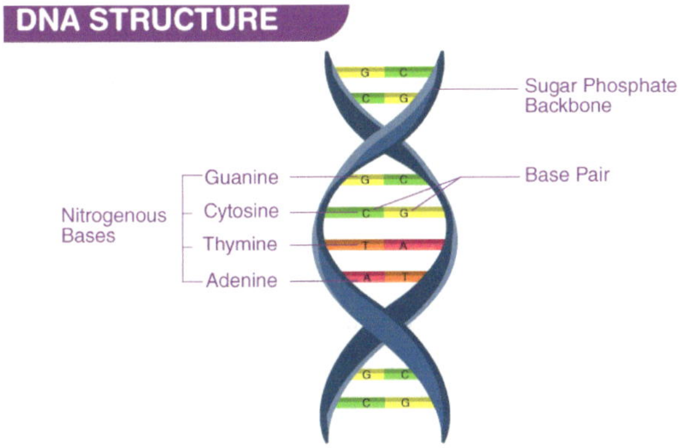

Figure 7.5. DNA structure and function of internal medicine.

Source: https://cdn1.byjus.com/wp-content/uploads/2023/07/DNA-Structure-Updated-1.png.

For instance, gene mutations such as PADI6 and TLE6 have been linked to embryonic development arrest, underscoring the importance of understanding genetic causation in clinical contexts (Liu et al., 2021). Examining such specific genetic alterations improves diagnostic and treatment plan precision, facilitating better management of reproductive health conditions. With growing access to DNA sequencing, the possibility of charting genetic susceptibilities will fundamentally change reproductive medicine and represents yet another example of DNA structure, function, and genomic medicine's broader context (Baranov, 2021) (Figure 7.5).

7.2.2. Genes and Alleles

Genes and alleles are the fundamental units of heredity and carry essential information that determines an organism's traits. A gene has a specific position on a chromosome and encodes instructions for protein production, which contribute to an organism's phenotype. Presence of different alleles—alternative versions of a gene—allows genetic diversity within a population. This diversity is necessary for evolution and adaptation, as it provides a reservoir of traits for natural selection to act upon. For instance, common single-nucleotide polymorphisms (SNPs) are predicted to collectively explain 40–50% of the variation in human height, demonstrating the role of genetic diversity in external attributes. This genetic variation not only distinguishes the individual but is also instrumental in unravelling intricate traits and their genetic determinants in genomic medicine (Loïc et al., 2022). Ongoing research on gene and allele function also elucidates their connections to a vast array of health conditions and to tailored medicine. Genomic medicine research is increasingly linking alleles to disease susceptibility and drug response. This correlation enhances our prognostic capacity for health risks and the development of treatment regimens based on individuals' genetic makeup. For example, specific alleles are implicated in diseases such as cancer, cardiovascular diseases, and metabolic syndrome. Knowing this enables early intervention and the enhancement of management strategies. The integration of genetic information into practice is evidenced by initiatives that promote the responsible sharing of genomic data, the importance of which lies in fostering cooperation to untangle the complex relationship between genes and alleles in disease and human health (Heidi et al., 2021). As we press forward in the field of genomics, the influence of genes and alleles extends from individual health to public health initiatives aimed at improving population health. The Global Alliance for Genomics and

Health (GA4GH) urges the adoption of uniform processes to unravel the complexities of genomic information sharing. By enabling the unification of diverse genomic information, scientists and doctors can conduct deeper research that accounts for population diversity and the multi-factorial nature of health conditions. Not only does this collaborative effort more adequately inform gene-allele interactions, but it also makes genomic medicine more democratic. Thus, it is critical that every population can tap into advances in genomics, illustrating the sheer magnitude of alleles and genes' impact not only on personal health but also on global health equity (Heidi et al., 2021) (Figure 7.6).

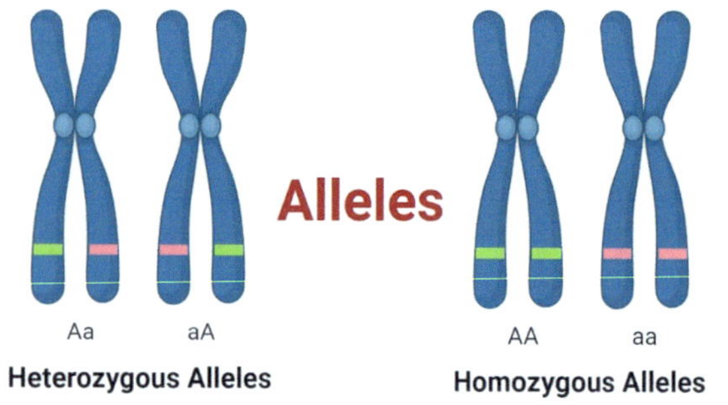

Figure 7.6. Genes and alleles serve as the fundamental units of heredity.

Source: https://microbenotes.com/wp-content/uploads/2023/05/Alleles.jpg.

7.2.3. Genetic Variation and Inheritance Patterns

Genetic variation is a unifying principle that underlies patterns of inheritance and exerts a tremendous influence on phenotypic expression and disease susceptibility. Variety is generated by mechanisms such as mutations, gene flow, and genetic recombination, each of which contributes to a vast gene pool in populations. Diversity is crucial in evolutionary processes as it allows populations to adapt to new environments and resist disease. In genomic medicine, it is essential to understand how variations result in specific phenotypes. For instance, the identification of rare mutations can illuminate the genetic etiology of complex traits and diseases and highlight the importance of precise genetic mapping and construction of extensive genetic databases enabling exploration of these differences in human populations, as determined by recent studies utilizing missense depletion analysis to uncover novel associations with neurodevelopmental disorders (Dumas et al., 2016). Inheritance patterns describe the mode by which genetic traits are passed from generation to generation and vary with the mechanism of inheritance—e.g., autosomal dominant, autosomal recessive, or X-linked. Each pattern provides a foundation for predicting how the traits will be expressed in offspring, allowing geneticists to translate family patterns of disease and relative risks. For instance, in autosomal dominant conditions, a single copy of a gene mutation is sufficient to express the disease or trait, whereas in autosomal recessive conditions, an individual requires two copies of the gene mutation to express the trait. These are complexities that necessitate the application of advanced genomic techniques to isolate the causative genetic factors in clinical cases. By studying these patterns of inheritance, genomic medicine can facilitate precision interventions and risk prediction for patients, enabling personalized treatment plans based on their individual genetic backgrounds (Bellone et al., 2019). Moreover, the understanding of genetic variation and inheritance patterns has been significantly improved by the publication of high-quality reference genomes, such as that of the Thoroughbred horse. Completion and refinement of reference genomes enable researchers to explore genetic variation more deeply and correlate it with specific traits or diseases. In equine genomics, for example, the use of whole-genome sequences (WGS) and single-nucleotide polymorphism (SNP) arrays has enabled scientists to explore the genetic architecture of traits affecting not just athletic performance but resilience to disease in horses. Such work not only illuminates the molecular mechanisms of genetic disease but also provides valuable information on the conservation of genetic diversity among species. Such research is a tangible illustration of how genetic and genomic science can translate knowledge into practical applications in medicine and animal breeding, ultimately enhancing health and performance outcomes (Bellone et al., 2019) (Figure 7.7).

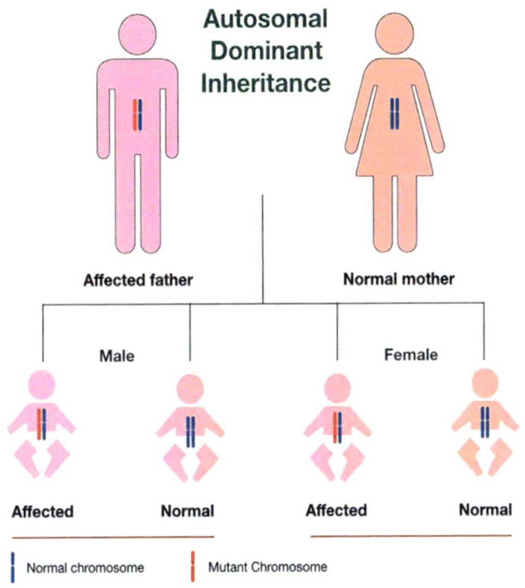

Figure 7.7. Genetic variation and inheritance patterns.

Source: https://geneticeducation.co.in/wp-content/uploads/2018/08/Genetic-inheritance-.001-e1580965422437.jpeg.

Test Your Knowledge

1. What are the basic components of DNA, and what is its primary function in the cell?
2. What is the difference between a gene and an allele?

7.3. Advances in Genomic Medicine

Learning Outcome

1. Next-generation sequencing technologies
2. CRISPR and gene editing
3. Personalized medicine and targeted therapies

The latest advances in genomic medicine have significantly transformed the healthcare industry, moving personalized medicine to the forefront of disease prevention and treatment. The ability to sequence genomes at a high speed and low cost created avenues for customized therapies based on individual genetic profiles. The advancements have enabled the detection of genetic variants predisposing a person to the disease, facilitating accurate risk assessment and targeted intervention. Furthermore, population-scale transcriptome analysis has revealed the role of alternative splicing in disease susceptibility and phenotypic variation. The information illustrates how genomic technologies not only increase our understanding of genetic contributions to disease but also enhance clinical outcomes through patient-specific therapeutic interventions grounded in the individual's stable genome (Lin et al., 2018). The addition of advanced computational technologies 'to genomic medicine has further accelerated discoveries that inform clinical practice. With the help of advanced technologies such as massively parallel reporter assays and deep learning algorithms, researchers can now parse genomic variants and their impact on splicing. This capability has completely revolutionized our understanding of mechanisms of alternative splicing and, by extension, of the genetic variability associated with specific disease pathways. As a result, therapeutic applications are being developed that use genomic data to inform treatment approaches in coordination with patients' unique biological profiles. The harmonized incorporation of these data into medical systems can enhance the precision of interventions, moving beyond one-size-fits-all models to more flexible and effective treatments tuned to unique genetic variation (Lin et al., 2018). Lastly, personalized medicine's vision depends on continued advances in genomic science and the expansion of its applications in the clinic. Enhanced genetic discoveries not only provide predictive glimpses of health trajectory but also enable a personalized model of care. As these genetic insights are increasingly translated ++into functional intervention strategies, genetics' relationship to disease is more clearly defined. Countries like Estonia demonstrate how these national genomics programs are being converted into systematic implementations in medicine that leverage these advancements, paving the way for preventive care based on genetic vulnerability. Through bridging the gap between discovery and use, genomic medicine has the potential to revolutionize individual and collective health paradigms.

7.3.1. Next-Generation Sequencing Technologies

The arrival of next-generation sequencing (NGS) technologies is a revolutionary era in genetics and genomic medicine. In addition to conventional sequencing techniques, NGS enables rapid and comprehensive examination of whole genomes or exomes at greatly reduced cost and time. This technology has facilitated faster diagnosis of a wide range of genetic diseases and complicated ailments. Therefore, clinicians can now make more precise therapeutic options based on an individual patient's own unique genetic blueprint. The impact of NGS extends to personalized medicine, in which treatments can be made more effective by leveraging careful knowledge of a patient's genetic makeup, thereby enhancing medicine's overall efficacy (Bale et al., 2013). However, this technological leap also raises the question of how to manage, read, and ethically use such vast amounts of genetic data in the clinic. While the benefits of

NGS can be staggering, the deployment of such technologies in routine clinical use is fraught with numerous difficulties. One of the chief concerns is the validation and uniformity of the sequencing output from various platforms, along with the necessity for standardized protocols. The American College of Medical Genetics and Genomics has recognised the need to define professional standards to enable quality control of NGS protocols in clinical labs. This includes ongoing monitoring of testing protocols and the interpretation of genetic variants found in patients. The challenge, therefore is not just how to take advantage of the speed and scalability of NGS but also to ensure that the outputs are clinically relevant and actionable to avert misinterpretation (Bale et al., 2013). As technology continues to evolve, it is essential that medical professionals also monitor these matters and uphold high standards. Moreover, the growth of NGS also widens the reach of genetic testing across diverse populations, including children, raising issues regarding informed consent and the right not to know. As NGS becomes increasingly accessible, particularly through direct-to-consumer portals, the implications for children—many of whom may not fully understand the ramifications of genomic data—are staggering. The individual's right to choose whether to know about genetic risks must be carefully considered, especially in pediatric populations. Early testing of children can violate their autonomy and their right to wait until they are older, more mature, and able to provide fully informed consent. It is therefore essential to meet this challenge with sensitivity to prevent ethical guidelines lagging behind technological developments, allowing the rights and welfare of all patients, but especially vulnerable ones, to be left unprotected (Figure 7.8).

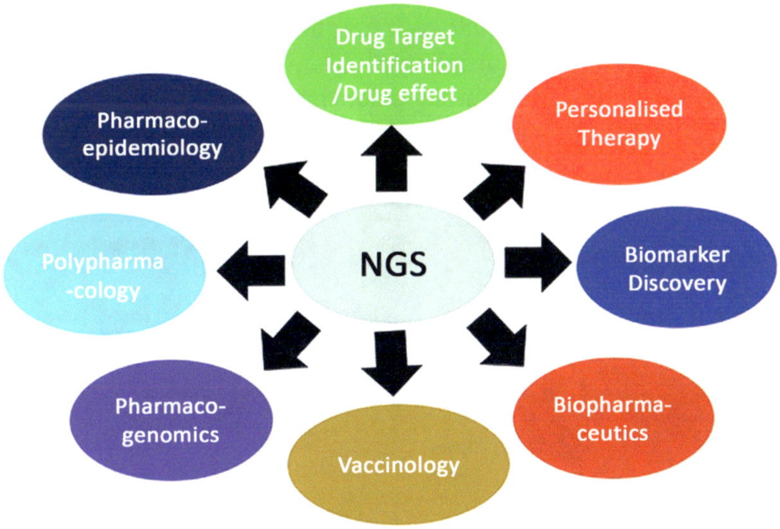

Figure 7.8. The advent of next-generation sequencing (NGS) technologies.

Source: https://encrypted-tbn0.gstatic.com/images?q=tbn:ANd9GcR95NxGvdjkXpFUTJLPxEvik6E_bXovCS1AQQ&s.

7.3.2. CRISPR and Gene Editing

The discovery of CRISPR technology has transformed gene editing by enabling unprecedented precision in genetic modification. This is a potent tool, and CRISPR/Cas9 can be used to add, delete, or modify DNA segments in a wide variety of organisms, including plants and animals. It is enabled by engineered RNA molecules that direct the Cas9 enzyme to specific locations in the genome, leading to edit-specific modifications. Its potential is enormous, particularly in the field of genomic medicine, where applications range from curing genetic illnesses to enhancing agricultural yields to the possibility of developing disease-free crops. With such capabilities, ethical debates are emerging as the prospect of germline editing raises concerns about long-term implications and social obligations in deploying such powerful tools (Beccari et al., 2017). Moreover, CRISPRs complementarity with cutting-edge technologies, such as artificial intelligence, further advances its potential. Artificial intelligence is at the heart of optimizing CRISPR operations by enhancing design effectiveness, minimizing off-target effects, and enabling real-time tracking during gene-editing procedures. The convergence of AI and genomic tools is creating opportunities for more precise and targeted approaches in genetic medicine. These advancements enable scientists to sift through large volumes of genomic data more quickly, leading to improved variant detection and functional genomics. The use of AI within CRISPR pipelines can further advance scientific research and clinical applications, enabling a greater understanding of complex diseases and patient-specific genomics (Aknazarov et al., 2024). Apart from its scientific merit, CRISPR also sparks critical discussions about policy regulations and ethical matters related to gene editing technology. The question of whether gene-edited organisms should be considered genetically modified organisms (GMOs) is of great importance to policy regulation and social acceptance. Further, international controversies surrounding human germline editing highlight the importance of clear ethical principles that guide efforts to address the potential consequences of such changes. As social attitudes toward genetic manipulation are formed, stakeholders must address the multifaceted issues of such technologies, including equity, access, and intellectual property rights within genetic innovations. As CRISPR and genomic medicine expand, collaboration among scientists, ethicists, and policymakers is crucial to ensure that these technologies are applied responsibly and effectively for the benefit of humankind (Beccari et al., 2017) (Figure 7.9).

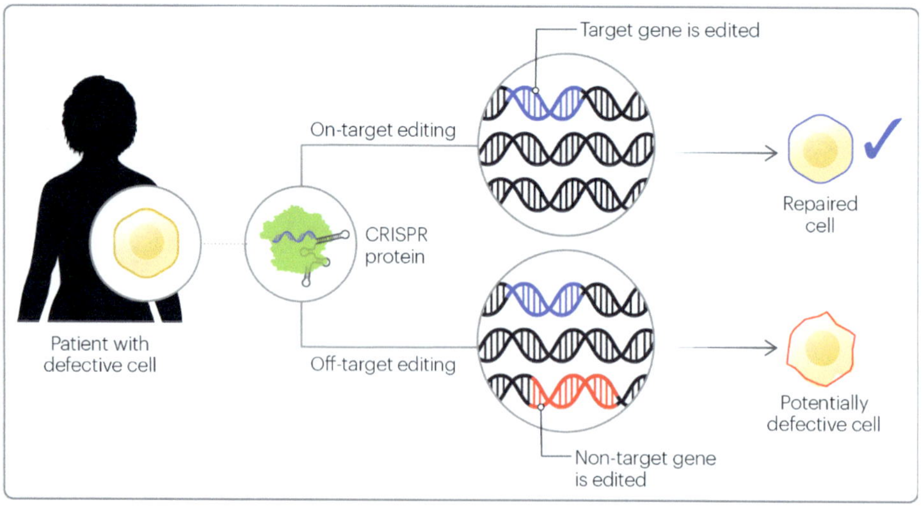

Figure 7.9. CRISPR and gene editing.

Source: https://innovativegenomics.org/wp-content/uploads/2024/10/Safety-Concerns-1.png.

7.3.3. Personalized Medicine and Targeted Therapies

The dawn of personalized medicine is a paradigm change in the provision of healthcare, particularly in oncology. The use of genomic information to tailor therapies to patients' unique molecular profiles has significantly improved treatment efficacy. This approach not only enhances the outcome of therapy but also minimizes toxicities associated with traditional one-size-fits-all therapy. For instance, advances in next-generation sequencing (NGS) have enabled us to detect specific genetic mutations, such as epidermal growth factor receptor (EGFR) in non-small cell lung cancer, which can be explicitly targeted with appropriate therapies. As a result, clinicians can take more strategic and informed treatment decisions based on the patient's distinct genetic profile, ushering in a new era of personalized, efficacious cancer treatment (Jamalinia et al., 2025). Furthermore, integration of genomic medicine into practice has enabled the development of new therapies that target the underlying genetic basis of diseases. This advancement can be seen across a number of medical specialities, including cardiology and genetics, where genomic profiling has made it possible to identify individual risk factors for disease onset and treatment response. Bioinformatics tool amplification maximizes the utility of genomic data, enabling healthcare providers to inform treatment plans. With precision medicine, clinicians can devise targeted therapies targeting specific pathways deregulated in disease, further enhancing patient outcomes. This crossing of genomics and therapeutic intervention demonstrates the revolutionary potential of personalized medicine to improve healthcare delivery and patient satisfaction (Khan et al., 2025). Despite progress in personalized medicine, numerous challenges limit its full integration into clinical care. The high cost, the complexity of interpreting data, and the requirement for genomic literacy on a large scale by healthcare providers are strong deterrents. In addition, ethical issues, equitable access to genomic testing, and regulatory frameworks for novel therapies complicate the personalized medicine scenario. While genetic technology shows no signs of slowing down, the medical community must act on these as a whole. Interdisciplinary collaboration and investment in infrastructure will be key to overcoming such obstacles, ultimately enabling personalized medicine to thrive and extend to all patients, thereby maximizing its game-changing potential in genetic and genomic medicine (Jamalinia et al., 2025; Khan et al., 2025).

Test Your Knowledge

1. What is next-generation sequencing (NGS), and how has it improved genetic analysis?
2. What is the role of CRISPR in gene editing, and why is it considered a breakthrough technology?
3. How does personalized medicine use genomic information to guide targeted therapies?

7.4. Applications of Genomic Medicine

Learning Outcome

1. Disease prevention and risk assessment
2. Treatment of genetic disorders
3. Pharmacogenomics and drug response

The revolutionary power of genomic medicine has increasingly been demonstrated across clinical scenarios, most notably through precision medicine. Genomic medicine uses individual genetic data to make disease prevention and treatment more personalized, thereby providing highly tailored healthcare. The technique is especially effective for treating complex conditions such as cancer, where genomic sequencing can detect mutations that lead to tumour formation. With targeted therapies, physicians can now deliver treatments precisely designed to counter these mutations, maximizing patient outcomes while reducing side effects. The addition of artificial intelligence (AI) to genomic data analysis also complements these applications by enabling health practitioners to extract valuable information from large datasets, ultimately leading to faster and more accurate diagnosis and treatment planning (Chen et al., 2025). Furthermore, genomic medicine extends beyond oncology to infectious diseases, where it is playing a pivotal role in outbreak tracing and containment. For instance, genomic sequencing techniques have been used to discern pathogens' genetic profiles, giving insight into their transmission patterns and virulence determinants. This not only increases understanding of disease mechanisms but also informs public health interventions, such as vaccine development and targeted therapeutic approaches. Genomic medicine's application in this setting is particularly valuable for addressing emerging infectious diseases, as it has been with developing vaccines against severe acute respiratory syndrome coronavirus 2 (SARS-CoV-2). As evidenced in the COVID-19 pandemic, genomically rapid sequencing allowed real-time surveillance of viral mutations that affected vaccine effectiveness and public health policies (Fakhkhari et al., 2024). Finally, applications of genomic medicine are not restricted to disease control alone but extend to preventative health. Genetic screening programs are now widely used to identify individuals at risk of inherited diseases, thus allowing early intervention strategies. Familial hypercholesterolemia, for instance, is a genetic disorder with an extremely high risk of cardiovascular disease; early detection using the application of genomic screening allows early treatment to prevent grave health repercussions. Additionally, in light of advances in genome editing technologies such as CRISPR, there are possibilities of curative therapy for genetic disorders by directly correcting pathogenic mutations.

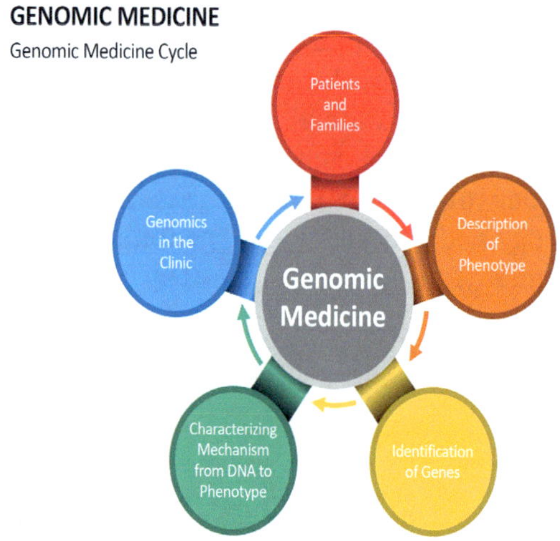

Figure 7.10. The transformative potential of genomic medicine.

Source: https://media.licdn.com/dms/image/v2/D4D12AQG9BqqkzdzyEw/article-cover_image-shrink_600_2000/article-cover_image-shrink_600_2000/0/1677135964428?e=2147483647&v=beta&t=JJsi6QcPcvesTjlxMpKg2nLxmHiz6nZBh91vNjepjTg.

This proactive approach to health care not only improves the well-being of people but also has important population health implications, thereby culminating in the overall aim of relieving healthcare systems globally of the genetic disorder burden (Chen et al., 2025) (Figure 7.10).

7.4.1. Disease Prevention and Risk Assessment

The intersection of disease prevention and genetics is a principal component of modern healthcare. Knowing the genetic elements that influence disease susceptibility can significantly enhance risk assessment models. With the identification of unique genetic markers for specific conditions, medical professionals can formulate more effective individualized prevention strategies than generic strategies. As an example, those with a genetic predisposition to certain diseases can be screened for those diseases, enabling early intervention and reducing the health system burden in the long term. The greater use of genetic testing, however, presents significant issues around regulation and ethics. Loose regulation in the genetic testing market can lead to unnecessary patient harm and wasteful expenditure, necessitating a well-defined policy to guide the application of such technologies in clinical settings (Michael, 2011). In the management of chronic diseases, risk assessment is key to managing conditions such as hypertension. Current strategies are generally based on a reductionist approach that focuses on single risk factors, without regard for the multifactorial nature of chronic illnesses. Research has identified that taking into account particular genetic phenotypes, environmental, and lifestyle aspects permits a more advanced assessment of an individual's health risk. This individualized approach to disease management points toward the inclusion of genomic data in disease management and thus the optimization of therapeutic interventions. Through the use of systems biology and high-throughput technological innovation, healthcare professionals can shift from a generic to a highly individualized practice in dealing with patient particularities, and consequently enhance chronic disease outcomes such as that of hypertension (Borghi et al., 2017). Moreover, the development of precision medicine places greater emphasis on the role of genetic information in disease prevention. With the evolution of genomics, the ability to personalize prevention and therapeutic strategies based on a patient's genetic profile will most likely transform the delivery of health care. Not only will individual patients benefit from , customized medicine, but public health returns will also be higher. By intervening on genetic risk factors, health systems will be able to optimize resource allocation and direct targeted public health interventions to high-risk populations. However, with the growing uptake of genetic testing and individualized treatment regimens, ongoing debate over ethical standards and data protection remains imperative. Therefore, the integration of genetics into disease prevention and risk stratification is of immense promise, provided it navigates the ethical landscape that such advancement engenders (Michael, 2011).

7.4.2. Treatment of Genetic Disorders

The treatment of genetic diseases has been significantly improved with the incorporation of genetics and genomic medicine. Gene therapy, by introducing, changing, or removing genes in a person's cells to fix genetic diseases, has also demonstrated success in clinical trials. For monogenic mutation diseases such as cystic fibrosis and haemophilia, targeted therapies can correct the genetic defect. The introduction of CRISPR technology has further revolutionized the field of medicine, enabling precise genome editing that can repair mutations at their roots. As such, as new techniques evolve, the ethical concerns about their use, especially regarding children and their genetic information, must be tackled squarely. A balanced strategy that prioritizes respect for the autonomy and "right not to know" of adolescent patients is essential as we move through this revolutionary period in genetic medicine (Borry et al., 2014). As promising as existing genetic therapies are, there are still a number of issues with their broader application. The growing practice of genetic testing, particularly in direct-to-consumer settings, raises concerns about the accuracy and interpretation of test results, which could lead to unnecessary worry and unwarranted clinical interventions. Because the regulation of genetic tests is relatively lax, patients are at risk of harm from inaccurate or misleading interpretations, contributing to current health disparities. Therefore, detailed guidelines and regulations are required for assessing the safety and efficacy of genetic tests and therapies. This calls for an immediate requirement of ongoing research to adequately evaluate and provide information on the most promising technology so that healthcare professionals can make informed choices while maintaining patient safety and health (Michael, 2011). The future treatment of genetic disorders largely hinges on the collaboration between advanced genetic technologies and patient-centred approaches. As genomic medicine continues to evolve, personalized medicine has the potential to provide therapy tailored to an individual's genetic makeup. This shift not only underscores the significance of genetic information within therapeutic regimens but also suggests the importance of informed consent and ethical considerations in treatment selection. For instance, the balance between providing state-of-the-art treatments and maintaining the "right not to know" regarding some genetic dangers is particularly tenuous in pediatric populations. Thus, the healthcare providers, policymakers, and researchers must collaborate in formulating a vision for the treatment of genetic disorders that reconciles scientific progress and ethical responsibility, which ultimately results in a fairer system of health care in the face of rapidly advancing genetic therapies (Borry et al., 2014) (Figure 7.11).

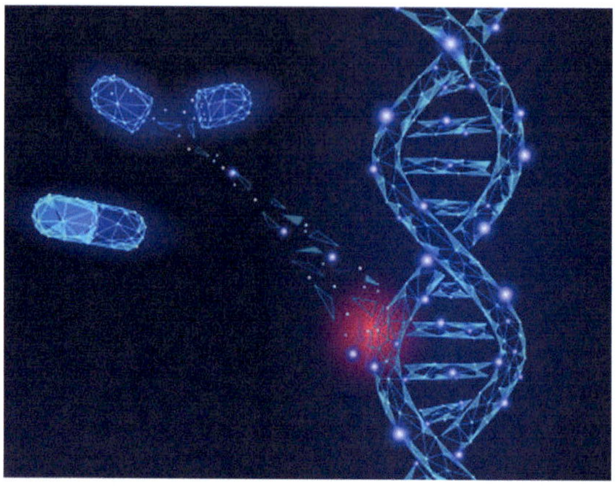

Figure 7.11. The treatment of genetic disorders.

Source: https://geneticsinindia.com/blog/wp-content/uploads/2020/08/genetic-disorders.jpg.

7.4.3. Pharmacogenomics and Drug Response

Pharmacogenomics, the study of how genes affect a person's response to drugs, has been a critical part of personalized medicine. Through genetic testing, physicians can individualize drug therapies for specific patients, substantially improving treatment outcomes and minimizing side effects. This customized approach is highly relevant in the treatment of complex diseases, such as cancer and cardiovascular disease, where drug response is most probably highly variable between patients. Literature has shown that integrating genetic tests into clinical care not only improves patient outcomes but also reduces healthcare costs by reducing trial-and-error medication use and subsequent complications. However, the ethical and normative implications of genetic testing remain debated and require special consideration before the full potential of pharmacogenomics is realized in clinical practice (Michael, 2011). Clinical application of pharmacogenomics is exemplified by recent technological advancements in genetic testing that enable detection of polymorphisms that influence drug metabolism. For example, differences in genes such as CYP450 can create significant disparities in patients' ability to metabolize drugs, directly impacting drug efficacy and safety. With more and more healthcare providers relying on genetic tests to guide their prescriptions, it is more important than ever to understand the meaning of these tests for patient care and health outcomes. International meetings such as the Golden Helix Pharmacogenomics Days reflect growing international interest in the exchange of knowledge on the use of pharmacogenomics and personalized medicine among both researchers and clinicians. The forums offer an opportunity for discussion and collaboration, and thereby foster an enhanced understanding and application of genetic testing in medical practice (Borg et al., 2012). While pharmacogenomics holds considerable promise for improving drug therapy, its incorporation into practice is hindered by several factors. The regulatory framework for genetic testing remains fragmented, creating uncertainty about test accuracy and quality accessible to patients. There is also a risk of increased healthcare costs due to unwarranted testing without evidence-based recommendations. As stated in the current literature, the need for hard evidence and tighter regulations is essential to reduce potential harms and inefficiencies in the health system (Michael, 2011). An advanced yet conservative implementation of pharmacogenomics can help improve patient care without exacerbating existing healthcare disparities. This balance will be necessary to realize the full potential of genetics and genomic medicine in maximizing therapeutic interventions (Figure 7.12).

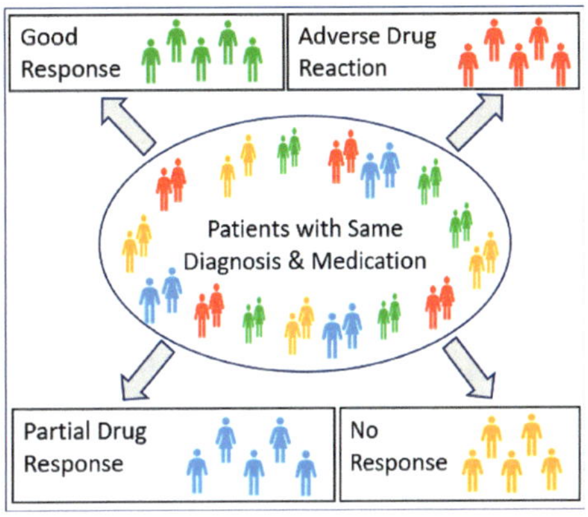

Figure 7.12. Pharmacogenomics and drug response.

Source: https://www.mdpi.com/jpm/jpm-11-00394/article_deploy/html/images/jpm-11-00394-g001.png.

Test Your Knowledge

1. How can genomic medicine help in assessing an individual's risk for inherited diseases like breast cancer or cardiovascular disease?
2. Give one example of how genomic information is used to treat a specific genetic disorder.
3. What is pharmacogenomics, and how does it influence a patient's response to medications?

7.5. Ethical Considerations in Genetics

Learning Outcome

1. Genetic privacy and data security
2. Ethical implications of gene editing
3. Discrimination based on genetic information

Advances in genetic and genomic medicine have provoked intense ethical controversy surrounding the use of genetic manipulation and data. Behind all the arguments lies the question of reductionism, which asserts that complex biological phenomena can be attributed to genetic determinants only. Opponents of this reductionist strategy believe that it leads to an oversimplistic understanding of life and brings a diminution of attention to the subtle interplay between genomics and the environment. In post-genomic sciences, scientists are now faced with the need to appreciate the complexity of biological interactions—integrating the contributions of genes to ecosystems. This shift in perspective gives rise to an ethical duty to consider the broader implications of genetic research and its uses, particularly regarding the potential effects on communities and individuals (Davies et al., 2011). Moreover, ethical considerations in genetics also encompass the management and interpretation of genetic information, particularly in precision medicine. The use of genomic nutritional profiling, for example, offers new potential for individualized health interventions, but also raises unprecedented ethical issues. Misuse of personal genetic information raises privacy and consent issues when third parties, such as insurance companies or employers, gain access to these genetic profiles. Through these ethical waters, regulatory systems must be established that protect individuals' rights and ensure that the benefits of genomic advancements are distributed equitably. The complexities of genetic data call for integrity among scientists, ethicists, and the general public so that rules can be formulated touching on innovation and ethics in genetics (Castle et al., 2007). Beyond privacy issues, ethical concerns also need to address the broader societal impact of genetic technologies, namely their implications for equity and justice. Unequal access to genomic medicine risks exacerbating existing health disparities, particularly among already disadvantaged populations. As advancements in genomic technologies proceed, there is a strong imperative to ascertain that these advances do not inadvertently accrue to already advantaged populations at the expense of others. This poses critical questions about policymakers' and researchers' obligations to foster inclusiveness in genetic research and to disseminate its benefits. By playing an active role and involving stakeholders and communities in the discourse on genetic breakthroughs, a more moral framework could develop, mandating that genetics is for humanity as a whole rather than for enhancing the driving forces of inequality (Davies et al., 2011).

7.5.1. Genetic Privacy and Data Security

The rate of innovation in genomic sequencing technology has transformed the study of genetics and individualized medicine. With cheap sequencing of very detailed genotypes now available, applications in medicine appear to be limitless. But this availability of the genomic information raises fundamental issues of genetic privacy and data security. The genome inherently possesses unique characteristics, such as associations with particular phenotypic traits and disease conditions, potential for forensic identification, and the revelation of familial connections. Thus, increased access to such sensitive information has led to a fine balance between expanded opportunities for customized medical treatment and the protection of the individual's privacy rights. Addressing these concerns requires a multifaceted approach involving not just technological solutions but robust public policy to control the use of genetic information as well as ensure informed consent. With the growth of direct-to-consumer genetic testing, the threat of genomic information being transferred to less-regulated environments increases. This trend is very concerning for genetic privacy, particularly given that individuals may unwittingly provide personal health data to a variety of stakeholders, including for-profit companies. The intersection of computer science, medicine, and public policy is key to understanding these challenges. Research has made clear that while protections for data privacy have been extensively studied across a variety of data types, the uniqueness of genomic data has been under-examined. Systematic threat analysis of genomic privacy, including privacy attacks and the effectiveness of existing countermeasures, is needed to safeguard individuals' rights and ensure the proper use of genetic information. Ayday et al. (2015) state that there are significant benefits as well as severe threats posed by the genomics revolution, and it is important that these challenges be addressed comprehensively. In addition, as the era of universal genetic knowledge arrives, protecting the confidentiality of data authors becomes increasingly essential.

The vast amounts of data generated not only serve to advance research and medical breakthroughs but also present an intriguing challenge to confidentiality and ownership. Mapping vulnerabilities is key to planning effective strategies for the safe release of genetic information. Acquisti et al. (2013) highlights the need for privacy-protecting systems that will be able to share genetic information without compromising individuals' rights to privacy. Creating these frameworks by combining technological progress with ethical considerations will be crucial to ensuring that genetic information can be used to advance science without jeopardizing personal privacy. By prioritizing data security, the sciences of genetics and genomic medicine can lay the groundwork for innovations that respect people's rights while expanding our understanding of human health (Figure 7.13).

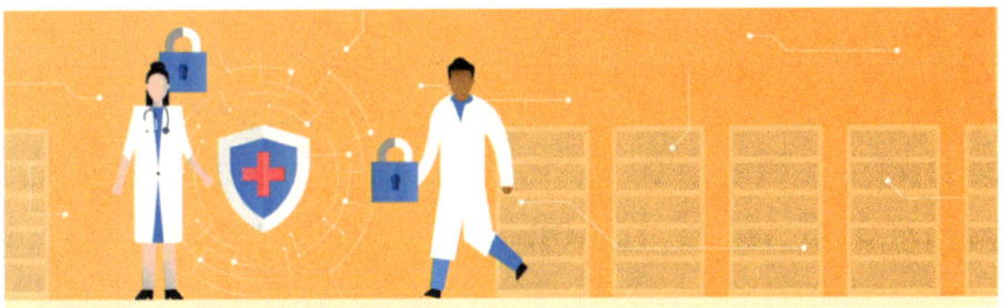

Figure 7.13. Genetic privacy and data security.

Source: https://healthcaretransformers.com/wp-content/uploads/2021/09/Roche_Brynn-Roberts-Data-privacy-security-Internal-Roche_Header-1440x450.png.

7.5.2. Ethical Implications of Gene Editing

The advent of gene editing technologies, particularly CRISPR/Cas9, has sparked widespread ethical debate about their use in human genetics. With human genome editing potentially a step closer, ethical arguments become more than technical feasibility. These concerns include issues of consent, long-term impact on genetic diversity, and potential unforeseen consequences. For instance, while CRISPR/Cas9 offers promising solutions for genetic diseases by enabling precise alterations in a patient's genome, it raises ethical concerns about the manipulation of hereditary traits and germline therapy. If gene editing is employed for these reasons, subsequent generations would carry the changes that were made without their consent, making the moral landscape of personal autonomy and genetic integrity convoluted (Ferreira et al., 2020). In addition, the socio-economic effects of gene editing technologies cannot be overlooked. The prospect of the creation of designer babies or the enhancement of physical and mental traits is a slippery slope towards socio-genetic disparity. Although gene editing has the potential to eradicate disabling genetic disorders and bring public health benefits, it may also exacerbate existing inequalities in access to healthcare and genetic technologies. This can lead to a social divide in which money alone can access the fruits of genome changes, ushering in a new form of inequality through genetic enhancement. This outcome underscores the necessity of institutional frameworks that enshrine access to genetic technologies on a just basis and their rational application, with the aim of curing and improving (Fox et al., 2020). Finally, the intersection of gene editing and human rights cannot be ignored in any ethical consideration. As scientists harness such tools to explore human genetics, the possibility of their abuse raises serious human rights issues. As an ethical imperative, scientists ought to engage with affected communities openly and take into consideration the cultural significance of genetic heritage. Surveys of particular groups must be conducted sensitively to avoid reinforcing stereotypes or exploiting vulnerability. Building alliances between geneticists, ethicists, and community members will then play a central role in buttressing the conviction that gene editing will serve humanity's best interests, promoting an integrated approach to genetics and genomic medicine that safeguards both individual rights and collective values (Ferreira et al., 2020).

7.5.3. Discrimination Based on Genetic Information

The growth of genomic medicine, on the other hand, has raised concerns about discrimination based on genetic information. With the improvement of genetic tests in providing better information on an individual's genetic predisposition to diseases, the risk of discrimination and stigmatization of people in healthcare insurance and employment coverage increasingly emerges. Individuals are presented with adverse options based on their genomic information alone, and this has been linked to conditions such as type 2 diabetes and cardiovascular disease. Such encounters pose ethical concerns over autonomy and privacy, with the worries that personal genetic information will be used to act in an unfavorable discriminatory manner, ultimately dictating health care coverage and job prospects disproportionately. With the complexities of genomic data outpacing societal norms, addressing these ethical dilemmas becomes necessary to ensure that progress in genomic medicine does not compromise basic rights and protections. In accepting these difficulties, imposing stringent legal measures is necessary to safeguard against discrimination. Laws such as the Genetic Information Nondiscrimination Act (GINA) have attempted to protect people from discrimination in employment and health insurance based on their genetic information. However, the usefulness of such a law can be questioned, especially given the complexities of diseases with multiple factors. With the addition of genomic profiling to a clinical framework, the concern is that discriminatory processes may extend beyond the protections afforded by existing legislation. The distinction between monogenic and multifactorial disease in genetic tests means that existing policy needs to be rethought, as the predictive value of multifactorial tests is often elusive and less precise, thereby complicating legal recourse for those afflicted (Janssens et al., 2009). Furthermore, the shift toward personal genomic data sharing programs raises questions about individual consent and privacy. While sites where individuals openly share their genomic information with scientists facilitate innovation and advance medical progress, they also expose individuals to significant privacy risks and potential abuse of their personal information. The awareness of the implications of such activities is crucial as persons must tread the thin line between furthering scientific research and protecting their own genetic information from unintentional disclosure or prejudice (Borry et al., 2015). As individuals decide whether to publish their genomic data, the need for extensive education and awareness records necessitates balancing investigation objectives with robust ethical considerations and provisions (Figure 7.14).

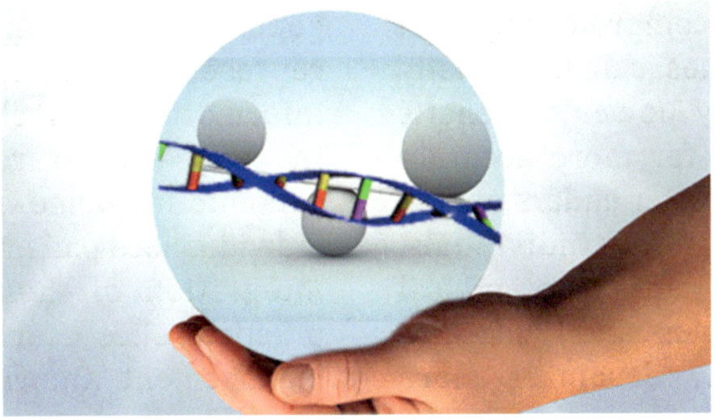

Figure 7.14. Discrimination based on genetic information.

Source: https://blogs.cdc.gov/genomics/wp-content/uploads/sites/20/2022/09/2022-09_blog_misuse.jpg.

Test Your Knowledge

1. Why is genetic privacy important, and what are the potential risks if genetic data is not securely protected?
2. What are two major ethical concerns related to the use of gene editing technologies like CRISPR in humans?
3. How might genetic information be misused in ways that lead to discrimination in employment or insurance?

7.6. Future Directions in Genetics and Genomic Medicine

Learning Outcome

1. Emerging technologies and research
2. Potential for curing genetic diseases
3. Global health implications and accessibility

The future of genetics and genomic medicine is to bring revolutionary innovation across different areas, particularly in understanding disease mechanisms and generating targeted therapeutics. For instance, new paradigms in research into melanocytes outline possible avenues for the treatment of disorders and cancers of the skin, such as melanoma. Researchers are implementing cutting-edge technologies, including genomics and systems biology, to gain insights into the genetic determinants of melanoma (Birlea et al., 2018). With the advancement of the field, more than ever before, it is imperative to address the challenges posed by genetic diversity in patients, which impacts the efficacy of personalized medicine approaches. These advances can enhance clinical outcomes and provide individualized therapies that maximize patients' quality of life. Moreover, the integration of epigenetics and proteomics into genomic medicine represents a paradigm shift with a highly promising future for research and applications. By employing epigenetic biomarkers, scientists are developing methods to refine genetic profiling methods further, which could become a game-changer for forensic applications and medical diagnosis. For example, these biomarkers can allow forensic scientists to estimate biological samples with critical data for criminal proceedings (Eilerts et al., 2016).

Similarly, enhanced proteomics, particularly through mass spectrometry, has enabled the identification of biological tissues derived from forensic samples without compromising DNA evidence. Such technologies can potentially amplify the discriminatory power of genetic evidence, paving the way for more accurate forensic techniques and a greater understanding of biological variation among individuals. Beyond these advances in technology, ethical concerns involving genetics and genomics medicine are increasingly becoming more pressing as the speciality advances. The employment of next-generation sequencing and gene-editing technologies raises serious issues regarding privacy, consent, and equitable access to genetic therapy. As healthcare systems embrace such new technologies, it becomes important to design frameworks that preserve ethical standards and ensure equitable patient access to genetic testing and treatment. The implications of genetic discoveries are not limited to clinical settings but extend to public health policy and cultural norms. Stakeholders such as researchers, clinicians, ethicists, and community members must continue to discuss the complications of genetic advances to navigate them and establish a setting in which innovations can be responsibly integrated into healthcare systems.

7.6.1. Emerging Technologies and Research

The rapid pace of development in new technologies has significantly altered the genetics and genomic medicine landscape, enabling previously unimaginable advances. These technologies, such as whole genome sequencing (WGS) have enabled scientists and clinicians to study genetic blueprints at previously unimagined resolution levels. Such capabilities are necessary to identify genetic mutations that contribute to most diseases, thereby enabling the development of individually tailored therapeutic strategies. Therefore, genomic data can enhance diagnostic accuracy and improve patient outcomes by enabling targeted therapy based on patient-specific genetic profiles. In general, these advances represent the integration of biotechnology, informatics, and clinical practice, changing the way healthcare professionals approach genomic medicine, ultimately toward a more individualized patient experience. Yet, the proper integration of these new technologies into practice relies heavily on effective knowledge management. Knowledge integration is critical, according to recent publications on translating genomic studies into actionable information that doctors can use. It incorporates several iterative steps, including knowledge management, synthesis, and translation, that collectively construct a framework for the use of genomics in medicine. For instance, horizon scanning uses new methods to monitor real-time advances in genomic technologies and keep clinicians and stakeholders updated on the latest developments. This proactive approach not only enhances the evidence base for decision-making but also prepares healthcare providers to better navigate the subtleties of genomic medicine, ultimately improving care delivery for patients with genetic disorders (N/A). Initiatives such as the MedSeq Project also demonstrate the deployment of novel sequencing technologies into everyday clinical practice, signaling their ability to inform patient care. Through an evaluation of the effects of WGS in primary care and cardiology, this project seeks to systematically review how genomic data influences clinical decision-making, patient education, and healthcare use more generally. The project design anticipates the communication challenges inherent in conveying complex genetic data to doctors and patients. It thereby closes a significant knowledge gap regarding the utilization and interpretation of genomic test results. With a variety of methods such as surveys and semi-structured interviews, the MedSeq Project aims to make meaningful contributions regarding the integration of genomic medicine within clinical practice, paving ways for future studies and furthering the role of genetics in patient care (Amy et al., 2014) (Figure 7.15).

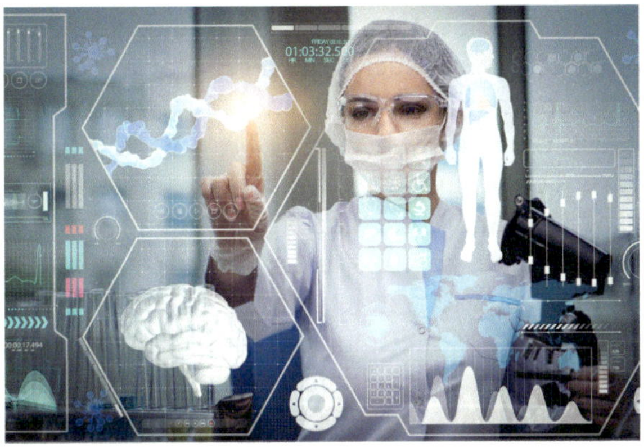

Figure 7.15. Emerging technologies and research.

Source: https://electronicsmaker.com/wp-content/uploads/2021/02/Healthcare.jpg.

7.6.2. Potential for Curing Genetic Diseases

Genetic disease discovery has accelerated due to advancements in genomic medicine, offering unprecedented hope of cures. Gene therapy is one such therapeutic potential that includes modifying genes to prevent or cure diseases. Efficiency has been demonstrated through experiments targeting specific genetic mutations responsible for diseases such as muscular dystrophy and cystic fibrosis. These targeted interventions, which might include the introduction of normal genes via viral vectors, can cure the disease or even eliminate the underlying cause altogether. The complexity of the human genome necessitates a systemic solution that goes beyond manipulating genes. Thus, there is an urgent need for a theoretical framework to understand the interactions among genomics, phenotypes, and the environment to optimize the use of these advances (Arnold et al., 2013). With gene therapy, targeted medicine has been a central aspect of the discussion on the management of genetic disorders. Personalized medicine is medical treatment tailored to each patient's unique characteristics, particularly their genes. Personalized medicine has the potential to improve through the detection and management of some of the causative genetic factors in disease that can yield more efficient treatment with fewer adverse effects. However, critics argue that the focus on genomic information could overshadow the need to prioritize ecological and developmental methods that could supplement our knowledge of disease and health. This is a testament to wariness towards the kind of speculation involved in relying on genomic information to the point that other explanatory structures needed in the medical sciences are lost (Gilbert et al., 2018). In the years to come, the hope of eradicating genetic disease hinges on an interdisciplinary effort that marries genomics with a transdisciplinary understanding. While advances in genomic technologies and access to information have opened the door to new paradigms in therapy, we must beware of the temptation to believe that genetics is the silver bullet for all disease. Distinguishing between the interplay of genetic susceptibility and environmental stress can help develop more thorough treatment programs. With the incorporation of new scientific paradigms, including genomic medicine, scientists can construct a more robust framework for understanding and treating genetic disorders. Thus, as we proceed toward an era when genome-informed approaches guide discussion, being balanced with ecological and phenomenological views will be crucial to achieving maximal therapeutic gain and genuinely reaching the depths of genetic disorder (Arnold et al., 2013).

7.6.3. Global Health Implications and Accessibility

The rapid advancement of genetics and genomic medicine has profound implications for global health, particularly in terms of access to biobanks and genetic data. Biobanks are valuable collections of biomedical research resources that hold essential human biological materials and data. Their efficient use depends on the facility of access to these resources. Though some biobanks provide access to their samples and data, genuine, unreserved access is not common. For example, a recent poll showed that although 95.7% of biobanks made sample access available, such as describing proposed uses and traversing funding realities, often got in the way of easy sharing. Such tension between cooperation and restriction can stifle innovation and limit the potential benefits of genomic research for society as a whole, suggesting the need for improved models of accessibility that balance public health interests with academic and economic incentives (Anagnostou et al., 2016). Beyond this, sharing phenotypic and genotypic data between individuals adds more elements to the global health implications. Initiatives to encourage the sharing of individual genomic data are increasing in momentum, driven by advances in technology and public engagement. Platforms like Consent to Research and Genomes Unzipped allow the public to voluntarily contribute their health and genomic data to facilitate larger studies. This approach not only engages the public but also provides access to genomic data that can inform health care practice. However, as individuals consider sharing their data, issues of privacy, consent, and abuse arise. Ensuring individuals know the repercussions of such sharing is crucial because it affects the face of genomic medicine and its access on a global level (Borry et al., 2015). Moreover, disparities in access to genomics resources and information between low- and high-income regions cannot be overlooked. Often, populations in low-resource settings have significant restrictions on accessing genomic therapies and technologies, further exacerbating overall health inequities. The globalization of genomic medicine, without an equitable response, would result in a situation in which only affluent populations benefit from genetic advancements, while needy populations fall even further behind. Accessibility improvement efforts must consider the socio-economic, moral, and legal context of different areas. Through facilitating international collaborations and harnessing the combined platforms, the stakeholders can move toward an inclusive model that aligns genomic research advances with real health benefits for all, thereby ensuring a fair distribution of the dividends of genetic research across the globe.

Test Your Knowledge

1. What are some emerging technologies in genetics that could transform diagnosis and treatment in the next decade?
2. What are some challenges to ensuring global accessibility to genomic medicine, especially in low- and middle-income countries?

SUMMARY

The discovery of genetics and genomic medicine has opened doors to greater progress with profound implications for ethics. As the field evolves, it is crucial to weigh the advantages of genetic knowledge against the possible effects on individual rights. The principle of the "right not to know" highlights the individual's autonomy, particularly that of children, in deciding whether to be informed about their genetic susceptibility. The increased likelihood of genetic testing, particularly through direct consumer routes, complicates this terrain and necessitates urgent discussion of ethical measures and regulatory interventions. In keeping with recent peer-reviewed literature, respecting this right is crucial to maintaining the integrity of the informed consent and genetic counselling procedures (Borry et al., 2014). These factors affect how healthcare providers navigate the delicate tension between formulating genetic information and safeguarding patients' rights. Further, the hope of improved health results from genetic testing is also marred by regulation and implementation challenges. With the spread of genetic testing, the risks include not only financial costs and burden to the healthcare system but also physical and psychological injury to patients. Lack of rigorous regulation in the area leads to uneven test quality and misinterpretation of test results. The significance of greater regulation and transparency is clear, as is the need to make evidence-based recommendations regarding the use of these technologies (Michael, 2011). These barriers will be overcome through a concerted effort from policymakers, healthcare professionals, and geneticists to create systems that protect patients but also maximize the potential of genomic medicine. Ultimately, the future of genetics and genomic medicine hangs on our ability to reconcile the multifaceted ethical and practical issues posed by the development of technologies. The dual imperative of empowering patients while avoiding abuse of genetic knowledge is paramount. This will require not just legislative action but also a commitment from the scientific community to ensure ongoing debate on ethical practice and patient protection. As we proceed in de-mystifying the human genome, patient-centered and integrated approaches will be instrumental in building the world of genomic medicine. Sustaining both scientific integrity and individual freedom will ultimately result in a more knowledgeable and equitable health system in which the benefits of genetic achievement can be shared by everyone (Borry et al., 2014; Michael, 2011).

The intersection of genomic medicine and genetics is a paradigm-breaking frontier in healthcare with immense potential for disease prevention, diagnosis, and treatment. The general trend in research today is to identify genetic variants with pleiotropic effects across several organs. A proteomics and imaging-based multiorgan in-depth analysis revealed intricate interactions among the brain, heart, and eye, shared pathways, and the necessity of a unified biological program in systemic disease. In addition to clarifying basic mechanisms in human ageing and chronic diseases such as Alzheimer's disease and heart failure, this cross-organ study underscores the utility of integrated genomic data for predicting disease risk. The cumulative evidence supports a multimodal approach beyond single-organ investigations in genomic science, as reflected in the incorporation of variances across organ systems, thereby facilitating improved clinical outcomes in genomic medicine (Boquet-Pujadas et al., 2025). Advances in genomic technology have also driven the evolution of personalized medicine, particularly among underrepresented communities. Recent initiatives, such as the Ghana Genome Project and Nigeria's 100K Genome Project, aim to leverage the potential of genetic research to deliver personalized healthcare solutions. The projects reflect growing appreciation for the contribution of gene diversity in understanding disease mechanisms and the development of individually effective therapies. Besides, the translation of gene editing therapies for diseases like sickle cell disease to the clinic is a giant step towards minimizing health inequities. Nevertheless, the equitable distribution of such innovations remains a chief challenge, particularly in low and middle-income countries. To eliminate such disparities, collaborative frameworks that include government, academic, and industry stakeholders are needed to ensure the equitable provision and delivery of genomic gains (Munung, 2025). In the coming times, genetics and genomic medicine will be governed by ongoing efforts to make data sharing and worldwide collaboration more accessible. Science diplomacy will play an increasingly important role in enforcing policies that make genetic resources equally accessible across borders. By such collaborative efforts, it is possible to minimize the likelihood of monopolizing genomic discoveries, which may disproportionately benefit advanced nations at the expense of others labouring in settings with poor resources. Promoting ethical sharing of data and the creation of international treaties to enable equitable access to genomic advantages is essential. Bridging financing gaps and promoting an inclusive research paradigm are ways stakeholders can create a sustainable system to realize the benefits of genomic medicine globally, making the solution sensitive to culture and adaptable to the global diversity of healthcare concerns (Munung, 2025).

KEY TERMS FROM THIS CHAPTER

- Gene
- Genome
- Chromosome
- Mutation
- Polymorphism
- Genotype
- Phenotype
- Inheritance
- Mendelian Disorder
- Autosomal Dominant
- Autosomal Recessive
- X-Linked Disorder
- Epigenetics
- Gene Expression

CRITICAL THINKING QUESTIONS

1. **Which of the following conditions is most commonly associated with a mutation in the LDL receptor gene?**
   a. Type 2 diabetes mellitus
   b. Familial hypercholesterolemia
   c. Polycystic ovary syndrome
   d. Cystic fibrosis
2. **A patient with atrial fibrillation is prescribed warfarin. Genetic testing reveals a polymorphism in the CYP2C9 gene. What is the clinical relevance of this result?**
   a. It predicts poor absorption of warfarin
   b. It indicates increased risk of thromboembolism
   c. It affects warfarin metabolism and dosing
   d. It confirms drug resistance
3. **Which genetic test is most appropriate for evaluating inherited cancer risk in internal medicine?**
   a. Karyotyping
   b. BRCA1/2 gene testing
   c. ELISA
   d. CT scan
4. **Which of the following is a key advantage of using genomic medicine in internal medicine practice?**
   a. It eliminates the need for family history
   b. It enables population-wide vaccination
   c. It allows personalized risk prediction and targeted treatment
   d. It replaces physical examination
5. **In pharmacogenomics, which gene is commonly tested before initiating clopidogrel to assess antiplatelet response?**
   a. CFTR
   b. CYP2C19
   c. BRCA2
   d. HLA-B27

Short Answer Questions

1. How can genomic information assist in the diagnosis of hereditary conditions in internal medicine, such as familial hypercholesterolemia or polycystic kidney disease?
2. What is the role of pharmacogenomics in prescribing medications like warfarin or clopidogrel in internal medicine?
3. Name one example where genetic testing influences cancer risk assessment and screening strategies in internal medicine.
4. How can whole exome or genome sequencing aid in solving complex, undiagnosed cases in internal medicine?
5. Why is genetic counseling important before and after ordering genetic tests in internal medicine practice?

Answers to Critical Thinking Questions

1. (b); 2. (c); 3. (b); 4. (c); 5. (b)

REFERENCES

1. Erlich, Y., Narayanan, A. Routes for breaching and protecting genetic privacy. *Nat Rev Genet* **15**, 409–421 (2014). https://doi.org/10.1038/nrg3723Aknazarov, S., Makambaev, A., Osmonaliev, K., Rehman, M., et al. (2024). The role of artificial intelligence in genetic: Current and future perspective. https://core.ac.uk/download/640070154.docx (accessed on 17th July 2025).
2. Alexander, M., Bell, C. M., Burke, W., Calvillo, J., Clark, M. M., Coady, D., Daniels, N., et al. (2020). "What if there's something wrong with her?"—How biomedical technologies contribute to epistemic injustice in healthcare. https://core.ac.uk/download/231877365.pdf (accessed on 17th July 2025).
3. Anagnostou, P., Bisol, G. D., Capocasa, M., D'Abramo, F., et al. (2016). Samples and data accessibility in research biobanks: An explorative survey. https://core.ac.uk/download/188827024.pdf (accessed on 17th July 2025).
4. Arnold, S. J., Bejerano, G., Brodie, E. D., Hibbett, D., et al. (2013). Evolutionary biology for the 21st century. https://core.ac.uk/download/12174890.pdf (accessed on 17th July 2025).
5. Aultman, J. (2006). Eugenomics: Eugenics and ethics in the 21st century. https://core.ac.uk/download/46955287.pdf (accessed on 17th July 2025).
6. Ayday, E., Clayton, E. W., Fellay, J., Gunter, C., et al. (2015). Privacy in the genomic era. https://core.ac.uk/download/148015081.pdf (accessed on 17th July 2025).
7. Babian, C., & Kumar, S. (2024). Visualizing genomic medicine: An introduction to general biology. *The American Biology Teacher, 86*, 265–273. https://www.semanticscholar.org/paper/e767a43664efff6b370b19bd4df87afb9aa55c4f (accessed on 17th July 2025).
8. Bale, S. J., Bayrak-Toydemir, P., Berg, J. S., Brown, K., et al. (2013). ACMG clinical laboratory standards for next-generation sequencing. https://core.ac.uk/download/345209090.pdf (accessed on 17th July 2025).
9. Baranov, V. (2021). Genomics and predictive medicine. *The Siberian Journal of Clinical and Experimental Medicine*. https://www.semanticscholar.org/paper/dd084e814ef6701ef442f2b3463cf760e37c4b70 (accessed on 17th July 2025).
10. Beccari, T., Dundar, M., Gartland, J. S., Gartland, D., et al. (2017). Advances in biotechnology: Genomics and genome editing. https://core.ac.uk/download/293859551.pdf (accessed on 17th July 2025).
11. Bellone, R., Finno, C., Petersen, J., Raudsepp, T., et al. (2019). Ten years of the horse reference genome: Insights into equine biology, domestication and population dynamics in the post-genome era. https://core.ac.uk/download/323069762.pdf (accessed on 17th July 2025).
12. Birlea, S., Bosenberg, M. W., Box, N. F., Brash, D. E., et al. (2018). Frontiers in pigment cell and melanoma research. http://arxiv.org/abs/1808.01869 (accessed on 17th July 2025).
13. Boquet-Pujadas, F., Anagnostakis, M., Duggan, C., Joynes, A., Toga, A., Yang, Z., Walker, K. A., et al. (2025). Brain-heart-eye axis revealed by multi-organ imaging, genetics and proteomics. *medRxiv*. https://www.semanticscholar.org/paper/6df4ac5e4718ba0a0794d65cbe17af2dfb7e4014 (accessed on 17th July 2025).
14. Borg, J. J., Fenech, A. G., Grech, G., Patrinos, G. P., et al. (2012). Conference scene: Golden Helix Pharmacogenomics Days: Educational activities on pharmacogenomics and personalized medicine. https://core.ac.uk/download/46603880.pdf (accessed on 17th July 2025).

15. Borghi, C., Grassi, G., Rosei, E. A., Savoia, C., et al. (2017). Personalized medicine—A modern approach for the diagnosis and management of hypertension. https://core.ac.uk/download/96884785.pdf (accessed on 17th July 2025).

16. Borry, P., & Shabani, M. (2015). Challenges of web-based personal genomic data sharing. https://core.ac.uk/download/237011211.pdf (accessed on 17th July 2025).

17. Borry, P., Howard, H., & Shabani, M. (2014). Is there a right time to know? The right not to know and genetic testing in children. https://core.ac.uk/download/237011214.pdf (accessed on 17th July 2025).

18. Cabré, J. A. (2017). Personalized medicine of cystic fibrosis. https://core.ac.uk/download/83830434.pdf (accessed on 17th July 2025).

19. Castle, D. (2007). Genomic nutritional profiling: Innovation and regulation in nutrigenomics. https://core.ac.uk/download/28966982.pdf (accessed on 17th July 2025).

20. Chen, Y. M., Hsiao, T. H., Lin, C. H., & Fann, Y. (2025). Unlocking precision medicine: Clinical applications of integrating health records, genetics, and immunology through artificial intelligence. *Journal of Biomedical Science, 32*. https://www.semanticscholar.org/paper/83f27e603e672f2c17b7c8c6aad7f50f11290739 (accessed on 17th July 2025).

21. Davies, G. F. (2011). Writing biology with mutant mice: The monstrous potential of post genomic life. https://core.ac.uk/download/1682653.pdf (accessed on 17th July 2025).

22. De Paepe, A., & Vanakker, O. (2013). Pharmacogenomics in children: Advantages and challenges of next generation sequencing applications. https://core.ac.uk/download/55848729.pdf (accessed on 17th July 2025).

23. Dumas, K., Ge, X., Gong, H., Grody, W. W., et al. (2016). Missense-depleted regions in population exomes implicate RAS superfamily nucleotide-binding protein alteration in patients with brain malformation. https://core.ac.uk/download/323063504.pdf (accessed on 17th July 2025).

24. Eilerts, D. F. (2016). Beyond DNA: Epigenetics and proteomics in forensic science. https://core.ac.uk/download/70427288.pdf (accessed on 17th July 2025).

25. Ellard, H., Clarke, A., Wynn, S. L., Pichini, A., & Lewis, C. (2024). Written communication of whole genome sequencing results in the NHS Genomic Medicine Service: A multi-center service evaluation. *European Journal of Human Genetics, 32*, 1436–1445. https://www.semanticscholar.org/paper/c46501cf84d2c682407390ae81f62f34e4cd6471 (accessed on 17th July 2025).

26. Fakhkhari, M., Salih, I., Maazaz, N., Nembaware, V., Munung, N. S., Matimba, A., Chala, S., et al. (2024). Application of genomic medicine in Africa: 14th Conference of the African Society of Human Genetics and the 2nd International Congress of the Moroccan Society of Genomics and Human Genetics, Rabat, Morocco 2022. *The American Journal of Tropical Medicine and Hygiene*. https://www.semanticscholar.org/paper/35adfe1ab6f33947adbb167ded3c93a326c31f6f (accessed on 17th July 2025).

27. Ferreira, B. I., Jacinto, F., & Link, W. (2020). CRISPR/Cas9-mediated genome editing: From basic research to translational medicine. https://core.ac.uk/download/288958587.pdf (accessed on 17th July 2025).

28. Fischer, K., Haller, T., Leitsalu, L., Metspalu, A., et al. (2021). Advances in genomic discovery and implications for personalized prevention and medicine: Estonia as example. https://core.ac.uk/download/429667327.pdf (accessed on 17th July 2025).

29. Fox, K., Komor, A. C., & Rallapalli, K. L. (2020). Rewriting human history and empowering indigenous communities with genome editing tools. https://core.ac.uk/download/323064893.pdf (accessed on 17th July 2025).

30. Gilbert, S. F. (2018). Health fetishism among the Nacirema: A fugue on Jenny Reardon's *The Postgenomic Condition: Ethics, Justice, and Knowledge After the Genome* (Chicago University Press, 2017) and Isabelle Stengers' *Another Science Is Possible: A Manifesto for Slow Science* (Polity Press, 2018). https://core.ac.uk/download/215477887.pdf (accessed on 17th July 2025).

31. Huss, J. E., & Juengst, E. T. (2009). From metagenomics to the metagenome: Conceptual change and the rhetoric of translational genomic research. https://core.ac.uk/download/237182407.pdf (accessed on 17th July 2025).

32. Jamalinia, M., & Weiskirchen, R. (2025). Advances in personalized medicine: Translating genomic insights into targeted therapies for cancer treatment. *Annals of Translational Medicine, 13*. https://www.semanticscholar.org/paper/c3e7ad865aff18da2ec9d11167bac6dea1b8145c (accessed on 17th July 2025).

33. Janssens, A. C. J. W., & Khoury, M. J. (2009). Predictive value of testing for multiple genetic variants in multifactorial. https://core.ac.uk/download/19184379.pdf (accessed on 17th July 2025).

34. Khan, A., Barapatre, A. R., Babar, N., Doshi, J., Ghaly, M., Patel, K., Nawaz, S., et al. (2025). Genomic medicine and personalized treatment: A narrative review. *Annals of Medicine and Surgery, 87*, 1406–1414. https://www.semanticscholar.org/paper/a48c7f88008ee3f6f5e730cd7155fc1a412d588b (accessed on 17th July 2025).

35. Lin, L., Pan, Z., Park, E., Xing, Y., et al. (2018). The expanding landscape of alternative splicing variation in human populations. https://core.ac.uk/download/323076946.pdf (accessed on 17th July 2025).

36. Liu, J., Tan, Z., He, J., Jin, T., Han, Y., Hu, L. Z., & Huang, S. (2021). Two novel mutations in PADI6 and TLE6 genes cause female infertility due to arrest in embryonic development. *Journal of Assisted Reproduction and Genetics, 38*, 1551–1559. https://www.semanticscholar.org/paper/d0d6de6d39c45efc28f32de4e07b640043696dab (accessed on 17th July 2025).

37. Manickam, P., Mariappan, S. A., Murugesan, S. M., Hansda, S., Kaushik, A., Shinde, R. B., & Thipperudraswamy, S. P. (2022). Artificial intelligence (AI) and Internet of Medical Things (IoMT) assisted biomedical systems for intelligent healthcare. *Biosensors, 12*, 562–562. https://doi.org/10.3390/bios12080562 (accessed on 17th July 2025).

38. McGuire, A. L., MacRae, C. A., Ho, C. Y., Seidman, C. E., Lautenbach, D. M., McLaughlin, H. M., Rehm, H. L., et al. (2014). The MedSeq Project: A randomized trial of integrating whole genome sequencing into clinical medicine. https://core.ac.uk/download/28950190.pdf (accessed on 17th July 2025).

39. Miethke, M., Pieroni, M., Weber, T., Brönstrup, M., Hammann, P., Halby, L., Arimondo, P. B., et al. (2021). Towards the sustainable discovery and development of new antibiotics. *Nature Reviews Chemistry, 5*, 726–749. https://doi.org/10.1038/s41570-021-00313-1 (accessed on 17th July 2025).

40. Millenson, M. L. (2011). How can we move clinical genomics beyond the hype? https://core.ac.uk/download/71357266.pdf (accessed on 17th July 2025).

41. Munung, N. S. (2025). Science and society: Pathways to equitable access and delivery of genomics medicine in Africa. *Current Genetic Medicine Reports, 13*. https://www.semanticscholar.org/paper/6fc3895a08b17522fc38c5f597e25ee9aaeeaf24 (accessed on 17th July 2025).

42. N/A (2025). *Genet Med.* https://core.ac.uk/download/144166694.pdf (accessed on 17th July 2025).

43. Reemtsen, B., Finn, J. P., Alejos, J., Touma, M., Halnon, N., Nelson, S. F., et al. (2017). A path to implement precision child health cardiovascular medicine. https://core.ac.uk/download/323077346.pdf (accessed on 17th July 2025).

44. Rehm, H. L., Page, A., Smith, L., Adams, J., Alterovitz, G., Babb, L., Barkley, M. P., et al. (2021). GA4GH: International policies and standards for data sharing across genomic research and healthcare. *Cell Genomics, 1*, 100029–100029. https://doi.org/10.1016/j.xgen.2021.100029 (accessed on 17th July 2025).

45. Terzic, A., & Waldman, S. A. (2017). *Clinical Pharmacology & Therapeutics*: Past, present, and future. https://core.ac.uk/download/83049656.pdf (accessed on 17th July 2025).

46. Yengo, L., Vedantam, S., Marouli, E., Sidorenko, J., Bartell, E., Sakaue, S., Graff, M., et al. (2022). A saturated map of common genetic variants associated with human height. *Nature, 610*, 704–712. https://doi.org/10.1038/s41586-022-05275-y (accessed on 17th July 2025).

MUSCULOSKELETAL AND ORTHOPEDIC MEDICINE

8

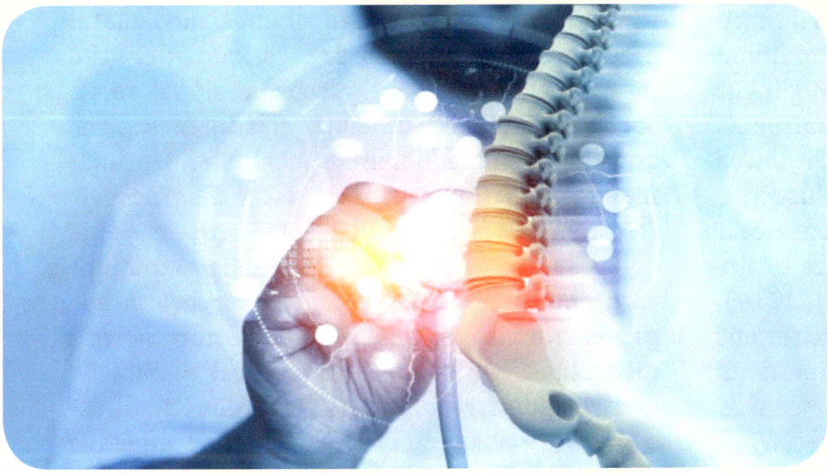

LEARNING OBJECTIVES

After studying this chapter, you will be able to:

1. Discuss the anatomy of the musculoskeletal system
2. Explain the common musculoskeletal disorders
3. Understand diagnostic techniques in orthopedic medicine
4. Know treatment modalities in orthopedic medicine
5. Describe the rehabilitation in orthopedic care
6. Focus son current trends and innovations in orthopedic medicine

Introduction

Musculoskeletal and orthopedic medical practice involves a wide range of disorders of bones, joints, muscles, and connective tissue. The speciality is not just at the core of the diagnosis and management of trauma but also in optimizing patient quality of life through adequate handling. A strong foundation orthopedic in human anatomy and biomechanical principles is integral to orthopedic practice, guiding the clinician in assessing a patient's musculoskeletal system. Advances in imaging modalities, such as MRI and CT scans, have improved diagnostic accuracy, allowing healthcare providers to devise customized treatment plans. With a foundation for successful orthopedic care, elaborate education in musculoskeletal anatomy, pathology, and biomechanics is essential to develop both surgical and non-surgical competence. Pain management of musculoskeletal disorders is also part and parcel of orthopedic medicine. Evidence has shown that inadequate pain education in health care curricula is an ongoing issue that can have a detrimental effect on treatment outcomes. A survey of Doctor of Physical

Therapy programs revealed that, although many institutions teach important content on pain, a high percentage of instructors remain unaware of current guidelines and educational resources specific to pain management (Bement et al., 2015). This knowledge gap highlights the need for additional training programs to equip prospective healthcare professionals with the skills needed to effectively assess and manage pain in orthopedic patients. Through reinforcing a heightened insight into pain mechanisms and management, the field can trend toward more effective and integrated patient care. In addition, diseases such as Morquio A syndrome highlight the challenges of orthopedic treatment, particularly in managing deformities of the lower and upper limbs. The latter syndrome illustrates the relationship between genetic disease and orthopedic complications, and this calls for interdisciplinary care (Bache et al., 2014). Existing recommendations for the treatment of extremity problems in Morquio A patients were the result of multidisciplinary consensus among specialists, emphasizing the necessity of early diagnosis and treatment to avoid further progression. These recommendations emphasize the importance of individualized orthopedic management based on the features of patients with specific syndromes, emphasizing that ongoing research and practice should mirror the evolving paradigms in musculoskeletal disease. In summary, the musculoskeletal and orthopedic medicine introduction serves as a bridge between theory and practice, ultimately enhancing patient care in different situations.

Definition and Scope of Musculoskeletal Medicine

Musculoskeletal medicine is a broad spectrum of musculoskeletal conditions affecting bones, muscles, ligaments, tendons, and joints. The specialty deals with the etiology, diagnosis, and management of a broad range of conditions that impair mobility and decrease quality of life. Arthritis, osteoporosis, and overuse sports injuries are some of the problems encountered by clinicians in this specialty. Furthermore, musculoskeletal medicine also extends beyond management, typically encompassing prevention and rehabilitation methods to maximize patient outcomes. As the population ages and the incidence of musculoskeletal disorders rises, there is an even greater need for multidisciplinary treatment in this specialty that demands effort on the part of healthcare professionals in all the disciplines in order to manage these conditions effectively. In establishing the scope of musculoskeletal medicine, it is necessary to consider the interaction among various professional roles, such as orthopedic surgeons, physical therapists, and pain management specialists. Optimal management of musculoskeletal disorders is frequently a multidisciplinary process. This collaboration enables individualized patient care and underscores the need for healthcare professionals to share information across disciplines. For instance, a physical therapist's knowledge of rehabilitation can directly affect a patient's postsurgical recovery, and effective pain management procedures derived from core competencies can make treatment as a whole more effective (Bement et al., 2013). Therefore, the musculoskeletal medicine practice not only involves explicit treatment interventions but also knowledge of the patient's overall needs to deliver effective and patient-centered care. Emerging trends in musculoskeletal medicine highlight the need for emerging models of care delivery, particularly in specialty centerscenters. Emerging developments have reported an increasing number of speciality hospitals and ambulatory surgery centers owned by physicians focusing on musculoskeletal care. These centers promise greater efficiency and improved patient outcomes as a result of focused attention to individual conditions and procedures (Annemans et al., 2013). However, the impact of such specialty care on healthcare systems as a whole, and on full-service general hospitals in particular, must be carefully investigated. With musculoskeletal medicine advancing as it is, it is essential to consider how these new venues will interact with current models of care so as to enhance proper access and comprehensive service delivery to all musculoskeletal patients (Figure 8.1).

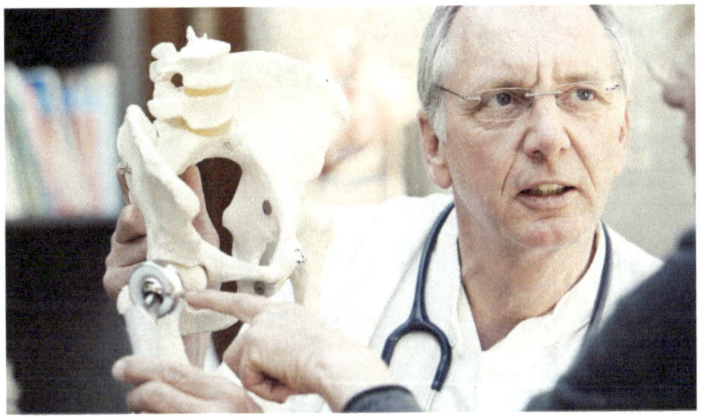

Figure 8.1. Musculoskeletal medicine encompasses a broad spectrum of disorders affecting the musculoskeletal system.

Source: https://brettgilbert.emergeortho.com/wp-content/uploads/2023/03/iStock-471393540-1-957x540-1.jpg.

Importance of Orthopedic Care in Healthcare

The importance of orthopedic treatment in healthcare cannot be overstated, particularly as it relates to musculoskeletal disorder management. Such disorders consist of a range of injuries and diseases affecting bones, joints, and associated soft tissues, and are prevalent among athletes and the elderly. Effective care for these disorders alleviates not only pain but also enhances overall functional mobility and quality of life. For instance, surgical procedures, such as open versus endoscopic gluteal tendon repair, have been effective in alleviating pain and restoring function. Studies reveal that the two approaches yield significant clinical benefit, though variations in patient history and tear complexity may influence procedural choice and outcome (Bini et al., 2020). With the emphasis on orthopedic care, health systems are able to optimize therapeutic processes aligned to patient needs, eventually yielding healthier statuses in different populations. The integration of advanced modalities of treatment in orthopedic care has also seen improved patient outcomes for chronic disease management and post-surgical recovery. Application of evidence-based practice, such as Spa therapy for musculoskeletal disorders, represents the increasingly interdisciplinary nature of orthopedic treatment plans. Expert opinion regarding the appropriateness of such treatments impacts treatment outcomes, providing an overall response to patients' health (Bernetti et al., 2017). Being able to apply a wide range of interventions not only promotes recovery but also empowers patients by simply involving them in their care routines. This commitment to overall orthopedic care does a great deal to reduce the long-term effects of musculoskeletal afflictions, relieving the aches and stresses for patients and health systems alike. In general, orthopedic treatment is an essential part of the health system, treating a wide array of musculoskeletal disorders that affect individuals at various stages in the life cycle. Its value is greater than mere pain relief; it is a multifaceted approach to understanding health that values function and quality of life. With surgical techniques and rehabilitative therapy only continuing to evolve, focus on orthopedic care will have to double, becoming a key component of prevention models of healthcare. Lastly, highlighting the importance of orthopedic treatment is not only important for maximizing individual results but also for ensuring overall health system performance and efficiency in managing musculoskeletal disorders. As a preventive measure, this is most important, as society is about to experience the rising burden of such conditions among its ageing and working populations.

Overview of Common Musculoskeletal Disorders

Musculoskeletal conditions are a broad category that affects bones, joints, muscles, and connective tissues. Musculoskeletal conditions have a profound impact on quality of life and mobility. Osteoarthritis, rheumatoid arthritis, and low back pain are among the most common conditions. Joint cartilage and the bone beneath it break down in osteoarthritis, resulting in pain and stiffness, particularly in weight-bearing joints. Rheumatoid arthritis, an autoimmune disease, causes chronic joint and related soft-tissue inflammation, which may eventually lead to joint deformity and systemic symptoms. Low back pain, a frequent complaint among adults, can result from various causes, including muscle strain, disc degeneration, and structural disorders, and generally requires a multidisciplinary approach to effective management. In addition to the more prominent disorders, disorders such as Morquio A syndrome illustrate the heterogeneity and variability of musculoskeletal disorders. Morquio A syndrome is a lysosomal storage disorder with skeletal and joint deformities as well as many non-skeletal manifestations, such as respiratory manifestations and cardiac disease. Because of the heterogeneity of the condition, patients present with varying rates of progression and degrees of symptom severity. Treatment of Morquio A involves a multidisciplinary approach across multiple specialities, underscoring the importance of a multidisciplinary strategy in addressing the diverse needs of patients with complex musculoskeletal conditions. Multidisciplinary management guidelines are crucial to improving patient outcomes and quality of life. The presentation role of myofascial pelvic pain (MFPP), which is frequently underdiagnosed in chronic pelvic pain syndromes, is among the significant musculoskeletal disorders. MFPP is characterized by the presence of myofascial trigger points within the pelvic floor muscles that refer pain to adjacent regions. Unfortunately, MFPP is frequently underdiagnosed or inadequately treated, which attests to the need for increased provider awareness. Efficacious interventions, such as myofascial trigger point release and biofeedback, can reduce pain and improve patient function. The management of MFPP is conducted by an interdisciplinary team of professionals to effectively diagnose the condition and deliver comprehensive treatment, thereby enhancing the general model for managing chronic pain in musculoskeletal and orthopedic medicine (Figure 8.2).

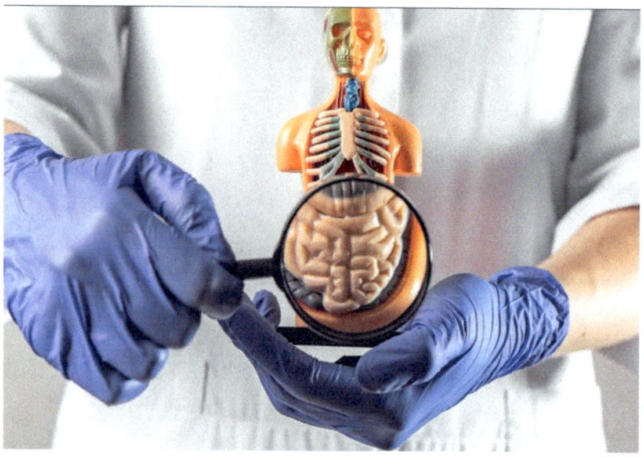

Figure 8.2. Musculoskeletal disorders encompass a wide range of conditions affecting bones.

Source: https://burtominternational.com/wp-content/uploads/2023/09/Internal-Medicine.jpg.

8.1. Anatomy of the Musculoskeletal System

Learning Outcome

1. Structure and function of bones
2. Role of muscles and tendons
3. Importance of ligaments and joints

The musculoskeletal system's anatomy underpins the modulation of movement, stability, and general physiological function. It is a complex system composed of bones, muscles, tendons, ligaments, and cartilage, which work in unison to enable physical exercise. Bones form the fixed structures that provide the body's shape and act as levers for muscle forces. Muscles, made up of skeletal, smooth, and cardiac, enable voluntary and involuntary movements. Ligaments connect bones to bones to support the stability of joints, and tendons connect muscles to bones to facilitate movement. This interplay of these components underscores the intricacy of the musculoskeletal system, underscoring its essential role in everyday function and sporting performance. An understanding of this anatomy is paramount in specialties such as orthopedic medicine, where diagnosing and treating musculoskeletal trauma and disease begins with a deep appreciation of these components. The inclusion of advanced treatments such as cupping therapy is indicative of ongoing progress in orthopedic medicine in terms of flexibility and injury prevention. New studies indicate that treatments can enhance the flexibility of the musculoskeletal system, which is important for reducing the risk of injury during exercise. For instance, research has confirmed that cupping can be effective on an injured group by enhancing flexibility, although this may be highly variable between subjects. In clinical trials, ten-minute passive cupping was found to significantly increase hamstring range of motion relative to control, with implications for clinical practice. Yet further investigation into the placebo effects of these treatments should be conducted to ascertain their effectiveness in practice. Such results highlight the importance of using more than one treatment modality in the orthopedic clinic to achieve optimal patient outcomes (Schafer et al., 2018). The functional and anatomical interactions in the musculoskeletal system are more than mere mechanical properties; they include intricate physiological processes that affect health and function. Acute or chronic musculoskeletal disorders can significantly disrupt mobility and quality of life. The specificity of muscle fibers, joint tissues, and connective tissues can provide precise diagnostic information and treatment options in orthopedic practice. Effective treatment programs are commonly multifaceted and include physical therapy, strengthening programs, and, in some cases, supportive treatments such as cupping. These therapies are not only designed to repair damaged areas but also to extend global flexibility and range of motion, hence preventing future complications. As science continues to uncover, the best approach to musculoskeletal health through a range of interventions remains the emphasis in the search to maximize athletic performance and prevent injury in orthopedic medicine (N/A, 1997).

8.1.1. Structure and Function of Bones

It is important to understand the bone structure to understand its function in the musculoskeletal system. Bones consist of a predominantly collagen fiber matrix, which confers tensile strength, and mineralized components, mainly hydroxyapatite crystals, which confer compressive strength. This unique composition allows bones to sustain various mechanical loads without being excessively heavy. Bones are also classified into various types—long, short, flat, and irregular—and each has a different function in the body. Long bones, such as the femur, act as levers to facilitate movement, whereas flat bones, like the skull, act as coverings for vital organs. The intricate composition of bone, comprising its cortical outer and spongy inner texture, maximizes its strength without adding too much weight, demonstrating how structure will forever predetermine function in musculoskeletal and orthopedic medicine. Bone functions extend far beyond providing a rigid structure; they also play crucial roles in metabolism. The bones are involved in maintaining mineral equilibrium in the body, such as calcium and phosphorus. The bones act as reservoirs for these minerals, releasing them into the bloodstream when required to maintain homeostasis. The bone marrow contained in certain bones is also vital for hematopoiesis, the production of blood cells. This dual role is indicative of the versatility and complexity of the skeletal system, as highlighted in recent literature. Recent studies have recognized the effects of some conditions, including prolonged weightlessness in space, which are known to cause significant adaptive changes in bone structure and function, compromising musculoskeletal well-being during long-duration missions (N/A). The advent of technologies such as computer-aided orthopedic surgery (CAOS) systems has revolutionized orthopedic practice by enhancing the understanding of bone structure and function. The systems use advanced imaging technologies such as CT and MRI to create accurate three-dimensional models of bones, facilitating effective surgical planning and intervention. Their introduction enables surgeons to navigate challenging anatomy with greater accuracy, significantly improving recovery and patient outcomes (Kalová et al., 2019). Furthermore, ongoing research into the biomechanical properties of bones has illuminated the bone adaptation process as dynamic, emphasizing the role of mechanical loading in controlling bone structure and density. These findings are at the forefront of the formulation of effective treatment regimens for bone diseases and trauma, cementing the inseparable relationship among structure, function, and orthopedic medical innovations (Figure 8.3).

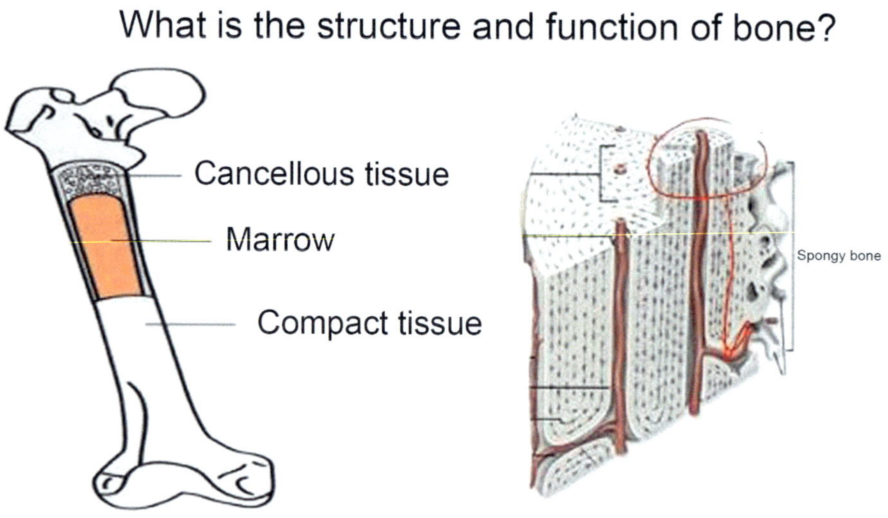

Figure 8.3. The structural composition of bones.

Source: https://i.ytimg.com/vi/-oQ2BtKmb8Q/hq720.jpg?sqp=-oaymwE7CK4FEIIDSFryq4qpAy0IARUAAAAAGAElAADIQj0AgKJD8AEB-AH-CYAC0AWKAgwIABABGGUgZShlMA8=&rs=AOn4CLAhbCGPJIPTUpi8hf-aywqrzHqLfQ.

8.1.2. Role of Muscles and Tendons

Muscles and tendons belong to the musculoskeletal system and are crucial for movement mechanics and stability. Muscles, composed of elastic fibers, shorten to produce motion, while tendons connect muscles with bones to facilitate force transmission for movement. The harmonious operation of the two structures enables a range of physical activities, from simple daily functions to advanced sports. Notably, the health of both tendons and muscles are interdependent; tendon robustness is determined by muscular strength, and robust tendons facilitate efficient muscle function. This intricate relationship underscores the importance of training and rehabilitation programs in both sporting and clinical settings, where muscle and tendon health can significantly impact an individual's overall physical ability and quality of life. Injuries to the tendons and muscles can lead to extreme impairment, not just of movement, but also of a person's capability to carry on with regular daily activities. Rotator cuff tears are a widespread injury that exemplifies the destruction that such injuries can cause in a person's life. Epidemiological literature indicates that although rotator cuff tears are most commonly the result of degenerative alterations with age or repetitive use, they may also cause significant pain and functional compromise that prevents regular activity (Loccisano et al., 2016). As such, treatment of the injury often becomes an integral part in orthopedic medicine. The choice of treatment ranges from conservative treatments like injections and physical therapy to more invasive surgical methods, each with uncertain success.

Treatment strategies can be chosen with the utmost care and attention, weighing the risks and benefits of each method to achieve the best possible recovery and restoration of function. In addition, tendons play an out-of-proportion role in maintaining overall musculoskeletal health, as they not only transmit forces but also accommodate physical loads. Current studies have elaborated on how training and detraining contribute significantly to determining tendon structure and function, as well as their susceptibility to physiological changes (Aldini et al., 2016). An acute reduction in training, for instance, can compromise tendon integrity to the extent that structures and mechanical properties alter, placing them at risk of injury. Therefore, embracing a systematic rehabilitation protocol following injury is paramount to realizing tendon functionality and health. Understanding the relationship between training, detraining, and tendon health is vital to designing effective prevention and rehabilitation strategies that positively impact sporting performance and the long-term health of participants in physical activity.

8.1.3. Importance of Ligaments and Joints

The role of ligaments and joints in musculoskeletal and orthopedic medicine cannot be overstated, as they are essential to mobility and stability. Ligaments connect bones to other bones at the point of the joints and are stabilizers of great importance that allow for functional movement through a number of activities. In their absence, people are susceptible to joint instability, increasing the risk of sprains and tears. Furthermore, ligament integrity has significant implications for the mechanical function of the joints they stabilize, affecting the body's capacity to absorb shock and distribute load during movement. Interdisciplinary research in biomechanics, as indicated by advances in model and simulation techniques, has yet to elucidate the complex dynamics of such soft tissues, thereby shaping novel understanding of injury mechanisms and rehabilitation treatment strategies effective in boosting clinical efficacy (Harris et al., 2012). Joints, on the other hand, are critical to the formation of movement and to the smooth interaction of bones. Comprised of various tissues like cartilage, synovial membranes, and ligaments, joints allow extensive ranges of motion while supporting and cushioning to prevent abrasion. Joint function is not only important for maintaining physical function but also for enhancing overall quality of life, as populations worldwide face the burden of degenerative joint disease, such as osteoarthritis. Evidence in the area clearly demonstrates that orthopedic injury prevalence increases with advancing age, and therefore there is an urgent need for preventive approaches as well as optimal treatment modalities. Involvement in cross-training intervention has been found to reduce swim-related injury among Masters athletes, demonstrating how targeted interventions can restrict joint-related injury and inform our understanding of joint-conserving strategies (Baker et al., 2019). In musculoskeletal and orthopedic medicine, the connection between ligaments and joints is critical in designing global treatment protocols. Realizing that damage or dysfunction of these structures can have a significant effect on function and mobility is most vital in promoting healing in the patient. Rehabilitation protocols are not just for restoring strength and range of motion but also for maintaining good joint alignment and intact ligaments. Progress in biomechanical research is opening doors to new therapeutic techniques and surgical interventions that address the origins of failure in ligaments and joints, thereby emphasizing the importance of a holistic approach to musculoskeletal medicine. As it continues to advance, continuing research will bring more insight and practical applications that will continue to enhance the prevention and therapy methods as they pertain to such crucial aspects of the human musculoskeletal system (Harris et al., 2012) (Figure 8.4).

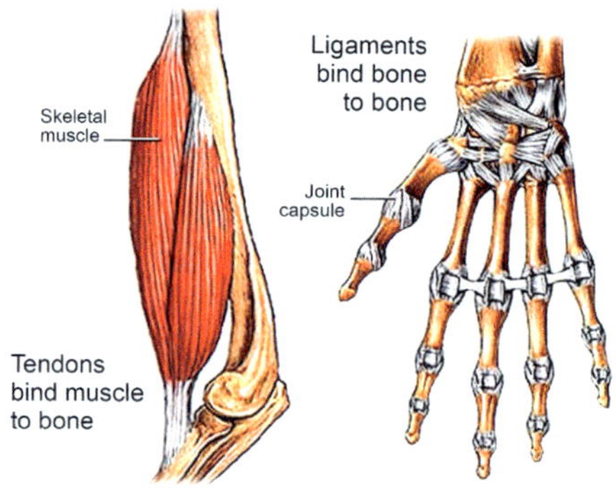

Figure 8.4. The importance of ligaments and joints.

Source: https://medlineplus.gov/ency/images/ency/fullsize/19089.jpg.

Test Your Knowledge

1. What are the main functions of bones in the human body besides providing structural support?
2. How do muscles and tendons work together to move?
3. Why are ligaments and joints essential for stability and mobility in the skeletal system?

8.2. Common Musculoskeletal Disorders

Learning Outcome

1. Osteoarthritis and its impact
2. Rheumatoid arthritis and treatment options
3. Fractures and their management

Musculoskeletal disorders encompass a wide range of conditions affecting the muscles, joints, and connective tissue, leading to pain and functional impairment. The most prevalent among these are osteoarthritis, rheumatoid arthritis, and myofascial pain syndromes. Osteoarthritis, characterized by degeneration of cartilage and bone beneath, is predominantly seen in elderly individuals as pain, stiffness, and reduced mobility. Rheumatoid arthritis, on the other hand, is an autoimmune disorder that primarily affects synovial joints and, if left untreated, causes inflammation, swelling, and deformity. The role of the psychological and emotional factors in coping with both of these disorders cannot be overemphasized, as chronic pain usually leads to anxiety and distress, complicating subsequent treatment and rehabilitation procedures. Myofascial pelvic pain (MFPP) is another leading cause of musculoskeletal disorders and is most often underdiagnosed clinically.

This condition is diagnosed through the presence of myofascial trigger points in the muscles of the pelvic floor, which refer pain to nearby regions. Katzman et al. (2012) highlight the importance of detecting these trigger points because they are the cornerstone of MFPPs diagnosis. It is most commonly treated effectively and in a combined manner, utilizing manual therapy modalities such as the myofascial trigger point release, alongside adjunct therapies such as biofeedback and electrical stimulation. Multidisciplinary team involvement is required for holistic assessment and tailored treatment strategies, maximizing the potential for favorable patient outcomes and improved quality of life. Morquio A syndrome, an inherited but rare condition, most aptly characterizes the complexity in managing musculoskeletal disease due to its heterogeneous clinical presentation. The patients of this condition have very severe skeletal and joint abnormalities, along with several systemic complaints impacting the patients' overall well-being, including respiratory disease and spinal cord compression. The heterogeneity of the onset, severity, and progression of symptoms makes diagnosis and treatment plans challenging, requiring a multidisciplinary approach for optimal management. Berger et al. (2014) emphasize the necessity for interaction among professionals in pediatrics, genetics, and orthopedics in addressing the different problems faced by individuals with Morquio A syndrome. Drafting international guidelines for diagnosis and symptom-oriented treatment is important for promoting continuity of care and responding to patients' needs, thereby establishing the advantage of multidisciplinary practice in musculoskeletal and orthopedic care.

8.2.1. Osteoarthritis and Its Impact

Osteoarthritis (OA) is a chronic arthritis condition in which the progressive degeneration of articular cartilage leads to pain, stiffness, and impairment of function. OA predominantly affects weight-bearing joints such as the knees and hips, and is highly prevalent in the older population. It has been observed by research that the increased prevalence of OA is coinciding with a growing number of elderly, who desire to be active and hence impose a significant burden on healthcare systems. OA's influence does not stop at the physical limitation level; instead, it affects mental well-being and quality of life, as chronic pain may lead to depression and loneliness. Thus, an understanding of the dynamic and intricate nature of OA is critical to developing effective treatment strategies that address not only the physical but also the psychological needs of individuals involved. Treatment of osteoarthritis has evolved significantly over the years, with an emphasis on integrating both conventional and complementary treatments. Traditional management techniques most commonly include NSAIDs and physical therapy, which aim to diminish pain and improve the function of the joint. However, as demand for improved treatment increases, new therapies are being explored. Among these, biologic therapies such as platelet-rich plasma (PRP) and bone marrow aspirate concentrate (BMAC) are emerging as new options for the existing management of knee pathologies, including OA. These treatments capitalize on the body's own internal healing processes, yet how well they perform remains under investigation. The literature indicates that while there is much interest in these biologic agents, strong evidence for their best preparation and composition are largely lacking in the literature (Chahla et al., 2017). The ability to combine biologic agents with biomaterials has opened new avenues for osteoarthritis treatment. Various biomaterial formulations, including natural and synthetic polymers, have been investigated as carriers of

PRP and BMAC in clinical trials. The strategy aims to enhance regenerative processes within the joint environment by offering a multimodal solution to address the causes of OA. Incorporation of such orthobiologic therapies into clinical routine may revolutionize patient outcomes, particularly for those seeking to return to an active lifestyle after injury or in the treatment of OA. With ongoing research into these new therapeutic strategies, it is important to critically assess their effectiveness and establish universally accepted protocols for their application (Shams et al., 2019). Ultimately, the integration of advanced therapies into the management framework for OA has the potential to redefine the landscape of orthopedic and musculoskeletal medicine, underscoring the necessity of continued research and clinical surveillance (Figure 8.5).

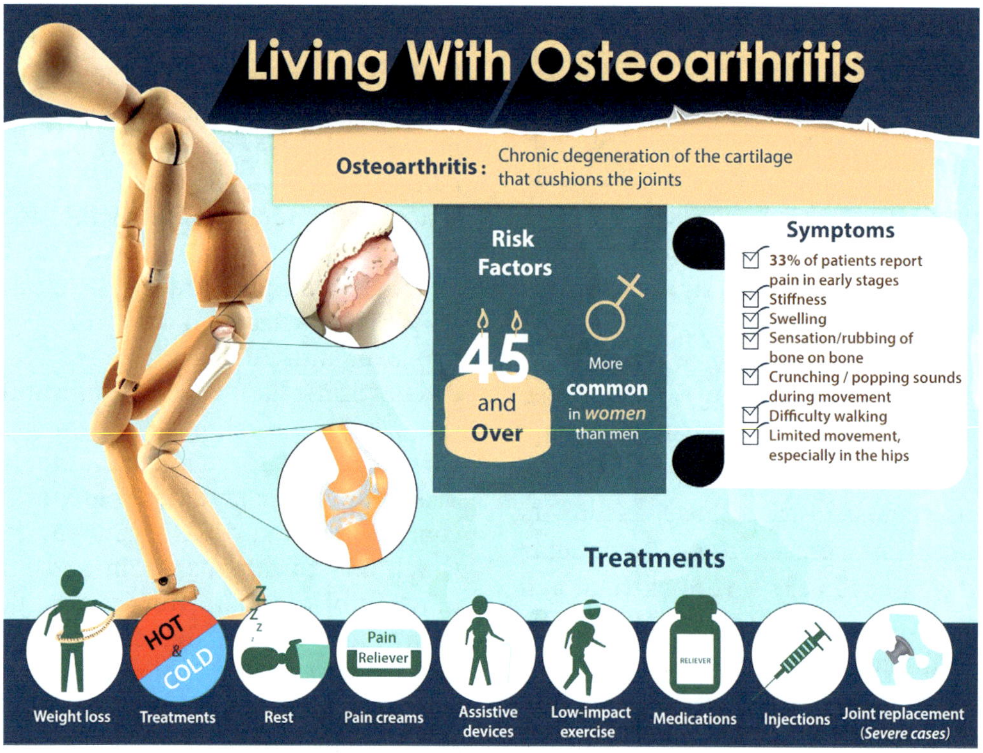

Figure 8.5. Osteoarthritis and its impact.

Source: https://lh6.googleusercontent.com/proxy/BTo50fJMYnPb2Zua4NGFoX0ngIyUx6sxbNadNvE37JmFomcypZT6HUmoYgFwPRFVwSjuP4BXQyUTRmFraMhrgIrOeqqr0RWI18EKhwo9Vd4Eyuyg-hz2rvyAZH1y.

8.2.2. Rheumatoid Arthritis and Treatment Options

Rheumatoid arthritis (RA) is an inflammatory disease that affects the joints predominantly and is associated with high morbidity and reduced quality of life in those who are affected. As a result of chronic synovitis, RA can lead to joint damage and disability. The pathophysiology of RA results from the complex interplay between environmental determinants and genetic susceptibility, culminating in an autoimmune response. Accurate diagnosis, in most instances, relies on administrative data algorithms that are highly sensitive and specific. For instance, the latest reports indicate the most effective algorithm for RA case identification requires at least a single hospital diagnosis code or three doctor diagnosis codes, with resulting sensitivity of 78% and specificity of 100% (Bombardier et al., 2014). These machines are vital for early interventions and for improving patient outcomes, particularly in the initial stages of the disease. Rheumatoid arthritis treatment has improved significantly over time and is now progressing towards an aggressive and integrated policy. Disease-modifying antirheumatic drugs (DMARDs) are the foundation of management, aiming at slowing the disease process and preventing joint destruction. Methotrexate remains the first choice for most patients, but biologics have redefined treatment strategies. Biologics, such as tumor necrosis factor (TNF) inhibitors, target specific pathways within the inflammatory pathway. Janus kinase (JAK) inhibitors introduce a new oral therapy with flexibility and patient convenience for nonresponders to traditional agents. Regimen optimization is important in that individualized treatment yields better disease control and more patient-reported outcomes, underscoring patient participation in therapeutic decision-making. In spite of treatment improvements, RA management continues to be complicated by complications and calls for a multiaxial approach. Replacement of joints, particularly with extensive joint destruction, is often performed for the recovery of function and relief of pain. Shoulder prosthesis implantation, for instance, is common owing to its favorable clinical outcomes and high patient satisfaction (Buck et al., 2018). However, caution should be taken regarding the risks of the operation because loosening of the prosthesis or rotator cuff rupture are amongst the potential complications. Also, the management of RA is not only drug therapy but also physical rehabilitation and lifestyle modifications, which are critical in enhancing quality of life overall. Ongoing research into both medical and surgical treatments will play a significant role in enhancing techniques for caring for patients with rheumatoid arthritis.

8.2.3. Fractures and Their Management

Fracture management is a central aspect of orthopedic and musculoskeletal medicine, requiring advanced knowledge of anatomical concepts and the body's physiological response to trauma. The unique needs of the growing skeleton, as seen in children at the time of fracture, must be addressed. The expanding pediatric skeleton, which undergoes periods of accelerated growth, also presents specific challenges; in injury, some issues significantly affect long-term function and mobility and require careful evaluation and planning (Clark et al., 2013). In adults, conventional fracture management methods involve stabilizing maneuvers such as casting or surgical fixation that restore the bone to anatomic position and promote healing. The nature of the intervention depends on the type of fracture, patient age, and overall health. Surgery is typically indicated in complicated fractures with significant displacement or damage to key anatomical structures. In these cases, techniques such as open reduction and internal fixation (ORIF) are used to optimize the alignment and stability of the fractured bone. This is particularly relevant in high-energy fracture, which has the potential to be complicated by the introduction of such phenomena as post-traumatic radioulnar synostosis—a disabling but less frequent outcome. This entity, involving the development of a bony connection between the radius and ulna, may have the potential for significant loss of motion and disability following injury. Surgical excision of synostosis, usually scheduled six months to two years after the onset of trauma, is rooted in patient-by-patient analysis and the readiness of involved bone elements, highlighting fracture management challenges and the necessity of customized care protocols (Arief et al., 2017). Postsurgical rehabilitation is an essential component of fracture management, facilitating functional restoration and reducing complications. Early mobilization and targeted physiotherapy are to maintain the range of motion and strengthen the surrounding musculature, hopefully reducing stiffness and contractures after injury. In selected high-risk patients—i.e., those with a history of previous traumatic brain injuries or significant comorbidities—adjuvant therapies may be applied to enhance recovery and optimize outcomes. This comprehensive approach emphasizes the value of patient-specific rehabilitation efforts, considering the unique needs of each patient and psychosocial issues that can impact patterns of recovery, as fracture consequences entail more than physical rehabilitation in the context of orthopedic and musculoskeletal practice (Figure 8.6).

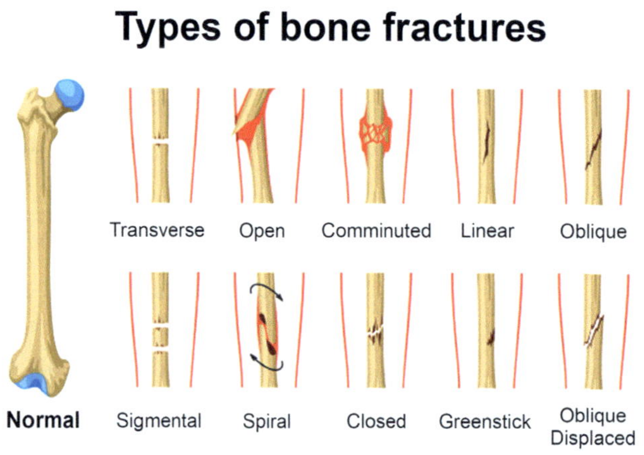

Figure 8.6. The management of fractures is a critical aspect of musculoskeletal and orthopedic medicine.

Source: https://www.manipalhospitals.com/uploads/image_gallery/types-of-bone-fracures.png.

Test Your Knowledge

1. How does osteoarthritis affect joint function, and what are the common symptoms experienced by patients?
2. What are two commonly used treatment options for managing rheumatoid arthritis?
3. What factors determine the choice between surgical and non-surgical management of fractures?

8.3. Diagnostic Techniques in Orthopedic Medicine

Learning Outcome

1. Imaging technologies: X-rays, MRIs, and CT scans
2. Physical examination methods
3. Laboratory tests and their relevance

Orthopedic diagnosis is essential for appropriate evaluation and care of musculoskeletal disease. Among the tremendous variety of imaging modalities available, magnetic resonance imaging (MRI) stands out as superior because of its singular ability to depict soft-tissue anatomy. MRI is particularly valuable for assessing ligament injury, cartilage loss, and spinal cord disease, making it a valuable tool in both preoperative and postoperative settings. Unlike other imaging techniques that utilize ionizing radiation, MRI provides a safer alternative, allowing for repeated evaluations without the associated risks of radiation exposure. This characteristic is especially pertinent in pediatric patients and those requiring ongoing monitoring, emphasizing MRI's integral role in orthopedic diagnostics. In contrast, computed tomography (CT) has established itself as a powerful imaging tool, particularly in complex cases where detailed bony anatomy is paramount. CT scans are more specific and sensitive for diagnosing fine fractures, especially in complex regions such as the spine and pelvis. There has been a significant escalation in follow-up imaging with CT following complicated spinal surgery, with the potential for overuse and associated patient damage from exposure to ionizing radiation, according to recent studies. For instance, the prevalence of postoperative CT can rise hugely in the post-surgical period, typically more than 40% within the five-year time frame, a reminder of the necessity of proper application in surveillance of orthopedic conditions (Andersson et al., 2017). This emphasizes the need to balance patient safety and diagnostic efficiency in the practice of orthopedics. Ultrasound has emerged as an increasingly valuable diagnostic imaging modality in orthopedic medicine, particularly for real-time imaging and radiation avoidance. It is commonly utilized for guiding injections into joints, evaluating soft tissue structures, and detecting of fluid collections. The advantages of ultrasound include dynamic assessment, i.e., observing muscle contractions or joint motion, which are crucial in sports medicine. On the other hand, advances in ultrasound technology have enhanced image quality and diagnostic sensitivity, making it a valuable adjunct to traditional imaging methods. Although restricted in imaging structures beyond the transducer, the beneficial aspects of ultrasound, including cost-effectiveness and immediate availability, solidify its position as an essential diagnostic in the orthopedic armory. As medicine evolves, the complementary use of various imaging modalities will optimize patient care and treatment outcomes in musculoskeletal and orthopedic practice.

8.3.1. Imaging Technologies: X-Rays, MRIs, and CT Scans

The establishment of imaging technologies, particularly X-rays, MRIs, and CT scans, has a profound influence on orthopedic and musculoskeletal medicine. X-rays, being the most common imaging tool, enable fast confirmation of bone fractures and other skeletal ailments. With the advent of digital imaging, X-ray techniques have advanced to enable near-simultaneous image assessment after exposure, significantly reducing diagnostic time and making workflows more efficient. In addition, the use of automatic exposure systems minimizes radiation exposure to the lowest possible level, maintaining patient health and maximizing imaging efficiency. The technologies serve as a shining example of how technology enhances patient care and outcomes in the orthopedic field by enabling health professionals to make timely, informed decisions with precise imaging results (Gregory et al., 2023). Magnetic Resonance Imaging (MRI) provides an alternative for musculoskeletal imaging, particularly for soft tissues, ligaments, and cartilage, which may not be adequately visualized with X-rays. The non-invasive nature of MRI, coupled with no ionizing radiation, renders it an attractive alternative in most clinical cases. Novel synthetic CT technologies offer a promising solution, generating CT-like images from MRI scans to further minimize radiation exposure while maintaining the necessary diagnostic capabilities. As in recent publications, these new technologies hold great promise in orthopedic surgery, where precise imaging of anatomical details is paramount for procedures like pedicle screw placement. With accurate diagnosis and improved treatment planning, MRI and newer technologies validate their role in enhancing orthopedic management (McDonnell et al., 2024). Computed Tomography (CT) scan complements the function of X-ray and MRI, particularly for complex situations where precise visualization of bone anatomy is essential. CT scan is particularly useful for fracture evaluation, assessment of degenerative changes, and surgical planning. But radiation exposure that goes with it continues to be a problem, and so alternatives such as synthetic CT have been explored. Synthetic CT technology, in fact, generates CT images from existing MRI data, dramatically reducing radiation exposure while maintaining high imaging accuracy. How enormous a step these developments are for orthopedic medicine cannot be overstated, for they represent a massive leap towards safer diagnosis. With advances in technology and increasingly sophisticated imaging capabilities, musculoskeletal and orthopedic medicine is poised to keep pace with developments, enhancing patient care in terms of safety and accuracy and laying the foundation for future innovations (McDonnell et al., 2024) (Figure 8.7).

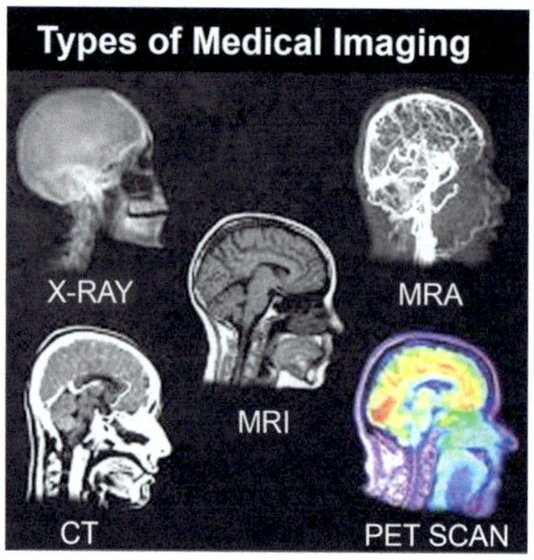

Figure 8.7. Imaging technologies: X-rays, MRIs, and CT scans.

Source: https://encrypted-tbn0.gstatic.com/images?q=tbn:ANd9GcTc-IxC0NXakXC5DncS1ddmahXcyPJr5U5_JA&s.

8.3.2. Physical Examination Methods

The physical examination techniques used in musculoskeletal and orthopedic medicine play a crucial role in proper diagnosis and successful treatment planning. These techniques are often used in combination with patient history assessment, visual observation, palpation, and range-of-motion measurement. A proper patient history is significant in providing information about the onset, location, and character of symptoms and in directing subsequent examination procedures. Visual examination allows the clinician to observe any deformity, swelling, or asymmetry that would indicate underlying pathology. Palpation is also critical for assessing tenderness, crepitus, or temperature variations in the affected area, enabling localized evaluation of potential conditions or injuries. The of range of motion—active and passive—provides information on functional limitations and assists in isolating specific deficits that can guide rehabilitation interventions. Over the past decades, new methods have been incorporated into traditional examination procedures, enhancing the overall accuracy of the tests. Therapies such as Cupping therapy are now widely accepted by clinicians as adjuncts for physical examination and treatment techniques. Evidence indicates that although Cupping therapy is well-researched in non-orthopedic contexts, it may offer benefits for increased flexibility and recovery in injured groups, though its efficacy remains uncertain, with studies showing negligible long-term effects on hamstring flexibility (Schafer et al., 2018). Synthesizing alternative methods, when applied alongside conventional measures, may provide a greater indication of a patient's musculoskeletal function. As clinical practice changes, it is significant that clinicians be familiar with both traditional methods and those that are newer to provide the optimal patient outcomes. Further, the disparity that exists concerning physical therapists' levels of comfort and applications of thrust joint manipulation (TJM) across different spinal regions demonstrates the complexities that exist with physical examination methods. A survey of therapists ascertained that a clear majority feel comfortable with the use of TJM to the thoracic and lumbar regions but exercise caution in using it on the cervical spine due to perceived safety concerns and variable levels of training (Reilly et al., 2016). This variation suggests the necessity of ongoing education and consistent training in orthopedic care to ensure proficient evaluation and treatment. This training can ultimately close the gap between theory and practice and enhance clinical decision-making. It is essential that one values nuances in physical examination methods and the significance of knowledge of these methods by practitioners in offering high-quality musculoskeletal care.

8.3.3. Laboratory Tests and Their Relevance

In orthopedic and musculoskeletal medicine, laboratory tests are pivotal in the diagnostic process. Laboratory tests support clinicians in the diagnosis of a variety of conditions that would be impossible to identify with physical examination alone. By examining biological specimens, such as blood and synovial fluid, these tests can detect underlying abnormalities, including inflammatory markers, evidence of infection, and signs of metabolic disturbance. Furthermore, laboratory tests provide for the discrimination of complex musculoskeletal disorders and facilitate individualized interventions. The use of diagnostic decision support software as part of conventional methods for interpreting these laboratory tests ultimately enhances diagnostic precision and patient outcomes. These advances address the issue of insufficient specialists in the specialty, making generalists more capable of efficiently managing musculoskeletal complaints and reducing the risk of diagnostic errors (Athreya et al., 2016). In addition to diagnosis, laboratory testing is not limited; it is also crucial for tracking the disease's course and the effectiveness of therapy. For example, in the case of rotator cuff-related shoulder pain (RCRSP), laboratory studies can be beneficial in identifying inflammatory processes which can guide treatment strategies (Lewis et al., 2016). Routine testing can help the clinician assess the response to therapy, whether surgical or conservative, thereby allowing modification of treatment plans. Therefore, an integrated approach to patient care considers both laboratory findings and clinical presentations in order to present an overall picture of the patient's health status. As knowledge in the field of musculoskeletal disease advances, the use of laboratory tests to personalize treatment protocols and optimize patient satisfaction becomes increasingly vital. By keeping pace with the real-time advancements in laboratory technology and techniques, the influence on musculoskeletal and orthopedic medicine is profound. New diagnostic technologies, including more advanced imaging and biomarker research, provide more insight with routine laboratory testing. With these devices, clinicians can better understand osteoarthritis and rheumatoid arthritis, among others, informing clinical decisions along the way. The more scientists investigate the complexities of musculoskeletal diseases, the more laboratory-clinical outcome correlation will only be more refined. This overlap between clinical evaluation and laboratory testing provides a more robust foundation for diagnosing and managing orthopedic conditions, ultimately improving the delivery of health care in this critical area of medicine (Athreya et al., 2016; Lewis et al., 2016) (Figure 8.8).

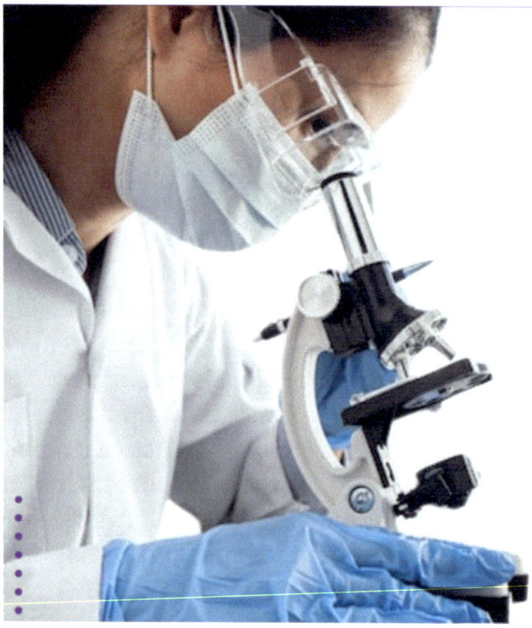

Figure 8.8. Laboratory tests and their relevance.

Source: https://www.sriramakrishnahospital.com/wp-content/uploads/2024/05/Clinical-laboratory.png.

Test Your Knowledge

1. What are the primary differences between X-rays, MRI, and CT scans in diagnosing orthopedic conditions?
2. How can laboratory tests support the diagnosis of orthopedic conditions such as infections or inflammatory arthritis?

8.4. Treatment Modalities in Orthopedic Medicine

Learning Outcome

1. Non-surgical interventions: Physical therapy and medications
2. Surgical options: Arthroscopy and joint replacemen
3. Emerging treatments: Regenerative medicine and stem cell therapy

The treatment options available in orthopedic medicine encompass a broad range of techniques designed to address various musculoskeletal disorders and dysfunctions. These are non-surgical methods, such as physical therapy, pharmacologic management, and bracing, aimed at symptom relief and functional restoration without surgery. Physical therapy, for example, is most crucial in rehabilitation because it enables strength gains, improved range of motion, and pain reduction through exercise and modalities. Pharmacologic interventions, including nonsteroidal anti-inflammatory drugs (NSAIDs) and corticosteroids, are also widely used to manage inflammation and pain, thereby making other therapies more effective. This multi-modal strategy sets the precedent for individualized treatment plans tailored to patient demand and condition to achieve optimal outcomes in orthopedic treatment. Surgical interventions remain a core component of orthopedic treatment, especially when conservative measures fail to provide adequate relief. Technically, they can range from arthroscopic interventions for the repair of soft-tissue injuries, e.g., SLAP tears in the shoulders, to total joint replacements for degenerative conditions such as osteoarthritis. In a recent study involving an investigation into the prevalence of SLAP tears by age, there was a high rate of occurrence among individuals aged 50 years and above, highlighting the importance of surgical procedures in advancing ages, where conservative options can achieve little (Bendich et al., 2018). This trend underscores the importance of early diagnoses and appropriate surgical interventions in maintaining function and preventing long-term disability in patients suffering from acute musculoskeletal disorders. Beyond traditional surgery, alternative therapies have become increasingly popular in orthopedic medicine, particularly spa treatments, which have shown promise in the management of some musculoskeletal disorders. There is professional consensus that spa therapy can be highly effective for patients with chronic musculoskeletal pathologies, relieving symptoms through hydrotherapy and therapeutic exercises in a specific environment (Bernetti et al., 2017). The treatment is typical of the growing acceptance of integrative treatments applied in addition to conventional treatments. As knowledge in the practice of orthopedic medicine continues to advance, there is a need to continue researching and validating the effectiveness of both traditional and novel treatments to ensure patients are provided with comprehensive care tailored to their unique clinical presentation and preferences.

8.4.1. Non-Surgical Interventions: Physical Therapy and Medications

In musculoskeletal and orthopedic medicine, drug and non-surgical treatment are essential in the management of many conditions. Physical therapy constitutes a wide variety of modalities that promote healing, mobilize joints and muscles, and enable overall function. Modalities include therapeutic exercises, manual therapy, and methods such as ultrasound and electrical stimulation. By focusing on tailored treatment programs, physical therapists aim to address the individual needs of patients who suffer from injuries, chronic pain, or post-operative conditions. Not only does this approach eliminate pain but also motivates patients to play an active role in their own rehabilitation, thereby enhancing their quality of life. Moreover, the addition of exercise is essential for preventing subsequent injury and maintaining musculoskeletal health, and thus physical therapy is a valuable component of a comprehensive treatment regimen. Medication management in the treatment of musculoskeletal disorders is also relevant, particularly in pain modulation and inflammation reduction. Nonsteroidal anti-inflammatory drugs (NSAIDs) and acetaminophen are most commonly employed as first-line pharmacologic options for conditions such as arthritis and tendinitis. Apart from conventional oral pills, corticosteroid injections can provide localized symptom relief for inflammatory conditions by targeting areas such as the shoulder, for example, in rotator cuff tears. New guidelines also emphasize a multimodal approach to pain management, where the pharmacologic interventions are complemented by physical therapy to prevent reliance on opioids and other narcotics. This paradigm change attempts to ease the opioid crisis outlined in recent medical literature, where overprescription has led to serious problems with pain management (Hsu et al., 2019). By exploring other medications and therapies, clinicians can enhance patient care while minimizing risks of narcotic addiction. As conditions of the musculoskeletal system often require individualized management plans, the inclusion of new treatments is also gaining prominence. For instance, the use of autologous platelet-rich plasma (PRP) injections is emerging as an extremely valuable nonoperative treatment for conditions such as partial rotator cuff tears. PRP therapy leverages the body's natural healing mechanisms, using growth factors to accelerate tissue repair and regeneration (Loccisano et al., 2016). This approach not only reduces the need for more disruptive surgery but also provides patients with choices that honor their preferences for less invasive interventions. The diversity of clinical outcomes for such therapies supports the need for continued investigation to identify optimal protocols and efficacy. As interventional techniques improve, there is a potential to revolutionize musculoskeletal care by providing patients with a strong arsenal of options for controlling pain and restoring function (Figure 8.9).

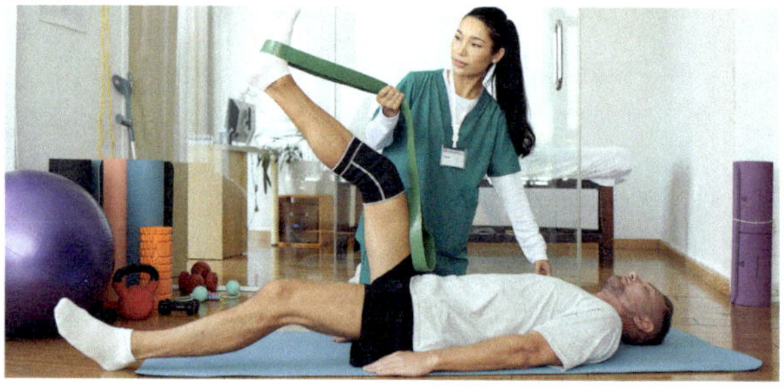

Figure 8.9. Non-surgical interventions: Physical therapy and medications.

Source: https://kineticptgreenville.com/wp-content/uploads/2024/09/Why-Non-Invasive-Treatment-is-Often-the-Better-Choice-17.jpg.

8.4.2. Surgical Options: Arthroscopy and Joint Replacement

Surgical interventions for musculoskeletal disorders have advanced significantly, offering the patient a variety of options to select from based on the illness and personal need. Two of the most prominent surgical techniques are arthroscopy and joint replacement. Arthroscopy is a minimally invasive procedure that uses small incisions and specialized instruments to diagnose and treat joint problems. Recovery is quicker and postoperative discomfort is minimal with this method compared to traditional open surgery. Its application in the knee, shoulder, and hip has changed orthopedic surgeons' approach to managing rotator cuff tears, meniscus injury, and articular cartilage lesions. The benefits of arthroscopy even extend to its diagnostic value. It facilitates precise visualization of the interior of the joints, thus ensuring that treatment regimens become effectively customized. In contrast, joint replacement is a more complex procedure typically recommended for individuals with widespread joint damage due to disorders such as osteoarthritis or rheumatoid arthritis.

It involves replacing a deformed joint with an artificial component, thereby diminishing pain and regaining function. Advances over the past few decades in implant materials and techniques have improved the success and durability of joint replacements, making them a lifelong solution for the majority of patients. Moreover, the utilization of patient-specific models for preoperative planning, as emphasized in a recent review of orthopedic simulators, underscores the importance of individualized treatment approaches to ensure accurate positioning of replacements (Abbaszadeh et al., 2015). As a result, joint replacement remains a cornerstone of orthopedic practice. It offers substantial benefits to patients with lower extremity disorders. Importantly, more recent research has also assigned a role to specialized training and simulation in maximizing surgical outcomes. The development of virtual reality-based simulators for surgeries such as joint replacement has been highly promising in maximizing surgeons' abilities and ultimately improving patient safety. These simulators can replicate real-world situations that challenge surgeons, allowing them to practice and hone their skills before operating on real patients. In conditions such as Morquio A syndrome, which is characterized by considerable musculoskeletal complexity, the use of such training tools can be exceptionally beneficial for the management of upper and lower extremity deformities (Bache et al., 2014). With ongoing improvements in surgical techniques and educational materials, the practice of musculoskeletal and orthopedic medicine has the potential to enhance patient outcomes and the overall quality of surgical practice.

8.4.3. Emerging Treatments: Regenerative Medicine and Stem Cell Therapy

The musculoskeletal and orthopedic medicine practice is being transformed by novel treatments that rely on stem cell therapy and regenerative medicine. The conventional methods in orthopedic treatment have relied on surgery and traditional therapy. The emergence of regenerative techniques, particularly those that harness the power of stem cell technology, has revolutionized the field toward a greater understanding of biological mechanisms of repair. Such therapies aim to restore damaged tissue by harnessing stem cells' natural regenerative mechanisms. Novel technologies, such as AI-driven self-evolving stem cell therapies, are optimized using machine learning to deliver personalized, real-time improvements in cure rates. This use of advanced technology represents a paradigm shift in the treatment of chronic musculoskeletal disorders and is ushering in more patient-focused care (Khan et al., 2025). In addition to stem cell therapy, the study of elastin-focused treatments holds immense potential under the paradigm of musculoskeletal rehabilitation. Elastin is responsible for maintaining the structural integrity and function of tendons and ligaments, but it can lose its effectiveness, leading to tissue dysfunction and increased susceptibility to injury. Emerging therapies such as platelet-rich plasma (PRP), bioengineered scaffolds, and microRNA-based therapies target elastin synthesis to enhance tissue strength and healing. Research indicates that such new methods are not only capable of improving tissue pliability but also of overcoming degenerative processes associated with injuries such as Achilles tendinopathy and rotator cuff tears. This convergence of regenerative medicine and elastin-focused therapy underscores the urgent need to further refine treatment techniques that prioritize long-term healing and joint stability in orthopedics (Banyś et al., 2024). The combined impact of regenerative medicine and rising technologies provides tremendous potential to the future of orthopedic care. As researchers continue to explore the therapeutic use of stem cells and biologic agents, there is an increasing emphasis on developing precision-based and proactive therapies. Future innovations, such as autonomous nanorobotic tissue generation and AI-driven musculoskeletal construct generation, are paving the way for the next generation of orthopedic solutions. The integration of cellular therapy with bioengineering protocols will drive enhanced regenerative capacity and improved patient outcomes in musculoskeletal disorders. In this way, the future of orthopedic medicine awaits further development, with an even greater focus on enhancing healing and restoring function through such advanced modalities (Khan et al., 2025) (Figure 8.10).

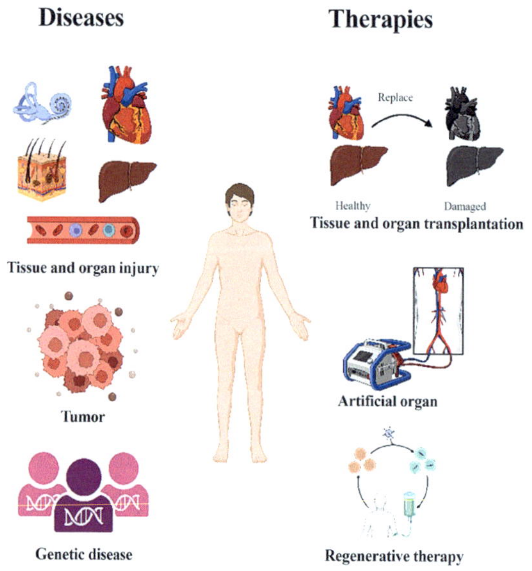

Figure 8.10. Emerging treatments: Regenerative medicine and stem cell therapy.

Source: https://www.frontiersin.org/files/Articles/1269577/fnins-18-1269577-HTML/image_m/fnins-18-1269577-g001.jpg.

Test Your Knowledge

1. What are two common non-surgical treatments used for managing orthopedic conditions such as osteoarthritis or back pain?
2. How do surgical procedures like arthroscopy and joint replacement differ in terms of indications and invasiveness?
3. What is the role of regenerative medicine, including stem cell therapy, in the future treatment of orthopedic injuries?

8.5. Rehabilitation in Orthopedic Care

Learning Outcome

1. Importance of rehabilitation post-surgery
2. Role of physical therapy in recovery
3. Strategies for preventing re-injury

Rehabilitation of orthopedic treatment is a critical phase with far-reaching consequences regarding patient recuperation and general life quality following musculoskeletal trauma or surgery. Following an injury or operation, such as a gluteal tendon repair, rehabilitation aims to restore normal function, reduce pain, and improve mobility. Various rehabilitation methods have been developed, aimed at individualized treatment programs tailored to patients' specific requirements. For instance, patients who underwent open repair of gluteal tendons showed varying degrees of fatty degeneration in their recovery; those with higher Goutallier-Fuchs Classification (GFC) scores demonstrated worse limping and lower functional scores. Therefore, understanding how surgery and rehabilitation procedures interact is essential to enhancing patient outcomes in orthopedic care, as the findings show that both open and endoscopic procedures can be used effectively regardless of the nature of the injury (Bini et al., 2020). The integration of digital health technologies into orthopedic rehabilitation is a paradigm shift in the provision of patient care, particularly during the COVID-19 pandemic. With traditional rehabilitation methods disrupted, telehealth and online platforms have come to facilitate remote monitoring and engagement for orthopedic patients. This transition guaranteed care continuity and allowed clinicians to track progress effectively remotely while improving accessibility. The successful rollout of these technologies not only validated that they could sustain or improve recovery outcomes but also underscored their long-term usefulness beyond the pandemic. Both the clinicians and the patients have come to appreciate the advantages of digital health solutions, and therefore, there exists a potential shift in orthopedic rehabilitation practices prioritizing convenience and patient-centred care (Ast et al., 2020). The future holds that orthopedic rehabilitation will also keep changing as clinicians embrace innovations that enable treatment success and patient participation. Incorporating digital health technologies can speed therapeutic interventions through real-time feedback and monitoring, thereby improving protocol compliance. Facilitated access to data can enable customized rehabilitation programs, allowing healthcare providers to make evidence-based modifications in accordance with patient progress. With the continuous evolution of practice in orthopedic medicine, future research on the effectiveness of varying rehab strategies and tech-enabled solutions will be critical. This approach emphasizes the need for a combined rehabilitation process using traditional and new strategies to ensure improved outcomes for patients in musculoskeletal well-being (Bini et al., 2020).

8.5.1. Importance of Rehabilitation Post-Surgery

The contribution of postoperative rehabilitation in musculoskeletal and orthopedic medicine cannot be overemphasized, as it is at the core of recovery and ultimately of patient outcomes. Postoperative rehabilitation is necessary to restore function, build strength, and enhance flexibility, which are essential to a successful return to daily function. The rehabilitation process can usually be initiated shortly after surgery to control pain and prevent complications such as stiffness or muscle atrophy. It is during this period that a customized rehabilitation program, with possibly physical therapy and some therapeutic modalities, can really oversee the recovery process. These rehabilitation programs are not only directed towards physical rehabilitation but also address mental issues, ensuring that patients are adequately cared for during the healing process, thereby ensuring more holistic post-operative care. Second, the effectiveness of rehabilitation programs is enhanced by consensus among the medical fraternity on their ability to heal various musculoskeletal conditions. A recent study outlined that adequate rehabilitation techniques significantly improve function and minimize the danger of complications during the post-surgical period. Specifically, consensus statements developed by a rheumatology and rehabilitation expert panel emphasize individualized treatment strategies according to pathology and patient condition (Bernetti et al., 2017). This underscores the necessity of a patient-centric strategy that incorporates physician expertise and interdisciplinary management. Effective rehabilitation not only reduces recovery time but also aims to prevent musculoskeletal disease formation, rendering long-term patient health benefits through surgery feasible. Lastly, the postoperative recovery process, and specifically for common injuries such as rotator cuff tears, demonstrates the revolutionary role that rehabilitation can have in patient outcomes. Surgery, though it is needed in severe cases, is typically accompanied by extended recovery periods, and during this time rehabilitation forms the basis of the treatment process. Studies have shown that although surgery for reconstruction addresses the immediate structural deformity, postoperative rehabilitation with conservative measures, such as physical therapy and more sophisticated treatments such as platelet-rich plasma (PRP), significantly improves the patient's quality of life (Loccisano et al., 2016). Moreover, a well-planned rehabilitation program facilitates stepwise return to normal activities, diminishes the perceived intensity of pain, and enhances global function. The introduction of rehabilitation following surgery thus emerges as a significant factor in achieving optimal recovery and long-term success of orthopedic procedures (Figure 8.11).

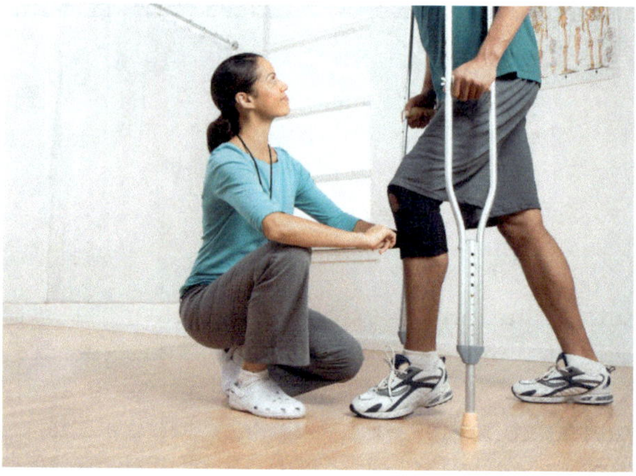

Figure 8.11. The significance of rehabilitation following surgery in the realm of musculoskeletal and orthopedic medicine.

Source: https://images.squarespace-cdn.com/content/v1/56257cd5e4b046286a8a63f4/1487806599285-AB51LIFM156R4CIDAVB4/Physical-Therapy-After-Surgery.

8.5.2. Role of Physical Therapy in Recovery

The integration of physical therapy significantly augments the orthopedic and musculoskeletal medical rehabilitation. With customized exercise regimens and manipulative treatment techniques, physical therapy plays a critical role in restoring function, reducing pain, and improving overall physical health. Injured, surgical, or chronic patients enjoy increased mobility and strength through customized therapy sessions. Functional movement assessment allows physical therapists to identify deficits and design interventions tailored to each patient's specific needs, facilitating a more timely and effective recovery. This systematic approach to rehabilitation honors the complex interaction between physical movement and healing, allowing patients to be secure in their physical capability once again as they return to day-to-day function. There is strong evidence of the effectiveness of physical therapy in rehabilitation, and its worth to the health care continuum is reaffirmed. Various studies indicate that consistent attendance at physical therapy is associated with improved outcomes after surgery and reduced pain medication use. For example, studies show that patients undergoing various procedures experience marked improvements in pain control and function after a comprehensive physical therapy program.

These findings suggest that incorporating physical therapy into treatment protocols not only accelerates recovery but also leads to better long-term outcomes, including reduced reinjury rates and improved quality of life. The uniform incorporation of physical therapy into recovery stories reaffirms its integral role in musculoskeletal and orthopedic care. Physical therapy's influence extends beyond the short-term recovery, determining long-term management of musculoskeletal disease. Progressive rehab techniques, such as neuromuscular reeducation and functional training, empower patients to develop healthier movement patterns. This is especially relevant to chronic illness patients who often have recurring pain or functional impairments. By emphasizing posture, biomechanics, and self-management, physical therapists empower patients to be active participants in their health. Also, the interdisciplinary physical therapy intervention, typically arranged in conjunction with other medical experts, encourages a coordinated approach to treatment aligned with contemporary practices endorsed in orthopedic and musculoskeletal medicine. Healthcare professionals agree that integrated thinking improves treatment outcomes and engages patients in their care, leading to long-term rehabilitation outcomes (Bernetti et al., 2017; Bini et al., 2020).

8.5.3. Strategies for Preventing Re-Injury

Safe prevention of re-injury in musculoskeletal and orthopedic environments is critical in optimizing post-injury rehabilitation and maximizing athletic performance. Progressive rehabilitation protocols to restore strength, flexibility, and coordination are perhaps the most vital of these. Return to activity in a stepwise fashion allows adaptation of injured tissues and strengthens support structures, minimizing the risk of re-injury. Moreover, integrating sport-specific drills during rehabilitation helps condition the body to the stresses of the selected sports and prepares athletes effectively for the physical demands of those sports. With an emphasis on strength and eccentric training, this aligns with a preventive approach that addresses biomechanical and muscular adjustments required to sustain athletic function after rehabilitation (Devon et al., 2008). Another practical approach is to monitor and modify training loads to avoid overuse and physiological overload, two of the most common precursors to re-injury. Applying principles of periodization training, athletes can utilize repeated cycles of different training intensity and volume, with adequate rest to maintain a balance between re-injury avoidance and preserving fitness. Ongoing monitoring by sports medicine professionals can provide early indications of a likely re-injury, allowing for prompt intervention. Secondly, they must be informed about rest and recovery needs, and encouraged to listen to their bodies and report pain. Active management of training is crucial in preventing the high recurrence rates of specific injuries, such as distal radioulnar heterotopic ossification, where specialized therapy will have to address the underlying causes (Bakhshi et al., 2019). Lastly, biomechanical interventions, such as proper footwear, orthotic devices, and ergonomic interventions, can significantly reduce the risk of re-injury in patients and athletes recovering from musculoskeletal injuries. Gait and movement pattern analysis will identify flaws that cause re-injury. Custom orthotics used as interventions will enhance foot and ankle alignment and thus overall kinetic chain biomechanics. Besides, educating patients on body mechanics—e.g., proper lifting and the need for warm-up exercises—may help prevent reinjury. These strategies promote a culture of prevention, eventually resulting in longevity in sports careers and overall physical activity (Devon et al., 2008) (Figure 8.12).

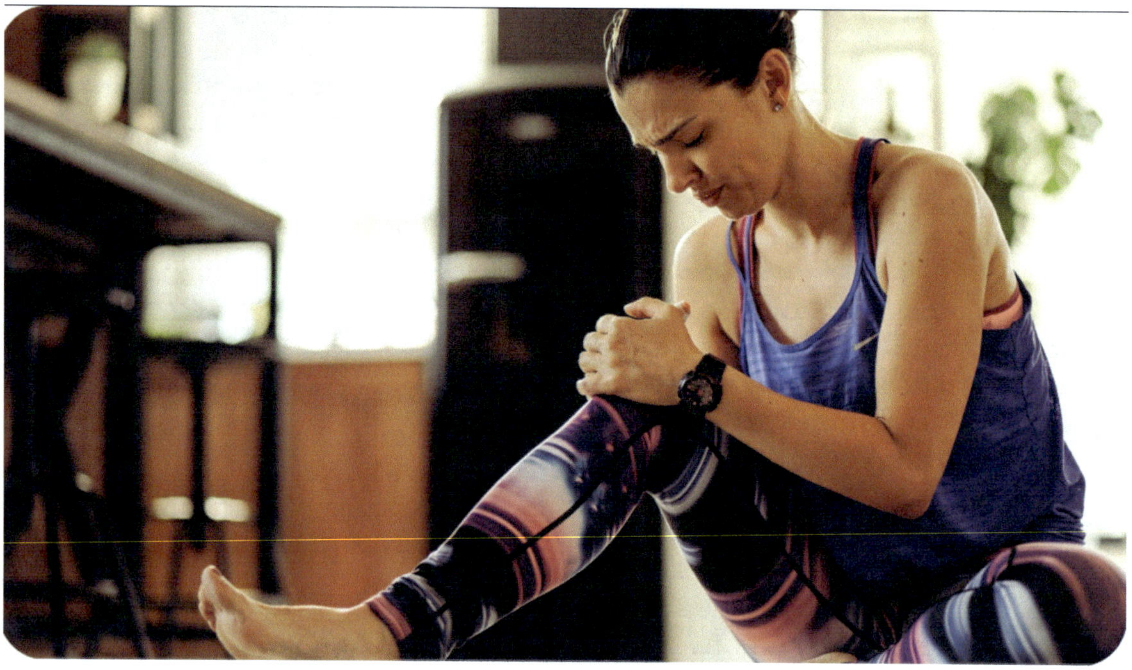

Figure 8.12. Effective strategies for preventing re-injury in musculoskeletal.

Source: https://cdn.prod.website-files.com/64686418489e82e99a49f4c8/66fe3e152b520db33b803c2b_5-strategies-for-preventing-sports-related-injuries-img.jpg.

Test Your Knowledge

1. Why is rehabilitation important after orthopedic surgery such as joint replacement or ligament repair?
2. How does physical therapy contribute to functional recovery following a musculoskeletal injury?
3. What are two common strategies used in rehabilitation programs to prevent re-injury during and after recovery?

8.6. Current Trends and Innovations in Orthopedic Medicine

Learning Outcome

1. Advances in minimally invasive surgical techniques
2. Use of technology in orthopedic practice
3. Research on biomaterials and implants

The face of orthopedic medicine is undergoing a dramatic transformation, driven by persistent trends and technologies that enhance patient care and surgical outcomes. One of the biggest trends is the use of advanced imaging technologies, such as 3D printing and AR, in preoperative planning and during surgery. These technologies enable orthopedic surgeons to create precise, patient-specific implants and models that accurately reflect anatomic structures, enabling them to plan and perform surgeries more accurately. These advances not only improve the authenticity of surgery but also reduce the chances of complications and enable more tailored interventions. Furthermore, AR utilization supports surgery by providing real-time overlay data that enhances visibility and decision-making, thereby optimizing patient safety and efficiency in orthopedic operations (N/A, 2002). In addition to technological advances, there is a noticeable increase in minimally invasive surgical methods in orthopedic practice. These methods try to reduce the trauma of the traditional open procedures, resulting in quicker recovery periods and minimal postoperative pain for patients. As a result, orthopedic procedures such as arthroscopy and robotic-assisted surgery are becoming more common. This is particularly important in the management of chronic musculoskeletal conditions, allowing patients to return to their normal lives quickly. In addition, the establishment of more efficient recovery processes following such minimally invasive surgeries underscores an emphasis on improving overall patient experiences and outcomes. The establishment of such protocols represents a yet broader shift toward patient-centred care, with individual needs and wants prioritized in treatment approaches (Silver et al., 2002). A fourth growing trend in orthopedic medicine is the increasing visibility of personalized medicine and its future implications for musculoskeletal well-being. This technique applies genetic profiling and biomarker analysis to determine treatment strategies based on individual patients' distinctive biological traits. This precision is particularly valuable when devising individually optimized rehabilitation programs and determining the most appropriate action in cases of osteoarthritis or musculoskeletal trauma.

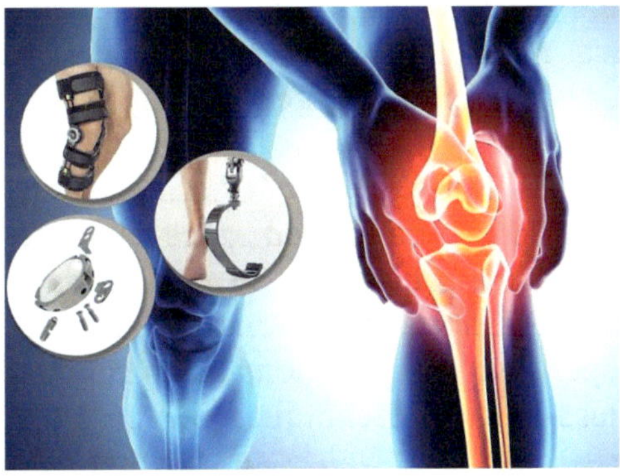

Figure 8.13. Current trends and innovations in orthopedic medicine.

Source: https://www.santacruzortho.com/wp-content/uploads/2022/09/7-Must-Know-Orthopedic-Technology-Trends.webp.

The integration of artificial intelligence and machine learning in practice also takes treatment personalization to the next level by predicting patients' responses to various treatments based on prior data. Overall, the integration of cutting-edge technologies with treatment plans tailored to individual needs is a paradigm shift in orthopedic medicine, which allows practitioners to make well-informed decisions that optimize patient outcomes and facilitate the development of this dynamic specialty (N/A, 2002; Silver-Thorn et al., 2002) (Figure 8.13).

8.6.1. Advances in Minimally Invasive Surgical Techniques

In orthopedic and musculoskeletal medicine, advances in minimally invasive surgery have revolutionized patient treatment and surgical outcomes. The technique emphasizes minimal incisions that are less traumatic to the adjacent tissues and lead to quicker healing for patients. A significant step forward has been the development of computer-assisted orthopedic surgery (CAOS) systems, which enhance surgical accuracy by integrating varied imaging modalities such as CT and MRI. These modern navigation systems directly influence the surgical process, enabling precise planning and execution. By coupling advanced imaging with real-time information, surgeons can make informed decisions that significantly improve the efficacy and safety of interventions, representing a great advance in orthopedic capabilities (Kalová et al., 2019). Another major advance in minimally invasive techniques is the use of new prosthetic technology in limb salvage procedures. For such patients faced with the predicament of bone tumors, particularly in the hip and knee regions, the development of personally crafted megaendoprostheses is an acceptable solution against amputation. Through thorough preoperative diagnosis and planning, this method enables more individualized therapy and significantly enhances functional outcomes. Improved techniques in the repair of soft tissues and minimal invasive procedures lead to fewer complications and enhanced overall recovery rates. Such developments underscore the importance of tailored surgical methods for the management of complex musculoskeletal disorders and the promise of modern orthopedic surgery to improve patients' quality of life (Barjaktarović et al., 2011). Also, the incorporation of robotic assistance in surgery is critical to reducing invasiveness as surgical capabilities rise. Robotic devices give surgeons greater dexterity and precision, enabling precise manoeuvres in the limited space characteristic of minimally invasive techniques. Robotic-assisted surgeries are proving to be vital in various orthopedic applications from joint replacement to fracture fixation. Practitioners can offer greater precision for aligning implants and reducing postoperative complications using robotic technology. With advancing technology, robotic systems and less-invasive techniques will be a synergy to redefine surgical standards, ushering in an era of unparalleled efficiency and patient safety in orthopedic and musculoskeletal medicine, thereby improving patients' long-term outcomes (Kalová et al., 2019) (Figure 8.14).

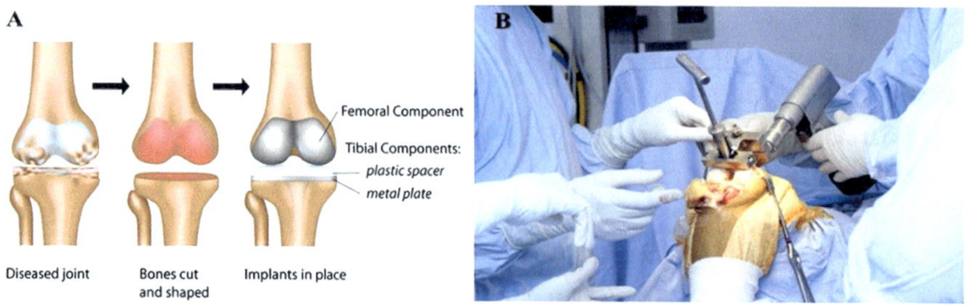

Figure 8.14. Advances in minimally invasive surgical techniques.

Source: https://www.frontiersin.org/files/Articles/1328997/fbioe-12-1328997-HTML/image_m/fbioe-12-1328997-g002.jpg.

8.6.2. Use of Technology in Orthopedic Practice

The incorporation of technology into orthopedic practice has significantly influenced patient outcomes and treatment paradigms. Minimally invasive surgeries, robot-assisted surgeries, and advanced imaging modalities have enhanced the accuracy and efficacy of orthopedic treatment. For instance, a study comparing open gluteal tendon repairs (OGR) and endoscopic gluteal tendon repairs (EGR) revealed that despite the perceived severity commonly associated with open surgery, both procedures resulted in clinical improvement. The study proved that EGR recorded a higher reduction in opioid use, citing the potential of technology to curb postoperative pain and rehabilitation (Bini et al., 2020). These advancements not only enhance the surgeon's technical expertise but also offer the patient the opportunity for faster rehabilitation, in contrast to previously observed complications with more invasive procedures. Additionally, the COVID-19 outbreak catalyzed a record-breaking convergence of digital health technologies into orthopedic practice. The enforced telehealth models, including virtual visits and remote monitoring, allowed orthopedic physicians to provide continuity of care while maintaining pace with safeguards in place. Consequently, regulatory reforms in support of digital health opened the door to the adoption of such technologies, which were pivotal in the treatment of musculoskeletal disorders at a time when face-to-face visits were limited. In the post-pandemic period, the digital orthopedic reality promotes greater patient satisfaction and engagement, likely recalibrating expectations for care among all stakeholders (Ast et al., 2020). This transformation underscores how technology not only addresses existing issues but also shapes the future of orthopedic patient management. Finally, the role of artificial intelligence (AI) and machine learning in the practice of orthopedics should not be underestimated, as these technologies have the potential to improve the accuracy of diagnosis and treatment individualization. AI algorithms can handle large amounts of data and identify patterns in patient presentations, thereby enabling clinicians to make more informed treatment decisions. Furthermore, predictive analytics can be essential for forecasting complications or outcomes, enabling proactive care interventions tailored to individual patients. As more orthopedic experts embrace these advanced tools, the emphasis will remain on ensuring that technology supports clinical expertise rather than supplanting it. In achieving this equilibrium, the orthopedic specialty will have a lot to benefit from new technologies that will eventually translate into better patient outcomes and operational effectiveness in other environments within healthcare (Bini et al., 2020) (Figure 8.15).

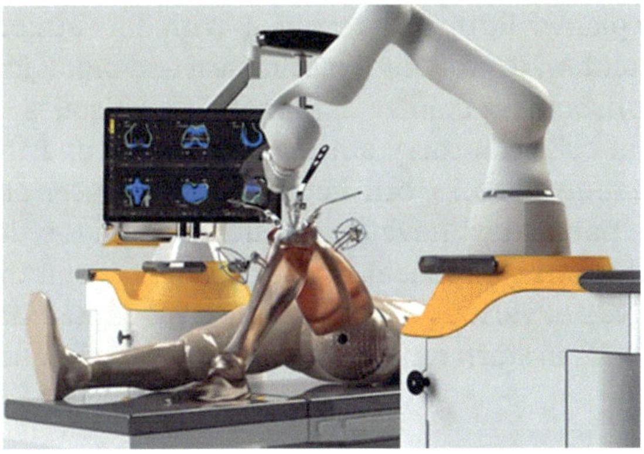

Figure 8.15. Use of technology in orthopedic practice.

Source: https://drpraneethreddy.com/wp-content/uploads/2023/09/Robotics-and-Computer-Assisted-Surgery-Blog-1-Small-Image.jpg.

8.6.3. Research on Biomaterials and Implants

The evolving biomaterials and implants market is a cornerstone of advancement in musculoskeletal and orthopedic medicine. Their design and application are intricately intertwined with optimizing patient outcomes following surgery, particularly in complex spinal surgery. Representative research demonstrates increased anxiety surrounding postoperative imaging, such as computed tomography (CT) scan, which, while crucial for monitoring surgical effectiveness, is risky due to ionizing radiation exposure (Andersson et al., 2017). In light of growing awareness of such risks, there is a need to optimize imaging protocols, stratify essential scans, and develop new monitoring methods to minimize radiation-related complications in patients undergoing complex spine surgery. Thus, integration of new biomaterials that can be compatible with less invasive imaging modalities, such as MRI, is essential in minimizing long-term health consequences and ensuring successful patient care. Of these, polymers and hybrid materials have emerged as solid contenders for application in tissue engineering and orthopedic implants. Both are designed with the utmost attention to creating a mechanical and biological environment similar to that of native tissues so that cells can carry out their functions and the healing process can begin. Hybrid materials, in particular, have a unique advantage: the inorganic component can be designed to suit the needs of various tissue types. Such adaptability stands in stark contrast to traditional techniques that use homogeneous biomaterials, with the innovation a radical shift towards more adaptive solutions for tissue repair. Researchers are working to simplify the makeup and structure of the materials while also probing their drug delivery potential, adding to their functionality with active pharmacologically active components and growth factors being encapsulated to fulfil specific therapeutic needs (Abalymov et al., 2020). Outside the laboratory, the research outcomes also have implications for clinical practice and the management of musculoskeletal and orthopedic medicine patient care. The fact that sophisticated biomaterials are being implemented in clinics underscores the need for interdisciplinarity among material scientists, biologists, and doctors to make innovations effective and biocompatible. Furthermore, the focus on developing one-size-fits products—a foundational concept in the field—helps address the varied needs of patients with different tissue types, including connective tissue, vascular tissue, and musculoskeletal tissue. Through this process, such interdisciplinary research not only enhances material properties and interactions with the biological system but also prepares researchers for upcoming breakthroughs in regenerative medicine to further improve patients' overall quality of life during convalescence from orthopedic ailments.

Test Your Knowledge

1. What are two key advantages of minimally invasive surgical techniques in orthopedic procedures compared to traditional open surgery?
2. How is technology, such as computer-assisted navigation or robotics being used to improve orthopedic surgical outcomes?
3. What are biomaterials, and how are they used in the development of orthopedic implants like joint prostheses or bone graft substitutes?

SUMMARY

In musculoskeletal and orthopedic medicine, the incorporation of more recent evidence underscores the need for a more comprehensive approach to patient care, particularly in pain management and surgery. The evolving landscape of pain education in the health professions requires greater emphasis on ensuring that practitioners are well grounded in pain mechanisms and pain management strategies. As highlighted in the findings of a survey on pain education in Doctor of Physical Therapy programs, there remains significant scope to further develop the curriculum to enhance practitioners' expertise in pain management. This is essential not only for effective treatment but to build a comprehensive understanding of patient experience within orthopedic practice (Bement et al., 2015). Moreover, the variations in surgical technique, for instance, open gluteal tendon repair (OGR) versus endoscopic gluteal tendon repair (EGR), are an indication of the complexity of orthopedic surgery. Analysis of clinical outcomes shows that both techniques can have good results; however, procedural variations can influence postoperative discomfort and functional recovery. The retrospective review revealed that while both methods showed significant improvement, EGR showed a statistically greater reduction in opioid use, indicating a difference in pain management methods following surgery (Bini et al., 2020). This finding calls for continued studies to refine surgical methods further and ultimately improve patient outcomes for orthopedic care. Cumulatively, these discoveries demonstrate the significant intersection of education, surgical innovation, and pain management in musculoskeletal and orthopedic medicine. As professionals strive to enhance clinical practice and adopt evidence-based practices, embracing ongoing education and data collection regarding multiple surgical approaches will be imperative. The challenge is not merely to improve surgical competency but to establish the capacity of healthcare providers to navigate the subtleties of pain management. Therefore, a comprehensive, multidisciplinary strategy for pain education and surgical effectiveness can significantly improve care standards and achieve a patient-focused approach in the evolving era of orthopedic medicine.

The orthopedic and musculoskeletal medicine specialty has a vast array of conditions, injuries, and treatment options. A landmark review of several weight-training sports reveals the most prevalent injury epidemiology in these sports. Research has demonstrated that even though these sports, including bodybuilding and strongman, involve heavy loads, they have relatively low injury rates compared to other common team sports. For instance, bodybuilding's injury rates are 0.12 to 0.7 injuries per annum per lifter, whereas more demanding sports like strongman have higher rates of 4.5 to 6.1 injuries per 1,000 competition hours (Eberhardt et al., 2017). This finding highlights the importance of a comprehensive explanation of risk factors for different sports, which could direct prevention strategies and enhance athlete safety. Also, symptomatic adult spinal deformity (SASD) health consequence is a significant area of study in orthopedics. Evidence indicates that SASD patients experience lower health-related quality of life compared to similar normative U.S. populations. For instance, SASD patients' mean physical component summary (PCS) scores are below the national average, indicating severe limitations in activities of daily living (Akbarnia et al., 2016). Research has found that the impact of lumbar scoliosis and increased sagittal vertical axis (SVA) can increasingly deteriorate such scores, underscoring the complex relationship between spinal deformities and overall well-being. Data such as this are valuable for clinicians to diagnose better and treat SASD, ultimately improving patient outcomes through targeted interventions. In summary, musculoskeletal and orthopedic medicine is a multifaceted field that reviews injury epidemiology and degenerative disease, both of which affect quality of life in distinct ways. The evidence of weight-training sport proposes a compelling rationale for sustained research to generate evidence-based prevention initiatives at various levels of competition. Similarly, the disabling implications of SASD necessitate increased awareness among healthcare professionals regarding its impact on disability and management possibilities. Together, these emphasis points underscore the function of systematic research in guiding clinical practice, shaping effective management, and promoting overall patient well-being in the context of musculoskeletal health (Akbarnia et al., 2016; Eberhardt et al., 2017).

KEY TERMS FROM THIS CHAPTER

Musculoskeletal System
Bone
Muscle
Tendon
Fracture
Osteoarthritis
Osteoporosis
Orthopedics
Joint
Ligament
Cartilage
Dislocation
Rheumatoid Arthritis
Sprain

CRITICAL THINKING QUESTIONS

1. **Which of the following is the most common site of osteoporotic fractures?**
   a. Humerus
   b. Femoral shaft
   c. Vertebrae
   d. Tibia
2. **A positive Lachman test suggests injury to which ligament?**
   a. Posterior cruciate ligament
   b. Medial collateral ligament
   c. Lateral collateral ligament
   d. Anterior cruciate ligament
3. **Which imaging modality is most sensitive for detecting early osteomyelitis?**
   a. X-ray
   b. CT scan
   c. MRI
   d. Ultrasound
4. **The most common primary malignant bone tumor in children is:**
   a. Chondrosarcoma
   b. Osteosarcoma
   c. Multiple myeloma
   d. Ewing's sarcoma
5. **What is the first-line treatment for a patient with acute gout?**
   a. Allopurinol
   b. NSAIDs
   c. Colchicine
   d. Probenecid

Short Answer Questions

1. Describe the pathophysiology, clinical features, diagnostic workup, and management of rheumatoid arthritis.
2. Discuss the evaluation and treatment of a patient presenting with acute low back pain. Include red flags, differential diagnoses, and criteria for imaging.
3. Explain the mechanisms, types, and clinical implications of bone fractures.
4. Describe the causes, clinical presentation, and treatment options for rotator cuff injuries.
5. Explain the anatomy and biomechanics of the knee joint. What are the common ligamentous injuries, and how are they assessed and managed clinically?

Answer to Critical Thinking Questions

1. (c) 2. (d) 3. (c) 4. (b) 5. (b)

REFERENCES

1. Abalymov, A., Parakhonskiy, B., & Skirtach, A. (2020). Polymer- and Hybrid-Based biomaterials for interstitial, connective, vascular, nerve, visceral and musculoskeletal tissue engineering. *Polymers, 12*(3), 620. https://doi.org/10.3390/polym12030620Abbaszadeh, A., Akhtar, M., Assassi, P., Barrow, C., Bliss, R., Blyth, P., et al. (2015). A review of virtual reality-based training simulators for orthopedic surgery. https://core.ac.uk/download/42143364.pdf (accessed on 17th July 2025).
2. Akbarnia, B., Ames, C., Bess, S., Burton, D., et al. (2016). The health impact of symptomatic adult spinal deformity: Comparison of deformity types to United States population norms and chronic diseases. https://core.ac.uk/download/323069856.pdf (accessed on 17th July 2025).
3. Aldini, N., Nicoli, D., Della Bella, E., Fini, M., Frizziero, L., et al. (2016). The role of detraining in tendon mechanobiology. https://core.ac.uk/download/53528699.pdf (accessed on 17th July 2025).
4. Andersson, G. B. J., Block, J. E., Garfin, S. R., Patel, V., et al. (2017). Utilization of CT scanning associated with complex spine surgery. https://core.ac.uk/download/323065336.pdf (accessed on 17th July 2025).
5. Annemans, L., De Regge, M., Duyck, P., Gemmel, P., et al. (2013). Physician-owned specialized facilities: Focused factories or destructive competition? A systematic review. https://core.ac.uk/download/55777137.pdf (accessed on 17th July 2025).
6. Arief, M. S., & Osterman, A. L. (2017). Optimal management of post-traumatic radioulnar synostosis. https://core.ac.uk/download/155271801.pdf (accessed on 17th July 2025).
7. Ast, M. P., Bini, S. A., Chung, C. C., Kalore, N., et al. (2020). Digital orthopedics: A glimpse into the future in the midst of a pandemic. https://core.ac.uk/download/323308683.pdf (accessed on 17th July 2025).
8. Athreya, B., Newgard, C. D., Correll, C. K., Deal, C. L., Zurakowski, D., Vittinghoff, E., Ang, E. Y. N., et al. (2016). Evidence-based decision support for pediatric rheumatology reduces diagnostic errors. https://core.ac.uk/download/83049477.pdf (accessed on 17th July 2025).
9. Bache, C. E., Harmatz, P. R., Jester, A., Mackenzie, W. G., et al. (2014). Orthopedic management of the extremities in patients with Morquio A syndrome. https://core.ac.uk/download/323062594.pdf (accessed on 17th July 2025).
10. Baker, B. D., Jr. (2019). The role of cross-training in swim-related injuries in master's swimmers. https://core.ac.uk/download/227521250.pdf (accessed on 17th July 2025).
11. Bakhshi, S., Breuing, K., Dohn, A., Ellis, J., Failla, J., Fernandez, H., Friedrich, J., et al. (2019). Use of acellular dermal matrix to prevent recurrence of radioulnar heterotopic ossification. https://core.ac.uk/download/323066682.pdf (accessed on 17th July 2025).
12. Banyś, F., Bochen, K., Czyżewski, F., Dziegciarczyk, M., et al. (2024). The role of elastin in tendon and ligament disorders: Therapeutic interventions in orthopedics and sports medicine. https://core.ac.uk/download/636385462.pdf (accessed on 17th July 2025).
13. Barjaktarović, R., Popović, Z., & Radoičić, D. (2011). Mega endoprosthesis in the treatment of bone tumors in the knee and hip region. https://core.ac.uk/download/pdf/26893915.pdf (accessed on 17th July 2025).

14. Bement, M. K. H., & Sluka, K. A. (2015). The current state of physical therapy pain curricula in the United States: A faculty survey. https://core.ac.uk/download/213078620.pdf (accessed on 17th July 2025).
15. Bement, M. K. H., Christensen, N., Fishman, S. M., Koebner, J., et al. (2013). An interprofessional consensus of core competencies for prelicensure education in pain management: Curriculum application for physical therapy. https://core.ac.uk/download/213085442.pdf (accessed on 17th July 2025).
16. Bendich, I., Feeley, B. T., Lansdown, D. A., Motamedi, D., et al. (2018). Imaging-based prevalence of superior labral anterior-posterior tears significantly increases in the aging shoulder. https://core.ac.uk/download/323073381.pdf (accessed on 17th July 2025).
17. Berger, K. I., Giugliani, R., Harmatz, P., Hendriksz, C., et al. (2014). International guidelines for the management and treatment of Morquio A syndrome. https://core.ac.uk/download/323073271.pdf (accessed on 17th July 2025).
18. Bini, S. A., Jäger, M., Maslaris, A., Patel, V., et al. (2020). Equivalent mid-term results of open vs endoscopic gluteal tendon tear repair using suture anchors in forty-five patients. https://core.ac.uk/download/323073887.pdf (accessed on 17th July 2025).
19. Bombardier, C., Butt, D. A., Green, D., Thorne, J. C., Paterson, J. M., Young, J., Widdifield, J., et al. (2014). An administrative data validation study of the accuracy of algorithms for identifying rheumatoid arthritis: The influence of the reference standard on algorithm performance. https://core.ac.uk/download/pdf/81865692.pdf (accessed on 17th July 2025).
20. Buck, F., Hodler, J., & Jost, B. (2018). Shoulder arthroplasty. https://core.ac.uk/download/159152401.pdf (accessed on 17th July 2025).
21. Chahla, J., Cinque, M. E., Engebretsen, L., Laprade, R. F., et al. (2017). Biological treatment of the knee with platelet-rich plasma or bone marrow aspirate concentrates. https://core.ac.uk/download/212863427.pdf (accessed on 17th July 2025).
22. Clark, T. J., Cleary, M. A., & Eberman, L. E. (2013). Physeal growth plate fractures: Implications for the pediatric athlete. https://core.ac.uk/download/46946337.pdf (accessed on 17th July 2025).
23. Devon, O., Horner, M., Jain, N., Lauencin, C., et al. (2008). Understanding sports hernia (athletic pubalgia)–The anatomic and pathophysiologic basis for abdominal and groin pain in athletes. https://core.ac.uk/download/46965603.pdf (accessed on 17th July 2025).
24. Eberhardt, A., Junge, A., Raske, A., Faigenbaum, A. D., Lopes, A. D., Kluitenberg, B., Gabbe, B. J., et al. (2017). The epidemiology of injuries across the weight-training sports. https://core.ac.uk/download/196601696.pdf (accessed on 17th July 2025).
25. Gregory, D. (2023). Innovations of radiology. https://core.ac.uk/download/619747458.pdf (accessed on 17th July 2025).
26. Harris, G. F., & Slavens, B. A. (2012). *Biomechanics*. https://core.ac.uk/download/213080657.pdf (accessed on 17th July 2025).
27. Hsu, J. R., Jahangir, A. A., Miller, A. N., Mir, H. R., et al. (2019). Confronting the opioid crisis: Practical pain management and strategies: AOA 2018 critical issues symposium. https://core.ac.uk/download/286537307.pdf (accessed on 17th July 2025).

28. Kalová, M., Kubíček, J., Oczka, D., Tomanec, T., et al. (2019). Recent trends, technical concepts and components of computer-assisted orthopedic surgery systems: A comprehensive review. https://core.ac.uk/download/287649034.pdf (accessed on 17th July 2025).

29. Katzman, W. B., & Pastore, E. A. (2012). Recognizing myofascial pelvic pain in the female patient with chronic pelvic pain. https://core.ac.uk/download/305124272.pdf (accessed on 17th July 2025).

30. Khan, A., Khan, A., Makki, F., & Albeez, S. F. (2025). AI, robotics, and next-generation biologic therapies in orthopedic regeneration: The future of autonomous musculoskeletal healing. https://core.ac.uk/download/647976397.pdf (accessed on 17th July 2025).

31. Lewis, J. (2016). Rotator cuff related shoulder pain: Assessment, management and uncertainties. https://core.ac.uk/download/132614159.pdf (accessed on 17th July 2025).

32. Loccisano, A. (2016). Platelet-rich plasma for the treatment of partial rotator cuff tears. https://open.bu.edu/bitstream/2144/14355/9/Loccisano_bu_0017N_10415.pdf (accessed on 17th July 2025).

33. McDonnell, J. M., Butler, J. S., Sankar, S., & Darwish, S. (2024). The potential role of synthetic computed tomography in spinal surgery: Generation, applications, and implications for future clinical practice. https://core.ac.uk/download/656981062.pdf (accessed on 17th July 2025).

34. N/A. (1997). *Focal Spot, Spring 1997*. https://core.ac.uk/download/129069307.pdf (accessed on 17th July 2025).

35. N/A. (2002). *Focal Spot, Summer 2002*. https://core.ac.uk/download/129069324.pdf (accessed on 17th July 2025).

36. N/A. (2025). *Musculoskeletal Discipline Science Plan*. https://core.ac.uk/download/pdf/42808673.pdf (accessed on 17th July 2025).

37. Reilly, S., Slaughter, R., & Ventura, E. (2016). Thrust joint manipulation utilization by US physical therapists. https://digitalscholarship.unlv.edu/cgi/viewcontent.cgi?article=4549&context=thesesdissertations (accessed on 17th July 2025).

38. Schafer, M. (2018). The acute effects of cupping therapy on hamstring range of motion compared to sham. https://digitalscholarship.unlv.edu/cgi/viewcontent.cgi?article=4327&context=thesesdissertations (accessed on 17th July 2025).

39. Shams, S., Silva, E. A., Stilhano, R. S., Yamaguchi, D. T., et al. (2019). PRP and BMAC for musculoskeletal conditions via biomaterial carriers. https://core.ac.uk/download/323068821.pdf (accessed on 17th July 2025).

40. Silver-Thorn, M. B. (2002). A rehabilitation engineering course for biomedical engineers. https://core.ac.uk/download/213072188.pdf (accessed on 17th July 2025).

OBSTETRIC AND GYNECOLOGIC MEDICINE

9

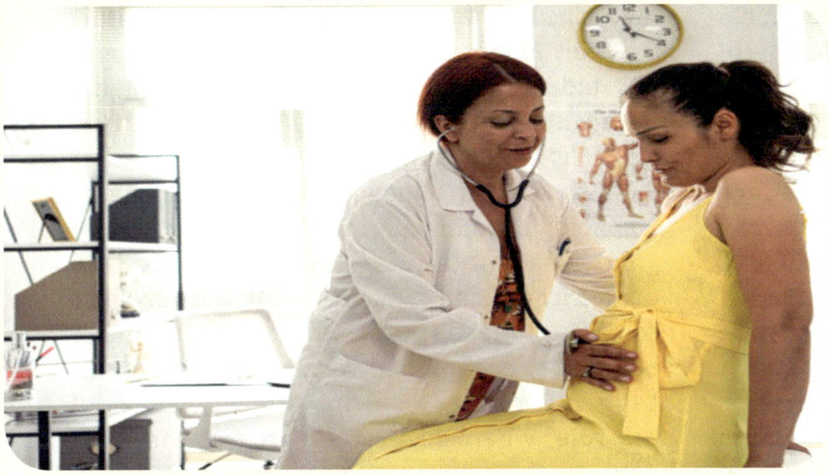

LEARNING OBJECTIVES

After studying this chapter, you will be able to:

1. Explain the historical development of obstetrics and gynecology
2. Discuss the significant areas of focus in obstetrics
3. Understand major areas of focus in gynecology
4. Discuss the common conditions treated in obstetric and gynecologic medicine
5. Understand advances in technology and treatment
6. Know challenges in obstetric and gynecologic medicine

Introduction

The specialty of obstetric and gynecologic medicine plays a crucial role in the provision of special care to women at various phases of life. Throughout their lives, from puberty to menopause, women experience tremendous physiological changes that influence their health outcomes. Obstetric care is primarily concerned with pregnancy, delivery, and postpartum recovery. At the same time, the domain of gynecologic medicine encompasses other issues of women's reproductive health, including menstrual disorders, contraception, and management of menopause. Understanding the interface between these fields of science is crucial for developing comprehensive healthcare policies that address the needs of women. The constantly changing nature of women's health requires professionals to stay up to date on recent studies, best practices, and guidelines to deliver high-quality care. One of the key complexities of obstetric and gynecologic medicine is the heterogeneous population that it serves. Age, ethnic origin, and socioeconomic status differences could be primarily responsible for differences in women's health outcomes. For instance, studies have established that pregnant adolescents, particularly those who are between the ages of 15 and younger, are at increased risk of having medical complications due to the reasons of low gynecologic age and lower pre-pregnancy weight (Felice et al., 1984). The importance of considering these variables cannot be emphasized enough, as they not only affect the mother's health but also may have enduring consequences for the developing fetus. This multifaceted model of care considers the social determinants of health to ensure that practitioners understand how these variables affect access to and the quality of care available. Furthermore, emerging technology and increased knowledge concerning reproductive healthcare options are changing the obstetric and gynecologic practice environment. Natural family planning is now an accepted option for women, particularly those within their perimenopausal period and who do not wish to become pregnant in their current state (Fehring et al., 2014). The effectiveness of these practices when appropriately used attests to empowering women to be in charge of their reproductive lives. By merging patient-centred care and evidence-based practice, healthcare practitioners can enhance women's health. As the profession evolves, the need to address the complex needs of women and employ new interventions will remain paramount to overall health and well-being.

Definition of Obstetric and Gynecologic Medicine

The specialty of obstetrics and gynecology, often intertwined, encompasses an enormous span of medicine dedicated to the reproductive well-being of women. Obstetric and gynecologic medicine is divided mainly into two subspecialties: obstetrics, pregnancy and childbirth care for women, and gynecology, in regard to the health of the female reproductive system in non-pregnant states. Thus, practitioners in this specialty must possess extensive knowledge of both the disease and physiological processes affecting women's health. The need for this medical specialty is also emphasized by increased interest in preventive medicine, educational assistance, and scientific research aimed at improving the course of motherhood and reproduction. Obstetric and gynecologic medicine is thus tasked with promoting women's health across the life span. Furthermore, the evolution of obstetric and gynecologic medicine reflects societal and medical scientific transformations and advancements. The practice has undergone significant alteration during the last centuries through both shifting cultural patterns and technological innovations. For instance, the introduction of advanced imaging technologies, minimally invasive procedures, and greater patient-centrism has transformed how obstetricians and gynaecologists deliver their services. Educational programs, such as nurse education, exemplified by Charlotte Seymour Yapp, reflect the increasing professionalism of the role, where her career progression from nursing through to infant health inspection illustrates the central role of nurses in assisting obstetric and gynecologic services (Chatterton et al., 2013).

The developments reflect ongoing efforts to accord women's health issues due attention and input. Furthermore, the adjective obstetric and gynecologic medicine is ever defined by evolving needs of the populations it serves. Issues like reproductive rights, access to complete care, and advances in fertility therapies highlight the dynamic nature of the specialty. Providers face complex ethical dilemmas and must advocate for policies that protect women's health as societal attitudes evolve. The ongoing controversy surrounding practices such as the employment of female labour in male clinics—evident in historical periods, such as the 1920 Wakefield demonstration—is indicative of social tensions influencing current care provision (Chatterton et al., 2013). Finally, an understanding of the definition and scope of obstetric and gynecologic medicine is based on its historical development, its evolution in practice, and ongoing advocacy to address the broad range of women's needs today (Figure 9.1).

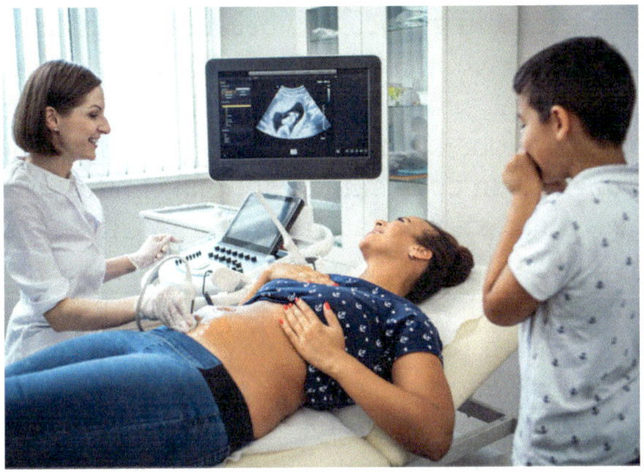

Figure 9.1. The field of obstetric and gynecologic medicine.

Source: https://www.aucmed.edu/sites/g/files/krcnkv361/files/styles/atge_default_md/public/2022-03/OB-GYN.jpg?itok=kC6zCG5y.

Importance of Women's Health

The role of women's health cannot be overstated, particularly in the field of obstetric and gynecologic medicine. Women's health concerns extend beyond reproductive well-being to encompass a comprehensive appreciation of physical, emotional, and mental well-being. Concerns like polycystic ovary syndrome, endometriosis, and the impact of pregnancy require specialist expertise and management. Women's health also encompasses knowledge of social determinants that lead to health inequalities. For instance, oppressed women might experience a deficiency in access to care, and this can result in delayed diagnosis and suboptimal treatment. Healthcare practitioners must adopt a holistic approach, not just the biological, but also the sociocultural, since it can influence women's health outcomes. The prevalence of sexual violence against women also underscores the necessity of a robust women's health system. One in three Australian women will experience some form of sexual violence during their lifetime. This is a traumatic experience that has a high correlation with chronic illness issues, including chronic pain, anxiety, and depression, which can complicate gynecological illness. Health professionals must identify and respond to a patient's history of sexual violence. If they fail to provide this information, it leads to insufficient awareness of ongoing health issues, ultimately resulting in suboptimal care. For this reason, creating an environment where women can provide such histories with confidence allows for better treatment and care, making it essential to use trauma-informed care in obstetrics and gynecology (Coles et al., 2012).

Additionally, women's greater role in society has implications for their healthcare needs and access to care. Historically, economic and social changes, e.g., women's increased labor market engagement and shifting family roles, have redirected care demands. For instance, in the early 20th century in England, the employment of women in what were previously men's professions posed challenges of working conditions and health risks for women, as seen in protests against women's work in men's wards of mental asylums (Chatterton et al., 2013). Women nowadays, as they struggle to contend with the complex balance between professional and reproductive roles, have their healthcare needs complicated. This calls for an integrated approach to gynecologic and obstetric care that not only addresses short-term reproductive health problems but also takes into account long-term health trajectories shaped by gender roles and societal expectations.

9.1. Historical Development of Obstetrics and Gynecology

Learning Outcome

1. Ancient practices and beliefs
2. Evolution of medical techniques
3. Key figures in the field

The development of obstetrics and gynecology is a tale of revolutionary change propelled by scientific, medical, and cultural progress. Childbirth mainly was the domain of midwives and family members in ancient times and had little formal education or awareness of the physiological process involved. With the development of civilizations, the need for a more organized medical practice became apparent. By the Middle Ages, universities began establishing medical faculties, where formal education in surgery and medicine was born. The emergence of specialist practices such as obstetrics and gynecology was a milestone in history, marking a transition towards evidence-based approaches to childbirth and women's healthcare. This shift is reflected in the increasing sophistication of instruments used during delivery and the rising incidence of surgical procedures, providing a platform for modern obstetric and gynecologic practice. The American College of Obstetricians and Gynecologists (ACOG) has a profound impact on the practices and regulations in obstetrics and gynecology. A review of ACOG's practice bulletins published during the 1998 to 2004 period illustrates that although a high percentage of recommendations are underpinned by high-level evidence, there remains a significant percentage of recommendations that are reliant on lower-level guidelines, indicating an area for remediation in the standardization of care. In particular, advice is classified as level A, which has solid scientific evidence, in 29% of instances. Different intensities of advice supplied subtlety in understanding between gynecologic and obstetric practices. These findings underscore the importance of continued research and prompt reflection on clinical advice to ensure that treatment protocols remain responsive to current evidence in patient care (Berghella et al., 2006). Knowledge of the reproductive health timeline is central to the development of obstetrics and gynecology because it highlights the issues women struggle with during their childbearing years. It appears that physiological considerations, such as pelvic morphology, play a strong role in determining optimal childbearing ages, suggesting that factors beyond simple societal influences are involved. Research indicates that women tend to want children at age 27, with real patterns of childbirth closely mirroring such desires, thus demonstrating a rational reproductive strategy based on physical capability and social conditions. These findings highlight the importance of integrating physiological knowledge into medical practice, promoting a more holistic approach to women's health that respects both past patterns and contemporary realities (Brewer et al., 2014) (Figure 9.2).

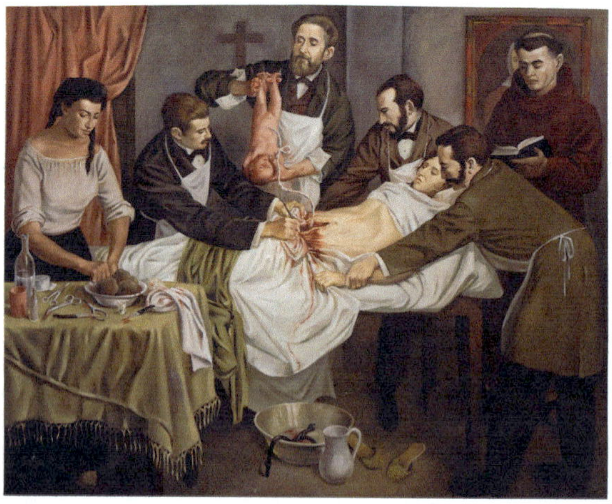

Figure 9.2. The historical development of obstetrics and gynecology.

Source: https://i0.wp.com/imss.org/wp-content/uploads/2024/05/img_6629.jpg?ssl=1.

9.1.1. Ancient Practices and Beliefs

When considering the historical background of obstetric and gynecologic medicine, it is essential to be mindful of the ancient customs and attitudes that shaped early understandings of childbirth and women's health. The majority of ancient cultures, including the Egyptians and Greeks, cultivated a holistic model of healthcare that integrated physical, spiritual, and emotional wellness. They believed that a woman's capability to become pregnant and give birth was under the influence of the cosmos and the coordination of bodily humours. The use of herbal remedies, rituals, and midwives was central to practices designed to support women during pregnancy and childbirth. These historic practices show a high level of sensitivity to women's unique health needs and an appreciation for the intricacies of female reproductive anatomy that have persisted across cultures and centuries. Such wisdom contextualizes the modern issue of obstetric care complications, particularly among disadvantaged groups, as seen in recent studies (Clair et al., 2020). Furthermore, the convergence of ancient ideology and mothering reveals the persistence of cultural storylines that have influenced women's health practices over the centuries. Childbirth is considered a public process in some native cultures, enveloped by cultural rituals meant to intensify the support network for the mother in labor. These customs not only make the body healthier but also help reinforce social relationships and intergenerational information transfer between older generations and young mothers. For example, customs such as unique birthing positions and consultations with skilled elders demonstrate public interest in safe delivery. Despite this, tales of race and maternal healthcare access, particularly for Black women, are starkly different from these beneficial traditions based on the current society's inability to overcome systemic barriers that continue to undermine equity in care (Zapalo et al., 2006). These obstetric and gynecologic practice patterns, again, are adapting to the uptake and application of knowledge from bygone days. As cultures advanced in medical knowledge, they came to embrace sound methodologies and reject unsafe or outmoded beliefs. The transition, for instance, from supernatural explanations of difficulties in birthing to a more scientific framework is an important shift in knowledge of female anatomy and physiology. The evolutionary history highlights the importance of evidence-based practices in modern obstetrics and gynecology. But it is still necessary to critically analyze practices from yesteryears because they are likely to contain valuable knowledge related to gender-specific healthcare and well-being. Incorporating such historical knowledge into contemporary medical practices, we work towards developing a more inclusive and holistic system for women's healthcare that honors the past while addressing today's disparities (Clair et al., 2020).

9.1.2. Evolution of Medical Techniques

The evolution of medical practices in obstetrics and gynecology has been strongly influenced by socio-political and historical determinants. The early 20th century was a defining period in which traditional practices began to evolve significantly, particularly influenced by greater advocacy for women's participation within healthcare. The Wakefield 1920 demonstration, for example, encapsulates the sociocultural forces at work on women's work in medical settings, particularly within the male-superior clinical sections. The motion at that time captured a concern about women healthcare workers' roles and indicated a changing perception of the need for specialty care in obstetrics and gynecology, thereby encouraging progress in these areas as women became further engaged in healthcare roles. Thus, this change provided foundational support for the slow evolution of women's health-focused medical procedures (Chatterton et al., 2013). Future advances in obstetric and gynecologic medicine can be mapped out through the careers of figures such as Charlotte Seymour Yapp, whose professional life reflects the expanding horizons of women's medical practice. After her nurse training in 1903 and midwifery certification, Yapp directed her professional life towards infant health and community welfare. Her forays from other regions of the country—Keighley, Halifax—rendered a more developed background in the study of maternal and infant health. As a leading figure, Yapp's professional trajectory reflects not only the evolving status of women medical professionals but also a broader acknowledgment of their essential contributions to obstetric care during a time when such developments were critical to improving maternal and child health results (Chatterton et al., 2013). With the evolution of the medical environment, techniques in obstetrics and gynecology kept pace with advances in technology and medicine.

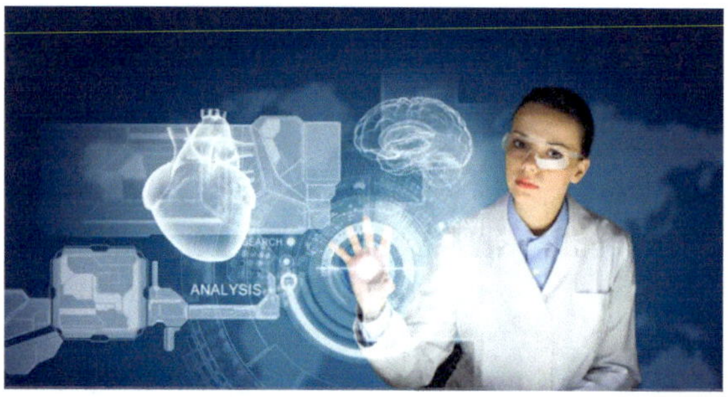

Figure 9.3. The evolution of medical techniques.

Source: https://i0.wp.com/nancy-rubin.com/wp-content/uploads/2015/09/medicine.jpg?fit=750%2C391&ssl=1.

From humble practices like asepsis and the establishment of maternity units, the increased reliance on evidence-based practice transformed ancient care practices. Innovations such as ultrasound scanning and minimally invasive surgery have changed diagnostics and treatment in obstetric practice, presenting a safer experience for mothers and babies. The technological developments represent a continued evolution that draws from the history of women's healthcare. The acknowledgment of medical innovations by women doctors and the adoption of traditional methods are manifestations of an active response to societal needs, ultimately evolving into a more comprehensive practice of obstetric and gynecologic medicine over the decades (Figure 9.3).

9.1.3. Key Figures in the Field

In Obstetric and Gynecologic Medicine, several key individuals have contributed to shaping our present practice and knowledge. Often leading the charge in research and clinical practice, these figures have helped advance our outcomes in maternal and fetal well-being. In addition to advancing medical knowledge, they also contribute to the development and implementation of practice guidelines. For instance, studies on the best reproductive age have been essential, as evidenced by findings that show women prefer to have their firstborn at an age of around 27 years. This observation, documented in both current studies and historical census records, underscores the overlap between physiological maturity and social forces in reproductive choice, in which women's reproductive aging is a turning point in successful gynecological practice (Brewer et al., 2014). Moreover, powerful characters have highlighted the rarity and subtleties of conditions such as placental site trophoblastic tumors, which pose challenges for healthcare providers due to their devious presentation and treatment issues. The evaluation of landmark cases provides an overview of ideal diagnosis and management, emphasizing the importance of correlating the medical history with laboratory testing. This level of accuracy not only improves clinical practice but also enhances the training of new practitioners in the field. A case involving a gravida 1 para 1 patient with a history of amenorrhea describes these challenges. It underscores the significant role of surgery as well as potential chemotherapy in managing such cases. As the body of work grows, these advances become increasingly important for developing effective treatment strategies for uncommon gynecological pathologies (Cunha et al., 2015). The influence of these pioneers extends to educational contexts, impacting curricula that educate future healthcare providers. Their research and clinical experiences are distilled into medical education, equipping future obstetricians and gynecologists with an in-depth understanding of the nuances of women's health. This general educational foundation is critical in addressing emerging problems in gynecologic and obstetric medicine, including reproductive health disparities and the application of technology in healthcare provision. As the specialty evolves, their ongoing contributions will remain key in addressing the subtleties of women's health, enhancing evidence-based care, and offering optimal care for populations with heterogeneous demographics. The outcome of their labor is not only to improve individual patient outcomes, but also to create an informed and responsive health environment for women (Brewer et al., 2014).

Test Your Knowledge

1. What were some common beliefs or practices related to childbirth in ancient civilizations such as Egypt or Greece?
2. How have medical techniques in obstetrics, such as cesarean sections or prenatal care, evolved?
3. Name one key historical figure who significantly contributed to the development of obstetrics or gynecology and describe their impact.

9.2. Major Areas of Focus in Obstetrics

Learning Outcome

1. Prenatal care and monitoring
2. Labor and delivery practices
3. Postpartum care and recovery

The field of obstetrics comprises an expansive range of indispensable disciplines, and maternal-fetal medicine is among the most prominent. The subspecialty itself encompasses the complexities of pregnancy, particularly those involving risky situations. Maternal-fetal medicine specialists not only track the well-being of the mother and fetus but also anticipate complications such as gestational diabetes, hypertension, and premature labor. These specialists perform extensive ultrasound examinations, prenatal evaluations, and genetic counselling to deliver the best outcomes. Interestingly, studies have reported striking differences in the quality of clinical advice on obstetric treatment, with only 29% of the American College of Obstetricians and Gynecologists recommendations at level A, which signifies strong evidence (Berghella et al., 2006). This underscores the need for continued research and advances to improve obstetric practice so that all women have access to high-quality, evidence-based care. Labor and delivery management is another key area of concern in obstetrics, aside from maternal-fetal medicine. Obstetricians are charged with monitoring labor progress, pain management, and life-and-death decisions on interventions such as cesarean delivery or instrumental deliveries. The complexity of these decisions is also aggravated by maternal condition, fetal distress, and patient preference. Moreover, the ongoing evolution of labor management strategies underscores the need for obstetricians to stay current on advances in technology and methods that can improve the safety of delivery. Given that labor complications remain very risky, evidence-based recommendations must be applied. This is particularly important when examining the type of recommendations issued by professional bodies, as exemplified by the comparative study of obstetric and gynecologic bulletins, which shows varying levels of adherence to best practices (Berghella et al., 2006). Finally, postpartum care is one such primary area of concern in obstetrics with immediate implications for maternal health outcomes. Postpartum conditions such as hemorrhage, infection, and psychiatric disorders require explicit attention and intervention strategies.

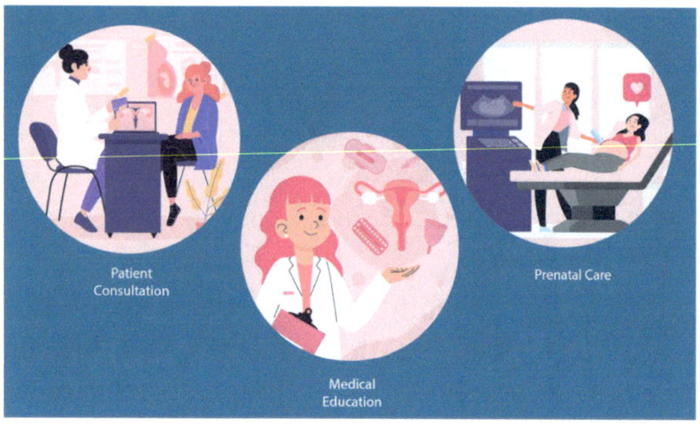

Figure 9.4. Major areas of focus in obstetrics.

Source: https://cdn.shortpixel.ai/spai/q_glossy+ret_img+to_webp/www.auamed.org/wp-content/uploads/2023/11/What-Does-a-Gynecologist-Do_-1024x683.png.

Furthermore, effective postpartum care entails enhancing the motherhood transition and supporting emotional well-being, thereby necessitating a holistic approach. Interprofessional collaboration among care providers, including obstetricians, midwives, and mental health services, is key to addressing such multifaceted issues. Research verifies that conditions like myofascial pelvic pain can exacerbate postpartum complications if left untreated. The interdisciplinary model is therefore imperative in the diagnosis and treatment of such conditions. Prioritizing postpartum care has the potential to improve recovery processes and long-term health outcomes among mothers, as seen in the requirement for comprehensive obstetric care in general women's health (Figure 9.4).

9.2.1. Prenatal Care and Monitoring

Prenatal care and monitoring are pillars of obstetric care, with a significant impact on both the mother's and the fetus's health status. Regular prenatal examinations allow healthcare providers to monitor the progression of the pregnancy, identify potential complications, and provide counsel on diet and lifestyle. Contacts like these make it possible to recognize gestational diabetes, hypertension, and infection that can affect both mother and fetus early on. Furthermore, the psychological well-being of expectant mothers is also considered as equally important as it may influence pregnancy outcomes. Through continuous assessment and treatment, health providers can ensure a holistic model of prenatal care with attention to the mother's as well as the developing fetus's health. Also, recent research has pointed to the application of probiotics in prenatal care, specifically for GBS colonization. A pilot trial indicated that an oral prenatal probiotic reduced GBS colony counts in pregnant women. Patients who received the probiotic regimen had healthier gastrointestinal tracts and lower rates of GBS colonization, thereby demonstrating the potential of nutritional interventions to be integrated into prenatal care. These findings not only highlight the importance of individualized care plans in obstetrics but also suggest that probiotics may aid in a healthier pregnancy. The resultant enhanced awareness of drug-free interventions necessitates a closer look at the role of food supplements in antenatal care. Interoperability of electronic health records

(EHR) is another essential characteristic of effective prenatal surveillance. The development of the Obstetric and Neonatal Ontology (OntONeo) aims to enable the sharing and continuity of prenatal care data among heterogeneous healthcare systems. Clinical and translational data representation standardization, OntONeo, enables better communication among clinicians, ensuring that essential information on maternal and fetal health is readily available at all times. This information exchange is critical to clinical decision-making, particularly in the treatment of complicated or high-risk pregnancies. Finally, the development of EHR interoperability, as outlined in projects such as OntONeo, has the potential to significantly enhance the quality of prenatal care and monitoring, leading to healthier outcomes for both mothers and their infants.

9.2.2. Labor and Delivery Practices

Practices in delivery and labour have evolved significantly over time, fueled by numerous factors such as medical technology, cultural beliefs, and the inclusion of patient-centered care. Classical childbirth had the woman being on her own, with minimal support during labor and delivery. In present practice, there is increased understanding of professional labor support (PLS) as a key component of the childbearing experience. A research study suggests that intrapartum nurses play a central role in providing this assistance, as their attitudes, behaviors, and individual experiences can strongly impact the labor experience. Positive attitudes among nurses regarding PLS enable them to provide a supportive environment for emotional support and reduction of anxiety, ultimately enhancing maternal satisfaction and birth outcomes. These findings underscore the necessity of incorporating in-depth PLS education into nursing curricula to better equip healthcare professionals to address the multifaceted needs of laboring women (Aschenbrenner et al., 2016). Delivery and labor dynamics also come under the impact of interactions between medical interventions and pregnant women's preferences. Choice of analgesia, such as epidural anesthesia, further dominates the debate around labor practice. While pain-reducing interventions like epidurals do lower pain levels, they may also introduce mobility and labor progression complications. Understanding the outcomes of pain-relief interventions enables healthcare professionals to provide care appropriate to individual patients' needs and desires. Access to support systems like doulas and individual birth plans is likely to enhance the positive experiences of childbirth by providing the illusion of control to mothers. However, bureaucratic barriers such as budget shortages and hospital policies can bring to a halt the effective implementation of such supporting interventions.

The combat of such challenges plays a critical role in shaping better labor environments (Chatterton et al., 2013). Lastly, social and cultural factors cannot be ruled out when making decisions regarding labor and delivery practices. Variations in cultural beliefs and practices related to childbirth may impact women's preferences for labor experience, thereby impacting their choice of setting, provider, and pain relief. For instance, cultural beliefs in some societies may favor home birth or midwifery care to align with culturally preferred views of motherhood and family. Intrapartum care should therefore respond to these various cultural perspectives while maintaining safe practice. The research highlights the need to close the gap between traditional practice and modern medical guidelines to facilitate comprehensive care. Integrative care is equally significant not only for facilitating favorable birth experiences but also in fostering trust between the practitioners of care and the populations they serve. Enhancing the relationship can eventually translate to better maternal and neonatal well-being (Aschenbrenner et al., 2016) (Figure 9.5).

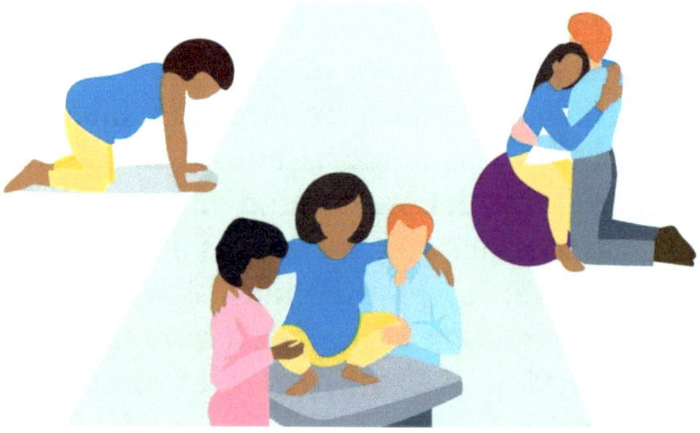

Figure 9.5. Labor and delivery practices.

Source: https://assets.clevelandclinic.org/transform/LargeFeatureImage/7c232732-9e12-451f-9bd2-0c3618b1cb51/childbirth-positions-1167672019.

9.2.3. Postpartum Care and Recovery

Post-childbirth recovery and postpartum care are crucial aspects of obstetric and gynecologic practice, requiring sustained support during the weeks following childbirth. A period of enormous physical and emotional transformation for the mothers as they move into a new life. Effective postpartum care involves monitoring for physical healing, e.g., perineal healing, pain control, and the management of delivery-related complications. Furthermore, the attention of the mother's emotional state is vital because many women are struck by postpartum depression and anxiety. Effective counselling at this time can help mothers adapt more smoothly to motherhood, enabling them to perform well in their new role while maintaining optimal health for both mother and child. The integration of nursing practice into postpartum care substantially enhances recovery for new mothers. Nurses are uniquely positioned to provide education and assistance through the aspects of postpartum health. In healthcare today, nurse-managed programs are a modern approach to assisting women with fertility management and postpartum recovery. For instance, one Internet-based natural family planning program showed high rates of pregnancy prevention among breastfeeding women, emphasizing the value of tailored educational interventions. This indicates that information provided by healthcare professionals can significantly impact a mother's ability to make informed decisions in the postpartum period, again highlighting the importance of individualized support in enhancing maternal and infant health (Bouchard et al., 2017). Further, understanding adaptation to motherhood is essential to support women through their postpartum journey best. Recent studies show that many women have trouble with physical, emotional, and social components during the early weeks after giving birth. Research studies on this adaptation process have revealed that the complexity of influencing factors to a mother's recovery, involving both demographic and perinatal factors, has been implicated. The results prove that the adaptation experience is not uniform but rather shaped by individual circumstances and community settings, necessitating a less one-size-fits-all approach to postpartum care. By aligning supportive interventions with mothers' unique experiences, healthcare workers can enhance resilience and maintain well-being at this crucial moment, thereby enhancing care continuity in obstetric and gynecologic practice (Aber et al., 2013).

Test Your Knowledge

1. What are the key components of routine prenatal care during pregnancy?
2. What are some important aspects of postpartum care to ensure the mother's physical and emotional recovery?

9.3. Major Areas of Focus in Gynecology

Learning Outcome

1. Routine gynecological exams
2. Management of menstrual disorders
3. Reproductive health and family planning

Gynecology is a multidisciplinary field that encompasses many crucial areas of women's health care throughout the life cycle. Reproductive health is one of the primary fields of concern, which involves evaluating and managing menstrual problems, infertility, and birth control options. Gynecologists have a critical role in providing integrated reproductive health care because they not only diagnose disorders but also help patients make decisions regarding their reproductive life. Notably, sexually transmitted infections (STIs) care is also integral to gynecological practice in integrating prevention and treatment for the overall health of the patient. According to the literature, organizational guidelines from organizations such as the American College of Obstetricians and Gynecologists offer many recommendations that can be applied to these domains, which are crucial for evidence-based practice in the field (Berghella et al., 2006). Another serious area of gynecology is the management of diseases of the female reproductive system, including cancers of ovarian, cervical, and endometrial origin. Early diagnosis and management are particularly important for the patient's recovery, with a focus on regular checkups such as Pap smears and HPV vaccinations. Gynecologists must guide patients through the complexity of diagnosis, treatment, and follow-up, addressing all areas of their health. Use of existing research evidence is fundamental to enhancing patient care. Reading through practice bulletins reveals that the vast majority of gynecological guidance is based on solid scientific evidence, highlighting the importance of gynecologists staying up to date on advances in the field (Berghella et al., 2006). Management of chronic pelvic pain (CPP), particularly myofascial pelvic pain (MFPP), is a significant area of concern in gynecology since it is a multifaceted condition and significantly affects women's quality of life. MFPP is either neglected or misdiagnosed and can be caused by a myriad of underlying pathologies, making diagnosis challenging. It is characterized by myofascial trigger points in the pelvic floor muscles that can refer pain to adjacent areas. Effective management of MFPP calls for a multidisciplinary approach, with interventions such as myofascial trigger point release and biofeedback. By facilitating cooperation among practitioners, gynecologists can maximize outcomes for patients with this condition, addressing both physical and psychological aspects of pain control. As the understanding of CPP evolves, gynecologists must remain adept at recognizing and treating these complex presentations (Figure 9.6).

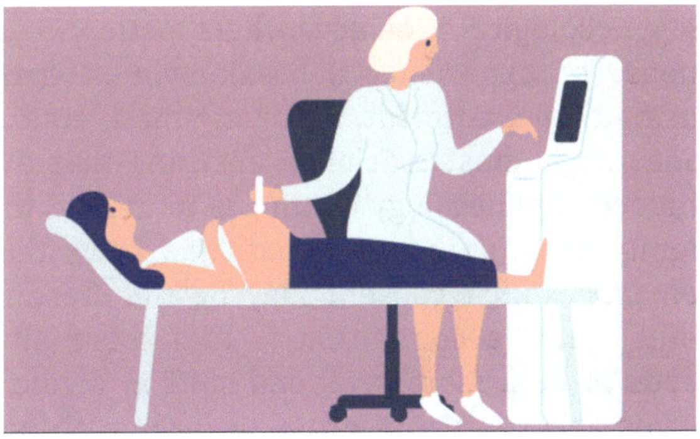

Figure 9.6. Major areas of focus in gynecology.

Source: https://buzzrx.s3.amazonaws.com/a366ea70-d563-4673-b305-366e9ca663cb/GynecologistvsObstetrician-WhatstheDifference_.png.

9.3.1. Routine Gynecological Exams

Routine gynecologic examination is an essential component of preventive women's health care, serving as both a diagnostic tool and a health education forum. These procedures provide the possibility to assess reproductive health without painlessly causing harm, for example, the breast examination, pap smear, and pelvic examination. These assessments allow the practitioner to diagnose pathology, screen for cervical cancer, and treat sexually transmitted diseases (STDs), thus facilitating long-term health dividends. Above all, women also form a rapport and trust relationship with gynecologists during visits, which is necessary for patients to openly communicate health issues and embrace medical advice. Regular gynecological examinations, therefore, not only play a clinical role but also help provide a proactive approach to women's health care. The moral considerations of regular gynecologic examinations have also become more common in recent years, particularly in the context of informed consent and patient autonomy. Consent is particularly applicable in situations such as when medical students perform pelvic exams and patients may not be aware of who their examiners are. Such unawareness can result in what has been termed as gynecological violence, where patients get uneasy or experience a breakdown in trust during their treatment. Resolving these ethical concerns is most crucial in ensuring that the practice of gynecology continues to uphold the dignity and autonomy of patients. Laws that demand explicit consent may be the starting point, but the contention is that there also needs to be a more profound shift in medical norms and culture in order to have a proper culture of respect and patient-centered culture in obstetric and gynecologic care (Parekh et al., 2022). In addition to the ethical issues, the routine gyn exams are necessarily part of the larger context of women's primary care. Given that obstetricians and gynecologists serve dual roles in both specialized surgical procedures and primary care, their training and practice patterns have significant consequences for women's health. Since curriculum reform was introduced in 1997, residency programs have emphasized the primary care elements in obstetrics and gynecology. However, there is a mismatch between how practitioners view their role in the primary care environment, particularly in screening and managing routine health conditions without referral to a specialist. It is valuable to understand the attitudes and practice patterns of obstetricians and gynecologists towards primary care to ensure that women's special health needs are addressed holistically and effectively within the scope of routine gynecological examinations (Patel et al., 2006). This approach focuses on the potential of these tests not only for the diagnosis and treatment of current situations but also for enabling women to be proactive about their health.

9.3.2. Management of Menstrual Disorders

The management of menstrual disorders encompasses several conditions that affect women's health and well-being. Some of the conditions, including dysmenorrhea, amenorrhea, and menorrhagia, require thorough knowledge of the participating hormonal and physiological mechanisms controlling menstruation. Effective management may include multidisciplinary treatment with medical, psychological, and lifestyle measures, depending on the patient's specifics. For instance, nonsteroidal anti-inflammatory drugs can relax dysmenorrhea pain, but hormonal contraceptives excel at regulating menstrual cycles and managing excessive bleeding in menorrhagia. Secondly, it is crucial to have information about the patient's lifestyle, such as stressors and diet, as part of holistic treatment methods that not only cure symptoms but also improve overall reproductive health. Accurate diagnosis of menstrual disorders involves a thorough clinical examination, patient history, and laboratory investigations. A range of diagnostic tests, such as pelvic ultrasound and hormone level tests, may assist medical professionals in diagnosing specific disorders and ruling out other causes of abnormal bleeding or pain. Patient education is also vital, with the majority of women benefitting from further information on their reproductive system and what the effects of their symptoms are. This education can enable the patient to be actively engaged in treatment and care planning. Additionally, health professionals must be vigilant in looking for complications of menstrual disorders, such as anemia due to excessive loss of blood, thereby offering complete care under the ambit of obstetric and gynecologic practice. Evidence of treatments in the form of medical treatment as well as surgery has dramatically revolutionized the management of menstrual disorders.

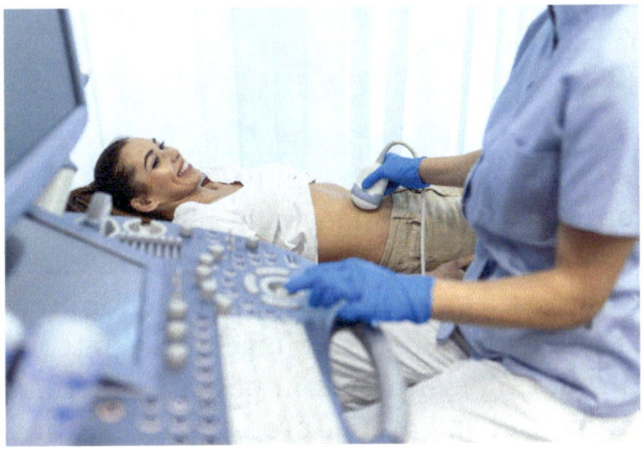

Figure 9.7. The management of menstrual disorders.

Source: https://buzzrx.s3.amazonaws.com/a366ea70-d563-4673-b305-366e9ca663cb/GynecologistvsObstetrician-WhatstheDifference_.png.

The coming of minimally invasive procedures, such as endometrial ablation, offers alternatives for women who are refractory to medical control of menorrhagia. Further, hormonal therapies, closely related to the treatment of menopause, have broadened the range of options offered for palliation of symptoms. Menopausal hormone therapy (MHT), for instance, is effective for associated symptoms and applicable to a broader age range if specific criteria are met (Davis et al., 2015). Patients can also talk to their doctor about non-hormonal treatments, such as dietary impact and complementary therapies, to add to an individually tailored treatment plan based on personal tolerance and medical history. Thus, the integrated strategy to treat menstrual disorders addresses not just the symptoms in the short term but guarantees long-term reproductive health in women (Figure 9.7).

9.3.3. Reproductive Health and Family Planning

The intricate relationship between reproductive health and family planning is paramount in the practice of obstetric and gynecologic care. Effective family planning not just facilitates responsible reproduction but also overall reproductive health by better enabling and informing individuals. Existing studies highlight education as a factor in this regard; for instance, an online natural family planning (NFP) service showed participants improved fertility knowledge after six months, with significant gains (8.96 to 9.46) reported among users participating in the program (Fehring et al., 2011). These educational interventions remain an important strategy in the realization of informed reproductive choices and reducing unwanted pregnancies that have a significant impact on maternal and child health outcomes. Moreover, the implementation of the NFP methods is proven to be very effective in preventing unwanted pregnancies among various groups of individuals. A secondary analysis of 40–55-year-old women revealed that there was a six per 100 typical use pregnancy rate over 12 months. With good instruction, NFP is a rightful method of contraception for older women (Fehring et al., 2014). This age group will usually have specific problems like diminished fertility and health disparities, which can render pregnancy difficult. The conclusions highlight the importance of comprehensive family planning services to meet women's diverse needs, particularly those entering perimenopause who seek to space their families as they take care of their reproductive health. With reproductive health becoming more and more caught up with sociocultural and economic factors, accessible family planning services are necessary. Innovative platforms, including online education models, have the potential to bridge gaps in traditional healthcare delivery, providing scalable resources for individuals without access to face-to-face services. The combination of nurse-managed online programs and in-person care is an integrated approach to reproductive health that fosters informed decision-making (Fehring et al., 2011). In addition, with the development of reproductive technology, ongoing research will be critical to adapting and refining family planning measures to maximize their effectiveness while addressing shifting requirements in society. Ultimately, integrating comprehensive reproductive health education and access to family planning interventions will be critical to healthier family and community outcomes."

Test Your Knowledge

1. What are the main components of a routine gynecological exam, and why are they important?
2. What are some key methods used in reproductive health and family planning counseling?

9.4. Common Conditions Treated in Obstetric and Gynecologic Medicine

Learning Outcome

1. Pregnancy complications
2. Gynecological cancers
3. Hormonal disorders

Obstetric and gynecologic medicine encompasses a range of conditions, one of which is most prevalent as chronic pelvic pain (CPP). It significantly impacts women's quality of life and may be caused by a range of underlying etiologies, one of which is myofascial pelvic pain (MFPP). MFPP is the occurrence of myofascial trigger points within the pelvic floor musculature, which refer pain to other regions of the body. Most clinicians also fail to make this diagnosis, and consequently the patient might not receive appropriate treatment. Interdisciplinary management techniques such as myofascial trigger point release, biofeedback, and electrical stimulation are needed for proper treatment of MFPP, enabling better outcomes and reducing symptoms in patients; therefore, awareness of and proper protocols for treatment are highlighted in obstetric and gynecologic practice (Katzman et al., 2012). One of the major conditions addressed in obstetric and gynecologic practice is infertility, which affects a high percentage of couples. Evaluation and treatment of infertility include a complete evaluation of female and male factors and may require more than one intervention to be applied. Natural family planning (NFP) instruction has become an alternative option for women who want to know about their fertility and obtain planned pregnancy outcomes. Recent studies show that internet-based NFP programs can enhance women's knowledge of fertility as well as reduce unwanted pregnancies by efficient charting methods. Internet-based platforms enable women to take charge of their reproductive health while providing the requisite support, and thus are striving to improve the field of family planning and reproductive health (Fehring et al., 2011). In addition, endometriosis and polycystic ovary syndrome (PCOS) are likewise frequent conditions encountered in obstetric and gynecologic practice. PCOS can be accompanied by several complications, including irregular menses, anovulation, and metabolic disturbances, necessitating a multidisciplinary approach to management. Endometriosis, however, presents unique challenges as it typically results in severe pelvic pain and is also capable of impacting fertility. Early treatment, most often with imaging investigations and possibly laparoscopic resection, is required for optimal management. Hormonal therapy, analgesia, or surgery are possible treatment options. Both syndromes illustrate the intricacies of women's health and the need for specialty care to address the unique challenges women face throughout their reproductive cycles (Figure 9.8).

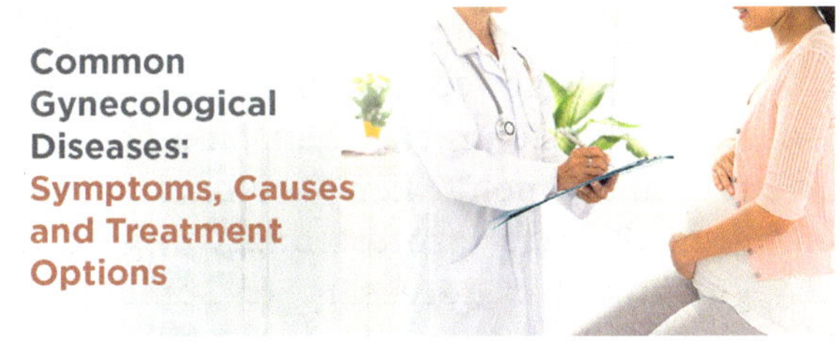

Figure 9.8. Common conditions treated in obstetric and gynecologic medicine.

Source: https://mmi.edu.pk/wp-content/uploads/2023/05/gynae3.jpg.

9.4.1. Pregnancy Complications

Complications of pregnancy are not only of various origins but also require intensive monitoring and control for the health of both mother and baby. Among the complications, adnexal masses are important, with an incidence ranging from 0.19% to 8.8%. Though the majority of the masses are benign, malignancy varies between 1% and 6%, and therefore, there is an urgent need for cautious examination. Proper evaluation differentiates patients requiring surgery from those who may be treated by a "wait-and-see" policy. An example of how complex it can be is a case study of a 36-year-old woman who was diagnosed with endometrioid ovarian adenocarcinoma and received widespread surgery, but later had no residual cancer on histopathologic examination. These conditions emphasize the importance of careful monitoring throughout pregnancy to detect potential complications early and address them accordingly, in accordance with the overall principles of obstetric and gynecologic care (Guarino et al., 2017). Another critical condition during pregnancy is acute abdominal conditions, which complicate the situation and lead to serious consequences unless addressed promptly. Acute cholecystitis and acute appendicitis are the most frequent causes of acute abdominal pain during pregnancy, with varied presentations that complicate diagnosis. There was one special case of a 33-year-old woman who, at 16 weeks pregnant, developed post-in vitro fertilization acute cholecystitis. Despite previous cycle failure, the patient required a laparoscopic cholecystectomy due to clinical worsening under conservative management. This intervention reflects the challenges of acute abdominal disorders in pregnant patients, necessitating surgical management despite known fertility issues. Perceptibility of the risk of such complications is thus required for obstetric practitioners to facilitate timely and efficient management, leading to improved pregnancy outcomes (Augustin et al., 2012). Prevention measures as well as risk reduction guidelines are also part of managing pregnancy complications beyond emergency medical intervention. Specifically, conditions such as ovarian hyperstimulation syndrome (OHSS) need to be monitored closely because they can lead to acute complications if they are not detected. For instance, the patient who presented with acute cholecystitis following IVF presented a high risk of thromboembolic complications—a topic not well addressed by existing guidelines for some subgroups. While protocols for the treatment of frequent complications like acute abdomen do exist, they are behind for the particular instance of IVF-ET patients and therefore require more research and development of specific protocols. A holistic approach to obstetrics and gynecology medicine thus requires not only acute management plans but also the formulation of all-encompassing protocols that address the special issues faced by different groups of patients during pregnancy. This multi-dimensional focus ensures that each aspect of maternal and fetal health is considered (Augustin et al., 2012) (Figure 9.9).

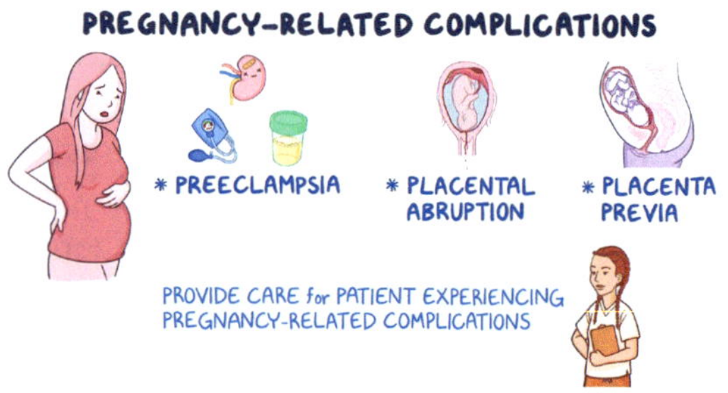

Figure 9.9. Pregnancy complications can arise from a variety of sources.

Source: https://www.osmosis.org/_next/image?url=https%3A%2F%2Fd16qt3wv6xm098.cloudfront.net%2FdKfQrXWBRfa04e01TWRJMpMJQ4SlclOh%2F_.jpg&w=3840&q=75.

9.4.2. Gynecological Cancers

Gynecologic cancers are a public health priority, particularly in obstetrics and gynecology. Gynecologic cancers are a collection of cancers of the female genital tract, such as cervical, ovarian, and uterine cancer. Among all cancers in developing countries, recent data show that approximately 25% are, which underscores the need for effective screening and early detection systems. Early diagnosis remains essential, as it is directly associated with improved survival rates. The application of advanced imaging modalities, such as positron emission tomography/computed tomography ([18F]FDG PET/CT), has proved beneficial for the effective detection of high-grade cancers and their metastases. Such diagnostic imaging developments are important for physicians to coordinate therapy regimens for affected patients, thereby enhancing outcomes of care for the gynecologic medicine branch (Vahidfar et al., 2022). Endometrial cancer, one of the most frequent endometrial forms of gynecologic neoplasia, requires personalized management strategies to achieve optimal therapy outcomes. Contemporary global agreement recognizes the importance of using histo-molecular characteristics and radiological data to inform clinical decisions. A Delphi poll of French and Swiss experts highlighted the complexity of defining endometrial cancer by risk factors, such as low- or high-risk. Such definitions guide therapy, including surgeries and adjuvant therapy, thus providing personalized treatment for patients. The integration of expert opinions into clinical practice recommendations is intended to reduce practice gaps and optimize patient management. Early communication among healthcare professionals regarding such guidelines is necessary to standardize care and improve clinical outcomes for patients diagnosed with endometrial cancer (Marti et al., 2022). Ovarian cancer presents additional challenges to the list of gynecologic malignancies, particularly given its tendency to occur in a delayed pattern and prove challenging to secure early diagnoses. Symptoms can be non-specific and readily misattributed as a cause of a benign process, resulting in delayed treatment and poorer prognoses. Thus, educating health professionals and the public on early warning signs of ovarian cancer is crucial in raising awareness and promoting early medical consultations. Emerging evidence is now showing that both public campaigns and organized screening programs can help reduce ovarian cancer mortality rates. Also, exploratory therapies such as targeted and immunotherapy offer promising future treatment options. Ongoing research and innovation in oncology and gynecology are critical to further develop knowledge and enhance resources invested in fighting these multifaceted cancers, ultimately improving patient care in obstetric and gynecologic practice (Figure 9.10).

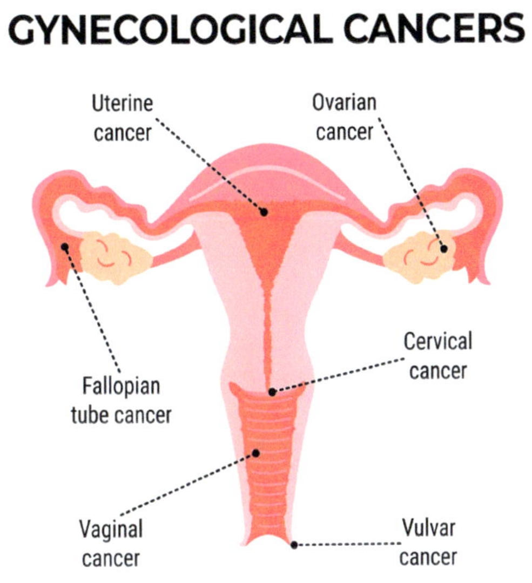

Figure 9.10. The topic of gynecological cancers.

Source: https://www.aurorahealthcare.org/-/media/Project/Health-System-Enterprise/AuroraHealthCareOrg/aurorahealthcare/images/images/services/gynecological-cancers.webp?h=1200&iar=0&w=1200&rev=3b255cde29e0467e9b9d91245c111160&hash=3FC676C030645E9A2C717C893E6E17A4.

9.4.3. Hormonal Disorders

Hormonal disturbances have a profound impact on women's reproductive health and often lead to situations that must be handled with tact in obstetric and gynecologic practice. Polycystic ovary syndrome (PCOS) is one of the complex interactions between hormones, metabolism, and reproductive function, manifesting signs and symptoms like irregular menses and infertility. Not only does this disease harm reproductive potential, but it also makes a patient vulnerable to other illnesses, like diabetes and vascular complications. The clinician must utilize a multimodal plan of diagnosis and management, mixing lifestyle modification, pharmacologic treatment, and repeated observation to optimize patient response. The relevance of treating these hormonal imbalances extends beyond gynecology, further underscoring the notion that hormonal well-being is integral to overall feminine health. The other crucial field of endocrine disorders of obstetrics is the occurrence of gestational trophoblastic tumors, such as the placental site trophoblastic tumors, which are exceedingly rare but have significant implications for maternal health. Abnormally formed trophoblasts cause the tumors and have the clinical presentation with manifestations like abnormal bleeding and elevated β-hCG, thus making them a diagnostic challenge with their idiosyncratic presentation. Because these tumors are relatively chemoresistant, surgery might be necessary, underscoring the need for an interdisciplinary approach between gynecologic oncologists and obstetricians. Additionally, the rarity of such tumors also emphasizes the need for continuous education and experience in the identification and management of hormonal disorders, to avoid misdiagnosis and to allow timely treatment options, thereby safeguarding women's health during pregnancy and beyond (Cunha et al., 2015). Apart from the pregnancy's implications on endocrine disorders, understanding the hormonal control of cycles is crucial in supporting couples' conception. Traditional methods, such as observing basal body temperature (BBT), were employed to indicate ovulation. New research has raised questions about BBT's effectiveness and reliability as an indicator of peak conception time. In parallel with advances in fertility awareness and reproductive medicine, medical professionals are obliged to critically evaluate the guidelines handed out to couples who want to conceive. Although BBT can hint at ovulatory cycles, its limitations must be discussed in detail to patients who wish to get advice on conception methods. This combined focus on both hormonal dysfunction and fertility counselling enhances the overall competence of practitioners in obstetric and gynecologic care so that women's reproductive health concerns are addressed comprehensively (Barron et al., 2005) (Figure 9.11).

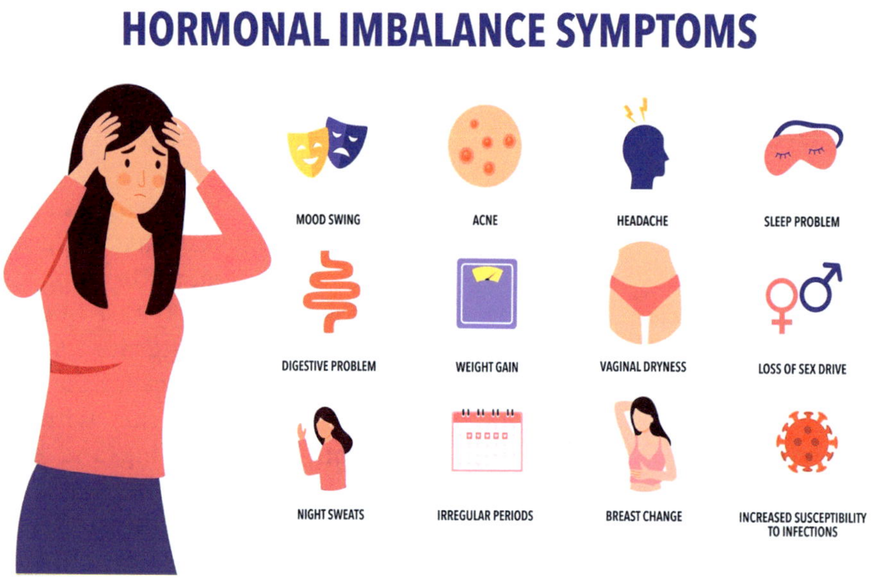

Figure 9.11. Hormonal disorders.

Source: https://www.manipalhospitals.com/uploads/image_gallery/hormonal-imbalance-infographics-1.png.

Test Your Knowledge

1. What are two common pregnancy complications, and how can they impact maternal or fetal health?
2. Name one type of gynecological cancer and describe a key symptom or method of detection.
3. What is a common hormonal disorder affecting women, and how is it generally managed?

9.5. Advances in Technology and Treatment

Learning Outcome

1. Imaging techniques in obstetrics
2. Minimally invasive surgical procedures
3. Telemedicine in women's health

The intersection of technology and treatment in obstetrics and gynecology has witnessed revolutionary advancements that overwhelmingly favor improved patient care. Among all the advancements, minimally invasive gynecologic surgery (MIGS) has transformed surgical procedures and set new standards for patient outcomes. With robotic-assisted surgery, patients enjoy enhanced precision and control that guarantees minimal injury to neighboring tissues. Such a technology-driven approach not only reduces recovery times but also limits postoperative complications, a necessary component in obstetric and gynecologic environments. While surgical techniques evolve, treatment personalization is increasingly approached with a greater emphasis on maintaining patient needs at the forefront, adapting treatment to personal health profiles to optimize recovery and satisfaction, thus positioning the patient-centered model as the core of contemporary healthcare approaches. A second essential challenge in gynecologic and obstetric medicine is addressing health inequities, which continue to hinder access to more advanced treatments. There exist significant disparities in outcomes across various populations, as challenges like distance to specialists, insurance disparities, and physician bias disproportionately affect underrepresented populations. These interruptions pose multiple levels of challenge to health inequities, leading to worse health outcomes. Therefore, addressing these problems requires a strategy of multi-dimensional approaches consisting of policy reform, community outreach, and increased access to care, particularly for regions with inadequate access to specialist care. The focus on equity ensures that technological advances not only enhance the quality of care overall but also become common, offering evidence-based solutions that actually have a meaningful impact on enhancing the care of patients for race, ethnicity, and socioeconomic status, as focused in ongoing discussions on the necessity of equity for specialty care (Carlson et al., 2016). Further, technological progress in imaging modalities and monitoring equipment for patients has played an important role in enhancing the effectiveness in the treatment of obstetric and gynecological conditions. With such technological progress, patient conditions can be monitored in real-time, enabling timely intervention and better outcomes. For instance, advances in ultrasound technologies permit more accurate prenatal diagnosis, a necessity to manage anticipated complications in pregnancy. These imaging technologies not only benefit clinicians in making well-informed choices but also empower patients by providing them with comprehensible information about their health status and treatment options. Furthermore, the adoption of telehealth platforms has enhanced access to care, particularly for women who reside in geographically remote or underserved areas. Embracing such technology propels us toward an integrated model of care that focuses on preventive and proactive treatment, ultimately guiding us toward healthier futures for obstetric and gynecologic health (Patange et al., 2023).

9.5.1. Imaging Techniques in Obstetrics

In gynecologic and obstetric practice, imaging modalities are valuable tools that enable accurate diagnosis and appropriate management of a multitude of conditions. Ultrasound, the most common imaging modality used in pregnancy, provides real-time imaging of the developing fetus and maternal organs. Its lesser invasiveness and ability to offer simultaneous results make it highly valuable for observing fetal growth, diagnosing abnormalities, and assessing amniotic fluid volumes. Additionally, advances in three-dimensional ultrasound technology have improved visual capabilities, enabling healthcare professionals to obtain precise anatomical detail, which is essential for prenatal care and intraoperative guidance. That blend of close observational skill, honed from working in the visual arts, can introduce a third dimension to the effectiveness of ultrasound examinations, helping the clinician pick up on tiny deviations from normal structures, particularly in sensitive areas of anatomy (Pien et al., 2025). Magnetic Resonance Imaging (MRI) is also an excellent alternative in some obstetric and gynecologic conditions, especially where increased anatomical detail is required. MRI can be particularly useful for evaluating complex conditions such as uterine leiomyosarcoma and placenta accreta, where standard imaging techniques would be inappropriate. Advances in artificial intelligence (AI) in recent years are revolutionizing MRI data analysis by improving segmentation and diagnostic performance across various pathologies. By leveraging large datasets and advanced algorithms, AI-based approaches are on the cusp of accelerating analysis to deliver personalized medical information, paving the way for individually tailored therapeutic interventions. Accordingly, the introduction of MRI to obstetrics and gynecology's armamentarium is a step towards more advanced diagnosis for these specialties since the increasing complexity of patient management requires (Saida et al., 2024). Even as imaging technologies such as ultrasound and MRI significantly enhance diagnostic potential, image interpretation remains highly dependent on the clinician's skill and perceptual capabilities. The cross-fertilization of art and medicine, demonstrated through the parallels between artistic observation and medical understanding, promotes an elevated state of awareness among professionals. As demonstrated by the analysis of historical depictions of medical disorders, extra observational training can fine-tune the clinical eye of medical professionals to the point where abnormalities that would otherwise go undetected can be identified. By offering multidisciplinary education, the field of obstetrics and gynecology can benefit from cross-pollination of ideas that inspire innovation in imaging interpretation and patient management. This union of science and art ultimately underscores the critical importance of imaging in achieving optimal outcomes in obstetric and gynecologic medicine (Pien et al., 2025) (Figure 9.12).

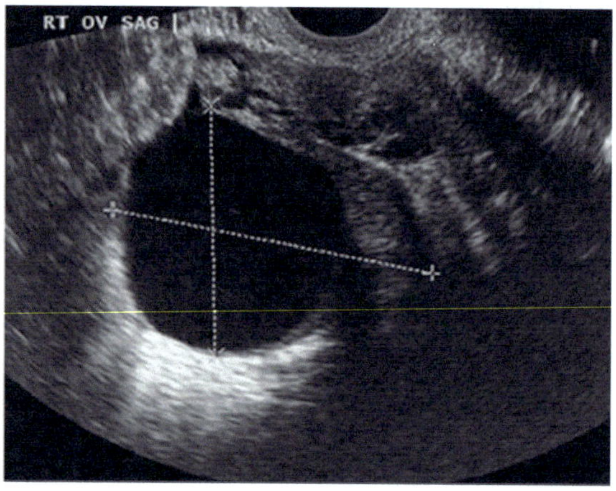

Figure 9.12. Imaging techniques in obstetrics.

Source: https://obgynkey.com/wp-content/uploads/2016/06/m_p9780071849081-ch002_f001.png.

9.5.2. Minimally Invasive Surgical Procedures

The environment of gynecologic and obstetric medicine has been drastically transformed by the introduction of minimally invasive surgical techniques (MISP). They are a collection of methods designed to reduce the trauma involved in surgery while also providing results equal to or better than those achieved through traditional surgery. By minimizing incisions and leveraging new technologies, such as robotic surgery and laparoscopy, MISP enables clinicians to perform complex surgeries with greater precision and less disruption to the patient's body. The evolution of the procedure has been marked by rapid advances in imaging and instrumentation, facilitating growing visualization and control during operation. Accordingly, patients experience less operative time, decreased postoperative pain, and earlier recovery to usual activities, thereby renovating surgical recovery expectations and patient outcomes in obstetrics and gynecology practice (Patange et al., 2023). One of the standout effects of minimally invasive surgical techniques is improved patient outcomes and safety profiles. After the use of advanced pain management methods and customized care regimens, the postoperative experience for patients has dramatically improved. Studies have indicated that MISP generally leads to more favorable blood loss and complications than traditional open procedures, which is especially crucial in obstetrics, where hemorrhagic events prove to be acutely dangerous. This is important in cases of morbidly adherent placenta (MAP), where the stakes are incredibly high, and routine procedures may be downright hazardous to mother and infant. Through the application of approaches such as early mobilization and psychological support, the speed of recovery increases further, cumulatively establishing the efficacy and popularity of MISP in practice (Chen et al., 2018). While the healthcare world gravitates increasingly toward the advantages of minimally invasive procedures, education programs and training courses are essential to making their broader adoption possible. Increased awareness and knowledge among doctors will make these advanced techniques become a part of mainstream practice, thereby optimizing surgical outcomes in obstetrics and gynecology. Further, ongoing research and development of emerging technologies will continue to enhance further the capability of minimally invasive methods to address the evolving needs of patients. Their inclusion in clinical guidelines will not only demonstrate dedication to patient care but also enhance overall standards of surgical practice in obstetrics and gynecology. Hence, critical funds and resources must be allocated to enhance practice and innovation in minimally invasive approaches to pay dividends to coming generations of patients (Patange et al., 2023).

9.5.3. Telemedicine in Women's Health

Telemedicine integration into women's health is a significant milestone in the practice of obstetrics and gynecology, particularly in addressing the looming challenge of unwanted pregnancies. In the United States, in 2018, nearly half of all pregnancies were unintended, with socioeconomic reasons being a predominant factor behind such a circumstance. Telemedicine provides a window for increasing the availability of contraceptive options through remote consultations, enabling professionals to give advice and prescriptions more conveniently. Such a shift would decrease the agony caused to low-income and uninsured individuals who typically have difficulty accessing prescription contraceptives due to issues of access. As in recent Tennessee movements, there is an immediate necessity for legislative reform to facilitate the over-the-counter accessibility of contraceptives, ultimately reducing unplanned pregnancies and associated abortion cases among vulnerable sections (Todd et al., 2021). Telemedicine is thus destined to play a crucial role in promoting women's reproductive health. The COVID-19 pandemic increased the use of telemedicine in maternal and newborn healthcare, highlighting opportunities and challenges in this rapidly evolving arena. In a worldwide survey of health professionals working in maternal and newborn health, 58% employed telemedicine during the pandemic to provide essential care services, ranging from antenatal consultations to psychosocial support via digital platforms. Despite its potential to increase access to and continuity of care, respondents identified significant impediments, including poor infrastructure and patients' distrust of online consultations. These are indications of the need for guidelines and ongoing training of healthcare practitioners on the application of telemedicine. That delicate balance between providing good care and addressing the growing inequities in healthcare access must be preserved so that telemedicine won't be an alternative but a complementary element to the conventional face-to-face interaction (Afolabi et al., 2021). In conclusion, telemedicine has the potential to transform women's health by increasing access to rudimentary services, particularly among the underserved populations, but its use must be exercised with caution. Support for policy updates to allow greater access to contraceptives and establishing firm guidelines for telemedicine practice will be crucial in facilitating better maternal health outcomes. Furthermore, ongoing research must evaluate the benefits and quality of telemedicine care for obstetric and gynecologic care compared with traditional modalities. By eliminating infrastructural and learning barriers, the healthcare system can attain a greater extent of using telemedicine in providing equal treatment for all women so that advances in technology enhance the delivery of women's health services rather than compromising them (Afolabi et al., 2021; Todd et al., 2021) (Figure 9.13).

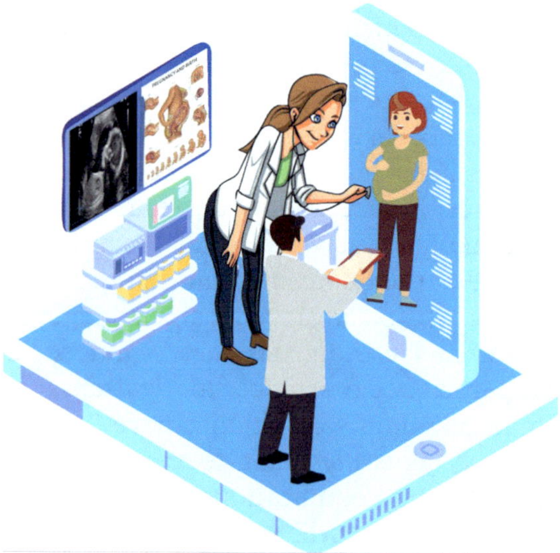

Figure 9.13. Telemedicine in women's health.

Source: https://www.technozo.in/wp-content/uploads/2021/04/telehealth-1024x977.jpeg.

Test Your Knowledge

1. What is the primary role of ultrasound imaging in obstetrics, and when is it commonly performed during pregnancy?
2. How has telemedicine improved access to women's health services, especially in underserved or remote areas?

9.6. Challenges in Obstetric and Gynecologic Medicine

Learning Outcome

1. Access to care and health disparities
2. Ethical considerations in women's health
3. Impact of societal attitudes on care

The obstetric and gynecologic health environment is littered with numerous challenges that have a significant impact on maternal and newborn health outcomes. Access to care, particularly among the disadvantaged, is a primary issue. Disparities in access to care are most likely to translate into delayed or inadequate prenatal care, which is one of the most crucial determinants for healthy pregnancies. Studies have indicated that women with restricted prenatal care are more likely to develop complications such as preterm labor, gestational diabetes, and hypertensive disorders. Furthermore, socioeconomic determinants, including income level, education, and geography, that also drive overall health inequities complicate the challenge. Overcoming these barriers requires a multi-faceted approach through education, outreach, and resources to ensure that all women, regardless of circumstance, receive the care they need throughout their reproductive lives. Another significant barrier in obstetric and gynecologic practice is integrating evidence-based and technological practices into daily care, particularly in the domain of fertility awareness and natural family planning (NFP). Though innovations such as internet-based fertility charting systems have shown promise in educating women about reproductive health, the acceptability and effectiveness of these programs across populations may vary. An example is a study of an online NFP educational program managed by nurses, in which, although participants showed increased fertility knowledge, the system's acceptability was unknown (Fehring et al., 2011). This highlights the need for greater research and targeted education strategies to ensure the maximum effectiveness of new technology across diverse demographic groups, so that women can use these tools to make decisions about their own reproductive health. The practice of immediate skin-to-skin contact after cesarean deliveries also raises other concerns in obstetric settings. Although there is considerable evidence of the benefits of SSC, including increased bonding and physiological stability in infants at the time of delivery, the possibility of implementing this practice after cesarean deliveries is generally not present. Research identifies a variety of perceived barriers from health professionals, particularly obstetric nurses, to implementing SSC in operating rooms (Balatero et al., 2018). Despite a general belief by nurses of the benefits of SSC, logistical constraints and safety concerns tend to impede routine utilization of SSC. These observations point to a pressing need for protocols and training that streamline the integration of SSC into birth practice for surgery, thereby enhancing mothers' and infants' outcomes in obstetric settings (Figure 9.14).

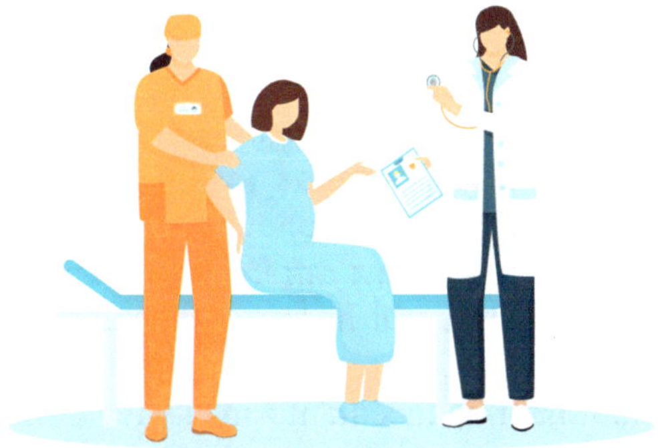

Figure 9.14. Challenges in obstetric and gynecologic medicine.

Source: https://media.healthecareers.com/wp-content/uploads/2023/04/11140631/OB-Gyn-2.png.webp.

9.6.1. Access to Care and Health Disparities

Access to care is a crucial determinant of health outcomes, particularly in obstetrics and gynecology. Variation in access to healthcare can lead to differences in maternal and neonatal health outcomes across population groups. In research on such variation, it has been found that specific populations, most frequently those of low socioeconomic status or with a greater percentage of racial and ethnic minorities, have high levels of barriers to prenatal care. Of special concern, a close examination of caesarean delivery rates in Georgia identified that wealthier counties with higher proportions of caesarean deliveries had fewer available midwives and higher proportions of Medicaid-covered births. Such findings highlight how health system organization and population factors interact to create settings in which access to appropriate care is limited, thereby increasing disparities in health outcomes among at-risk groups (Dunlop et al., 2020). Moreover, the lives of women with disabilities present a poignant description of how access to care intersects with health disparities. As the number of women of childbearing age with disabilities grows, evidence regarding their pregnancy outcomes and healthcare needs remains limited. Evidence indicates that, although there are specific perils from pregnancies in women with disabilities, such as increased rates of preterm birth and neonatal complications, the lack of significant differences in modes of delivery or maternal hospitalizations suggests that the availability of prenatal care is still paramount. Enhancements in health behavior and remediation of systemic barriers can have a significant impact on pregnancy outcomes for this group of women. Hence, one should determine and value the unique needs of women with disabilities in planning successful health care strategies that promote universal access to care (Mwachofi et al., 2017). Lastly, addressing health disparities in obstetric and gynecologic practice necessitates a multi-level strategy that combines community-based and systemic interventions. Effective strategies might include expanding access to midwife care, improving insurance coverage for low-income groups, and strengthening community health initiatives that address the specific needs of underserved groups. Decreasing barriers to care must also address socioeconomic determinants of health inequities, such as transportation challenges or limited awareness of available services. By prioritizing the provision of equal access to quality care for all women, especially those in vulnerable communities, health providers can help improve maternal and infant well-being outcomes and mitigate the persistence of health inequities (Mwachofi et al., 2017; Dunlop et al., 2020) (Figure 9.15).

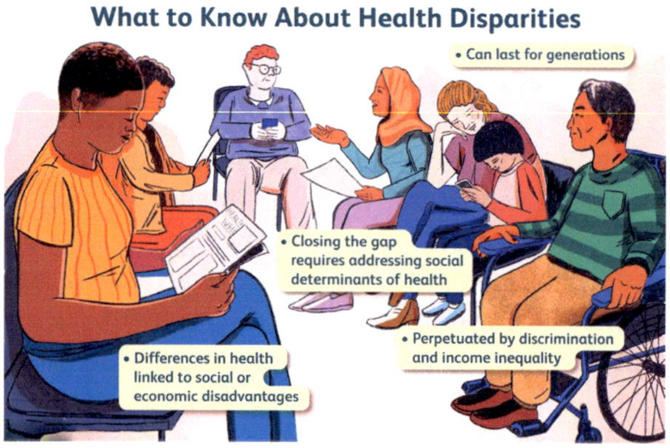

Figure 9.15. Access to care and health disparities.

Source: https://www.verywellhealth.com/thmb/CYVkCMe_-z5dlXxzqOYgAJZwdcE=/750x0/filters:no_upscale():max_bytes(150000):strip_icc():format(webp)/health-disparities-4173220_v1-e8914773af574e3d9f02b08d86835de5.jpg.

9.6.2. Ethical Considerations in Women's Health

The ethical problems of women's health, particularly in obstetric and gynecologic practice, must be addressed in an integrated manner, keeping both physical and psychosocial aspects of care in view. Exceptional experiences of women undergoing treatments for conditions like cervical cancer, which is an important problem of public health all over the world, must be dealt with. The treatments have long-term consequences like physical distress as well as sexual dysfunction. As emphasized in research on Indonesian women, such patients had a range of issues from distressing psychological conditions to disruption of intimate relationships following cervical cancer treatment, as they noted that extensive care from the health professionals is urgently needed. These findings indicate that ethical medical practice is not only focused on the disease but also on the broader implications of treatment, so that women's health is not merely clinical success but also relational and emotional (Afiyanti et al., 2014). In addition, employing effective screening approaches is vital to treat women's health issues ethically and comprehensively. For instance, widespread screening for postpartum depression has been advocated by such influential organizations as the American College of Obstetricians and Gynecologists and the United States Preventive Services Task Force. Such a move intends to routinely identify and treat mental illnesses, which previously were not given proper attention. Notably, a quality improvement study in the Alaska VA Healthcare System presented an 81% rate of screening for postpartum depression, which indicated the necessity for implementing standard procedures for maternal mental health care. Ethical issues of this type require health care systems to enhance their capacity and facilitate access to mental health care so that women can feel cared for during vulnerable postpartum situations (Brown et al., 2017). Lastly, the ethical realm of women's health encompasses patient autonomy and informed consent. Women must be adequately informed about treatment options and how these options will impact their health and well-being. Informed consent is not simply a matter of signing on the line; it is continued communication among healthcare providers and patients. This exchange allows women to make decisions from their own perspectives and within their own value systems and situations. Ethical dilemmas most often arise when patient interests conflict with clinical advice, particularly in challenging situations regarding reproductive choices or end-of-life care. Finally, patient autonomy must be given first importance, with assurance of wide-ranging, supportive, and empathetic care, to encourage ethical practice in obstetric and gynecologic medicine, ultimately creating trust and improving the health status of women (Afiyanti et al., 2014; Brown et al., 2017) (Figure 9.16).

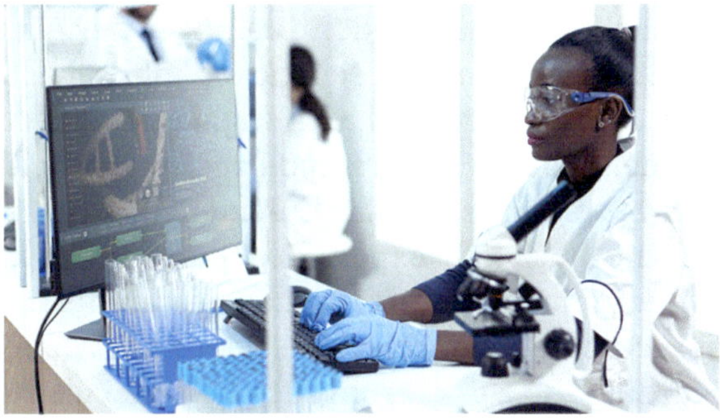

Figure 9.16. The ethical considerations in women's health.

Source: https://lpsonline.sas.upenn.edu/sites/default/files/2024-07/lpso-ethical-clinical-trials.jpg.

9.6.3. Impact of Societal Attitudes on Care

The impact of cultural beliefs is central to shaping the care provided in obstetric and gynecologic practice. Public opinion and cultural attitudes significantly impact attitudes toward pregnancy, childbirth, and reproductive health. For instance, emotional connections forming between expectant parents and their unborn babies have a significant impact on pregnancy-related maternal health habits. Studies have found that interventions that strengthen the parent-infant relationship can result in positive maternal outcomes, suggesting that societal support of emotional relationships between parents and infants might lead to healthier pregnancies and parent-child relationships. Nevertheless, it has proven difficult to obtain consistent results regarding these interventions, indicating that further research is needed to identify the societal factors that influence parental attachment. As highlighted by recent studies, the lack of acknowledgment and support for fathers in this evolving context reflects a broader cultural tendency to marginalize parental roles, particularly in prenatal engagement (Cunen et al., 2016). In obstetrics and gynecology, the consequences of social opinion overflow beyond pregnancy into the broader meaning of perinatal loss. Stillbirth, though a significant public health issue, is often burdened with stigma that affects how healthcare workers and society deal with bereaved parents. Available evidence indicates that the stillbirth experience places a great significant mental health burden on parents that is exacerbated by neglect or lack of knowledge regarding their grief from society. This cultural disposition can lead to inadequate support during periods of high emotional demand, and thus the work of healthcare professionals to deliver empathic, personalized interventions becomes especially significant. Through developing a culture that acknowledges the emotional toll of stillbirth, health systems can improve care provision and mental well-being for affected families, reinforcing the idea that societal attitudes are key to effective support mechanisms in obstetric and gynecologic medicine (Bhutta et al., 2016). Additionally, the impact of societal attitudes is further highlighted in the accessibility and affordability of care to marginalized groups. Socioeconomic inequality tends to dictate the level of care pregnant women and reproductive health patients receive, with societal biases still mirroring disparities in accessing health. This imbalance can also bleed into cultural competency in healthcare practices, wherein healthcare providers lack training or experience in diverse cultural practices in pregnancy and postpartum care. Thus, breaking down societal perceptions of these groups is paramount to providing equal care. Developing an inclusive healthcare setting that respects and values varied needs will not only enhance the quality of care but also health outcomes. Through education and awareness, the obstetric and gynecologic specialties can endeavor to dismantle prejudices, thereby establishing a more inclusive and supportive setting for all patients who require care during critical points in their reproductive health journey.

Test Your Knowledge

1. How do health disparities affect access to quality obstetric and gynecologic care among underserved populations?
2. What is one ethical challenge commonly faced in women's reproductive health decision-making?

SUMMARY

Obstetric and gynecologic medicine is paramount to understanding and optimizing women's health throughout every stage of life. The integration of advanced medical procedures, including web-based nurse-managed natural family planning (NFP) systems, demonstrates the burgeoning change towards patient-centered care. Research has shown that these systems can contribute a great deal positively towards a woman's level of awareness regarding her fertility, and evidence lies in the high increase in fertility awareness incurred throughout the study. Such programs empower women while promoting more informed family-planning decisions to ultimately improve reproductive health. The fact that relatively low rates of unintended pregnancy exist in this context points to the potential value of technology in facilitating responsible choice in obstetric care. It therefore represents a necessary area of emphasis in contemporary medical care (Fehring et al., 2011). Furthermore, intrapartum nurse attitudes and practices are crucial in shaping the experience of childbirth. Research findings have shown that personal experiences during birth significantly influence nurses' intentions to provide professional labor support (PLS). The association highlights the importance of continuous education and professional development in fostering favorable attitudes towards labor support among nurses. By removing obstacles such as staffing and documentation, healthcare systems can foster greater intrapartum nurse engagement in delivering quality care. This, in turn, will strengthen the labor experience of women, with beneficial birth outcomes and patient satisfaction and healthcare provider satisfaction (Aschenbrenner et al., 2016). Ultimately, the shifting landscape of advancement in obstetric and gynecologic practice requires an interactive plan that incorporates innovative technologies and professional development. Developing systems that are beneficial for both patients and healthcare providers can lead to improved educational gains for women regarding their reproductive health. In the future, it is essential to conduct more studies on effective training programs for healthcare providers and the integration of support mechanisms. This will not only improve clinical practice but also ensure that women's health is a priority in medical practice. By improving knowledge and support systems, obstetric and gynecologic medicine can continue expanding, and future generations of women will be enriched (Fehring et al., 2011; Aschenbrenner et al., 2016).

In the obstetric and gynecologic medical practice, understanding reproductive health and fertility is crucial to practitioners. One of the better-known aspects is the ability of basal body temperature (BBT) to help couples conceive. In the past, BBT was utilized as an indicator of ovulatory cycles, which allowed individuals to have better planning of intercourse. Recently, controversy emerged about the efficacy of using this method these days with the advances in research on reproductive health. The ramifications of such deliberations are significant, as they challenge healthcare providers to reflect carefully on the instruments they provide to expectant couples. Barron et al. (2005) also suggest that practitioners stay well-versed in both the strengths and limitations of conventional approaches such as BBT and embrace an evidence-based, integrative fertility counselling framework. Domestic violence (DV) is also a significant problem that crosses the boundaries of obstetric and gynecologic care, particularly for pregnant women. Systematic review of the prevalence of DV among pregnant women in Nigeria is informative, with a range of 2.3% to 44.6%. The review further points to the presence of high levels of exposure to risk factors for most women during pregnancy that have potential severe effects on maternal and fetal health. Further, the review lays out husbands as chief perpetrators in the majority of the reported cases, highlighting how healthcare providers must not neglect the warning signs of DV. The findings underscore the responsibility of obstetric and gynecologic care providers to foster safe, supportive environments for patients and to incorporate DV screening into routine obstetric care. Alo et al. (2017) emphasize the need for tailored interventions to address this pervasive issue competently. Lastly, the working knowledge of fertility, reproductive health, and domestic violence could be incorporated into practice to enhance the quality of care within the obstetrics and gynecology field significantly. Healthcare professionals must remain dedicated to ongoing education on upcoming research and policy implications for these disciplines. This involves constructing policies that address both the socio-cultural and clinical dimensions of issues like DV. Practitioners have to ensure holistic support systems that empower women educationally, in terms of resources, and in safe spaces. By synthesizing this rich method, obstetric and gynecologic practice can move toward more equitable, knowledge-based care, ultimately improving health outcomes for women and their families. In doing this, the profession can foster not only clinical excellence but also social justice in healthcare systems.

KEY TERMS FROM THIS CHAPTER

- Obstetrics
- Gynecology
- Menstrual Cycle
- Ovulation
- Fertilization
- Implantation
- Pregnancy
- Antenatal Care
- Labor
- Parturition
- Postnatal Care
- Menopause
- Amenorrhea
- Dysmenorrhea

CRITICAL THINKING QUESTIONS

1. **Which hormone is primarily responsible for maintaining the uterine lining during early pregnancy?**
   a. Estrogen
   b. Follicle-stimulating hormone (FSH)
   c. Luteinizing hormone (LH)
   d. Progesterone
2. **What is the recommended first-line treatment for bacterial vaginosis in non-pregnant women?**
   a. Clindamycin cream
   b. Metronidazole
   c. Fluconazole
   d. Amoxicillin
3. **Which of the following is a diagnostic criterion for polycystic ovary syndrome (PCOS)?**
   a. High prolactin levels
   b. Ovarian cancer markers
   c. Irregular menstrual cycles
   d. Endometrial thickening
4. **What is the most common site of ectopic pregnancy?**
   a. Ovary
   b. Cervix
   c. Fallopian tube
   d. Abdominal cavity
5. **Which of the following findings is suggestive of preeclampsia?**
   a. Hypertension and proteinuria after 20 weeks of gestation
   b. High blood glucose in early pregnancy
   c. Vaginal bleeding in the third trimester
   d. Preterm labor before 32 weeks

Short Answer Questions

1. What are the three trimesters of pregnancy and the general duration of each?
2. What is the purpose of a Pap smear in gynecologic screening?
3. How is gestational diabetes diagnosed during pregnancy?
4. What is the difference between preeclampsia and eclampsia?
5. List two common symptoms of polycystic ovary syndrome (PCOS).
6. What are the main hormonal changes during the menstrual cycle?

Answers to Critical Thinking Questions

1. (d); 2. (b); 3. (c); 4. (c); 5. (a)

REFERENCES

1. Aber, C., Weiss, M., & Fawcett, J. (2013). Contemporary Women's adaptation to motherhood. *Nursing Science Quarterly*, *26*(4), 344–351. https://doi.org/10.1177/0894318413500345Afiyanti, Y., Andrijono, A., Azwar, A., Setyowati, S., et al. (2014). Women's experiences of sexual problems after cervical cancer treatment: Lessons from Indonesian women. https://media.neliti.com/media/publications/150324-EN-womens-experiences-of-sexual-problems-af.pdf (accessed on 17th July 2025).

2. Afolabi, B. B., Asefa, A., Audet, C., Benova, L., et al. (2021). A double-edged sword: Telemedicine for maternal care during COVID-19: Findings from a global mixed-methods study of healthcare providers. https://core.ac.uk/download/395606337.pdf (accessed on 17th July 2025).

3. Almeida, M., Elkin, P., Farinelli, F., Smith, B., et al. (2016). OntONeo: The obstetric and neonatal ontology. https://core.ac.uk/download/131214730.pdf (accessed on 17th July 2025).

4. Alo, A. O., Ameh, N., Ansari, U., Arisi, R. O., Centre for Reviews and Dissemination, et al. (2017). The prevalence of domestic violence among pregnant women in Nigeria: A systematic review. https://core.ac.uk/download/153536469.pdf (accessed on 17th July 2025).

5. Aschenbrenner, A. P., Hanson, L., Johnson, T. S., Kelber, M., et al. (2016). Nurses' own birth experiences influence labor support attitudes and behaviors. https://core.ac.uk/download/213076331.pdf (accessed on 17th July 2025).

6. Augustin, G., Vrčić, H., & Župančić, B. (2012). Laparoscopic cholecystectomy due to acute calculous cholecystitis in 16 weeks' *in vitro* fertilization and embryo transfer pregnancy: Report of the first case. https://core.ac.uk/download/11700402.pdf (accessed on 17th July 2025).

7. Balatero, J. S. (2018). Obstetric nurses' perceived barriers to immediate skin-to-skin contact after cesarean birth. https://core.ac.uk/download/159401074.pdf (accessed on 17th July 2025).

8. Barron, M. L., & Fehring, R. (2005). Basal body temperature assessment: Is it useful to couples seeking pregnancy? https://core.ac.uk/download/213076060.pdf (accessed on 17th July 2025).

9. Berghella, V., Chauhan, S. P., Magann, E. F., Morrison, J., et al. (2006). American College of Obstetricians and Gynecologists practice bulletins: An overview. https://core.ac.uk/download/46972135.pdf (accessed on 17th July 2025).

10. Bhutta, Z. A., Blencowe, H., Burden, C., Cacciatore, J., et al. (2016). Stillbirths: Economic and psychosocial consequences. https://core.ac.uk/download/73982130.pdf (accessed on 17th July 2025).

11. Borg Cunen, N., Borg Xuereb, R., Jomeen, J., Poat, A., et al. (2016). A narrative review of interventions addressing the parental-fetal relationship. https://core.ac.uk/download/151162916.pdf (accessed on 17th July 2025).

12. Bouchard, T., Fehring, R., & Schneider, M. (2017). Effectiveness of an online natural family planning program for breastfeeding women. https://core.ac.uk/download/213089361.pdf (accessed on 17th July 2025).

13. Brewer, G., Hendrie, C. A., Lewis, H., Mills, R., et al. (2014). Contemporary and historical evidence to suggest that women's preference for age at birth of first child remains consistent across time. https://core.ac.uk/download/42138140.pdf (accessed on 17th July 2025).

14. Brown, E. L. (2017). Postpartum depression screening of women veterans in Alaska quality improvement project. https://core.ac.uk/download/286607496.pdf (accessed on 17th July 2025).

15. Carlson, C., Sholk, J., Nanni, J., Peterson, K., Smith, L. A., & Bhavaraju, N. (2016). Breaking the barriers to specialty care: Practical ideas to improve health equity and reduce cost–Striving for equity in specialty care. https://core.ac.uk/download/75785769.pdf (accessed on 17th July 2025).

16. Carugno, J., Della Corte, L., Di Guardo, F., Giampaolino, P., et al. (2020). Evaluation and treatment of the infertile women with Asherman syndrome: An updated review focusing on the role of hysteroscopy. https://core.ac.uk/download/323169526.pdf (accessed on 17th July 2025).

17. Chatterton, C. (2013). "An unsuitable job for a woman? Gender and mental health nursing." https://core.ac.uk/download/18306482.pdf (accessed on 17th July 2025).

18. Chatterton, C., & Wade, L. (2013). Charlotte Seymour Yapp. https://core.ac.uk/download/18306483.pdf (accessed on 17th July 2025).

19. Chen, H., Girda, E., Humphries, M. D., Kennedy, V. L., et al. (2018). Management of high-risk obstetrical patients with morbidly adherent placenta in the age of resuscitative endovascular balloon occlusion of the aorta. https://core.ac.uk/download/322437922.pdf (accessed on 17th July 2025).

20. Coles, J., Goodwach, R., Pugh, J., Taylor, A., et al. (2012). Sexual trauma in women: The importance of identifying a history of sexual violence. *No DOI provided.*

21. Cunha, T. M., Lucas, R., & Santos, F. B. (2015). Placental site trophoblastic tumor: A case report and review of the literature. https://core.ac.uk/download/62707709.pdf (accessed on 17th July 2025).

22. Davis, S. R., Gompel, A., Lumsden, M. A., Murad, M. H., et al. (2015). Treatment of symptoms of the menopause: An endocrine society clinical practice guideline. https://core.ac.uk/download/42367511.pdf (accessed on 17th July 2025).

23. De Ruiter, P. E. J., Bult, S. A., Dijkstra, J. R., & van Gulik, T. M. (2025). Erb's palsy: Visual diagnosis in art before medical history? *Gynecologic and Obstetric Investigation*. https://www.semanticscholar.org/paper/e50ca23156465e4aaedb51775c162499ec26d72f (accessed on 17th July 2025).

24. Dunlop, A., Edwards, J. A., & Vanderlaan, J. (2020). Geospatial variation in caesarean delivery. https://core.ac.uk/download/286130662.pdf (accessed on 17th July 2025).

25. Duster, M., Hanson, L., Safdar, N., VandeVusse, L., et al. (2014). Feasibility of oral prenatal probiotics against maternal group B *Streptococcus* vaginal and rectal colonization. https://core.ac.uk/download/213073262.pdf (accessed on 17th July 2025).

26. Fehring, R. J., Raviele, K., & Schneider, M. (2011). Pilot evaluation of an Internet-based natural family planning education and service program. https://core.ac.uk/download/213089353.pdf (accessed on 17th July 2025).

27. Fehring, R., & Mu, Q. (2014). Cohort efficacy study of natural family planning among perimenopause age women. https://core.ac.uk/download/213089348.pdf (accessed on 17th July 2025).

28. Felice, M. E., Hollingsworth, D. R., James, M., Shragg, P., et al. (1984). Observations related to chronologic and gynecologic age in pregnant adolescents. https://core.ac.uk/download/323069406.pdf (accessed on 17th July 2025).

29. Guarino, D., Caserta, L., Di Benedetto, M., Mallozzi, M., & Schimberni, M. (2017). Ovarian endometrioid adenocarcinoma diagnosed in pregnancy: A case report. https://core.ac.uk/download/154949756.pdf (accessed on 17th July 2025).

30. Katzman, W. B., & Pastore, E. A. (2012). Recognizing myofascial pelvic pain in the female patient with chronic pelvic pain. https://core.ac.uk/download/305124272.pdf (accessed on 17th July 2025).

31. Marti, E., Deluche, F., Jochum, S., Bendifallah, H., Azais, H., Deidier, J., Cockenpot, V., et al. (2022). Management of endometrial cancer: French Society of Onco-Gynecology 's evaluation through a Delphi survey. *Journal of Clinical Medicine, 11*. https://www.semanticscholar.org/paper/16984a0303c00975759666497f5b3a1f3217c0f6 (accessed on 17th July 2025).

32. Mwachofi, A. K. (2017). A comparative analysis of pregnancy outcomes for women with and without disabilities. https://digitalscholarship.unlv.edu/cgi/viewcontent.cgi?article=1453&context=jhdrp (accessed on 17th July 2025).

33. Parekh, M. (2022). A feminist analysis of pelvic exam violence. https://core.ac.uk/download/534957455.pdf (accessed on 17th July 2025).

34. Patange, R. P., et al. (2023). Innovations in minimally invasive gynecologic surgery: Improving outcomes and recovery gynecology. https://core.ac.uk/download/596247494.pdf (accessed on 17th July 2025).

35. Patel, S. (2006). Assessing obstetrician-gynecologist attitudes and knowledge of primary care. https://core.ac.uk/download/210607323.pdf (accessed on 17th July 2025).

36. Saida, T., Gu, W., Hoshiai, S., Ishiguro, T., Sakai, M., Amano, T., Nakahashi, Y., et al. (2024). Artificial intelligence in obstetric and gynecological MR imaging. *Magnetic Resonance in Medical Sciences: MRMS: An Official Journal of Japan Society of Magnetic Resonance in Medicine*. https://www.semanticscholar.org/paper/594f159097100abe0beabe8f411ae0494136095c (accessed on 17th July 2025).

37. St. Clair, M. (2020). "Disbelieving Black women to death"; the "double jeopardy": Racism and sexism affects Black women's access to and quality of care during pregnancy, birth, and postpartum. https://core.ac.uk/download/323029102.pdf (accessed on 17th July 2025).

38. Todd, P. M. (2021). Decreasing unintentional pregnancies for Tennesseans. https://core.ac.uk/download/491517591.pdf (accessed on 17th July 2025).

39. Vahidfar, N., Farzanefar, S., Ahmadzadehfar, H., Molloy, E. N., & Eppard, E. (2022). A review of nuclear medicine approaches in the diagnosis and the treatment of gynecological malignancies. *Cancers, 14*. https://www.semanticscholar.org/paper/8fd49c221aa46d44c7597a5a73e2a92784ddeedd (accessed on 17th July 2025).

40. Zapalo, B. (2006). Assessing the effect of a learning organization on change in levels of developmentally supportive care in the newborn intensive care unit. https://core.ac.uk/download/234047668.pdf (accessed on 17th July 2025).

CRITICAL CARE AND EMERGENCY MEDICINE

10

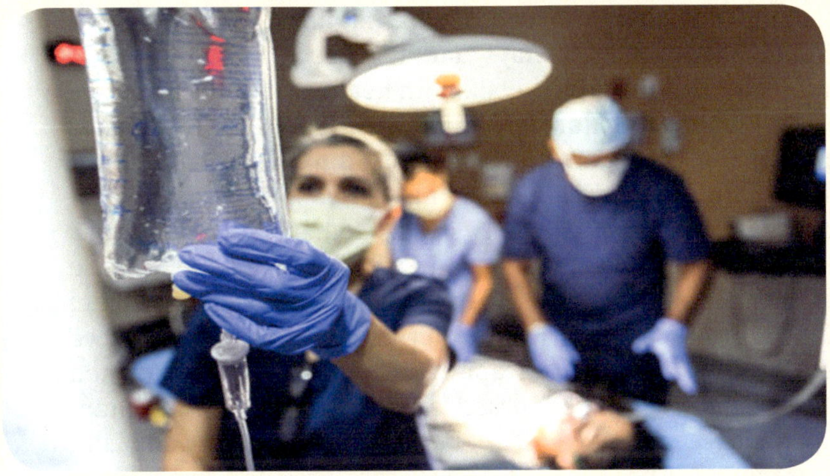

LEARNING OBJECTIVES

After studying this chapter, you will be able to:

1. Discuss the historical development of critical care
2. Explain the role of general practitioners in emergencies
3. Focus on common emergencies encountered
4. Understand training and skills required for general practitioners
5. Know challenges faced by general practitioners in emergency medicine
6. Focus on integration of technology in emergency medicine
7. Identify case studies and real-life applications
8. Discuss the challenges in critical care and emergency medicine

Introduction

In the healthcare arena, emergency medicine and critical care are two disciplines that address some of the most emergent and challenging patient demands. The ED serves as the initial line of care for assessing and stabilizing patients, particularly critically injured or ill patients. This rapid action is vital, as immediate intervention can significantly affect patient outcomes. Given that calls for emergency services continue to surge, with growing patient volumes and increasing care complexity, the subtleties of patient triage are imperative to understand. Emergency physicians (Eps) face significant challenges in effectively managing cases while ensuring urgently needed and appropriate treatment for critically ill patients (Mathews et al., 2020). The dynamic setting of these centers demands ongoing review and reconfiguration of protocols and practices to maximize the efficacy of care delivery. Further, the EMS role is central in the transfer of patient care from prehospital to appropriate acute care settings, for example, the ICU. Advanced Life Support (ALS) and Basic Life Support

(BLS) are crucial to triage, but can have serious consequences if there is miscommunication or misjudgment. A study found that approximately 2% of patients were misclassified during ALS to BLS triage (Mathews et al., 2020)., further indicating the importance of these evaluations being accurate. Patient demographics, such as presenting diagnoses like gastrointestinal or neurological complaints, further complicate triage decisions. Ensuring are well-armed with protocols and tools to guide their decisions is paramount for patient safety and optimal outcomes in critical care settings. With continued advancement in critical care and emergency medicine, collaboration between the insights of both prehospital services and emergency departments will be invaluable. Collaboration between EPs and EMS providers can lead to the formulation of more detailed, evidence-based algorithms that address the specific needs of patients being evaluated in the ED. Education and training in continuous triage decision-making and critical care management can improve emergency response times for patients. These efforts enhance the quality of care and address inherent capacity issues posed by high patient volumes and low-resource emergency care settings. Such healthcare systems must enable such collaborative efforts to solidify the chain of care of critically ill patients.

Definition of Critical Care

Critical care is a specialized clinical practice characterized by intensive monitoring and management of patients with life-threatening conditions. The specialty is characterized by its use of advanced technology and multidisciplinary approaches designed to stabilize patients' critical condition. Intensive care units, or critical care units, bring together medical experts such as intensivists, nurses, respiratory therapists, and pharmacists to collaborate and deliver end-to-end care tailored to specific patient needs. The acuity of the cases treated in such facilities forces healthcare systems to develop and refine protocols that prioritize early interventions and maximize outcomes for patients, particularly those facing severe medical emergencies. Boarding critically ill patients in the emergency departments (EDs) is a serious issue, reflecting the intricate dynamics of transitions of care. Boarding in the emergency department, or delivery of care to admitted patients in the ED due to ICU bed unavailability, is strongly correlated with adverse clinical outcomes. Research indicates that prolonged boarding will lead to increased ventilation times, increased hospital stays, and increased mortality rates in the critically ill. With healthcare settings unable to address the repercussions of this issue, organizations such as the Society of Critical Care Medicine and the American College of Emergency Physicians demand specific actions to minimize the effects of boarding and enhance the quality of care. These efforts are instrumental in ensuring that critically ill patients receive timely and appropriate interventions aligned with best practices in critical care (Al-Qahtani et al., 2020). Furthermore, definitions and practices of critical care are further confused by variations in care pathways that patients receive across hospital networks. Research has indicated that a fragmented view of hospitals is typically unable to explain the subtle interdependencies among departments involved in patient care. Utilizing a holistic approach, particularly through clinical pathway analysis, medical researchers are better positioned to realize how patients progress through intensive care systems. This unifying model not only de-mystifies the operational dynamics of care delivery but also equips health care deliverers with the knowledge necessary to maximize resource utilization and patient outcomes. Lastly, defining critical care necessitates accepting these dynamic relationships and resultant systemic issues, emphasizing the need for continuous improvement in care strategy at all levels of the health care continuum (Boucherie et al., 2009) (Figure 10.1).

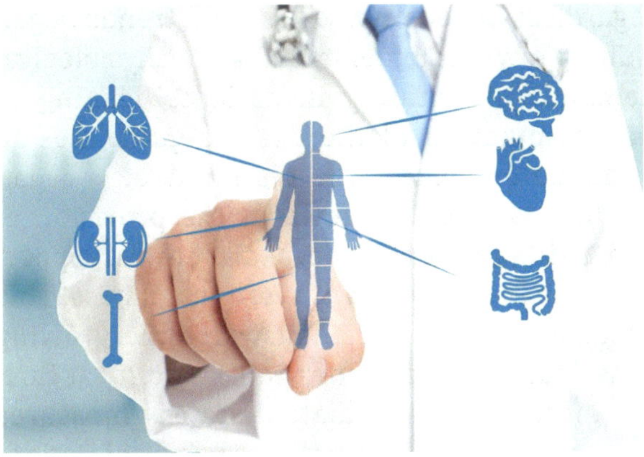

Figure 10.1. The critical care encompasses a specialized area of medical practice.

Source: https://productimages.withfloats.com/serviceimages/tile/645f44af4a1bc261491133cd27.

Importance of Emergency Medicine

Emergency medicine is vital to the healthcare system as the first line of response to acute medical emergencies. It is characterized by a focus on urgent, life-or-death problems that require immediate diagnosis and management. Emergency medical workers must have a broad foundation of knowledge, not just to provide management for a range of disorders from trauma to cardiac events, but also to initiate potentially life-saving interventions in high-pressure situations. Thus, the ability to perform efficiently in chaotic environments is a direct reflection of patient outcomes and indicates the relative importance placed on the establishment of skills and evidence-based practice in the emergency setting. The specialty needs to constantly evolve in response to advancing medical knowledge and technology, demonstrating the dynamic nature of emergency care and the need to minimize morbidity and mortality in the acute environment. A critical component of emergency medicine is procedural sedation and analgesia (PSA), which plays a central role in enabling pain relief during emergency procedures. According to guidelines described in current literature, PSA enables uncomfortable procedures to be performed while keeping the patient as comfortable and stress-free as possible, and overall improves treatment effectiveness in emergency departments. The importance of accurate assessment of patients can then be applied to at-risk groups, such as children and the elderly. This focus on patient-tailored sedation protocols not only improves outcomes but also prioritizes ongoing education and training for practitioners in safe management of sedation. The incorporation of new methods in sedation, based on current evidence, indicates a commitment to patient safety and to the delivery of high-quality emergency care pathways, as prioritized by recent overviews (Piccini et al., 2024). Moreover, the use of integrated models of care in emergency medicine shows its applicability in addressing complex patient needs. The prevalence of comorbidities during emergency presentations necessitate a multidisciplinary approach that addresses multiple health issues concurrently. This implies coordination among emergency medical personnel, specialists, and support staff to develop integrated care plans that address immediate and long-term patient health issues. By adequately diagnosing and controlling comorbidities, emergency medicine optimizes patient care and enhances recovery. Such intervention is crucial in improving health outcomes and facilitating smooth transitions to subsequent care, hence reflecting the critical role that emergency medicine plays in the healthcare system as a whole (Beyer et al., 2017).

10.1. Historical Development of Critical Care

Learning Outcome

1. Evolution of intensive care units (ICUs)
2. Key milestones in emergency medicine
3. Impact of technological advancements

The history of critical care dates back to the early 20th century, when the need for specialized medicine was recognized amid rising patient complexity. The treatment initially took place in general medical wards without advanced technology and strategies. The discovery of the first anesthetic drugs and the enhancement of surgical techniques formed the basis for the development of critical care. This was followed by the establishment of specialty centers for the treatment of patients with life-threatening conditions, paving the way for care to distinguish itself within medicine as a whole. Technological advances such as the iron lung of the 1920s for polio patients were a turning point in recognizing how desperately ill patients required targeted resources and specialist medical treatment, a trend that would grow throughout the century as diseases became more reliant on innovative care models (Denysova et al., 2024). By the middle of the 20th century, the field of critical care had come to recognize the importance of interdisciplinary care, which encompassed the services of other healthcare providers, such as nurses, respiratory therapists, and pharmacists. The collaboration facilitated a pivotal transition from primitive supportive measures to holistic care protocols aimed at patient stabilization and recovery. The evolution of intensive care units (ICUs) emerged at this time, in which specially trained staff treated severe cases such as trauma, respiratory failure, and cardiac arrest. Technology, such as mechanical ventilation and continuous monitoring equipment, also advanced patient management, enabling early intervention to improve outcomes. Therefore, critical care began to establish itself as a distinct medical specialty in its own right, and more effort was devoted to evidence-based medicine to guide treatment regimes (Arman, 2024). The second half of the 20th century witnessed a wave of further innovations that drove the field of critical care into new realms of efficacy. The growth of high-tech monitoring and telemedicine was pivotal in improving patient access to specialist knowledge regardless of geography. Research trends began shifting towards understanding the physiological demands of critically ill patients, leading to the formulation of therapeutic guidelines to optimize outcomes. The discipline also began to shift its attention towards the provision of end-of-life care and towards the ethical aspects of caring for patients with terminal illness. This expansion of focus demonstrates the growing consciousness of the finer points of critical care, not merely the immediate lifesaving measures required, but also the broader issues of patient autonomy and dignity (Denysova et al., 2024). As the specialty of critical care continues to evolve, its historical progress underscores the importance of continuing to learn and adapt to meet the ever-changing needs of patients in emergency medicine (Figure 10.2).

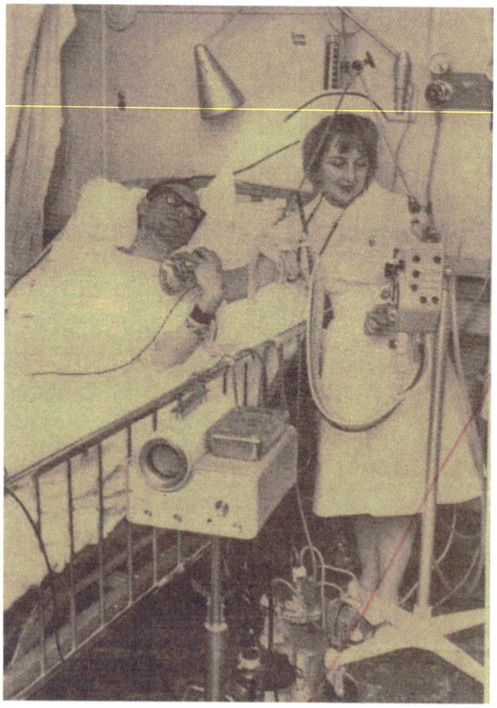

Figure 10.2. The historical development of critical care can be traced back to the early 20th century.

Source: https://rch150.wordpress.com/wp-content/uploads/2012/09/icu-command-post-1965.jpg.

10.1.2. Evolution of Intensive Care Units (ICUs)

The establishment of Intensive Care Units (ICUs) has played a significant role in enhancing outcomes for patients in the areas of critical care and emergency medicine. Intensive care initially emerged as a response to increased demand for specialized postoperative patient monitoring. Over time, the idea was further refined to accommodate more conditions, and it gave doctors a chance to treat critically ill patients in a special room with excellent facilities and cutting-edge technology. The ICU setting itself is designed to enable monitoring and immediate intervention, reflecting an interdisciplinary model that integrates diverse specialties for the best possible care. ICUs have therefore progressed from rudimentary arrangements to highly sophisticated units, employing modern technologies and practices that maximize recovery capacity for critically ill patients and reflect changing trends in critical care. Over the past few years, the ICU environment has continued to evolve in patient care, requiring the inclusion not only of technological innovation but also of techniques that meet the psychological and emotional needs of patients and their families. Grasping the intricacies of triaging and managing critically ill patients has led emergency physicians to emphasize the severity of illness and the interventions required, while working within systemic limitations such as ICU bed availability. A cross-sectional study found that systemic factors are less influential on admission decisions than patient-related factors (Mathews et al., 2020). The observation indicates greater acknowledgment of holistic patient care in ICUs, which is a key part of the overall treatment experience and outcomes in moments of urgency, reflecting a convergence of medical science and empathetic care. Additionally, ICUs have developed from responses to specific medical conditions, such as intra-abdominal hypertension and abdominal compartment syndrome (IAH/ACS). Clinical surveys report a widespread clinician unawareness and clinical management of these issues, and thus, this highlights the need for evidence-based guidelines (Keulenaer et al., 2014). In particular, the lack of standardized measurement procedures and management protocols poses challenges that can adversely affect patient recovery. With each new clinical update that becomes available, the necessity of ongoing education and adaptation among doctors is obvious. The development of ICUs is not only a measure of technological advancements but also an expression of the necessity for ongoing training and sensitization to prepare critical care teams to manage complex and dynamic medical conditions more effectively, ultimately leading to better patient outcomes and safety in emergency medicine.

10.1.2. Key Milestones in Emergency Medicine

: The emergence of emergency medicine has been marked by significant milestones that track the evolution of medical practice and the specialty's greater recognition. One of those milestones was the establishment of formal emergency medicine residency training programs during the 1970s, which formalized education and practice across the United States. Thus, emergency department (ED) physicians began to develop a distinct identity of their own, separate from other specialties such as internal medicine and surgery. The formative years saw the emergence of residency programs and board certification, which gave emergency medicine credibility as an integral component of healthcare. However, patient satisfaction metrics integration within emergency medicine has lagged, with studies finding that 27% of residencies report patient satisfaction (PS) data to their residents (Druck et al., 2016). This gap suggests an important area for improvement within the discipline. Beyond educational development, the evolution of emergency medicine is driven forcefully by the ever-present need for improved patient experience (PE) measures. The low rate of standardized implementation of these measures across various residency programs indicates a fragmented approach to medical education. A mere 35% of categorical emergency medicine residencies have an organized PE curriculum, reflecting a wide gap in preparing the future providers for the realities of a patient-centered care-driven healthcare system. The incorporation of several teaching modalities, such as didactic lectures and simulation workshops, reflects an evolving attempt to bridge the gap (Druck et al., 2016). As patient experience becomes more directly linked to hospital reimbursement and overall success, incorporating robust PE curricula is critical to advancing emergency medicine. Moreover, the worth of global views in emergency medicine cannot be overstated, particularly given the increasing differences in access to emergency care. In most low- and middle-income countries (LMICs), a lack of evidence on the acute disease burden greatly hinders the development of effective emergency care systems.

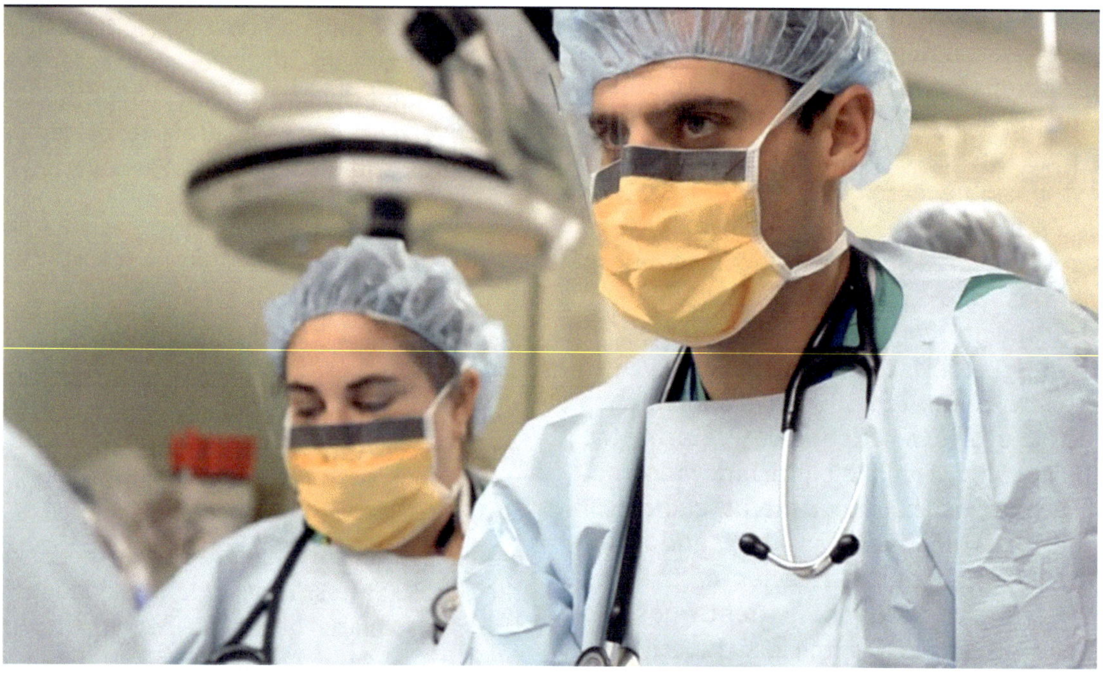

Figure 10.3. Key milestones in emergency medicine.

Source: https://pxl-evmsedu-v6.terminalfour.net/filters:format(webp)/prod01/channel_41/media/evms_public/departments/emergency_medicine/general_pictures/Emergency-med-possible-hero-2000X1149px.jpg.

Conquering barriers to emergency care evolution in these regions requires the establishment of consensus around prominent elements and the accumulation of data on which to evaluate intervention effects. Along with emergency medicine itself grows increasingly sophisticated, efforts to develop improved local and international emergency care will be necessary. By encouraging a research program focused on data gathering and management, the discipline is better able to understand and respond to the needs of diverse populations and ultimately improve the overall efficiency of emergency medicine (Figure 10.3).

10.1.3. Impact of Technological Advancements

The incorporation of innovations in critical care and emergency medicine has drastically changed the face of patient care. Innovative technologies such as AI, telemedicine, and advanced imaging modalities have enabled medical professionals to improve diagnostic yield and refine treatment strategies. The use of AI, especially, provides great benefits by breaking down large volumes of medical information to recognize patterns beyond the reach of traditional human observation. This not only reduces the frequency of diagnostic errors but also aids in developing customized treatment plans according to individual patient needs. Therefore, such developments provide avenues for improved patient results and streamlining clinical procedures, allowing medical professionals to focus on delivering quality care rather than administrative tasks (Shuroug et al., 2023). Moreover, the COVID-19 pandemic highlighted the fundamental role of technological innovations in emergency medicine. When healthcare systems faced extraordinary pressures, digital health interventions proved indispensable in ensuring uninterrupted access to care. The rapid implementation of telemedicine enabled healthcare practitioners to see patients remotely, reducing exposure risk while sustaining continuity of care. This shift has prompted a reconsideration of the integration of primary care with emergency services, with a focus on developing overall health policies that promote coordination during emergencies (Sultana et al., 2021). The pandemic highlighted gaps in current healthcare infrastructure, and the world demanded investment in technology to bolster both emergency and primary care systems to withstand future health emergencies. Moreover, technological advances in critical care units have increased the intensity of monitoring and management of critically ill patients. Wearable devices and smart technologies enable real-time monitoring of vital signs and physiological parameters, allowing healthcare professionals to respond proactively to patient needs. The technology does not only increase patient safety through continuous monitoring, but it also facilitates more efficient use of medical resources. With the development of the industry, embracing such innovations forms an active health environment with patient-centered approaches as its number one priority, and addressing disparities in health. The ultimate success will only be achieved through having the healthcare systems across the world embrace technological advancements and implement them as available and effective in diverse clinical environments (Shuroug et al., 2023).

Test Your Knowledge

1. Describe the evolution of Intensive Care Units (ICUs) from their inception. What were the key drivers for their development, and how have they changed in structure and function over time?
2. Identify and explain at least three major milestones in the development of emergency medicine as a specialty. How have these shaped modern emergency care delivery?

10.2. Role of General Practitioners in Emergency Situations

Learning Outcome

1. Understand initial assessment and triage
2. Focus on stabilization of patients
3. Deal with referral to specialized care

In emergency medicine, general practitioners' (GPs') services extend far beyond their routine clinical responsibilities. Their integration into emergencies, such as acute medical emergencies or sudden life-threatening conditions, enables the management of patients with a better understanding. Having gained a comprehensive understanding of patients' medical histories, GPs can quickly identify and prioritize, making them vital for triage during emergencies. By understanding the local health facilities and services, GPs have the expertise to plan follow-up treatment, including emergency referrals and continuity care. The role is most apparent in community healthcare settings, where GPs are likely to lead outreach to inform members of the public about the identification of emergency symptoms, ultimately contributing to community resilience against medical emergencies (Cribb et al., 2010). Furthermore, GPs' ability to cope with cultural and ethnic diversity during emergencies underscores their responsibility for ensuring equal access to healthcare. As communities grow more demographically diverse, GPs have an essential contribution towards serving racially and ethnically diverse patients. Racial and ethnic disparities have been observed to manifest in healthcare (Association of Public Health Observatories, 2014). When GPs are equipped with patient-specific information and cultural sensitivity, they can circumvent the impediments offered by language differences and cross-cultural miscommunication. Not only does this create trust between patients and clinicians, but it also improves diagnostic precision and clinical decision-making. When GPs work proactively with and understand the unique circumstances of their ethnically diverse patient populations, they can make potentially life-saving medical treatments appropriately tailored and well-executed under emergency conditions. In addition, the value of GPs during emergencies is also reflected in their capacity to perform immediate and lifesaving interventions. In time-sensitive cases, GPs can perform rapid diagnosis and treatment while waiting for specialized emergency services. Their exposure to emergency identification and management, as well as their ability to perform primary procedures such as airway management or cardiac resuscitation, render them critical first responders within the healthcare system. Additionally, GPs are sometimes engaged in emergency preparedness training to build skills critical to managing mass casualty incidents or public health emergencies. Such active participation not just strengthens personal GP ability but also the general emergency care system in communities, offering a unified approach to managing health emergencies (Cribb et al., 2010) (Figure 10.4).

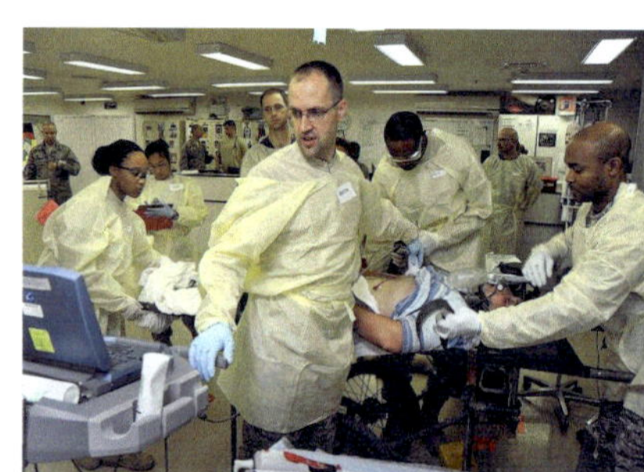

Figure 10.4. Medical personnel simulate emergency treatment.

Source: https://upload.wikimedia.org/wikipedia/commons/thumb/3/3b/Emergency_medicine_simulation_training_exercise_in_Balad%2C_Iraq.jpg/800px-Emergency_medicine_simulation_training_exercise_in_Balad%2C_Iraq.jpg.

10.2.1. Initial Assessment and Triage

In the practice of emergency medicine, triage and initial evaluation are key in managing patient care effectively. The process begins with a systematic evaluation of patients who present to emergency departments and are quickly sorted by healthcare professionals into serious and non-serious cases based on their conditions. Effective initial evaluation not only enhances patient prioritization based on the severity of their conditions but also improves overall workflow in healthcare facilities. Moreover, triage also has to adapt to the complexity of the healthcare environment to be more sensitive to diverse patient profiles. The application of structured triage systems ensures efficient use of resources to address the growing demands on emergency services in contemporary society. Triage strategies may vary significantly across health care systems, indicating strengths and weaknesses in implementation. For instance, in Indonesia, the majority of triage systems do not appear as robust as those of other countries because most hospitals have a reasonably primitive sorting process, one that might not satisfactorily perform re-triage. According to Morphet et al. (2016), regardless of the alignment in some segments of the Indonesian triage process with global best practices, the absence of systematic re-triage is an issue in terms of efficiency and patient outcomes. This calls for continually assessing and fine-tuning triage operations to keep pace with evolving healthcare needs and enhance the quality of patient care. One significant area of concern in triage is how health professionals recognize possible risk factors in which certain conditions are identified. For instance, identification of substance abuse, such as cocaine use, among patients who present with chest pain, is crucial in the delivery of particular interventions and management strategies. The discussion of the problem illustrates that a significant number of patients may present with drug-related complications that are not diagnosed, thus complicating their clinical presentation (Bandeeri et al., 2004). Therefore, the inclusion of appropriate assessments that assess such risk factors in triage is important to ensure an effective emergency response. With comprehensive evaluation, healthcare providers can promote patient health and safety and improve health outcomes, thereby supporting the underpinning principles of emergency medicine across general practice (Figure 10.5).

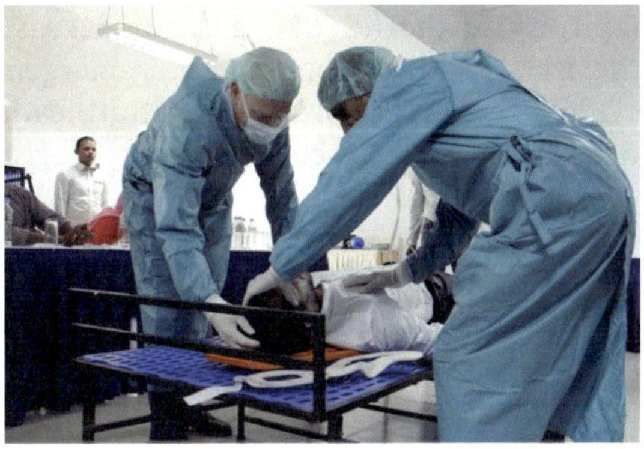

Figure 10.5. Initial assessment.

Source: https://www.icrc.org/sites/default/files/wysiwyg/Bangladesh/_mg_4880low.jpg.

10.2.2. Stabilization of Patients

In emergency medicine, stabilizing patients is a critical first response to acute medical conditions. It is the prompt assessment of life-threatening conditions and the treatment of the patient's immediate needs. An example is compliance with the Emergency Medical Treatment and Labor Act (EMTALA), which imposes legal and ethical obligations on health care providers to provide necessary treatment before patients are transferred to other facilities. The sheer volume of EMTALA cases presenting with obstetric emergencies illustrates stark inadequacies in the recognition and management of pregnant patient needs. Of 232 EMTALA settlements, nearly 40% were obstetric emergency-related, the majority citing neglect of administering adequate screening tests and stabilization treatment, indicating the urgency of education in the emergency department on to sufficient stabilization for avoiding negligence and ensuring patient safety (Arora et al., 2020). Similar effective stabilization of patients is also essential in cardiovascular emergencies, particularly non-ST-segment elevation myocardial infarction (NSTEMI). This condition calls for immediate treatment, including optimization of oxygen demand and supply to the myocardium. As the complexity of the NSTEMI patient increases, with possible multiple comorbidities, emergency providers must utilize precise risk stratification with adjunctive pharmacologic therapy. Current guidelines maximize the opportunity for beneficial outcomes for the patient and reduce the risk of readmission or recurrent events. By attaining competence in managing NSTEMI, emergency medicine practitioners can enhance care coordination and offer timely interventions, highlighting the importance of stabilization in enabling patients presenting with acute coronary syndromes (Amin et al., 2019). Given the central role of patient stabilization, there is a need for ongoing education and training among health practitioners involved in emergency medicine. Investment in rigorous training programs focused on adherence to emergency protocol and situational analysis can equip clinicians to respond optimally to a broad range of emergencies. This anticipatory process is most directly applicable in environments where resources are potentially limited and timely decision-making can critically improve patient outcomes. Additionally, advocating for an understanding of the legal aspects of patient stabilization, for example, for EMTALA violations, empowers healthcare professionals with the knowledge to move through the complexity of emergency care. Keeping such a lookout ensures that patients receive careful, efficient care in moments of need, thereby reinforcing the foundations of emergency medicine codes (Figure 10.6).

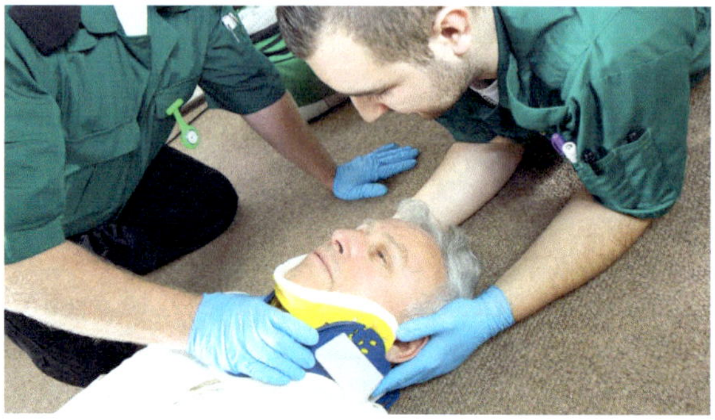

Figure 10.6. Manually stabilize a patient's head.

Source: https://www.c2cfirstaidaquatics.com/wp-content/uploads/2021/04/methods-to-manually-stabilize-a-patient-s-head-Coast2Coast-3-min.jpg.

10.2.3. Referral to Specialized Care

In emergency medicine, specialist referral is a critical factor in ensuring patients are properly diagnosed and treated with the most appropriate interventions for their conditions. GPs will need to handle complex cases that are outside their immediate competence and knowledge. Such instances require timely specialist referral, and it is not only crucial for patient care but also for a well-organized healthcare system. With such referrals, GPs can minimize treatment and diagnostic delays, thereby lowering morbidity and mortality from various medical conditions. There should be smooth coordination of care between specialists and general practitioners when attending to urgent health cases that require immediate care and intervention. Health disparities will, however, exert a significant influence on the referral to specialist care. Economic and insurance status often define the nature of care that is delivered to patients, particularly among racial and ethnic minorities. Literature shows that these disparities affect diagnosis and treatment for conditions like heart disease, in such a way that income-related factors and insurance coverage are determinants against receiving specialty care (Lara et al., 2006). Therefore, general practitioners must be acutely aware of these hurdles while negotiating the referral pathway, ensuring that patients are not only made aware of their specialist alternatives but indeed have clear channels access to such centers. This stratified structure underscores the importance of integrative and fair provision of care in the emergency medicine context. Furthermore, the changing landscape of specialty healthcare facilities has broader implications for emergency care and internal medicine. Although specialty hospitals and ambulatory surgical centers are formed with the intent of enhancing the efficiency and quality of care, evidence from the literature exists that their introduction might not always be beneficial to full-service general hospitals (Annemans et al., 2013). In fact, the claimed competitive edge of these specialty facilities deserves scrutiny, as their proliferation threatens to destabilize integrated healthcare systems unintentionally. General practitioners should be vigilant regarding such dynamics and ensure that referrals to specialty care do not compromise the overarching objective of an integrated healthcare system: to provide available, patient-centered care across levels. An appreciation of the sophisticated interaction between specialized and general care is essential in optimizing patient outcomes and sustaining the integrity of emergency medicine (Figure 10.7).

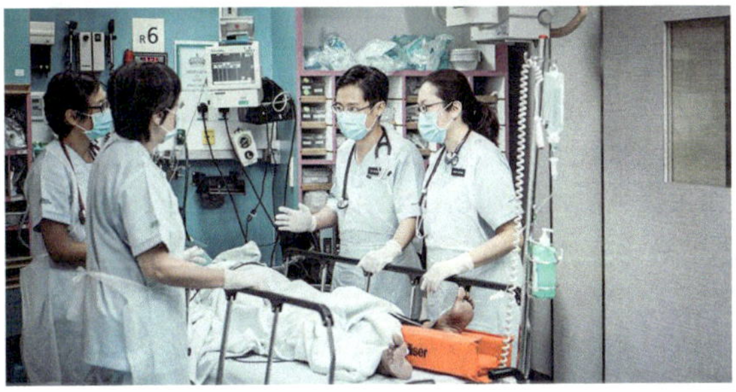

Figure 10.7. Doctors discussing for referral of patient to specialized care.

Source: https://www.sgh.com.sg/patient-care/specialties-services/PublishingImages/Dept-Banner/EmergencyMedicine.jpg.

Test Your Knowledge

1. How do general practitioners effectively prioritize patients in emergencies to ensure timely care and appropriate resource allocation?
2. What are the key steps a general practitioner should take to stabilize a critically ill or injured patient?
3. How do general practitioners coordinate referrals to emergency departments or specialists to ensure continuity and effectiveness of care?

10.3. Common Emergencies Encountered

Learning Outcome

1. Understand cardiac emergencies;
2. Discuss about respiratory distress;
3. Describe trauma and injuries.

Medical practitioners often face a range of emergencies that must be addressed immediately and efficiently. Routine conditions like acute asthma attacks, allergic reactions, and myocardial infarction often present to the general practitioner as emergency cases. Asthma attacks, in particular, can suddenly worsen, so timely intervention is essential to avoid respiratory failure. In the same way, allergic patients can present with symptoms ranging from mild urticaria to lethal anaphylaxis, for which there is a requirement of ready access to epinephrine as well as aggressive emergency measures. The ability to stabilize such patients within minutes can be life-changing and underscores the need for general physicians to be equipped to handle varied acute scenarios. Gastrointestinal emergencies are also an important part of internal medicine consultations. They encompass conditions such as appendicitis, bowel obstruction, and acute gastroenteritis that are sudden in onset and need urgent evaluation and treatment. Appendicitis involves pain in the abdomen and may need surgery if not addressed early. Patients with bowel obstructions can have a constellation of symptoms needing close evaluation and possibly lifesaving intervention. To navigate these challenges effectively, general practitioners must pursue continuous education and evidence-based practice, with the optimal routes of care for such severe ailments, such as the formulation of standardized guidelines for managing specific emergencies (Biega et al., 2024). Obstetrical emergency management is yet another specialty area of challenge for general practice, involving complications in labor and delivery. The Emergency Medical Treatment and Labor Act (EMTALA) mandates that all health care facilities provide required stabilizing treatment for urgent conditions, which is patently labor in an active state. Despite this, obstetric emergencies-related EMTALA violations have been rising to an alarming extent, and this suggests a lack of awareness and adherence on the part of health care providers (Arora et al., 2020). Examples such as failure to perform the appropriate screening test or initiating timely transfers for pregnant women in distress establish the imperative need for training and policy implementation so that practitioners become competent to handle the nuances of obstetric emergencies and thereby improve maternal and fetal outcomes.

10.3.1. Cardiac Emergencies

Cardiac emergencies constitute a severe category of events that occur and depict the critical need for professionals to possess sound knowledge and preparedness. These emergencies, including cardiac arrest, acute myocardial infarction, and unstable angina, necessitate immediate and appropriate interventions to enhance patient outcomes. Adequate cardiopulmonary resuscitation (CPR) training and the use of automated external defibrillators (AEDs) are necessary for healthcare providers. Notably, a critical reading of the literature shows that school nurses, for instance, are pretty sure to act in sudden cardiac arrest scenarios, thus making these kinds of training models applicable to all health care providers dealing with cardiac emergencies, with 44% of respondents reporting that they had adequate resources and assistance to manage such emergencies effectively (Dahlen et al., 2014). Familiarity with various presentations of cardiac emergencies is crucial for timely diagnosis and intervention. General practitioners must be able to recognize the prodromal signs of cardiac events in the presentation of chest pain, shortness of breath, and arrhythmias, since these are generally heading toward more severe complications. Given the elderly population, comorbidities can obscure the clinical presentation, making rapid assessment and intervention even more important. For instance, one study on the preparedness of dentists to handle medical emergencies found that recent graduates were more skilled in the diagnosis and treatment of such an episode than more experienced graduates (Blanchard et al., 2018). This brings to light how necessary it is to have continuous education and training in emergency medicine, not only in dental procedures but across all areas of medicine, because obsolescence can severely hinder treatment during an episode. Combining structured emergency response plans and regular training sessions can significantly enhance a practitioner's preparedness for cardiac emergencies.

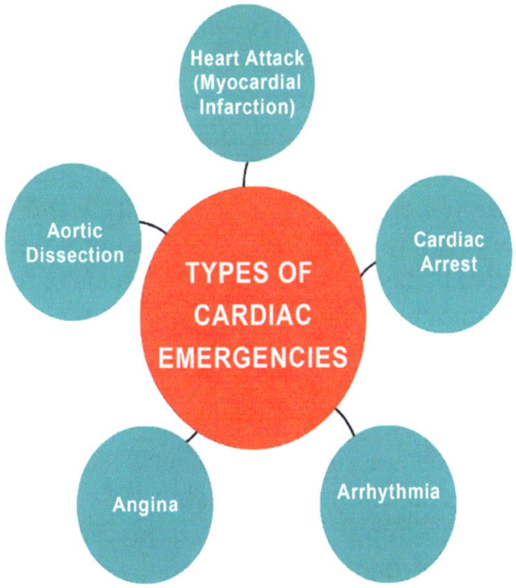

Figure 10.8. Types of cardiac emergencies.

Source: https://linkhospitals.in/blog/cardiac-emergencies:-symptoms-and-types.

A systematic process, as noted in healthcare institutions that emphasize emergency response plans, provides room for coordination and improvement in emergency response. For example, implementing policies similar to those used in schools to handle sudden cardiac arrest can be groundbreaking, establishing a preparedness culture. As alluded to in existing research, there is a need to evaluate such response systems regularly to ensure that medical practitioners are able to address new challenges in emergency medicine. Establishing a robust communication network and providing regular training not only equips practitioners but also enhances confidence among the healthcare team members, ultimately leading to better patient care (Dahlen et al., 2014) (Figure 10.8).

10.3.2. Respiratory Distress

Respiratory distress is an emergent illness that requires immediate intervention in emergency medicine practice. It is defined by clinical presentations of tachypnea, hypoxemia, and increased breathing effort and is due to a variety of underlying conditions, such as infections, allergic reactions, and chronic pulmonary diseases. In particular, the initial management of a patient with respiratory distress in internal medicine is critical. Clinicians must conduct a thorough evaluation, including clinical history, physical examination, and observation of vital signs, to determine the severity and possible cause of the distress. Early diagnosis and treatment will prevent not only complications, but can also significantly improve patient outcomes in the acute presentation, reinforcing the emergent status for determination of the condition in the emergency room. One of the significant causes of respiratory distress is acute respiratory distress syndrome (ARDS), which is characterized by widespread inflammation in the lungs, leading to impaired gas exchange. According to recent studies, such as the Large Observational Study to Understand the Global Impact of Severe Acute Respiratory Failure (LUNG SAFE), approximately 10.4% of ICU admissions are attributed to ARDS, indicating its prevalence in acute care (Alejandro et al., 2016). The clinically heterogeneous presentations of ARDS potentially complicate clinical identification, ranging from as low as 51.3% in milder cases to 78.5% in the most critical cases. Much of this disparity stems from differences in approach in clinical practice and varying levels of clinician awareness of the syndrome. Enhancing the capacity to identify ARDS quickly is thus imperative to maximizing treatment protocols and improving survival rates within those individuals who present with respiratory distress. Management of respiratory distress should be tailored, particularly for mechanical ventilation in patients with ARDS. Ventilation with low tidal volume should be used, particularly since fewer than two-thirds of patients with ARDS receive adequate tidal volume, as supported by new evidence (Alejandro et al., 2016).

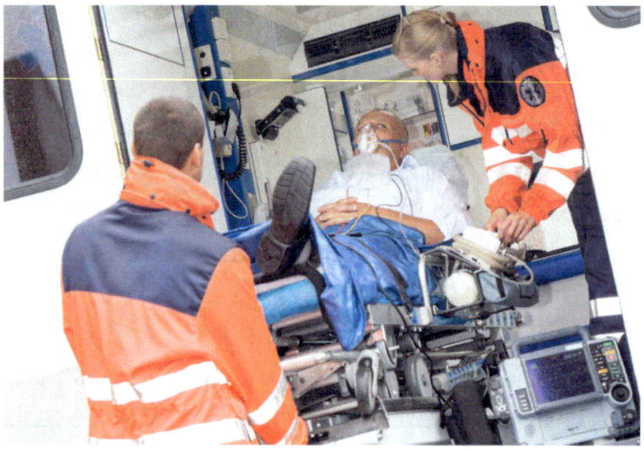

Figure 10.9. An illustration of respiratory emergency.

Source: https://blog.sscor.com/hubfs/Blog/rsz_gettyimages-154972130.png.

This underuse highlights a gap in practice that can make a significant difference in morbidity and mortality because ARDS carries a hospital mortality of 34.9% in mild illness and increases to 46.1% in severe disease. Moreover, adjunct therapies such as prone positioning have been shown to improve oxygenation but are underused, and just 16.3% of patients with severe involvement receive the treatment. Significantly, internal medicine healthcare providers remain current with these guidelines so that treatment for individuals with respiratory distress is enhanced, ultimately resulting in better clinical outcomes (Figure 10.9).

10.3.3. Trauma and Injuries

In the context of emergency medicine, the widespread nature of injury and trauma poses a considerable problem for general practitioners. The effects of traumatic injury are of particular concern in the elderly population, where prior health factors increase the trauma of injury. For instance, in a Tanzanian study in Shinyanga Regional Hospital, geriatric trauma was established to account for 22.7% of all admissions due to trauma at an average age of 68.5 years for the patients. The high injury rate—primarily attributable to violence, falls, and road traffic injuries—highlights the imperative need to implement interventions specifically for this vulnerable group. These results confirm that trauma in older individuals not only causes prolonged hospital stay but is also linked with high mortality, and there is an urgent need to implement preventive measures and early intervention to prevent such adverse effects (Chalya et al., 2012). The pathogenesis of trauma and injuries is multifactorial and generally comprises a combination of environmental and personal factors. In most cases, geriatric patients also have a higher rate of injury due to falls at home, which accounted for over 81% of cases in the aforementioned study. This raises pertinent questions about the safety and care systems in the community implemented to protect the elderly. In addition, the prevalence of high incidences of soft tissue injuries and fractures in the population calls for healthcare professionals to adopt an active role in preventing the same. By implementing community education programs and enhancing the living standards of vulnerable populations, healthcare professionals can be a key driver in reducing the incidence of such injuries, improving overall health outcomes, and lowering healthcare needs (Chalya et al., 2012). Furthermore, the inclusion of research networks in emergency care can significantly enhance knowledge for trauma treatment in internal medicine. The Pediatric Emergency Care Applied Research Network (PECARN) demonstrates how systematic research can improve treatment guidelines and outcomes for trauma patients. With its focus on new evidence and translation to practice, PECARN provides a strategy that can be applied across all ages, including older adults. Such research initiatives not only help develop maximally effective injury prevention strategies but also aid in establishing new researchers in the field. This emphasis on education and evidence-based practice is important, as it supports the sustainability and evolution of emergency medicine to ensure effective management of trauma and injury across diverse populations.

Test Your Knowledge

1. How should a GP assess and manage a patient presenting with acute shortness of breath?
2. What initial steps should a GP follow in managing a patient with suspected head trauma?

10.4. Training and Skills Required for General Practitioners

Learning Outcome

1. Discuss medical education and residency
2. Understand continuing medical education and certifications
3. Explain practical skills in emergency procedures

Training of general practitioners (GPs) is essential for managing the dynamic needs of emergency medicine within the context of primary healthcare. There should be an intensive educational program that includes extensive clinical practice and formal education in fields pertinent to emergencies. The current literature has reported a stark deficiency in coverage of specific sub-specialties, such as otolaryngology, which is significant, as 25% of complaints registered in primary care concern this specialty. By integrating specific modules of emergency management of otolaryngological disorders in the course of the curriculum, GPs can be made more capable of handling widespread disorders, thereby enhancing patient outcomes in emergencies. Besides this, new teaching approaches, such as simulation-based training and case-based learning, are crucial to research in order to bridge the knowledge gap between emergency care and the specialized fields, echoing the call for GP training program curriculum reform (Thal et al., 2016). To adequately equip GPs for the range of emergencies they will have to deal with, ongoing learning and skills development are necessary. With more emergency cases, GPs are more accountable for treating such emergencies in the most effective manner possible. Pre-graduation training must be intensified, with a strong focus on emergency medical care (EMC) protocols, to ensure professionals remain proficient in life-saving interventions. Analysis of professional literature has revealed that the training received directly influences the quality of emergency care provided by GPs. Long-term learning strategies, such as workshops, refresher training, and team training, can help ensure GPs stay up to date with changing practices and emergency treatment algorithms, thereby enhancing their preparedness to respond to emergencies in their communities (Гринзовський et al., 2022). Further, breaking from knowledge into practice application is essential in general practitioner training. In emergency cases, GPs are typically the initial contacts and must be equipped not only with knowledge but also with confidence to make quick decisions. The incorporation of hands-on practice sessions where the GPs can test real scenarios in the presence of seasoned mentors can be invaluable. These learning-through-experience sessions enhance practitioners' capabilities in conducting assessments and interventions that are critical to emergency medicine. By establishing a readiness culture and complementing theory with practice training, GPs' overall competence in emergency situations can be significantly enhanced, ultimately leading to improved patient outcomes in emergency medical conditions (Гринзовський et al., 2022).

10.4.1. Medical Education and Residency

The evolution of medical education and residency training, particularly in emergency medicine, has become increasingly crucial amid the evolving nature of health demands. Emergency medicine as a specialty has seen tremendous growth, particularly in countries like Oman, where a nascent national healthcare system is evolving extremely rapidly. The recent development of emergency nursing and residency training programs locally has strengthened the capacity of health practitioners to provide urgent care. This movement towards standardizing emergency medicine education not only enhances the practice sets of practitioners but also equips them aligned with international emergency care standards. The integration of formal training pathways ensures that new clinicians are sufficiently equipped to work in the fast-paced environment of emergency departments and, in turn, directly impact patient outcomes in internal medicine settings (Al-Harthi et al., 2009). Within emergency medicine scholarship, post-simulation debriefings have been considered for their potential to enhance residents' educational experience. Studies indicate that real-time, non-critical debriefing is an effective method for reinforcing educational principles, though little has been investigated regarding standard practices in emergency departments. It provides residents with a platform to reflect on what has taken place and, along with it, an environment of continuous improvement. The preliminary findings of a multicenter New York City study shows that clinicians recognize the value of these debriefing procedures within the educational setting, but most report no formal training in the performance of effective debriefings. Since emergency medicine is becoming increasingly embedded in primary care, it is essential that residency programs prioritize such training resources so that residents are adequately equipped to face the realities of practice (Bajaj et al., 2016). The meeting point between medical education and practical practice of emergency medicine can directly affect the overall effectiveness of internal medicine. As emergency medicine focuses on the immediacy of high-stakes decision-making, residency programs must put a high value on interprofessional teamwork and application. This includes training in high-stress, real-world simulation environments that allow residents to concentrate on clinical judgment and communication skills. Furthermore, the increasing focus on establishing educational infrastructure within emergency medicine provides opportunities for networking and mentorship, which are crucial for residents' early career development. Through the establishment of a robust learning system that incorporates practice skills with theoretical bases, medical education can ensure that future practitioners not only master situations but can also integrate their experiences into internal medicine, ultimately serving the patients (Al-Harthi et al., 2009; Bajaj et al., 2016) (Figure 10.10).

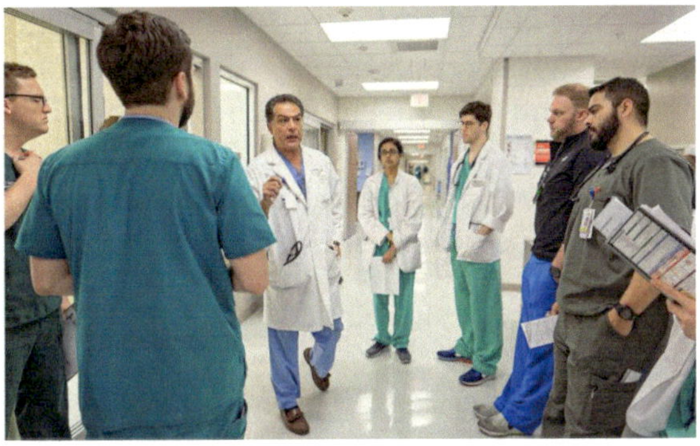

Figure 10.10. Briefing the staffs for emergency situation.

Source: https://lsom.uthscsa.edu/emergency-medicine/wp-content/uploads/sites/144/2020/12/EM-meded-1_2018_EmergencyRoomShots_001_39-800x486.jpg.

10.4.2. Continuing Medical Education and Certifications

Continuing Medical Education (CME) is essential to maintaining skilled, up-to-date, and knowledgeable healthcare professionals who can stay current with new practices in emergency medicine. Since medical knowledge is evolving at an unprecedented rate, internal medicine professionals need to make regular educational efforts to maintain licensure and certifications. These educational experiences not only enhance clinical skills but also promote the adoption of new technology and practices that may result in improved patient outcomes. The demand for CME is underscored by findings that practitioners who go to considerable lengths to obtain such education become more reliable in their decision-making, especially under high-stakes conditions such as emergency care. This ongoing training equips them to manage the complexities of emergencies with self-assurance and a degree of preparedness that is indispensable in life-or-death scenarios. Certifications are tangible evidence of a practitioner's commitment to his or her field of specialization, particularly in subspecialties such as emergency medicine. The credentials verify the physician's training and expertise in effectively managing acute medical conditions. For instance, ACLS or trauma life support certifications have been shown to significantly improve patient survival rates in emergency cases. Taking them would typically entail not only applying to quite rigorous training courses but also adhering to maintenance standards, infection control, and other standards, which could include periodic re-certification courses and skill testing. These strict learning frameworks ensure that general practitioners not only comply with current best practices but also react adequately to emergent medical events, thereby determining the overall quality of care provided in emergency cases.

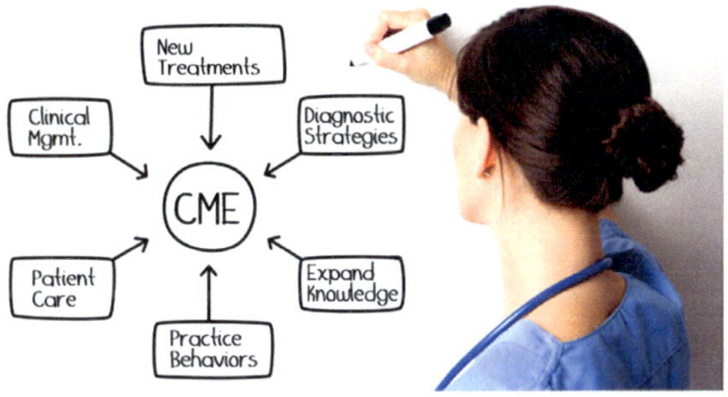

Figure 10.11. Continuing medical education (CME).

Source: https://www.medicalmagazine.in/wp-content/uploads/2020/04/cme-medical-equipment.jpg.

Further, the application of simulation-based training in CME and certification programs has been a novel way of preparing health professionals. Such a process allows practitioners to run realistic scenarios in a simulated environment, sharpening their skills without compromising patient safety. The "deliberate practice" process, as emphasized in current instructional methods, reiterates the "practice makes perfect" mantra and plays a pivotal role in learning complex procedures in emergency medicine. By utilizing low-cost simulation modalities, as outlined in recent research, training for emergency situations can be enhanced through experiential learning. By incorporating these technologies into CME programs, practitioners can be well-equipped for routine and critical incidents and thus develop a culture of excellence in emergency care (Reilly et al., 2016; Alinier et al., 2018) (Figure 10.11).

10.4.3. Practical Skills in Emergency Procedures

Practical emergency skills competence is vital for effective patient management in internal medicine settings, where the healthcare professional is often the first contact in acute situations. Skill competence in areas such as airway management, CPR, and wound management is essential for inpatient stabilization and the promotion of outcomes. Training exercises that combine simulation with hands-on practice allow professionals to rehearse in a simulated setting before facing the real-world ambiguity of emergencies. A study indicated, for instance, that patients who report chest pain most often have unsuspected substance abuse issues, which is an indication of how fast assessment and intervention procedures are essential in the emergency department (Bandeeri et al., 2004). Therefore, through rigorous training and practice in real settings, medical personnel can gain the proficiency to respond appropriately to a range of emergency conditions, thereby improving patient safety and continuity of care. No less critical in the area of emergency protocols is the establishment of guidelines for the recognition of specific cases, such as child abuse in the emergency department. Since general practitioners are first-line carers, they should know how to recognize and intervene in the presence of signs of abuse, as emergency departments are often the first contact for abused children (Biu et al., 2007). Surveys revealed that there is widespread compliance with written policies across child protection policies within emergency departments in England and Northern Ireland, with 91.3% possessing working guidelines. These standards ensure consistency and appropriate handling in cases of suspected abuse.

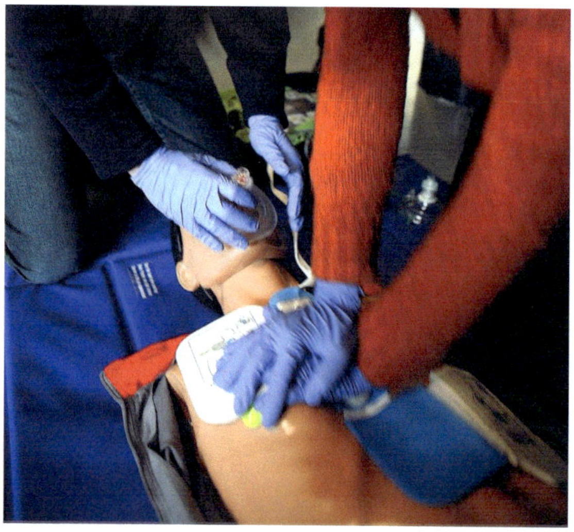

Figure 10.12. Cardiopulmonary resuscitation (CPR) being performed on a medical-training.

Source: https://upload.wikimedia.org/wikipedia/commons/thumb/5/58/CPR_training-04.jpg/800px-CPR_training-04.jpg.

Training courses must not only impart clinicians with technical expertise to administer emergency care, but also make them aware of the importance of identifying psychosocial variables so that an integrated approach to emergency medicine can be developed. Both skill and knowledge are highly crucial in the development of well-balanced practitioners capable of addressing the subtleties of child emergencies. Lastly, the worth of practical skills extends beyond a clinician's personal skill; it also encompasses the overarching emphasis on collaboration and communication during crises. Interagency collaboration among healthcare professionals is a requirement for a successful response during emergencies. For instance, an effective execution of a resuscitation procedure relies on efficient cooperation between doctors, nurses, and supporting staff. Simulated multidisciplinary training can significantly augment the potency of emergency care delivery. Through inter-professional skills rehearsal, healthcare teams will be more competent to handle the swift pace of emergencies with greater confidence and precision. Practice and strategy incorporated within training programs can help develop critical thinking and flexibility, enabling emergency medicine clinicians to respond both technically and to have the ability to lead and work together, ultimately enhancing patient outcomes in internal medicine settings (Figure 10.12).

Test Your Knowledge

1. What core emergency medicine competencies are typically included in the medical education and residency training general practitioners to prepare them for frontline emergency care?
2. Why is continuing medical education essential for general practitioners in maintaining proficiency in emergency care?

10.5. Challenges Faced by General Practitioners in Emergency Medicine

Learning Outcome

1. Explain how resource limitations in rural areas impact the delivery of emergency medical services (EMS);
2. Understand time constraints and patient volume
3. Discuss emotional and psychological stress

The emergency medicine environment within internal medicine is fraught with challenges that health practitioners must overcome daily. One serious challenge is the unpredictable nature of emergency cases, which often necessitate immediate, swift intervention, placing enormous pressure on general practitioners. These practitioners work under resource limitations, especially when handling acute cases. When access to specialized medical care is limited, the additional pressures can exacerbate general practitioners' workload, requiring them to handle a greater diversity of medical issues without full backup. This requirement to respond to complex emergencies also adds to the mental workload, with practitioners needing to rapidly assess and prioritize interventions while maintaining high standards of patient care. Moreover, communication barriers significantly hinder emergency care for diverse patient populations. General practitioners often encounter patients from various races and ethnicities, who possess unique health beliefs and varying levels of linguistic ability. Evidence indicates that differences in healthcare delivery arise as a result of ineffective cross-cultural communication, an issue that may lead to potential misdiagnosis or suboptimal treatment for minority patients (Association of Public Health Observatories, 2014). This condition is critical in emergency care, where the need is so compelling that there is little time at all for detailed patient histories or tailored communication plans. The ensuing disconnect between practitioner and patient expectations can undermine good clinical decision-making, ultimately impacting on patient outcomes through the provision of poorer quality care to vulnerable groups. Enhancing communication skills and cultural competence is thus paramount for general practitioners who practice in emergency contexts. Besides, the integration of emergency medicine into internal medicine tends to reveal training and preparedness gaps. Family physicians may not receive emergency training while focusing on training in preventive care and chronic disease prevention in primary care. The gap can foster doubt during life-threatening emergencies, ultimately affecting patient outcomes. Ongoing professional development and specific training workshops that impart significant emergency skills to general practitioners are important (Rogers et al., 2004). By creating a learning and adaptive system, healthcare systems can help enhance the emergency skills of general practitioners. Ultimately, patching up these training gaps in the system will enable general practitioners to address the demands of emergency care appropriately and provide quality services to their patients.

10.5.1. Resource Limitations in Rural Areas

Resource shortages among rural populations significantly affect the delivery of emergency medical services (EMS), creating demanding conditions in general practice. Rural populations lack access to the human and technological resources necessary to carry out effective emergency care. Specialists and sophisticated medical equipment are scarce, making it difficult to deal with critical cases. On top of that, rural areas tend to face logistical challenges in relocating patients to large medical centers, especially during emergencies. The consequences of these constraints go far and wide, for they can lead to delays in treatments, poorer patient outcomes, and an overall lower quality of care. Given these challenges, there is a strong rationale for new solutions to better allocate resources and deliver timely access to emergency medical care in these under-resourced areas, calling for ongoing research and development in this field. Blending education and training programs specifically designed for rural EMS providers can help mitigate some of these resource limitations. As considered in various EMS fellowship programs, such as those discussed by Colella et al. (2020), emerging pedagogies in curriculum provision are necessary in the education of medical professionals to deliver care effectively. Such programs integrate flexibility to meet the special requirements of rural society through distance-learning modules and hands-on training, further enhancing the emergency-response capabilities of professionals. Besides, such training initiatives can foster collaboration between healthcare providers and thereby improve the provision of emergency care. Through training professionals with the appropriate skills and expertise most suited to the needs of rural health care, these programs are best placed to bridge the gap in emergency medical care and address the outstanding concerns arising from limited resources. Apart from training and education, closing the financial gap rural healthcare facilities face is crucial in order to advance emergency medical services. The majority of clinics and hospitals in such environments go through tight budget constraints that leave them unable to purchase vital medical supplies or replace essential equipment. A survey by Tammy (2011) reflects these financial issues, finding that the costs of labs, equipment, and medications significantly constrain surgical capacity. Rural healthcare providers cannot accommodate a wide range of services with minimal finances and resources, leaving populations exposed during crises. Policy makers should give top priority to funding programs aimed at expanding rural healthcare facilities to enable them to respond adequately to emergencies and provide the care patients deserve and require.

10.5.2. Time Constraints and Patient Volume

The intersection of patient volume and time pressure exacts challenging demands in the emergency medicine environment. With increasing patient flow into emergency departments (EDs), the urgency that confronts emergency physicians (EPs) affects the quality of care as well as decision-making processes in triage, as a complex task. According to a recent study, EPs significantly consider patient severity of illness and requirement for ICU interventions over the procedural barrier of bed availability while deciding on intensive care unit admissions. Approximately 61.3% of EPs reported high patient volume as a foremost challenge in managing patients with pending ICU admission, highlighting a glaring contradiction between clinical needs and the pressures of busy ED environments (Mathews et al., 2020). It is thus important to understand the dynamics of time pressures under high patient volumes so that one can develop strategies to enhance patient outcomes without sacrificing the quality of care within the confines of emergency medicine. The COVID-19 pandemic has aggravated pre-existing time pressures and patient numbers of problems within emergency medicine. Emergency departments have been flooded with patients presenting acute infections, many of whom have increased emotional distress and fear about their health outcome. As a result, clinicians have the added task of not only meeting patients' physical demands but also their psychological needs. The traditional methods of empathetic communication have become more difficult, primarily due to the increasing number of patients and limitations in infection-prevention practices (Aaronson et al., 2020). However, it is still imperative to maintain the humanistic approach despite the challenges. By implementing techniques to enhance empathy and communication, emergency practitioners can establish a caring environment that mitigates patient anxiety while managing the exigencies of their clinical workload. With these issues in mind, the impact of time pressure and patient flow on emergency medicine extends beyond immediate clinical judgment to encompass patient and clinician experiences overall. The requirement to make rapid, effective decisions under duress can lead to clinician burnout and high levels of stress, which, in turn, can undermine the quality of care. Effective management of the factors requires creative measures that work towards balancing efficiency and patient-focused care. Emergency rooms can learn to integrate system reforms such as raising the staffing ratio, adopting telehealth technologies to triage less critical cases, and promoting connections with outpatient facilities. Such interventions are likely to help offset some of the burdens associated with high patient volumes, while not compromising emergency physicians' capacity to provide timely and compassionate care (Aaronson et al., 2020; Mathews et al., 2020) (Figure 10.13).

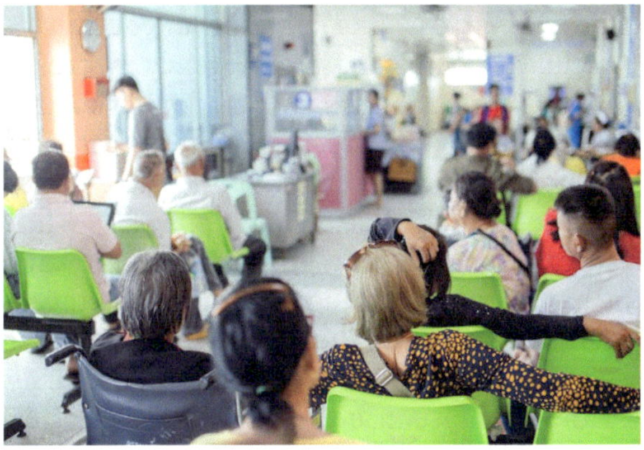

Figure 10.13. High patient volume at emergency cares.

Source: https://www.erexpress.com/wp-content/uploads/2023/03/shutterstock_1142067620-scaled.jpg.

10.5.3. Emotional and Psychological Stress

Emotional and psychological distress impacts healthcare professionals significantly, particularly emergency medicine physicians. The intense pressure of emergency care, where critical decisions must be made while being exposed to traumatic situations, is most likely to result in extreme stress and burnout among clinicians. Research has shown that healthcare professionals working in emergency settings have higher levels of emotional distress, which are mostly linked with long work hours and the gravity of patient outcomes. This culture can create a cycle of stress that not only affects individual physicians but also undermines the overall quality of patient care. This has been recognized as a problem by the Accreditation Council for Graduate Medical Education, which has resulted in initiatives to improve resident wellness and reduce burnout in residency programs. By applying individual-level and organizational interventions, institutions can foster a healthier workplace that may mitigate the adverse effects of psychological stress on care providers and enhance the delivery of care (Bailitz et al., 2020). The synergy between emotional stress and patient encounter is particularly significant in emergency medicine. Providers typically work with patients who have acute psychological stress from life-threatening conditions, which might trigger a heightened empathetic response. This empathy, while desirable for the best possible patient care, can be vicariously traumatizing to healthcare providers as well. They get weighed down by the emotional toll of their patients' lives and thus compromise their own psychological well-being. Laced with this is the increased prevalence of trauma disorders within some populations—such as Latino and African-American boys—documented in recent research, and it is essential that trauma-informed care protocols are adhered to. By recognizing and responding to the psychological impact of trauma on patients, emergency healthcare practitioners can not only improve patient outcomes but also create a more empathetic clinical atmosphere for themselves and their peers (Wilson et al., 2009). For emergency medicine physicians, managing emotional and psychological stress is as critical to individual well-being as to the best patient care. Effective means of addressing such stressors include mindfulness training, peer support groups, and organizational support systems aimed at promoting psychological well-being. Mental health programs that prioritize institutionalizing initiatives to address the unique stressors of emergency physicians are vital for healthcare organizations. By including holistic wellness programs and open discussions about mental health matters in the framework, it is possible to build clinician resilience. These types of efforts will instill a culture of care and comprehension, ultimately enhancing both provider and patient outcomes. As the profession adapts to these changing needs, the recognition of emotional and psychological stress as a primary driver of emergency medicine will spur advances in resilience and efficiency among healthcare providers (Bailitz et al., 2020) (Figure 10.14).

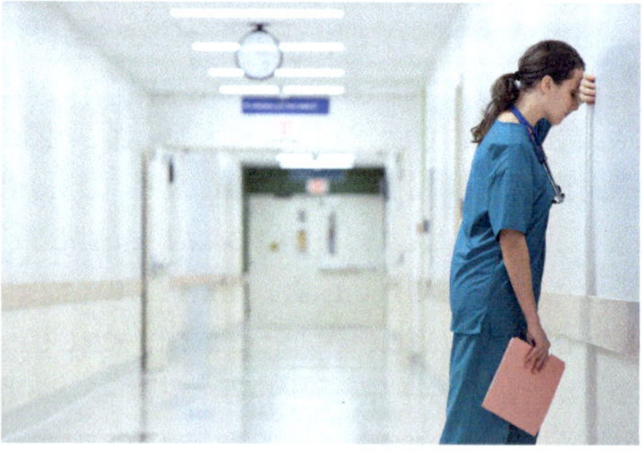

Figure 10.14. A lady doctor with psychological stress.

Source: https://s3-prod.modernhealthcare.com/s3fs-public/022221-feature-iStock-526223747_WEB.jpg.

Test Your Knowledge

1. How do limited medical supplies, equipment, and specialist access in rural or remote areas impact a general practitioner's ability to manage emergency cases effectively?
2. What strategies can general practitioners employ to manage high patient volumes and time-sensitive emergencies?

10.6. Integration of Technology in Emergency Medicine

Learning Outcome

1. Understand telemedicine and remote consultations
2. Discuss the role of electronic health records and data management
3. Explain the use of mobile applications for emergency protocols

The use of technology in emergency medicine has significantly altered the game of patient care, enhancing both the diagnostic process and treatment effectiveness. Examples include the implementation of Point-of-Care Ultrasonography (POCUS), which enables medical practitioners to perform bedside diagnoses. The technology enables rapid assessment of conditions such as trauma and acute respiratory distress, thereby accelerating clinical decision-making and improving patient outcomes. Evidence has shown that POCUS can increase diagnostic accuracy for conditions like acute dyspnea and heart failure, and is particularly valuable in pediatric emergencies where traditional imaging may be suboptimal. The key function of training emergency medicine residents in POCUS is crucial to ensure that the best advantages of this technology are attained in practice, ultimately transforming emergency departments into more effective care environments (Tamimi et al., 2023). Moreover, the incorporation of electronic health records (EHRs) has made it easier to manage patient information, enabling improved communication among healthcare providers. EHRs improve the availability of patient history, allergy, and drug interaction, especially critical in emergent cases where time is of the essence. Not only do they facilitate rapid access to patient data but also real-time documentation of care, taking away the possibility of errors that could compromise patient safety. In addition, the integration of EHRs with telemedicine capabilities facilitates expert consultations, enabling immediate expert assessment to guide treatment planning. Such integration is a paradigm for how technological innovation serves not just individual patient care but also overall health care systems by ensuring continuity of care and enhancing interprofessional practice among practitioners (Rosie et al., 2011). Finally, technologies such as machine learning and artificial intelligence are beginning to make an impact in emergency medicine through predictive analytics that can identify at-risk patients proactively. These technologies can sift through large datasets to identify trends or outliers that may go undetected by traditional methods, alerting clinicians to preventable disasters in advance. The predictive capabilities of AI help more effectively triage patients, so that the largest number of needy patients are reached in due time. As emergency medicine advances, the incorporation of such advanced technologies becomes increasingly necessary. The interplay between real-time data analysis and improved clinical tools results in more informed decision-making and can significantly contribute to enhanced patient safety and satisfaction in emergency settings (Tamimi et al., 2023).

10.6.1. Telemedicine and Remote Consultations

The integration of telemedicine and remote consultations into emergency medicine presents both opportunities and challenges, especially in internal medicine centers. Medical doctors use technology to extend their reach to patients who are unwilling or unable to visit a clinic in person. Such transformation is crucial for patients in rural or disadvantaged settings, where emergency services are typically lacking. Telemedicine adoption not only reduces barriers such as transport issues but also supports timely diagnosis and treatment, which are essential in emergencies. However, telemedicine development requires robust legislative and regulatory frameworks to support its widespread use, as seen by the issues explored in N/A (2010). Addressing these issues is pivotal to realizing the full potential of remote consultations to complement, not complicate, existing healthcare systems. Additionally, disparities in health care access significantly affect the effectiveness of telemedicine, underscoring the need for equitable solutions in the sector. Disadvantaged populations, including racial minorities and low-income groups, are disproportionately affected by access barriers to specialty care and emergency services, as indicated by Carlson et al. (2016). The disparities can be improved through better specialist access without geographic constraints. However, the root socio-economic causes of health inequities—such as the unavailability of internet access, shortcomings in health coverage, and provider biases—must be tackled programmatically. Remote consultations should therefore be integrated into broader efforts to augment health equity in emergency care. By promoting cross-coordination among policymakers, healthcare providers, and community organizations, telemedicine can considerably reduce gaps. Finally, the success of telemedicine in emergency settings calls for the development of specific protocols and training for healthcare professionals. As professionals adapt to new technologies, appropriate training ensures they can provide appropriate care while successfully using telemedicine applications. Appropriate patient consent guidelines, data protection, and remote triage procedures must also be developed, particularly in emergency cases where swift decision-making is of utmost concern. The synchronization of telemedicine is also made more challenging by different insurance policies and reimbursement strategies, which can make it sustainable and accessible to patients of diverse demographics, as seen in N/A (2010). Hence, building an environment conducive to the seamless integration of telemedicine into internal medicine not only improves patient care but is also central to addressing systemic inefficiencies within emergency medicine. Overall, the transition to remote consultations is a revolution in healthcare delivery that demands concerted efforts to overcome existing challenges (Figure 10.15).

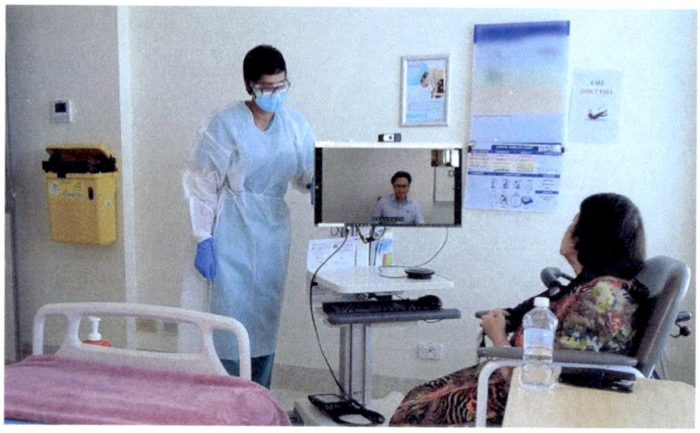

Figure 10.15. Telemedicine and remote consultations.

Source: https://dtresearch.com/blog/wp-content/uploads/2022/06/HPA_video3-1-1024x607.jpg.

10.6.2. Electronic Health Records and Data Management

In the emergency medicine setting in primary practice, the implementation of Electronic Health Records (EHRs) significantly enhances the accessibility and management of patient data. EHRs provide a single repository for storing patient information, allowing physicians to easily recover and modify critical medical histories, medications, and allergies. Instant availability is vital in emergency circumstances, where rapid decision-making can mean the difference between life and death. EHRs also enable care continuity by making it easier for clinicians to share information between providers and settings, thus reducing the risk of errors that could arise from disconnected information. Thus, the application of EHRs in emergency medicine underscores the need for a seamless healthcare delivery system so that evidence-based decisions made by practitioners fall within standardized treatment protocols established across facilities (Anne et al., 2008). Processes involved in managing data regarding EHR systems form part of improving care quality in emergency settings. Effective management is not merely the capture and warehousing of patient data, but also the analysis and structuring of the same to further enhance clinical outcomes. Through sophisticated data analysis, ultrasound clinicians can identify trends, track patient outcomes, and ultimately enhance treatment protocols. Further, EHRs encourage evidence-based practice through clinical decision support, which guides clinicians through evidence-based treatment protocols. This evidence-based practice not only enables timely patient care but also contributes to broader public health initiatives by enabling tracking of disease and outcomes (Cornet et al., 2017). Sophisticated data management under EHR systems is thus integral to the establishment of emergency medicine in general practice. Even with the recognized advantages of EHRs in emergency medicine, however, several issues must be addressed to realize their full potential. Some of these include issues related to interoperability between different EHR systems that may interfere with smooth data sharing, creating patient data gaps that may negatively impact care delivery in emergency situations. Moreover, patient confidentiality and data security concerns are also pressing issues which healthcare organizations face in their quest to comply with stringent regulations while dealing with sensitive health information. An effort must be made to enhance regulatory frameworks, improve infrastructure, and redesign payment structures to address these issues and improve data coordination among providers (Anne et al., 2008). Surmounting these challenges will empower healthcare systems to maximize the use of EHRs and, in turn, contribute to a more efficient and improved practice of emergency medicine in general practice.

10.6.3. Use of Mobile Applications for Emergency Protocols

Inclusion of mobile applications in emergency procedures significantly enhances the effectiveness and impact of emergency healthcare services. They are used as crucial resources for medical personnel across various roles, ranging from quick patient assessments to real-time communication with care teams. For instance, mobile applications can enable first responders to acquire and communicate vital patient information, such as medical history and vital signs, which could be life-saving during life-threatening emergencies. By making key information quickly accessible, such technologies improve informed decision-making in responding to emergencies so that patients are provided with proper care in a timely manner. In emergency care, the timely sharing of information helps bridge the communication gap between emergency staff and hospitals, ultimately leading to better patient outcomes. Besides, the use of mobile applications also encourages a heightened state of alertness among experts and the public at large. The apps may give comprehensive emergency protocols, guiding the user through the steps they must take in various emergencies, e.g., cardiac arrest or trauma. By offering users clear directions and instructions, mobile applications allow individuals to act with confidence in the critical moments and save lives. Emergency medicine democratization builds community resilience and capability by bringing more individuals into emergency response mechanisms. Therefore, the proliferation of smartphone technology and intuitive interfaces provides for more interaction and learning concerning emergency health procedures, such that the applications become a precious resource in internal medicine and emergency medicine. Moreover, the ongoing development of wireless technology enables the deployment of mobile healthcare applications that incorporate streamlined emergency protocols. The recent trend towards wireless and mobile solutions in healthcare provision has made it possible to transition from conventional models that involve continuous network connectivity. Healthcare providers can now view and exchange patients' information at any time and from anywhere, and this creates a more responsive emergency response system (Ayo et al., 2007). This kind of infrastructure facilitates the accurate collection and immediate exchange of essential patient data, leading to timely interventions and improved patient outcomes. Some roadblocks to implementing these technologies, including data security and the use of standards, must be addressed to realize the full potential of mobile applications in emergency medicine. Thus, as technology in mobile devices continues to advance, its integration into emergency protocols holds tremendous potential to enhance healthcare delivery within internal medicine (Eadie et al., 2015) (Figure 10.16).

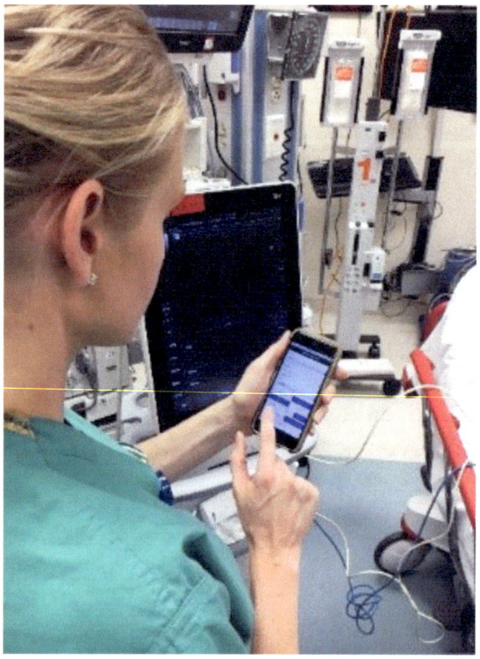

Figure 10.16. A clinical provider uses the Massive Transfusion Protocol mobile app to determine whether a trauma patient just admitted to the emergency room requires a massive blood transfusion.

Source: https://blogger.googleusercontent.com/img/b/R29vZ2xl/AVvXsEgN5myhbrsNd4PK_tO7V1-HSJ9Hy20ECB2uQBRdmNbvdM5qWg-tJ8MNieRDl1OnOr4ClKSe4lFILahuO4o2VumbjNJ34hxC2gvn8A4oapP8-SjUw8RosrNrQ6HMpOMoV1-481PfOEOofYwF/s1600/MTP+fig+02.png.

Test Your Knowledge

1. How can telemedicine support general practitioners in managing emergency cases in remote or underserved areas?
2. In what ways do electronic health records enhance the efficiency and accuracy of emergency care provided by GPs?

10.7. Case Studies and Real-Life Applications

Learning Outcome

1. Discuss successful emergency interventions by general practitioners
2. Focus on lessons learned from emergency scenarios
3. Understand the impact of emergency medicine on patient outcomes

Successful handover of patients in emergency medicine has important implications for outcomes in the wider general practice. For instance, studies of handover culture across three NHS emergency care pathways reported that most failures stem from the complexity of patient flow management and organizational goals. The research discovered that handovers could serve several functions, including passing the responsibility and the handling of capacity, but tended to be poorly communicated due to time constraints and variations in departmental priorities. It can be inferred from the findings that health care providers face built-in tensions in handovers, where urgency and detail are balanced. Hence, handover practices should be enhanced with these dynamics in mind to ensure patient safety and continuity of care, and to affirm the significance of effective communication in emergency situations, as the study's conclusions emphasize (Chessum et al., 2014). Realistic applications of enhanced handover strategies include hospitals using structured communication models, which significantly reduce handover failure. By employing models that integrate quantitative data and qualitative insights, hospitals will be able to gain better insight into patient care streams and interdepartmental dynamics. This can result in a more holistic view of patient management, as demonstrated in existing studies analyzing hospital department interrelationships. This integrated perspective can guide improvements in operational effectiveness and address the specific demands of emergency medicine. Thus, emergency departments that implement systematic and cooperative handover practices are likely to incur fewer mistakes in patient data handovers, eventually leading to better patient outcomes. They depict how clinical pathways can make patient flows less mysterious and enhance departmental cooperation, thereby embedding the role of emergency medicine within internal medicine more broadly (Boucherie et al., 2009). Moreover, embracing a sociotechnical approach to handover processes can potentially transform the provision of emergency care. Organizational culture and interdepartmental partnership focus, as the study indicates, support embracing an interdepartmental strategy that highly prioritizes communication within risky environments. With knowledge of the link between handover quality and patient flow management, healthcare organizations can create environments that foster better teamwork and communication, which are imperative for rapid decision-making in emergencies. This culture shift can help practitioners better manage the complexity of emergency care, providing critical patient information correctly. By doing so, medical practitioners can respond promptly to patients' needs, thereby improving the overall efficiency of emergency medicine in internal medicine institutions.

10.7.1. Successful Emergency Interventions by General Practitioners

The role of general practitioners (GPs) in emergency medicine is important, particularly in rural and deprived areas where access to specialist services in an emergency may be limited. In such environments, successful emergency intervention by GPs can have a significant impact on the patient's outcome. For instance, GPs are primarily involved in treating acute respiratory infections, trauma, and cardiovascular emergencies, which not only require medical expertise but also the capacity for quick decision-making. Their education prepares them to make initial diagnoses, stabilize patients, and identify the need for referrals to specialists when necessary. The ability to identify serious conditions early can prevent complications and improve recovery rates. Thus, the integration of emergency medicine training into the curriculum of GPs can enhance their capacity to give timely and effective care in emergencies and thereby accentuate their vital role in the healthcare system. Moreover, emergency care by GPs tends to spread beyond fast medical interventions. Successful interventions are usually a function of holistically addressing the social and psychological factors of a patient's health. GPs usually encounter patients with multifaceted healthcare needs stemming from socioeconomic factors, hence complicating their medical states. In addressing these issues, GPs implement care management interventions not only to treat acute conditions but also to improve long-term health outcomes. Care continuity and follow-up, for example, are critical in reducing hospital readmission and improving overall health. The delicate understanding of patients' backgrounds that comes from continuous contact enables GPs to perform customized interventions that match individual needs. Consequently, this approach underscores the importance of a comprehensive understanding of health in handling emergency cases humanely and compassionately. Finally, cutting-edge technology plays a vital role in supporting the capacity of GPs in delivering in emergency medicine. With the advent of digital technologies such as telemedicine and home monitoring, GPs now address emergencies differently. Virtual consultation technologies enable GPs to analyze and treat patients in real time, significantly enhancing access to care for patients in remote areas. However, as seen in existing research, there are specific challenges inherent in integrating these technologies, primarily in involving patients in participation and sustaining them within care management. For instance, while digital interventions show promise in improving outcomes, patient literacy and access to technology can impede their implementation. It is, therefore, imperative for GPs to weigh the implementation of technology against patient-centered care such that the emergency interventions are not only successful but also equitable, enhancing the quality of healthcare delivery in routine practice as a whole (Berry-Millett et al., 2009; Darby et al., 2017) (Figure 10.17).

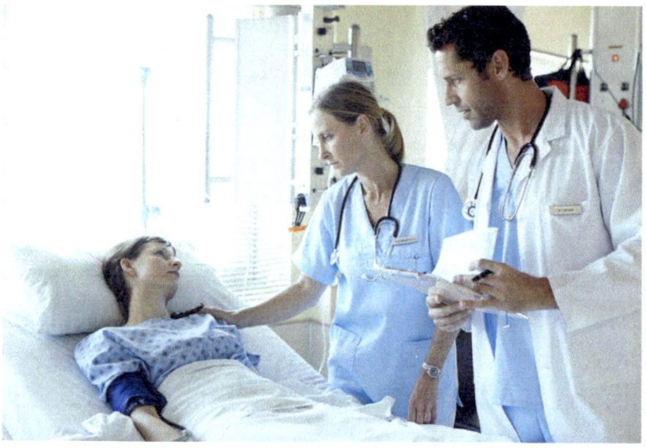

Figure 10.17. General practitioners (GPs) in emergency medicine.

Source: https://www.verywellhealth.com/thmb/wNRSrF2ctZbU3Csyx7_3-gqfSCo=/1500x0/filters:no_upscale():max_bytes(150000):strip_icc()/doctors-talking-to-patient-in-hospital-icu-493216255-583452e15f9b58d5b1b967c7.jpg.

10.7.2. Lessons Learned from Emergency Scenarios

In the context of emergency medicine, lessons learned from previous emergencies can be a valuable addition to making responses more effective in practice. As the experience of organizations such as Médecins Sans Frontières (MSF) can show, some of the lessons to be learned concern the management of urban health emergencies. MSF's realignment of response from reactive to proactive increases focus on the unique needs of vulnerable urban communities affected not only by natural disasters but also by violence and exclusion. The broad analysis enables a suitable medical approach and operational approach that can address the unique challenges in urban areas. These findings are precious to general practitioners who may well find themselves practicing in similar emergency settings, highlighting the need for adaptability and situational approaches to emergency medicine. In addition, integrating safety innovations in healthcare systems also reveals another lesson identified from emergency conditions. Case examples of health organization responses during crises indicate that systematic reviews of actions, effects, and learnings are crucial for designing safer clinical settings. For instance, initiatives aimed at promoting cross-learning between clinical teams have yielded innovative solutions to improve patient safety. The initiatives show that what is learned is meaningful only if it influences future best practices, enabling health care professionals to minimize risk and maximize patient outcomes during crises. The ability to learn from and adapt from past experiences in emergencies is essential to embedding a culture of safety in general practice, ultimately to the benefit of both practitioners and patients. It is equally important to highlight the significance of preparation in emergency medicine. The ability to make accurate assessments and implement measurable vulnerability standards is imperative for efficiently addressing health emergencies. Lessons derived from MSFs experiences in the field identify a call for situational security management and prompt closing of activities that were initiated under conditions of emergencies. Using such analysis, general practitioners can better anticipate and address their patients' special needs during crises. Thus, these lessons serve general practitioners of medicine as a reminder of the need for constant evaluation and adjustment in emergency response training so that they may be adequately equipped to address the diverse and changing demands that can arise.

10.7.3. Impact of Emergency Medicine on Patient Outcomes

The integration of emergency medicine into internal medicine has had a considerable impact on patient outcomes, particularly regarding the validity of diagnoses. Emergency conditions often require timely assessment to avoid lethal complications. In such settings, innovations such as Point-of-Care Ultrasonography (POCUS) have been critical. By enhancing diagnostic capability, POCUS enables clinicians to make the right treatment decisions in a timely manner, particularly for conditions such as acute dyspnea and Acute Decompensated Heart Failure (ADHF), where prompt intervention is paramount. The systematic review demonstrates that, in current studies, POCUS not only changes diagnostic impressions but also drastically influences the plan of management, thereby optimizing overall patient care and outcomes. In so doing, emergency medicine tools and practices contribute mainly to the optimal management of complex cases encountered in routine practice, emphasizing the need to incorporate such advancements in daily healthcare procedures (Tamimi et al., 2023). Leadership and collaboration among teams within emergency rooms are equally critical in informing patient safety outcomes. The perception of a supportive safety climate is well established to have profound effects on the effectiveness of medical care. As evidenced by a study in Southern Ontario, senior leadership support and teamwork climate were strongly associated with favorable overall PS perceptions. This suggests that when healthcare workers observe firm-level leadership support for safety, they are more engaged in safety improvement activities. Notably, the research also indicated that the existence of positive supervisory leadership can counteract poorer senior leadership, demonstrating the nuanced dynamics within emergency care settings. Thus, reinforcing these perceptions through practical leadership development and teamwork workshops can be critical in reasserting safety and improving patient outcomes in emergencies, illustrating the relationship between organizational culture and clinical effectiveness (Bain et al., 2018). Last but not least, ongoing training and education for emergency medicine physicians play a vital role in sustaining improvements in patient outcomes. The incorporation of POCUS into residency training has been shown to increase its use among emergency medicine residents, which is associated with improved patient management. This focus on training not only prepares practitioners with the abilities they require but also promotes a culture of continuous improvement and adaptability in emergency settings. Additionally, providing seminars on critical soft skills, such as conflict management, has been shown to boost interdisciplinary collaboration, thereby enhancing teamwork and communication in high-pressure settings. By confronting both technical ability and human interaction, hospitals can ensure emergency medicine is responsive to patient needs and optimizes the overall quality of care. Lastly, the advanced multi-faced learning, along with emerging technologies, facilitates the improving trend of patient outcomes in emergency medicine (Bain et al., 2018; Tamimi et al., 2023) (Figure 10.18).

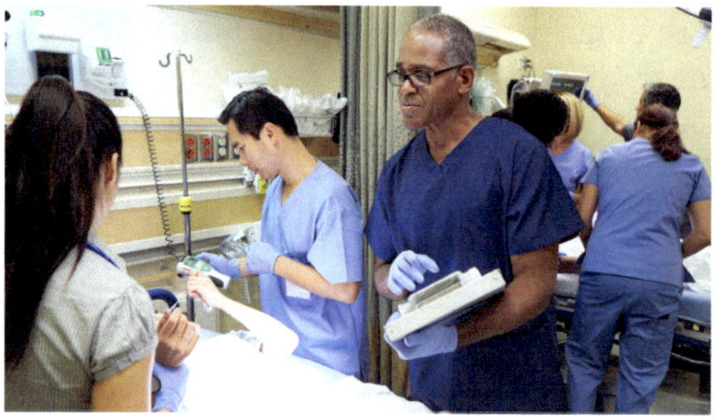

Figure 10.18. Impact of emergency medicine on patient outcomes.

Source: https://www.rmf.harvard.edu/-/media/Project/Rmf/CRICO/16x9images/em-contrib-factors16x9.jpg.

Test Your Knowledge

1. Can you describe a real-life case where a general practitioner successfully stabilized a patient in a life-threatening emergency before referral?
2. How have GPs adapted emergency care delivery during public health crises?

10.8. Challenges in Critical Care and Emergency Medicine

Learning Outcome

1. Staffing shortages and burnout
2. Access to care and health disparities
3. Evolving guidelines and best practices

The critical care and emergency medicine environment is riddled with complexities that complicate the treatment of patients following acute health emergencies. Most concerning is the increased reliance on diagnostic testing, which, though potentially efficacious, has not contributed to decreased rates of disease-related death. Instead, it is more likely to result in excessive healthcare costs and undesirable byproducts, such as incidental finding detection requiring further investigation or being exposed to harmful procedures. As clinicians address these concerns, integrating shared decision-making (SDM) can be a turning point in optimizing patient outcomes. By incorporating discussions of test harms and benefits, clinicians can better individualize care, enhance the partnership nature of patient-clinician relationships, and ensure that medical interventions align with patients' unique health outcomes and decisions (Arterburn et al., 2016). A second pressing concern in emergency medicine arises from the treatment of critically ill patients awaiting intensive care unit (ICU) admission in the emergency department (ED). The majority of emergency physicians feel overwhelmed by the pressure to provide prolonged critical care in the ED, particularly in high-volume settings. The boarding of ICU patients—patients who remain in the ED longer than needed—is one of the extra burdens assigned to the medical team. Studies have noted that patient illness severity and the need for ICU interventions have been precisely evaluated as triage criteria, with system-related factors such as bed availability. Such a dynamic seeks to capture the inherent conflict between patients' needs and the realities of healthcare system capabilities (Mathews et al., 2020). Finally, staffing shortages and patient volumes also add to the inherent dilemmas of critical care and emergency medicine. With the increased demands on emergency departments, inadequate staffing can compromise the quality of care and heighten provider stress. Emergency physicians have identified shortages in support staffing as a significant barrier to caring for critically ill patients. The inefficiencies that ensue can lead to suboptimal patient care, prolonged wait times, and a higher risk for adverse outcomes. Hence, issues of staffing and resource utilization in emergency departments need to be given high priority to enhance overall care delivery. Highlighting the relevance of systemic support frameworks will be vital in shaping the emergency medicine process to suit the needs of the current era and further optimize patient outcomes in critical care environments.

10.8.1. Staffing Shortages and Burnout

The impact of critical care and emergency medicine staffing shortages is a significant factor in the universal issue of burnout in healthcare professionals. The stressful nature of the working environment in these facilities heightens stress, leaving staff feeling exhausted, overwhelmed, and irritable. A 2024 survey of over 22,000 nurses across California, New York, and Texas found a significant connection between undue workload and negative emotional states (Okoronkwo et al., 2024). Particularly in emergency rooms where the throughput of patients easily exceeds available staff, continuous pressure on the nurses may render them unable to provide quality care and thus deplete their professional satisfaction as well as general well-being. This over-demanding cycle not only impacts individual performance but also demotivates, ultimately compromising patient care quality and safety in critical settings. In addition, ineffective support systems for health workers contribute to nurse shortages. Many nurses are reported to have insufficient preparation to manage their workloads, leading to increased turnover intentions (Faye et al., 2015). An alarming number of healthcare professionals are considering leaving their jobs due to unsustainable working conditions, further compounded by poor staffing. Interview data indicate that over 40% of staff identified staffing challenges as a prime reason for leaving employment, with impacts also observed in professional relationships and mental health (Faye et al., 2015). The ongoing stress resulting from inadequate staffing not only results in suboptimal patient care but also produces a potentially hazardous environment in which clinical staff are faced with elevated anxiety and diminished job satisfaction. This situation ultimately requires an urgent re-evaluation of resource management in critical care models. Creative interventions are needed to address the rising issues of burnout and staffing deficits. Implementing practices such as providing a dedicated serenity room, which is utilized to promote mindfulness and relaxation among critical care professionals, may bring positive outcomes. According to studies, providing such spaces can greatly enhance staff resilience and job satisfaction, thereby reducing burnout among nurses (Okoronkwo et al., 2024).

Further, applying flexible staffing models that are sensitive to the fluctuating nature of emergency care can temper some of the stress on healthcare professionals. By establishing a healthy work culture and acknowledging the psychological and emotional toll on staff, healthcare organizations can take their first steps toward reversing the attrition trend and enhancing the quality of care in critical care and emergency medicine settings. Inadequate investment in staffing and staff well-being programs is central to sustaining the healthcare workforce and delivering patient-centered care at patients' most vulnerable points (Figure 10.19).

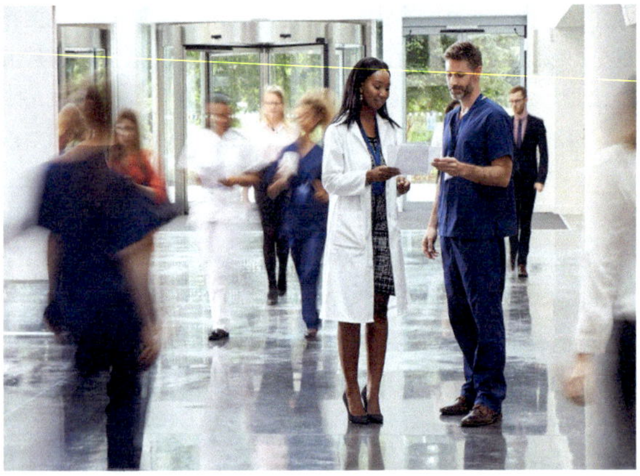

Figure 10.19. The phenomenon of staffing shortages in critical care and emergency medicine.

Source: https://www.taylor.com/hubfs/_Taylor.com%20-%20All%20files%20connected%20to%20main%20site%20and%20blogs/Blogs/Taylor%20-%20Blog/Staffing%20Shortages%20and%20Burnout%20Still%20Problematic%20for%20Hospitals/Blog%20Hero%20Image%20%E2%80%93%20Staffing.jpg.

10.8.2. Access to Care and Health Disparities

Access to care remains a high-priority concern in addressing health disparities, particularly in critical care and emergency medicine. There are many determinants, including socioeconomic status, geographical location, and racial/ethnic identity, which influence one's access to timely and appropriate healthcare. The barriers to access usually occur in the form of late emergency responses and inappropriate care, which exacerbate existing health conditions in underrepresented groups. Furthermore, marginalized groups are routinely faced with institutionalized inequalities that limit their ability to access healthcare services. The cumulative effect of these gaps is generating sharp ethical concerns about the fairness and effectiveness of the healthcare system, which require a thorough understanding of the complex problems that different populations face in seeking access to care. As regards emergency medicine, It is important to recognize that racial and ethnic disparities play a very critical role in determining patient outcomes and the quality of care delivered. Emergency services are a critical safety net, primarily for individuals living in ethnically diverse communities who are high utilizers of the services for their health requirements. The literature cites that the poor health status among some racial and ethnic groups is well documented, illustrating the persistence of the disparities. Many healthcare providers may lack the cultural competence to address the unique needs of minority patients, leading to ineffective and inequitable care. Patient ethnic data collection has come into focus, as recognize disparities and implement evidence-based, targeted interventions to address these inequities (Association of Public Health Observatories, 2014). Mitigating health disparities in emergency care requires broad-ranging actions that align with best practices in equity-focused healthcare delivery. Establishing a committee dedicated to addressing such disparities can foster a culture in which healthcare practitioners engage with their diverse patient populations. Some key recommendations include collecting disaggregated patient demographic information, setting realistic quality goals, and continually evaluating the effectiveness of implemented policies. These innovative strategies can help health organizations measure and monitor health disparities and encourage responsibility across emergency care systems. As health equity discourse evolves, healthcare professionals must listen to the voices of marginalized groups and dismantle the barriers that hinder their access to appropriate care, so that every patient receives the quality care they deserve (Alexander et al., 2009).

10.8.3. Evolving Guidelines and Best Practices

The emergency medicine and critical care environment is continually reshaped by new guidelines and best practices, improving patient outcomes and healthcare effectiveness. Evidence-based practices challenge healthcare professionals to adapt and refine their approaches to patient treatment. A prime example of this is the emphasis on reducing hospital readmissions for diseases such as pneumonia and heart failure. Investment in advanced practice nurses enables the hospitals to promote evidence-based practices as part of daily standard care, which has broad clinical outcomes and patient satisfaction effects (Lashbrook et al., 2011). Strategic alterations promote not only improved patient care but also optimize the use of resources by eliminating unnecessary hospital admissions and readmissions. The COVID-19 pandemic provided a real-world example of the necessity for immediate adaptation of guidelines and emergency medicine practices. The majority of healthcare institutions were compelled to realign hurriedly to address the unprecedented demand for services and scarce resources. The standardized leadership structure was key in facilitating communication and coordination among operating rooms. Prioritizing the protection of personal protective equipment and hospital bed capacity became critical in managing both COVID-19 patients and operative patients (Conte et al., 2020). The measures during this time demonstrated how departments were able to offer high-quality care amid crises and, therefore, established a precedent for future crises, emphasizing flexibility and resilience in operations. With each development in emergency medicine and critical care, the importance of staying responsive to ongoing education and training cannot be overstated. Health care professionals must remain responsive to emerging evidence from studies, clinical practice guidelines, and new technologies, which profoundly influence patient management strategies. Regular workshops, simulations, and inter-professional education programs foster a platform for continuous improvement and teamwork. Exchange of best practices learned in emergencies can also improve health care systems' general understanding of efficient patient care strategies. Such an initiative-driven educational approach not only improves the professional development of individuals but also makes the overall health system more resilient to looming threats and uncertainties.

Test Your Knowledge

1. Discuss the major challenges faced in Critical Care Medicine in managing critically ill patients.
2. Explain the challenges encountered in Emergency Medicine and their impact on patient outcomes

SUMMARY

The addition of emergency medicine as a component of internal medicine is a crucial reform in healthcare that focuses on patients' immediate needs and promotes a more comprehensive approach to care. As the health landscape continues to evolve, the need for primary care providers to receive emergency medicine training becomes the top priority. These trainings not only enhance the initial response to acute medical needs but also overall patient outcomes through prompt interventions. The emergency department providers' viewpoints illustrate significant facilitators and barriers to suicide risk screening, with the need for streamlined protocols and collaboration. These findings demonstrate the potential of interdisciplinary collaboration to address medically complex issues and improve the quality of care offered in emergency departments and internal medicine (Berlin et al., 2015). Moreover, this emphasis on integrated models of care becomes increasingly vital when addressing the complexities of medically at-risk populations. Severely mentally ill patients, for example, have higher rates of comorbid medical conditions but tend to utilize emergency resources for acute presentations rather than preventative care or utilization of primary healthcare. The lack of alignment results in inefficiency and adverse health effects, necessitating a comprehensive approach to managing their needs. The adoption of coordinated action between primary healthcare providers and mental health professionals can go a long way in remedying such challenges. By enhancing communication and planning in integrated care settings, health systems can improve access to care and patient satisfaction, and ultimately reduce pressure on emergency services (Read et al., 2016). Finally, the convergence of emergency medicine and internal medicine offers a promising model for addressing the healthcare needs of diverse populations. As principles of emergency medicine become more deeply rooted in the general practice model, practitioners can make significant strides in the treatment of acute and chronic illness, fostering a more proactive than reactive approach to patient care. The following recommendations, derived from current research and practitioner experience, can serve as a blueprint for future practice innovation and policymaking efforts. Through continuous enhancement and the effective use of strategies, health systems can improve service delivery, ensure the right and timely care for patients, and alleviate emergency department pressure (Berlin et al., 2015; Read et al., 2016).

The integration of emergency medicine into internal medicine is gradually becoming an urgent requirement for overall patient care. The core principle of integration concerns the effective training of medical professionals in the management of acute medical emergencies, particularly obstetric emergencies. The conditions demand unique skills and knowledge that might not often be encountered in routine practice and, as a result, create a gap in readiness among general practitioners. Active learning strategies, encouraging learning, such as labor and delivery situational board games, have been promising in the education of helpful knowledge and skills for residents effectively. Interactive learning materials used in this context facilitate collaboration and retention of useful information. As attested by learner feedback, these new pedagogical resources significantly improve learning outcomes compared with traditional lectures, as learners rate the educational value very highly and report that they effectively prepare practitioners for real-life applications (Chen et al., 2019). Additionally, effective debriefing competencies following simulated clinical education rely on principles guiding the fostering of ongoing improvement in emergency medicine training. Debriefing is an opportunity for students to reflect on their experience, thereby helping them better grasp and capitalize on their ability to handle comparable situations in real-life clinical practice. Reflective practice not only improves individual performance but also synchronizes team dynamics in the health care setting, guaranteeing safety and quality of care. Debriefing guidelines, as noted in expert literature, encompass a commitment to providing a respectful and supportive environment, and the relevance of acknowledging learner emotions in analyzing their decisions and actions. Encouraging a systematic debriefing strategy allows instructors to ensure the consolidation of learning, identify gaps and near misses in trainees' performance, and consequently contribute directly to enhanced patient safety (Alinier et al., 2017). With the ongoing evolution of healthcare, the interface between internal medicine and emergency medicine is critical. The application of cutting-edge learning techniques, including game-based teaching and systematic debriefing, is an innovative way of developing competencies in emergency response. Continuing to use and refine these teaching methods is necessary in preparing healthcare providers to respond appropriately to the acute presentations they may encounter in clinical practice. Notably, this training not only enhances technical proficiency but also critical thought and collaboration abilities, which are vital in high-stakes settings. Thus, this emphasis on emergency medicine within internal medicine training not only equips professionals with the necessary technical skills but also fosters a culture of safety and responsiveness, thereby indirectly enhancing patient outcomes across medical settings.

KEY TERMS FROM THIS CHAPTER

- Emergency Medicine
- Triage
- Airway Management
- Shock
- Cardiac Arrest
- Trauma
- Acute Respiratory Distress Syndrome
- Critical Care
- Resuscitation
- Mechanical Ventilation
- Sepsis
- Advanced Life Support
- Hemodynamic Monitoring
- Intensive Care Unit

CRITICAL THINKING QUESTIONS

1. **What is the primary role of a general practitioner (GP) in emergencies?**
   a. To provide long-term specialist care for chronic diseases
   b. To refer all emergencies to hospital-based emergency departments
   c. To assess, stabilize, and initiate management of acute conditions
   d. To perform complex surgical procedures in a primary care setting
2. **Which of the following is one of the most common emergencies encountered in general practice?**
   a. Cardiac tamponade
   b. Acute myocardial infarction
   c. Severe trauma with multiple fractures
   d. Stroke requiring neurosurgery
3. **What essential training or skill is most crucial for GPs dealing with emergencies?**
   a. Advanced neurosurgical training
   b. Specialized radiology certification
   c. Dialysis machine operation
   d. Basic life support (BLS) and advanced cardiac life support (ACLS)
4. **One of the main challenges faced by GPs in emergency medicine is:**
   a. Overstaffing in rural clinics
   b. Inadequate access to emergency diagnostic tools
   c. Too many ambulances in proximity
   d. Excessive training in emergency procedures
5. **How is technology increasingly integrated into emergency medicine within general practice?**
   a. By replacing GPs with fully autonomous AI systems
   b. Through paper-based records and faxes
   c. Via telemedicine consultations and portable diagnostic tools
   d. Through home visits, replacing clinic consultations

Short Answer Questions

1. What is the "golden hour" in trauma care, and why is it significant?
2. What are the key components of the primary survey in Advanced Trauma Life Support (ATLS)?
3. Define septic shock and list two early signs.
4. What is the role of lactate in assessing critically ill patients?
5. What are the indications for initiating mechanical ventilation in the ICU?

Answers to Critical Thinking Questions

1. (c); 2. (b); 3. (d); 4. (b); 5. (c)

REFERENCES

1. Sonis, J., Kennedy, M., Aaronson, E., Baugh, J., Raja, A., Yun, B., & White, B. (2020). Humanism in the Age of COVID-19: Renewing focus on communication and compassion. *Western Journal of Emergency Medicine, 21*(3), 499–502. https://doi.org/10.5811/westjem.2020.4.47596Al Tamimi, A. A. A., Alruwaili, A. M. S., Alruwaili, E. M., Alenazi, F. M., Almoammar, N. A., Alwayli, N. S., & Alfayer, T. A. (2023). The utility of point-of-care ultrasound (POCUS) in the emergency department: A systematic review. https://core.ac.uk/download/603897418.pdf (accessed on 17th July 2025).
2. Alinier, G. (2018). Cost-effective extracorporeal membrane oxygenation simulation. https://core.ac.uk/download/288394195.pdf (accessed on 17th July 2025).
3. Alinier, G., & Oriot, D. (2017). *Pocket Book for Simulation Debriefing in Healthcare*. https://core.ac.uk/download/159073196.pdf (accessed on 17th July 2025).
4. Allen, T. J. (2011). Addressing resource gaps in the U.S. health care safety net: An assessment of the free clinic network. https://core.ac.uk/download/71357645.pdf (accessed on 17th July 2025).
5. Amin, A., Cohen, M., Deitelzweig, S., DiLascia, J., et al. (2019). Contemporary NSTEMI management: The role of the hospitalist. https://core.ac.uk/download/322850160.pdf (accessed on 17th July 2025).
6. Annemans, L., De Regge, M., Duyck, P., Gemmel, P., et al. (2013). Physician-owned specialized facilities: Focused factories or destructive competition? A systematic review. https://core.ac.uk/download/55777137.pdf (accessed on 17th July 2025).
7. Arora, S., Burner, E., Menchine, M., Terp, S., et al. (2020). Penalties for Emergency Medical Treatment and Labor Act violations involving obstetrical emergencies. https://core.ac.uk/download/287622014.pdf (accessed on 17th July 2025).
8. Association of Public Health Observatories, BBC News, Department of Health (DH), Dorsett, R., DWP, et al. (2014). *Ethnic Minorities and Their Health Needs: Crisis of Perception and Behaviors*. https://core.ac.uk/download/20569137.pdf (accessed on 17th July 2025).
9. Ayo, C. K., & Omogbadegun, Z. O. (2007). Impact of mobile and wireless technology on healthcare delivery services. https://core.ac.uk/download/19447815.pdf (accessed on 17th July 2025).
10. Bailitz, J., Battaglioli, N., Chung, A. S., Clinton, W., et al. (2020). Evidence-based interventions that promote resident wellness from the Council of Emergency Residency Directors. https://core.ac.uk/download/287621996.pdf (accessed on 17th July 2025).
11. Bain, L., Ginsburg, L., Thomson, K., Wong, B., et al. (2018). Importance of safety climate, teamwork climate and demographics: Understanding nurses, allied health professionals and clerical staff perceptions of patient safety. https://core.ac.uk/download/288471195.pdf (accessed on 17th July 2025).
12. Bajaj, K., Bentley, S., Nadir, N. A., Papanagnou, D., et al. (2016). Characteristics of real-time, non-critical incident debriefing practices in the emergency department. https://core.ac.uk/download/83049577.pdf (accessed on 17th July 2025).
13. Bandeeri, N., Henry, J. A., Meredith, C., Treacy, M., et al. (2004). The prevalence of cocaine-associated chest pain in a London hospital. https://core.ac.uk/download/5230488.pdf (accessed on 17th July 2025).

14. Bangerter, A., Davis, D., Haroff-Tavel, H., Hauck, H., HPN (Humanitarian Practice Network), Koscalova, M., et al. (2012). Moving from the 'Why' to the 'How': Reflections on humanitarian response in urban settings. https://core.ac.uk/download/pdf/10674421.pdf (accessed on 17th July 2025).

15. Berlin, J. S., Gutierrez, P. M., Petrik, M. L., Saunders, S. M., et al. (2015). Barriers and facilitators of suicide risk assessment in emergency departments: A qualitative study of provider perspectives. https://core.ac.uk/download/213077361.pdf (accessed on 17th July 2025).

16. Berry-Millett, R., & Bodenheimer, T. (2009). Care management of patients with complex health care needs. https://core.ac.uk/download/71346306.pdf (accessed on 17th July 2025).

17. Biega, B. (2024). SCARES: A clinician guide to spinal cord awareness, response, and emergency support creation and implantation of SCARES protocol among hospitalist advanced practice providers. https://core.ac.uk/download/619611492.pdf (accessed on 17th July 2025).

18. Biu, T., Goldsworthy, L. L., & Sidebotham, P. (2007). Child protection procedures in emergency departments. https://core.ac.uk/download/45517.pdf (accessed on 17th July 2025).

19. Blanchard, S., de Bedout, T., Eckert, G. J., Hamada, Y., et al. (2018). Assessing the medical emergency preparedness of dental faculty, residents, and practicing periodontists: An exploratory study. https://core.ac.uk/download/188008401.pdf (accessed on 17th July 2025).

20. Blumenthal, D., & McCarthy, D. (2006). Committed to safety: Ten case studies on reducing harm to patients. https://core.ac.uk/download/71350251.pdf (accessed on 17th July 2025).

21. Boucherie, R. J., Hans, E. W., Hurink, J. L., Litvak, N., et al. (2009). A survey of health care models that encompass multiple departments. https://core.ac.uk/download/pdf/11471201.pdf (accessed on 17th July 2025).

22. Buchbinder, R., Underwood, M., Hartvigsen, J., & Maher, C. G. (2020). *The Lancet* series call to action to reduce low value care for low back pain: An update. *Pain, 161*, S57–S64. https://doi.org/10.1097/j.pain.0000000000001869 (accessed on 17th July 2025).

23. Carlson, C., Sholk, J., Nanni, J., Peterson, K., Smith, L. A., & Bhavaraju, N. (2016). Breaking the barriers to specialty care: Practical ideas to improve health equity and reduce cost–Increasing specialty care availability. https://core.ac.uk/download/75785770.pdf (accessed on 17th July 2025).

24. Chalya, P. L., Dass, R. M., Gilyoma, J. M., Mabula, M., et al. (2012). Geriatric injuries among patients attending a regional hospital in Shinyanga, Tanzania. https://core.ac.uk/download/pdf/18410878.pdf (accessed on 17th July 2025).

25. Chen, E. H., & Silverio, L. M. (2019). L&D in the ED: A game-based approach to learning high-risk obstetric emergencies. https://core.ac.uk/download/323074437.pdf (accessed on 17th July 2025).

26. Chessum, P., Cooke, M., Cross, S., Fitton, L., et al. (2014). Clinical handover within the emergency care pathway and the potential risks of clinical handover failure (ECHO): Primary research. https://core.ac.uk/download/19882629.pdf (accessed on 17th July 2025).

27. Colella, M. R., Gaither, J., Schulz, K., Smith, T., et al. (2020). Innovative approaches to emergency medical services fellowship challenges. https://core.ac.uk/download/287621995.pdf (accessed on 17th July 2025).

28. Cornet, R., McCowan, C., Peek, N., Scott, P., et al. (2017). Addendum to Informatics for Health 2017: Advancing both science and practice. https://core.ac.uk/download/132585011.pdf (accessed on 17th July 2025).

29. Cribb, A., Schutz, A., Thompson, A., Medina, A., McKinstry, B., Johnson, B., et al. (2010). A video life-world approach to consultation practice: The relevance of a socio-phenomenological approach. https://core.ac.uk/download/2707954.pdf (accessed on 17th July 2025).

30. Cross, K., Fallat, M. E., Laniewicz, M., Nti, N., et al. (2019). A novel streamlined trauma response team training improves imaging efficiency for pediatric blunt abdominal trauma patients. https://core.ac.uk/download/187423820.pdf (accessed on 17th July 2025).

31. Dahlen, P. (2014). School district assessment for sudden cardiac arrest preparation. https://core.ac.uk/download/162576263.pdf (accessed on 17th July 2025).

32. Darby, J., Jiwa, M., & Tambakis, G. (2017). What is the scope to test a smoking cessation intervention aimed at young people admitted to hospital? https://core.ac.uk/download/225151085.pdf (accessed on 17th July 2025).

33. Eadie, L. H., Mort, A. J., & Wilson, P. M. J. (2015). Technology to support rural health and well-being. https://core.ac.uk/download/29465861.pdf (accessed on 17th July 2025).

34. Gauthier, A. K., Shih, A., McCarthy, D., Davis, K., Nuzum, R., & Schoenbaum, S. C. (2008). *Organizing the U.S. Health Care Delivery System for High Performance.* https://core.ac.uk/download/71353608.pdf (accessed on 17th July 2025).

35. Kagioglou, M., Kobbacy, K. A. H., Lengu, D., Sapountzis, S., et al. (2012). Application of simulation and modelling in managing unplanned healthcare demand. https://core.ac.uk/download/12800084.pdf (accessed on 17th July 2025).

36. Kim, E., Kuppermann, N., & Tzimenatos, L. (2014). The Pediatric Emergency Care Applied Research Network: A history of multicenter collaboration in the United States. https://core.ac.uk/download/323069086.pdf (accessed on 17th July 2025).

37. Lara, A., Mead, H., & Regenstein, M. (2006). *The Heart of The Matter: The Relationship Between Communities, Cardiovascular Services and Racial and Ethnic Gaps in Care.* https://core.ac.uk/download/71346670.pdf (accessed on 17th July 2025).

38. Mathews, K. S., Nelson, J. E., Richardson, L. D., Rodriguez, R., et al. (2020). Triage and ongoing care for critically ill patients in the emergency department: Results from a national survey of emergency physicians. https://core.ac.uk/download/287622005.pdf (accessed on 17th July 2025).

39. Morphet, J., Plummer, V., & Rochana, N. (2016). Triage process in emergency departments: An Indonesian study. https://media.neliti.com/media/publications/155129-EN-triage-process-in-emergency-departments.pdf (accessed on 17th July 2025).

40. N/A. (2010). *Staying Connected: A Progress Report: Reimbursement Under the Telemedicine Development Act of 1996.* https://core.ac.uk/download/71355210.pdf (accessed on 17th July 2025).

41. O'Donnell, R., & Vijayaraghavan, V. (2011). *Sentara Healthcare: A Case Study Series on Disruptive Innovation Within Integrated Health Systems.* https://core.ac.uk/download/71358929.pdf (accessed on 17th July 2025).

42. Osborn, L., & Rossi, A. (2020). A case report of angioedema and anaphylactic shock induced by ingestion of polyethylene glycol. https://core.ac.uk/download/305124170.pdf (accessed on 17th July 2025).
43. Read, T. L. (2016). Emerging needs in behavioral health and the integrated care model. https://open.bu.edu/bitstream/2144/17694/1/Read_bu_0017N_11995.pdf (accessed on 17th July 2025).
44. Reilly, S., Slaughter, R., & Ventura, E. (2016). Thrust joint manipulation utilization by US physical therapists. https://digitalscholarship.unlv.edu/cgi/viewcontent.cgi?article=4549&context=thesesdissertations (accessed on 17th July 2025).
45. Risso, A. V., Alvarez, J., Bellani, G., Bettini, F., et al. (2016). Epidemiology, patterns of care, and mortality for patients with acute respiratory distress syndrome in intensive care units in 50 countries. https://core.ac.uk/download/54529633.pdf (accessed on 17th July 2025).
46. Rogers, W. A. (2004). Reducing health inequalities: Ethical issues in a Scottish child health home visiting program. https://core.ac.uk/download/14935808.pdf (accessed on 17th July 2025).
47. Skivington, K., Matthews, L., Simpson, S., Craig, P., Baird, J., Blazeby, J., Boyd, K., et al. (2021). A new framework for developing and evaluating complex interventions: Update of Medical Research Council guidance. *BMJ*. https://doi.org/10.1136/bmj.n2061 (accessed on 17th July 2025).
48. Thal, A., & Zapanta, P. (2016). Otolaryngology for internal medicine: Increasing exposure to otolaryngology using computer assisted instruction. https://core.ac.uk/download/230828860.pdf (accessed on 17th July 2025).
49. Wilson, A., Rich, J., Rich, L., Bloom, S., Evans, S., & Corbin, T. (2009). *Healing the Hurt: Trauma-Informed Approaches to the Health of Boys and Young Men of Color*. https://core.ac.uk/download/71360851.pdf (accessed on 17th July 2025).

INTERNAL MEDICINE FOR CLINICAL NUTRITION AND METABOLISM

11

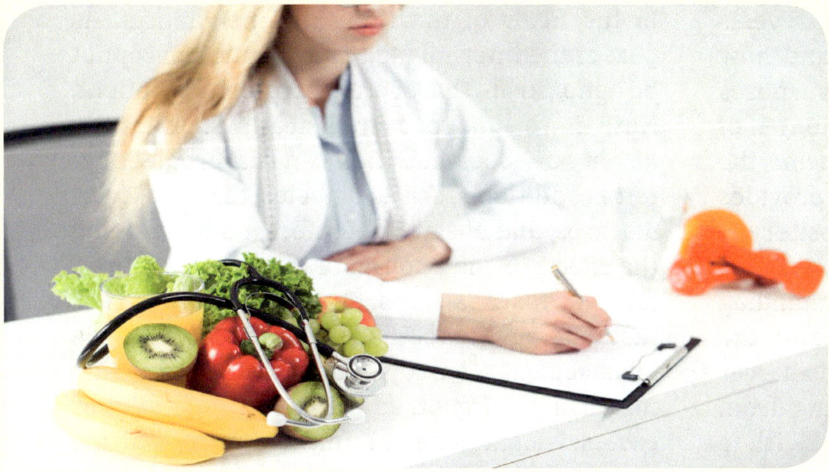

LEARNING OBJECTIVES

After studying this chapter, you will be able to:

1. Discuss the role of internal medicine in patient care
2. Explain the nutritional assessment techniques
3. Understand common nutritional disorders
4. Evaluate the therapeutic diets in internal medicine
5. Discuss the impact of lifestyle modifications
6. Learn about challenges in clinical nutrition

Introduction

It is highly essential to understand the relationship of internal medicine, clinical nutrition, and metabolism in addressing a wide range of health problems. Internal medicine delves into the intricacies of adult medicine and practices a whole-person approach to diagnosing, treating, and preventing disease. In this context, nutrition takes a central role in patient outcomes because it has a direct effect on metabolic function. As more medical facilities recognize the importance of diet as a treatment intervention for chronic disease management, the integration of clinical nutrition into internal medicine becomes imperative. With this focus, the emphasis shifts to healthcare professionals gaining a solid foundation in nutritional science as it relates to metabolic well-being, providing a foundation for informed food decisions to be used as treatment agents in disease management. The complex interplay between metabolism and nutrition continues to underscore the need for interdisciplinary practice in patient management. Metabolic pathways are central to how the body uses nutrients, and altering them can lead to major health problems. Recent developments in learning about the gut-brain axis continue to demonstrate the role that the gut microbiota may play in interacting with human metabolism and impacting mood and metabolic disease. The microbiota-gut-brain axis is a rapidly growing field of clinical research, opening new connections between dietary patterns and the psychological and physiological health of the individual. With ongoing dietary research examining these connections, practitioners must be attuned to evolving scholarship that reveals the role of diet in metabolic control and how this can be harnessed for therapeutic purposes (John et al., 2019). In looking to the potential of clinical nutrition to impact internal medicine, the Human Metabolome Database (HMDB) provides a valuable reference. As a scientific repository of the human metabolites and their functions in the body, the HMDB delivers depth of understanding and insight into metabolic disease and the impact of diet. As it expands to cover an ever more varied array of data—everything from metabolic pathways to interactions with a range of substances—the HMDB becomes an indispensable tool for researchers and clinicians (David et al., 2017). Health professionals can base nutritional interventions and treatment regimens on patients' metabolic profiles, making evidence-based decisions. With such accurate datasets, the future of internal medicine can become more integrated with the science of clinical nutrition and metabolism, paving the way for more sensitive, individually tailored management strategies.

Definition of Internal Medicine

Internal medicine is a fundamental medical specialty that primarily, but not solely, deals with the prevention, diagnosis, and treatment of internal illnesses. Unlike surgical specialties, internal medicine addresses a broad range of adult health challenges and provides comprehensive patient care. Specialists, or internists, use their techniques to treat complex diseases that typically affect more than a single organ system, thereby requiring a multidisciplinary approach to human physiology and disease. This specialty is a major part of the health care system because internists sometimes serve as primary care physicians, providing chronic disease management, acute illness care, and preventive care-oriented long-term care. The widespread engagement is required in caring for the complicated interactions between various health conditions and treatments, which is vast in the fields of nutrition and metabolism. As part of the internal medicines, nutrition cannot be ignored in the overall care of the patient. Nutrition's link to overall health significantly lies in how poor nutrition can exacerbate long-term conditions such as diabetes, cardiovascular diseases, and obesity. Therefore, understanding the effects on metabolism of various diet options for internists is important in this arena. For instance, evidence-based practices for the management of sarcopenic obesity are becoming increasingly urgent, as the condition combines excess weight with low muscle mass, putting the individual at greater risk for metabolic syndrome. The escalating incidence of sarcopenic obesity underscores the need for internists to address not only weight management but also muscle health as key components in a complete care plan (Choi et al., 2009). This general focus prioritizes the internist's role in achieving healthier outcomes through intensive nutritional interventions. Additionally, the definition of internal medicine is evolving in response to advances in medical science and increasing healthcare complexity. Internists today are not only responsible for disease management but also for educating patients regarding lifestyle behaviors, including diet and exercise, for the prevention and management of disease. This shift recognizes that patients decisions and behaviors result directly in their health outcomes. Internists are well-positioned to establish patient-centered care strategies that take into account patient preferences and needs, thereby enhancing adherence to regimens.

The emphasis on evidence-based practice in clinical nutrition is also consistent with internists' obligation to stay current on new research findings. For example, if the clinician understands the rate of universal growth in research impact, they can tap into studies applicable to them that inform practice (Kinney et al., 2007). Essentially, internal medicine's broad definition does contain a promise of whole care with a central role for nutrition and metabolism in their fostering of general well-being.

Importance of Clinical Nutrition and Metabolism

Clinical metabolism and nutrition are central to the treatment of a broad spectrum of medical illnesses and to enhancing overall patient health. Nutrition is no longer an adjunct to standard therapies but becomes more widely recognized as a cornerstone of management for numerous illnesses, including obesity, diabetes, and cardiovascular disease. A precisely formulated diet tailored to a person's requirements can influence metabolic pathways and influence the course of disease. Nonetheless, given its significance, numerous healthcare providers are poorly trained in nutritional science. The gap, therefore, calls for the incorporation of clinical nutrition in medical education so that healthcare professionals can accurately determine and treat patients' nutritional requirements. In this way, providers can help patients recognize the importance of food selection in maintaining health and avoiding disease (Al-Dujaili et al., 2016). Moreover, an understanding of metabolism also explains the body's response to food intake and physical activity. The metabolic pathways influence how nutrients are metabolized, utilized, and stored, thereby affecting energy levels, weight control, and susceptibility to disease. Altered pathways can evolve into severe health conditions such as insulin resistance, dyslipidemia, and chronic inflammation. For instance, research has identified oxidative stress to be increased in overweight patients, representing a complex metabolic-nutritional interaction with immediate implications for health outcomes (Arefiev et al., 2017). Management of these metabolic disturbances through dietary interventions can improve patients' health status and quality of life. As such, internal medicine practitioners ought to focus on these metabolic indices and incorporate nutritional guidance into treatment regimens. Finally, the applicability of clinical nutrition extends beyond individual health and has far-reaching implications for public health outcomes. With lifestyle conditions on the rise, healthcare expenses levied upon populations and healthcare systems increase tremendously. By promoting clinical nutrition, healthcare professionals can avert conditions such as obesity and metabolic syndrome, thereby reducing healthcare costs and improving population health.

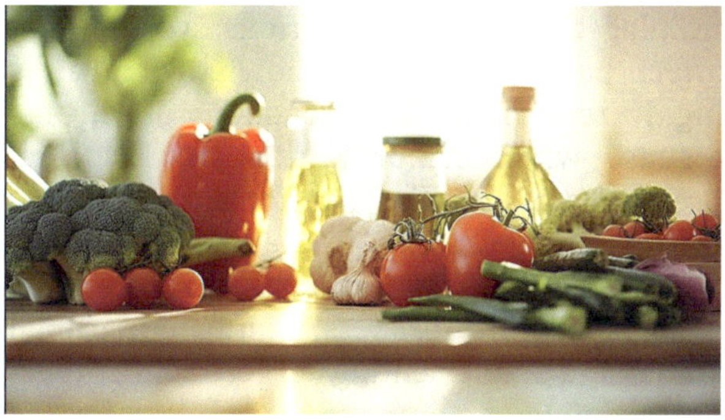

Figure 11.1. Clinical nutrition and metabolism.

Source: https://media.springernature.com/lw900/springer-cms/rest/v1/content/27123278/data/v1.

Nutrition education and access initiatives at the public health arena have the capacity to transform food consumption habits at the community level. Thus, fostering a keen appreciation of clinical nutrition among healthcare professionals can more effectively prevent ailments, ultimately enhancing the quality of life for individuals and communities

(Al-Dujaili et al., 2016). Emphasizing education in clinical nutrition and metabolism as a priority will equip healthcare professionals with what it takes to overcome the current challenges in medicine (Figure 11.1).

11.1. Role of Internal Medicine in Patient Care

Learning Outcome

1. Comprehensive patient assessment
2. Development of treatment plans
3. Coordination with multidisciplinary teams

Internal medicine plays a central role in patient care as the reference point for diagnosing, managing, and treating a variety of complex health conditions. Internal medicine physicians are well-versed in adult illnesses and undergo training to evaluate the various systems that affect patients' health. Knowledge level is highly relevant in the treatment of chronic disease when comorbidities are involved, presenting as a multi-dimensional complication in treatment planning. In the specific area of clinical nutrition and metabolism, internists are responsible for determining nutritional status and implementing targeted nutritional interventions. An example of such significance is the connection between nutritional supplementation and improved recovery rates in patient populations, demonstrating the importance of this specialty in promoting overall well-being and health. Internists usually advocate evidence-based treatments that optimize patients' metabolic response and well-being, offering a broad therapeutic strategy. Furthermore, the integration of clinical nutrition into internal medicine underscores the need for tailored dietary therapy for specific diseases management and prevention of conditions caused by lifestyle. By evaluating patients' nutritional needs based on their unique health status profiles, internist professionals can make a significant contribution to recovery patterns. For example, protein supplementation is found to enhance recovery periods, boost energy levels, and maintain immune function in individuals with existing nutritional deficiencies and undergoing other medical procedures (Patel et al., 2025). Internists not only monitor such patients' response to nutritional therapy but also examine other factors such as their psychological well-being and lifestyle determinants influencing health.

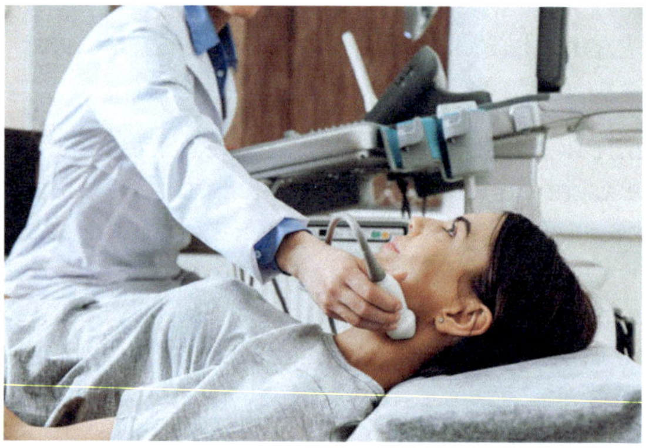

Figure 11.2. Internal medicine plays a critical role in patient care.

Source: https://www.aucmed.edu/sites/g/files/krcnkv361/files/styles/atge_3_2_crop_md/public/2022-03/Internal-Meds.jpg?h=cb35aeb6&itok=sqCcQMsl.

Thus, the role of internal medicine is not merely treatment but a comprehensive care plan, with an emphasis on prevention through diet to ensure long-term health outcomes. In acute settings, the role of internal medicine is even more prominent, as practitioners treat serious health conditions such as hepatitis and complex metabolic diseases systematically. Treatment for such conditions often entails intricate nutritional strategies in addition to standard medical treatment, with the clinician playing a central role in directing care pathways that optimally address different aspects of health. For example, internists offer nutritional support tailored to patients' individual needs, including enteral or parenteral nutrition for those unable to consume food orally, thereby enabling patients to receive the required nutrients despite compromised health. Moreover, the utilization of immune therapy and nutritional surveillance, such as pre-albumin values and global dietary assessment, is part of an integrated internal medicine management that maximizes patient outcomes (Wang et al., 2019). This multimodal treatment highlights the pivotal role of internal medicine in integrating and implementing patient-centered management that facilitates healing and helps achieve optimal health (Figure 11.2).

11.1.1. Comprehensive Patient Assessment

A thorough patient assessment is the cornerstone of effective internal medicine, particularly within the specialty practice of clinical nutrition and metabolism. This multimodal approach requires that clinicians assess virtually all aspects of a patient's overall health, including medical history, nutritional status, psychosocial factors, and metabolic disturbances. Through stepwise collection of this information, clinicians are in a position to make educated judgments about significant health dangers and modifiable nutritional inadequacies that are central to creating interventions tailored to the patient. The consolidation of findings from such appraisals not only enhances diagnostic accuracy but also contributes to the general management of complex conditions ranging from obesity to malnutrition. As a result, an emphasis on thorough patient assessment yields a more refined understanding of each individual's health trajectory and informs interventions that affect long-term outcomes in clinical practice and research. Tending to patients' nutritional requirements during a complete assessment is particularly crucial, as malnutrition can impact disease management and recovery significantly. For instance, screening tools such as the Mini-Nutritional Assessment can detect at-risk patients for malnutrition proficiently before clinical deterioration. Moreover, starting a dialogue about food lifestyle and eating habits can provide insight into a patient's willingness and adherence to required changes. Detailed patient evaluations must also consider comorbidities and their relevance to nutritional needs, as diseases such as diabetes or cardiovascular disease often require tailored dietary management. Seamless control of these complications leads to better health outcomes and allows the patient to take ownership of their health process, thereby promoting patient compliance with nutritional advice in internal medicine practices. In addition to the clinical assessment, the psychosocial elements of an individual's life cannot be overlooked, as they exert a tremendous influence on decision-making about health.

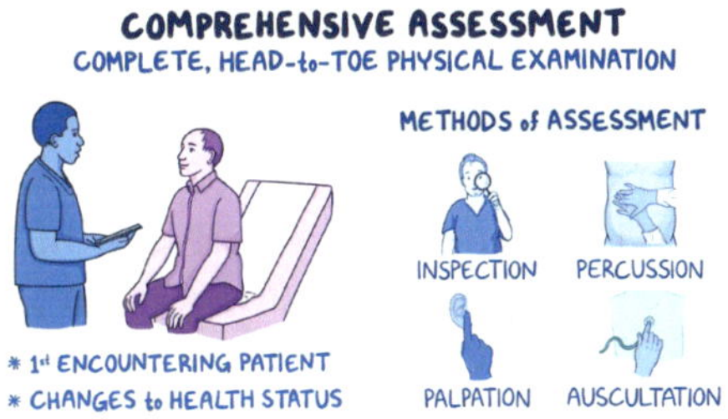

Figure 11.3. A comprehensive patient assessment.

Source: https://www.osmosis.org/_next/image?url=https%3A%2F%2Fd16qt3wv6xm098.cloudfront.net%2F-vU9gnHSRYGWxR3bjI1iOC5OQ3yy7kC6%2F_.jpg&w=3840&q=75.

Social support, mental status, and barriers to care are all essential elements that must be incorporated into comprehensive assessments. The realization that emotional and psychological health can significantly influence nutritional behavior and adherence to medical recommendations highlights the importance of addressing treatment holistically. For instance, an understanding of the patient's social situation may be used to customize education interventions that are more effectively embraced and lead to long-term change. As internal medicine evolves, integration of global assessments that encompass medical, nutritional, and psychosocial factors will be paramount in addressing the complexity of patient care and realizing maximal outcomes in clinical nutrition and metabolism (Figure 11.3).

11.1.2. Development of Treatment Plans

Treatment plan development in internal medicine, particularly with reference to clinical nutrition and metabolism, requires a keen understanding of each patient's unique health scenario. The treatment plans should be informed by a thorough assessment considering the medical history, eating habits, and metabolic requirements. An effective treatment strategy integrates clinical information and personalized experience in a way that makes interventions such as diet, supplements, and medication specific to the patient's lifestyle and interests. This active engagement of patients in treatment planning enhances adherence to treatment protocols and empowers individuals to be active participants of their own health. Thus, a meticulous process for developing a treatment plan is a cornerstone of efficient management in internal medicine, particularly for complex nutritional and metabolic disorders. An appreciation of the multidimensional nature of nutritional needs is critical to ensuring successful treatment plan development. For instance, diabetic patients may require holistic treatment incorporating calorie intake with the quality and amount of carbohydrates, with interventions specifically aimed at providing stable blood glucose control. Furthermore, obese and metabolic syndrome patients may be treated by programs that treat not only weight control but also comorbidities like hypertension or dyslipidemia. Based on the rich literature and clinical guidelines, healthcare providers can set outcome measures to assess treatment effectiveness, enabling ongoing improvement in patient care. This evidence-based approach aligns with current knowledge of health policy that supports the efficacy of evidence-based care, such as prevention and coordination of care, which can have a real,tangible impact on long-term patient outcomes. Furthermore, the treatment plan environment is continually evolving with advances in research and shifts in healthcare policy. As highlighted in recent studies, there is a significant need to prioritize palliative care and patient self-management in the context of aging populations. The integration of such perspectives into treatment planning can potentially enhance the quality of life for patients suffering from chronic nutritional and metabolic conditions. Such approaches to holistic care need an interdisciplinary process that involves coordination between physicians, dietitians, and other medical specialists. Last but not least, the development of treatment plans advances better health outcomes for the individual but can also translate into overall health policy initiatives to improve population health, as evidenced by an overwhelming number of studies with multiple promising policy concepts owed to clinical nutrition and overall metabolic health (N/A, 2006; Morton et al., 2015).

11.1.3. Coordination with Multidisciplinary Teams

The multidisciplinary nature of clinical nutrition and metabolism in internal medicine demands extensive coordination with expert groups to ensure optimal patient outcomes. All the specialties, such as endocrinology, gastroenterology, and dietetics, bring essential insights that contribute to extensive knowledge of nutritional needs and metabolic processes. Multidisciplinary practice provides an arena where diverse opinions challenge conventional wisdom, leading to innovative solutions for complex ailments. There is evidence that scientific collaboration enhances the quality of care, but many healthcare teams struggle to implement efficient multidisciplinary integration. By monitoring team dynamics through instruments such as the Organizational Culture Assessment Instrument (OCAI), it is evident that specific roles of individuals within these teams must be delineated and harmonized well to enhance overall performance and responsiveness to change, which is of utmost significance in addressing intricate healthcare problems (Lotrecchiano et al., 2013). Furthermore, collaboration among experts in a multidisciplinary setting is key to supporting patient care in internal medicine for clinical nutrition and metabolism. Continuous interaction strengthens teams, ensuring practitioners are informed of the latest evidence-based practices to simplify nutritional interventions and metabolic monitoring. Highlighting such interprofessional collaboration is essential in the coordination of shared problems, such as the management of chronic diseases and the facilitation of preventive care interventions. Research highlights coordination across specialties to improve patient self-management and reduce healthcare disparities (Morton et al., 2015). Successful information sharing across disciplines enhances decision-making and leads to a more integrative approach to patient care, particularly for elderly patients with multiple health issues. For clinical nutrition and metabolism, interdisciplinary practice efficiency is not merely communication; it demands a coordinated approach to treatment planning. Coordination between experts in intervention is essential to effective implementation, as it enables tailored strategies that fit the specific physiological and nutritional needs of a particular patient. For example, more active collaboration among physicians, dietitians, and pharmacy staff can lead to better control of conditions such as diabetes and obesity, where diet plays a central role. Furthermore, understanding the interplay between metabolic pathways among multidisciplinary staff can uncover novel therapeutic avenues and enhance coordination of care. Therefore, the establishment of collaborative platforms and fostering the culture of shared responsibility for healthcare teams is essential to addressing the complexities underlying the effective management of nutrition and metabolism (Morton et al., 2015) (Figure 11.4).

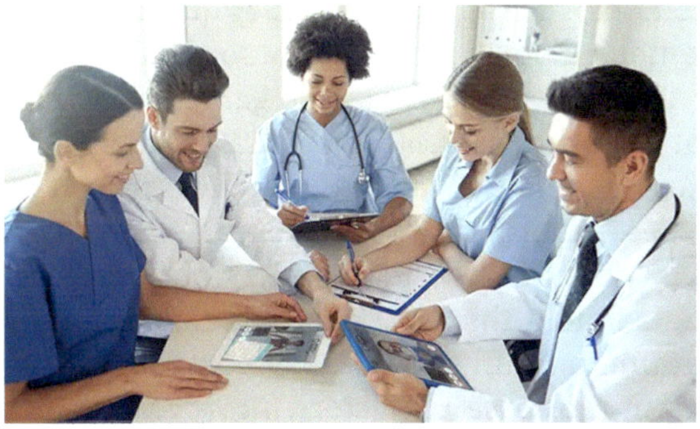

Figure 11.4. Coordination with multidisciplinary teams.

Source: https://bodyinteract.com/wp-content/uploads/2024/07/multidisciplinary-teams-healthcare-1.webp.

Test Your Knowledge

1. What are the key components of a comprehensive patient assessment in clinical nutrition?
2. How is an individualized nutrition treatment plan developed for a patient with chronic disease?
3. Why is coordination with a multidisciplinary team important in delivering effective nutritional care?

11.2. Nutritional Assessment Techniques

Learning Outcome

1. Dietary history and food frequency questionnaires
2. Anthropometric measurements
3. Biochemical and clinical evaluations

Understanding nutritional assessment tools is significant in clinical nutrition and metabolism, especially in internal medicine. The tools are broadly divided into dietary assessment, anthropometric measurements, and biochemical tests. Dietary assessment involves an analysis of the consumption of food through various methods, such as food frequency questionnaires, 24-hour dietary recalls, and food diaries. Each of these measures is used to gain insight into a patient's diet, which can be vital for diagnosing excesses and deficiencies that worsen medical issues. Anthropometric measurements, such as body mass index (BMI), waist measurement, and skinfold thickness, also provides objective data on an individual's body composition and potential disease risk factors. Incorporating these tests informs clinicians of necessary dietary modifications, allowing them to intervene more precisely. Use of biochemical tests cannot be overstated among assessment techniques in nutrition. The tests measure specific biomarkers present in blood or urine that reflect nutrient status and physiological adaptation of the body to various kinds of diets. For instance, serum albumin and prealbumin concentrations can indicate protein malnutrition, whereas concentration of other vitamins and minerals can indicate deficiencies related to specific dietary deficits. As highlighted in the current clinical controversy, integrating these biochemical assessments with dietary data yields a global view of a patient's nutritional status, facilitating better-informed therapeutic choices by health professionals. This symbiosis is particularly important when considering ailments such as alcoholic liver disease and inflammatory bowel disease, in which nutritional therapy can immensely impact disease course and management therapy, as argued in ongoing study endeavors (Allan et al., 2017; Feldstein et al., 2018). In general, a comprehensive approach to nutritional assessment techniques is important when tracking the complex interactions between nutrition and health in internal medicine. By combining dietary, anthropometric, and biochemical measures, clinicians can construct a precise image of the nutritional status of a patient. Close scrutiny is not only helpful in identifying areas of probable nutritional deficiencies but also in creating appropriate management plans for patients' needs. With clinical nutrition progress, study and training in these assessment methods remain pivotal. By integrating new nutritional assessment practices into daily practice, healthcare providers can enhance patient outcomes and foster a greater appreciation of the critical role nutrition plays in overall well-being and metabolic processes (Figure 11.5).

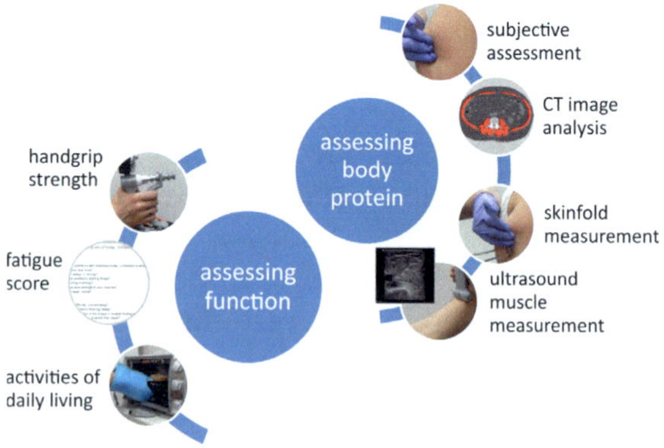

Figure 11.5. The nutritional assessment techniques.

Source: https://www.australiancriticalcare.com/cms/10.1016/j.aucc.2020.02.005/asset/8f593fc5-b8a4-4d47-9c27-048e3df989fa/main.assets/gr3_lrg.jpg.

11.2.1. Dietary History and Food Frequency Questionnaires

The application of Dietary History and Food Frequency Questionnaires (FFQs) is a basic advancement in clinical nutrition that provides extensive access to personalized information on eating patterns that may influence health. The tools allow clinicians to obtain detailed information on a patient's macronutrient and micronutrient intake over a target period. Through the analysis of this information, health practitioners can identify nutritional deficiencies or excesses that may result in disorders of health like obesity, cardiovascular disease, and diabetes. Furthermore, the data gathered from such questionnaires may be used to create individualized nutrition plans tailored to a patient's specific health needs and metabolic requirements, thereby enhancing the efficacy of treatment regimens in Internal Medicine for Clinical Nutrition and Metabolism. Aside from their utility in clinical practice, FFQs have been most important in epidemiologic research, connecting dietary habits with chronic disease outcomes. Investigations using FFQ can survey numerous individuals and thus permit examination of correlations between diet and measures of health. For instance, as is cited in more recent studies, increasing interest is being shown in the possible role of micronutrients like folate to alter health risk, say for asthma, and that nutritional assessment methods will uncover significant associations between disease prevalence and nutrient intake. The nuance captured by FFQs enables scientists to construct a more informed understanding of how certain dietary elements affect health within populations, providing a strong foundation for public health recommendations and nutrition interventions to maximize overall health outcomes. Second, the validity of Dietary History and FFQs also relies on accurate reporting and recall of food intake by patients. While these tools have the benefit of a number of advantages, they are susceptible to the frailties of self-reporting, like underreporting or misreporting of food consumption. To avoid these difficulties, clinicians should administer these questionnaires accurately and correctly interpret them, using strategies that ensure maximum participant participation and accuracy. As mounting evidence accumulates, most notably regarding micronutrients such as calcium and folate, assessment of food intake using these questionnaires becomes a key determinant in clinical decision-making. For example, the Panel on Dietetic Products would highlight that the new evidence does not necessitate revision of the tolerable upper intake levels of calcium, and there is a need for ongoing dietary evaluation in clinical practice to facilitate improved nutritional guidance (Abrams et al., 2012; Blatter et al., 2014).

11.2.2. Anthropometric Measurements

Anthropometric measurements are fundamental instruments in clinical nutrition and metabolism that provide critical information about a person's body composition and fat and muscle distribution. These measurements, such as body mass index (BMI), waist circumference, and skinfold thickness, are important for assessing nutritional status and the risk of obesity and malnutrition. These markers are used by clinicians not just to identify individual health profiles but also to track changes over time after dietary treatment or medical intervention. In this sense, anthropometric measures are included in establishing a baseline for patients that can guide individualized nutrition plans aimed at increased health gain. The significance of precise anthropometric measurements should never be discounted, as errors in their measurement will lead to misinterpretation of a person's nutritional and metabolic health. For instance, BMI, while a useful screening measure, is not always reflective of body fat percentage in all individuals, particularly those with higher muscle mass. In addition, waist circumference is an important indicator to evaluate visceral fat, which is linked to a greater risk of metabolic syndrome and cardiovascular disease. Based on studies, an awareness of the economic burden linked with obesity and other weight-related medical conditions through proper anthropometric data can be used in framing health policy initiatives toward public health promotion (Alston et al., 2025). Thus, the integration of precise anthropometric measurements into clinical practice has significant consequences for improving patient management and reducing total healthcare costs. Apart from their clinical usage, anthropometric measurements also play a relevant role in recent studies conducted on nutrition and metabolism. Recent studies have researched the impact of certain dietary treatments on oxidative stress condition, foremost in overweight and obese subjects. For example, evidence has revealed that antioxidant dietary intake, such as pomegranate juice, could minimize exercise-induced oxidative stress among these patients and thus enhance recovery and metabolic function overall (Al-Dujaili et al., 2016). Anthropometric measurements, in conjunction with food questionnaires, enable researchers to examine the relationships among metabolic health, diet, and body composition. This integrative perspective not only advances scientific knowledge but also informs clinical practice that prioritizes better health outcomes for multicultural groups, targeting evidence-based diet advice from anthropometric data (Figure 11.6).

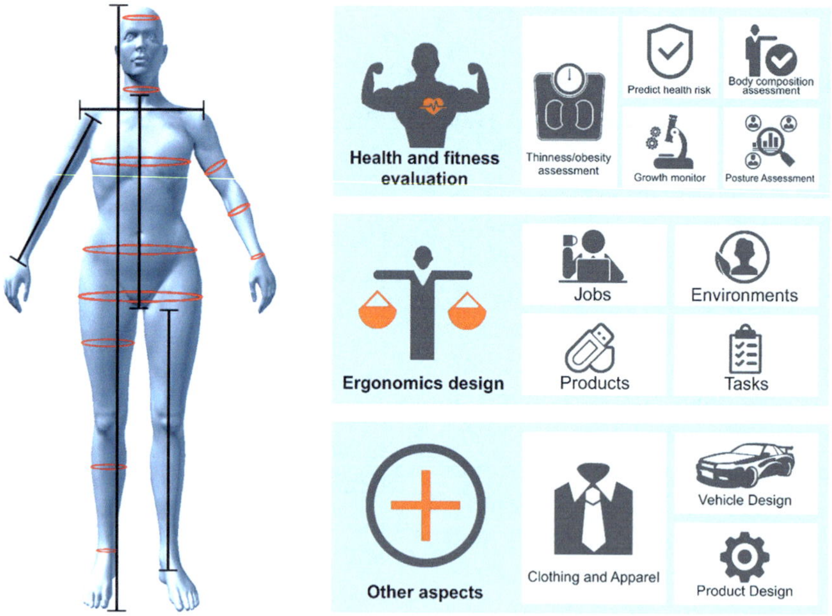

Figure 11.6. Anthropometric measurements.

Source: https://storage.googleapis.com/jnl-up-j-pah-files/journals/1/articles/379/66e19915727a9.png.

11.2.3. Biochemical and Clinical Evaluations

The function of biochemical tests in clinical nutrition and metabolism cannot be overstressed as they provide crucial information on the metabolic status and disease risk of an individual. Via the determination of biomarkers, such as blood glucose, lipid profiles, and vitamins, clinicians can identify metabolic dysfunction and deficiencies that may affect overall health. For instance, plasma amino acid analysis may identify inborn errors of metabolism such as phenylketonuria, thereby facilitating early dietary interventions that prevent dangerous complications. Additionally, biochemical testing enables individualized nutrition through dietary methods tailored to the patient's metabolic needs. Inclusion of these tests in the clinical setting thus not only aids diagnosis of conditions but also helps ensure the integrity of nutritional therapies tailored to individual patient needs, resulting in better health outcomes. In recent years, clinical testing beyond standard biochemical testing has been the focus in assessing patient health in terms of nutrition and metabolism. For example, the application of complete metabolic panels and advanced imaging modalities is able to further illuminate us on the physiological status of the patient. These modalities enable us to understand better the interplay between nutrient absorption, metabolic processes, and disease status. Also, the application of new therapies, such as stem cell transplantation, has produced promising results in the restoration of metabolic disease, e.g., in the management of β-mannosidase deficiency. Following one such intervention, there was some improvement in certain biochemical markers, but neurocognitive development problems still remained. This clearly indicates the requirement of periodic clinical evaluation to monitor and adjust treatment interventions to effectively impact change as well as to ensure that patients get the complete treatment for optimal cure and management of metabolic disorders (Eisengart et al., 2019). The importance of integrating rigorous research methodologies to the practice of internal medicine cannot be underestimated, particularly in evaluating the efficacy of clinical nutrition and metabolic therapies. Research techniques, such as the H-index, have been proposed to quantify the impact of scientific research, which is crucial for treatment-outcome-focused hospitals seeking excellence. By using benchmarks in measurement, such methods assist health care workers with establishing effective therapies and programs with strong scientific evidence (Kinney et al., 2007). This eventually means improved patient care with evidence-based therapy in clinical nutrition. Moreover, enhanced collaboration among clinicians and researchers improves the translation of new evidence into practice and, consequently, strengthens the link between biochemical examination and clinical assessment in the development of individualized therapeutic approaches for patients with metabolic disorders.

Test Your Knowledge

1. What is the purpose of taking a detailed dietary history or using a food frequency questionnaire in clinical nutrition?
2. How do biochemical and clinical evaluations support the diagnosis of nutritional deficiencies or metabolic imbalances?

11.3. Common Nutritional Disorders

Learning Outcome

1. Obesity and metabolic syndrome
2. Malnutrition and its consequences
3. Diabetes management and nutrition

The prevalence of overall nutritional disorders has been an emerging concern in the field of internal medicine because these disorders have the potential to influence health and wellness dramatically. Nutritional deficiencies such as vitamin D deficiency and iron deficiency anemia are prevalent among populations, influencing individuals' metabolic functions and immune systems. For example, iron deficiency anemia not only produces fatigue and decreased intellectual function but also speeds up chronic illness by disabling oxygen delivery to tissues. Similarly, less than optimum levels of vitamin D have been linked with osteoporosis, cardiovascular disease, and certain cancers.

These failures demand an understanding of both food sources of nutrients and the biological processes involved in the absorption and utilization of those nutrients, highlighting the intricate association among nutrition, metabolism, and health status, as highlighted in the literature on biochemistry and human physiology (Sarmidi et al., 2012). Moreover, the rising epidemic of obesity and its related metabolic derangements, including type 2 diabetes and metabolic syndrome, illustrates another dimension of nutritional derangements. These diseases are generally related to increased caloric intake and poor eating patterns, leading to inflammation and insulin resistance. Obesity is not merely the result of overeating but also leads to a variety of health issues, including cardiovascular disease and certain cancers. An all-encompassing approach emphasizing healthy eating patterns, activity, and behavior modification is needed in order to prevent and manage these disorders. Current research highlights that evidence-based interventions, drawing on both clinical nutrition and metabolism, should be used to develop strategies to address the enormous epidemic of obesity-related disorders (Eijck et al., 2003). Lastly, one must not forget the impact malnutrition, particularly in vulnerable populations such as the young and the elderly, has on health. Malnutrition, whether undernourished or overnourished, poses significant challenges to medical practitioners. Inadequate caloric intake can lead to stunted growth and retarded growth of children, while elderly malnutrition can increase the risk of frailty and lower disease resistance. Further, the socioeconomic status, availability of dietary nutrients, and health literacy form a complex interplay, making prevention and management of nutritional disorders more challenging. Conquering these hurdles requires an interdisciplinary approach that incorporates evidence from internal medicine, public health, and policy development to provide appropriate nutritional guidelines and interventions designed to achieve optimal health outcomes across different populations (Sarmidi et al., 2012) (Figure 11.7).

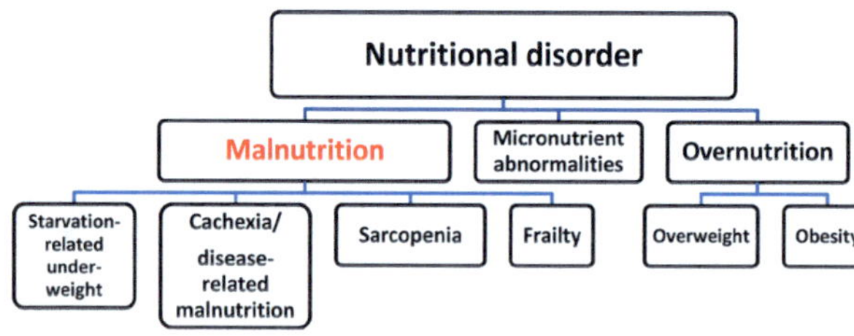

Figure 11.7. The prevalence of common nutritional disorders.

Source: https://www.researchgate.net/profile/Alison-Jesus/publication/308040914/figure/fig2/AS:1108565947351041@1641314126382/A-conceptual-tree-of-nutritional-disorders.png.

11.3.1. Obesity and Metabolic Syndrome

The rising prevalence of obesity and metabolic syndrome is a public health issue that requires significant attention in the practice of internal medicine. Obesity, which is an excess accumulation of body fat, is often accompanied by a variety of metabolic disorders collectively referred to as metabolic syndrome. This condition is primarily defined by insulin resistance, hypertension, dyslipidemia, and increased waist circumference, which all in sum refer to higher risks of cardiovascular diseases and type 2 diabetes. In contemplating the etiopathogeneses, it is evident that genetic as well as environmental factors, such as diet, dietary habits, and physical exercise, are essential. For instance, a diet rich in excess sugar and processed food may exacerbate insulin resistance to contribute to the metabolic condition of obese persons already afflicted with obesity. In addition, the interplay of sleep disturbances and metabolic wellness is a novel area of investigation that depicts the complexity of managing obesity and metabolic syndrome. It has been established through studies that disruption of sleep quality and the circadian rhythm can impede metabolic processes and, therefore, worsen insulin sensitivity and energy homeostasis. It was observed during a workshop at the National Institute for Diabetes and Digestive and Kidney Diseases that future studies must include sleep and circadian rhythm measures in the currently ongoing cohort studies of diabetes risk. Emphasizing this connection is likely to enhance the science of metabolic health through interdisciplinarity, integrating what is learned from sleep science with metabolic science (Arble et al., 2015). This can yield new approaches to mitigating the effects of sleep disorders on obesity and metabolic syndrome. A proactive strategy against obesity and metabolic syndrome needs a holistically integrated strategy with the focus on the central role of nutrition and dietary practices for metabolic homeostasis. Nutrient-rich foods have a significant impact on metabolic processes, not only on weight control but also on overall health. Integration of biochemistry, human physiology, and dietary behaviors is essential for the formulation of sound interventions in metabolic disorders. By focusing on whole foods and opting to note the intricate relationships between various nutrients, healthcare providers can create personalized nutritional approaches that address unique metabolic needs (Sarmidi et al., 2012). Through this, internal medicine is in a position to couple scientific discovery with practical application that translates into better health opportunities for victims of metabolic syndrome and obesity (Figure 11.8).

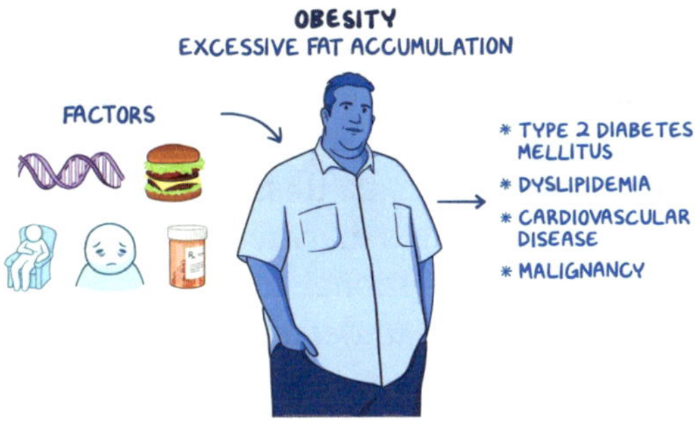

Figure 11.8. The rising prevalence of obesity and metabolic syndrome.

Source: https://www.osmosis.org/_next/image?url=https%3A%2F%2Fd16qt3wv6xm098.cloudfront.net%2FsWAJ01B6QyaJqO5oJuRrZpS7Qt26tRDp%2F_.jpg&w=3840&q=75.

11.3.2. Malnutrition and Its Consequences

Malnutrition remains an acute global health problem, impacting not only the health status of individuals but also the broader social dynamics. The implications of malnutrition are particularly severe in populations that must contend with chronic conditions, such as HIV/AIDS. The dynamics between malnutrition and these diseases both exacerbate the nutritional status of the affected and the food security status of the households. As the household loses purchasing power through the expenses on health and reduced working capacity, additional members of the household can become food-insecure in addition to people who are HIV-infected. The vicious cycle emphasizes the need for consistent food security interventions that address nutrition deficits associated with chronic disease and foster economic stability in the affected populations (Caesar et al., 2011). With an understanding of this complex interaction, health workers can better design interventions that not only address short-term dietary needs but also attain long-term food security outcomes. Environmental determinants have additionally emerged as a major role in malnutrition across the world, beyond chronic illnesses. Nutritional status relies critically on the availability of enhanced water, sanitation, and hygiene (WASH), especially in low- and middle-income contexts. Unsafety of water and poor sanitation lead to diarrhea, which weakens the process of nutritional intake and creates a vicious cycle of undernutrition. Research has revealed that improved WASH conditions help mitigate the effects of undernutrition and hence result in better overall health outcomes. Access to good sanitation and clean water improves the nutritional status of community members, especially vulnerable individuals such as women of childbearing age and children. This is underscored by the necessity of integrating WASH interventions with nutrition programs since they provide a base layer of health necessary for effective nutrition strategy (Mahmud et al., 2016). Malnutrition must be tackled in a multimodal approach incorporating medical, social, and environmental dimensions. Internal medicine healthcare professionals must strive to set comprehensive screening and treatment protocols for every patient with the broader socio-economic context in mind. For instance, nutritional assessment should evaluate not just intake but also household food security, socioeconomic status, and availability of healthcare resources. By advocating for policies of enhanced food security and nutritional support, practitioners can serve as catalysts in reversing the trends of malnutrition. This commitment to an integrated approach to health will not only improve patient outcomes but also generate healthier populations, ultimately helping eliminate the systemic deficiencies that lead to malnutrition and its catastrophic consequences.

11.3.3. Diabetes Management and Nutrition

Diabetes care, particularly Type 2 Diabetes Mellitus (T2DM), is a multi-modal therapy that is centered on diet and lifestyle modification. Modulation of macronutrient composition is its hallmark for control, which has been shown to be an important modulator of insulin sensitivity and glycemic control. Its epidemiologic evidence indicates that it is the chronic excess energy provision together with physical inactivity that leads to conditions of obesity and insulin resistance, both of which are critical predictors of T2DM. Therefore, energy-restricted diets are commonly prescribed for weight loss because they can effectively reduce abdominal fat mass and improve insulin sensitivity. Nonetheless, long-term weight reduction is hard to sustain, and further investigation into isoenergetic diet composition and its ensuing metabolic effect is essential; an area where randomized controlled trials are still lacking, yet insightful findings are emerging from both animal and short-term human studies (Weickert et al., 2012). With the need to individualize dietary interventions in mind, it is essential to consider the particular characteristics of PCOS patients, particularly as obesity and insulin resistance can each be prevalent in this population. Dietary weight management is important since minimal weight loss is sufficient to ameliorate several of the symptoms experienced in PCOS, including acne and infertility. An effective diet regimen involves reducing saturated fat intake while increasing the balanced consumption of unsaturated fats, carbohydrates, and proteins. The carbohydrate component is specially significant, considering that diets containing foods with high GI content may exacerbate insulin resistance and promote the likelihood of diabetes. Accordingly, current guidelines support a functional diet, not just in terms of macronutrient ratio but with an exercise program that, together, enhances insulin sensitivity and supports metabolic health (Ghazeeri et al., 2021). In diabetes and nutrition management, the interaction between physiological factors and food habits is central to patient management. As has been observed through various studies, the inclusion of nutrition education in diabetes management services is significant in allowing patients to make informed food decisions. Additionally, collaboration among healthcare providers and patients can also empower people to design personalized meal plans based on individual taste, metabolic responses, and cultural concerns. Personalized practices promote compliance as well as room for better health outcomes. The ongoing advancement of our knowledge of dietary effects on insulin resistance underscores the importance of evidence-based guidelines and underscores the need for ongoing research in this area. Finally, creating an encouraging environment in managing diabetes can lead to enhanced patient quality of life and metabolic well-being (Weickert et al., 2012) (Figure 11.9).

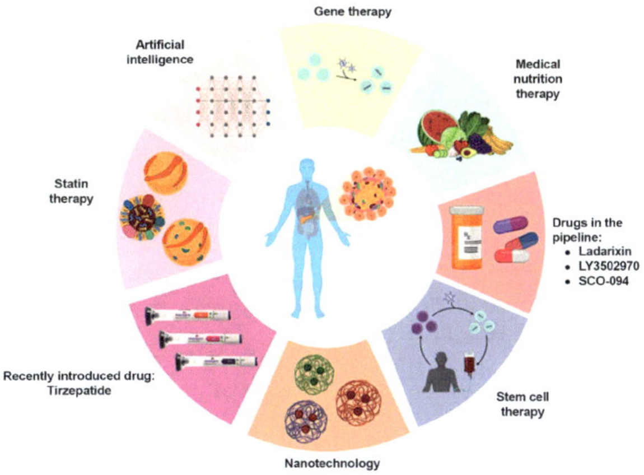

Figure 11.9. Diabetes management and nutrition.

Source: https://media.springernature.com/m685/springer-static/image/art%3A10.1038%2Fs41366-023-01369-3/MediaObjects/41366_2023_1369_Fig1_HTML.png.

Test Your Knowledge

1. What are the key components of metabolic syndrome, and how is obesity related to its development?
2. How does nutrition play a role in managing type 2 diabetes, and what dietary approach is commonly recommended?

11.4. Therapeutic Diets in Internal Medicine

Learning Outcome

1. Role of medical nutrition therapy
2. Specific diets for chronic conditions
3. Evidence-based guidelines for dietary interventions

Therapeutic diets are a unifying theme in the treatment of many internal medicine conditions. They are highly individualized to address the precise medical needs and are often the cornerstone of care for long-term disease conditions such as diabetes, obesity, and cardiovascular disease. Through the specific manipulation of macronutrient proportions, i.e., protein, carbohydrates, and fats, health workers can optimize patient outcomes through the support of metabolic processes and the modulation of disease pathogenesis. By way of illustration, a low-carbohydrate diet might improve blood glucose control in diabetic patients, while a Mediterranean diet rich in healthy fats and fiber consumption has been associated with reduced cardiovascular risk. Such nutrition intervention highlights the need for the incorporation of clinical nutrition in patient care, which is an indicator of the therapeutic potential present in tailored dietary programs. Recent studies have recognized the significance of nutritional treatment in managing illness from alcohol consumption. The symposium "Role of Nutrition in Alcoholic Liver Disease" at the European Society for Biomedical Research on Alcoholism Congress was tasked with food nutrient interactions and the pathogenesis of alcoholic liver disease (ALD) (Feldstein et al., 2018). The outcomes indicated that dietary manipulation of carbohydrate and fat could significantly influence the disease course of ALD, with some compounds, such as betaine and zinc, showing promise as novel dietary therapies. This note underscores the necessity of professionals in internal medicine not only to recognize the acute clinical effects of alcohol but also the capacity of specialized diets to abort undesirable results of alcoholic liver disease. Therefore, nutrition becomes a critical complement to the overall management of ALD and similar conditions. Apart from its application in the management of alcohol-related diseases, therapeutic diets are also crucial in the treatment of urolithiasis and other urinary disorders shared by human and veterinary medicine. The consensus towards the inclusion of modern dietary strategies indicates increased recognition of the significance of nutrition in the treatment and prevention of such disorders. An appropriately regulated diet can reduce the formation of stones in patients by offering adequate mineral balance and hydration. Recent guidelines recommend providing patient-centered guidance that considers individual food requirements and aims to improve treatment adherence (Adams et al., 2016). As internal medicine expands, application of therapeutic diets not only improves clinical outcomes but also facilitates more patient-specific treatment, demonstrating the long history of diet's relationship with health and disease management (Figure 11.10).

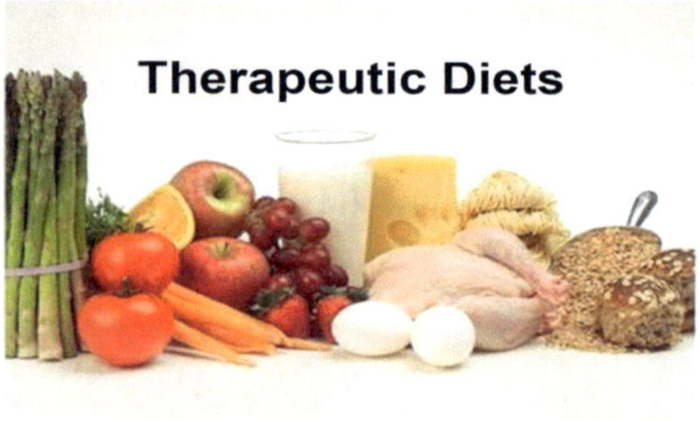

Figure 11.10. Therapeutic diets in internal medicine.

Source: https://cms.nutrical.co/uploads/diet_f795f768fd.jpg.

11.4.1. Role of Medical Nutrition Therapy

Medical Nutrition Therapy (MNT) is one aspect of managing a spectrum of health disorders with the use of food and nutrition. With its emphasis on the biochemical relationship between nutrition, metabolism, and homeostasis, MNT is an essential intervention in clinical practice. Defined in contemporary literature, MNT presents a solution for achieving cellular homeostasis and overall well-being, thereby managing metabolic syndromes that arise as a result of inappropriate food consumption or underlying pathology. This approach not only personalizes nutrition counseling based on physiological needs but also aligns it with more general clinical goals of stabilizing patients, promoting recovery, and preventing complications. Such is the incorporation of nutrition into clinical care, which is truly the acme of an understanding of diet's primary role in maintaining health and preventing disease, thus forming a good foundation for patient-centered practice in internal medicine. In critically ill patients, Medical Nutrition Therapy can completely alter the recovery process through proper nutrition support. For instance, parenteral nutrition (PN) is a vital factor when oral feeding is not possible or adequate because it effectively addresses the protein and caloric need of a patient. The recommended intake levels for amino acids and non-nitrogen energy substrates are crucial in preventing muscle catabolism and promoting anabolism, particularly under metabolic stress (Blumenstein et al., 2009). Through the implementation of individualized strategies, such as amino acid supplementation (in this case, glutamine), MNT enhances clinical outcomes. This adaptive approach guards nutritional approaches from the confines of being adjunctive but is skillfully designed to enable optimal recovery and metabolic balance in vulnerable groups. Outside critical care, MNT also encompasses a broad armamentarium of food interventions that impact the treatment of chronic conditions such as diabetes and hypertension. A concrete understanding of the role of nutrition in metabolic pathways and homeostasis empowers healthcare providers to customize dietary recommendations towards specific health outcomes. For example, by adjusting the macronutrient content of a diet or using therapeutic diets that target anti-inflammatory foods, healthcare providers can better manage chronic disease. According to the literature, the strategic use of food nutrients in conjunction with human physiology and biochemistry not only corrects metabolic syndromes but also enhances overall health (Sarmidi et al., 2012). Through ongoing education and research, MNT will remain a cornerstone of effective internal medicine and clinical nutrition, constantly evolving to meet the dynamic demand of patient groups (Figure 11.11).

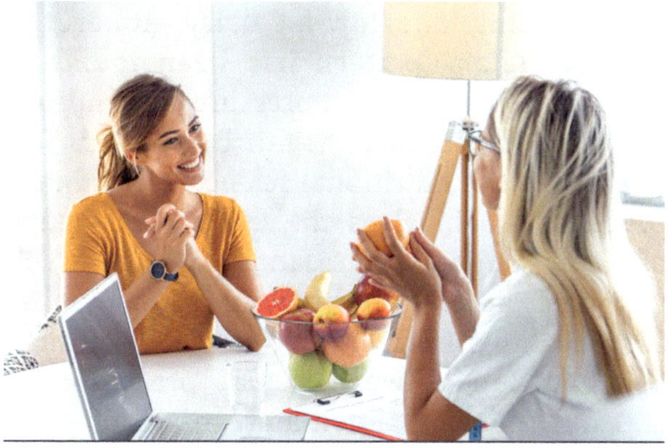

Figure 11.11. Role of medical nutrition therapy.

Source: https://protgold.com/cdn/shop/articles/prot-gold-medical-nutrition-therapy.jpg?v=1685877681&width=1024.

11.4.2. Specific Diets for Chronic Conditions

Chronic conditions such as diabetes, cardiovascular disease, and obesity need specific dietary adjustments to manage symptoms and improve overall health outcomes. A whole-food diet rich in fruits, vegetables, whole grains, lean protein, and healthy fat can slow the progression of these diseases. For instance, the Mediterranean diet, which is characterized by monounsaturated fats contained in olive oil and high fiber in fruits and vegetables, has been associated with reduced cardiovascular risk factors and improved glycemic control among diabetic patients. This is important because nutrition plays a pivotal role in the prevention and management of chronic diseases. Interestingly, identifying a patient's dietary requirements in the context of chronic diseases can guide clinicians in structuring interventions that align with their patients' health goals and enhance their quality of life through diet. Diets such as the DASH diet are a classic example of how certain diets can successfully manage chronic diseases such as hypertension. The DASH diet emphasizes reducing sodium while stimulating nutrient-dense foods like fruits, vegetables, whole grains, and low-fat dairy. Adherence to this dietary pattern has been found to significantly lower blood pressure and improve overall cardiovascular health by studies. The intersection of nutritional science with clinical practice also involves the use of knowledge of dietary supports in treating patients, which has also been found useful in managing complications from chronic disease. Through collaboration between health practitioners and nutritionists, patients are provided with personalized nutritional advice that addresses their particular health complications, hence allowing them to control their health and make proper nutrition choices. Furthermore, attention should also be paid to the effect of nutrition on unusual diseases such as alcoholic liver disease (ALD) and how nutrition choices influence the digestive system. Studies at symposia have shed light on the significant roles of dietary nutrients and malnutrition in ALD pathogenesis. For instance, the regulation of dietary fats and carbohydrates has been found to impact the progression of alcohol-induced disease, thereby underscoring the nutritional treatment in the clinic. Additionally, ongoing investigations into the effects of different diets on inflammation and organ condition further demonstrate the complexity involved in dietary management of chronic disease. As demonstrated by a study comparing diet type to markers of the gastrointestinal tract, whole prey diets among captive cheetahs have possible correlations in human health to validate an ever-growing body of evidence that highlights the significance of diet-specific management of disease (Depauw et al., 2014; Feldstein et al., 2018).

11.4.3. Evidence-Based Guidelines for Dietary Interventions

Management of the rising prevalence of chronic conditions such as Type 2 Diabetes (T2DM) calls for robust evidence-based nutritional strategies to help combat metabolic health. Central to these dietary strategies is the understanding of insulin resistance, a dysfunction recognized as an independent risk factor for the development of T2DM. The chronic mismatch between caloric intake and physical activity worsens metabolic impairment, leading not only to weight gain but also to corresponding fat deposition, particularly in visceral areas. All these lead to further insulin resistance, closing the cycle that sustains the disease. As shown in current research, energy-restricted regimens are able to facilitate weight loss and enhance metabolic abnormalities, although weight loss maintenance is an issue to be encountered by the majority. This is a point of emphasis in the investigation of dietary macronutrient composition changes during controlled intervention, which could be useful in offering further insights into optimal management regimens for insulin resistance in clinical nutrition (Weickert et al., 2012). Dietary fiber contribution to the regulation of various health conditions is a pointer to the intricacies of nutritional interventions. For example, in individuals with pancreatic diseases, the link between dietary fiber and disease outcomes is complex. While others show that a prebioticsupplemented diet is beneficial for the outcome in acute pancreatitis by enhancing intestinal health and reducing the infection rate, there is no data suggesting any drawbacks in the case of exocrine pancreatic insufficiency. In this regard, excessive fiber consumption may lead to increased fecal fat excretion via interference with pancreatic enzyme activity. It points to the necessity of individualized dietary interventions on the basis of a thorough assessment of each patient's unique metabolic status and clinical presentation. Lastly, an appreciation of these forces is at the core of creating integrative dietary recommendations counteracting the manifestations of patients with some pancreatic conditions (Badiali et al., 2019). Moreover, effective dietary interventions should be aided by a multitude of evidence-based procedures adjusted to the diverse statuses of patients. Marshaling of evidence from observational studies and randomized controlled trials is a major foundation upon which these guidelines are established. Control over postprandial blood glucose, for example, can be achieved through particular dietary practices that reduce glycemic index as well as enhance fiber intake. Here again, further research is required to identify mechanisms across various dietary systems, enabling more targeted nutrition plans. It is also crucial that health professionals receive constant education on the up-to-date evidence to enable them to make informed choices that deliver optimal outcomes for their patients. The constant growth of knowledge on diet and management of chronic diseases serves as a reminder that clinical nutrition and metabolism call for a dynamic, patient-centered approach (Figure 11.12).

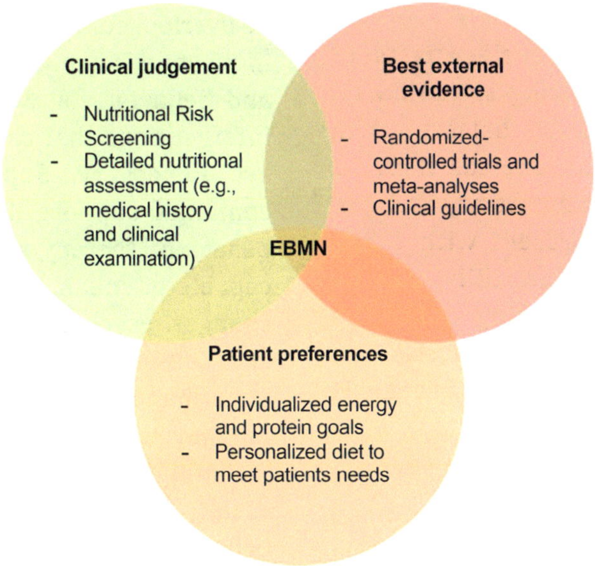

Figure 11.12. Evidence-based guidelines for dietary interventions.

Source: https://ars.els-cdn.com/content/image/1-s2.0-S0261561420300467-gr1.jpg.

Test Your Knowledge

1. What is Medical Nutrition Therapy (MNT), and how is it used in the management of chronic diseases like diabetes or kidney disease?
2. Why are evidence-based dietary guidelines important in formulating nutrition plans for patients with chronic conditions?

11.5. Impact of Lifestyle Modifications

Learning Outcome

1. Importance of physical activity
2. Behavioral changes for better nutrition
3. Role of patient education and support

Lifestyle modifications play a pivotal role in the management of many diseases, particularly those linked to metabolic syndromes. An example is Polycystic Ovary Syndrome (PCOS), which largely has the same link with insulin resistance and obesity. The evidence supports the fact that weight loss is the first-line management for PCOS, and dietary modification plays a pivotal role in achieving this.

By concentrating on specific parts of the diet, for example, reducing saturated fat while keeping unsaturated fats balanced with carbohydrates and proteins, one can increase insulin sensitivity. Through the dietary changes, manifestations typically present with PCOS, like hirsutism, acne, and infertility, can be reduced significantly. Embracing a healthy lifestyle, including regular physical exercise—30 minutes of exercise five times per week is recommended—is essential.

Therefore, diet and exercise behavioral interventions not only enhance metabolic health but also provide advantages in alleviating the multifaceted clinical symptoms of PCOS, establishing the role of lifestyle interventions in clinical nutrition and metabolism (Ghazeeri et al., 2021). In clinical disorders such as PCOS, apart from PCOS, lifestyle intervention is crucial to manage metabolic syndrome (MetS), an illness with a cluster of metabolic risk factors that pose an increased risk for cardiovascular disease. Studies on the lifestyle choices among MetS patients have revealed strong correlations of adverse behaviors—like unhealthy eating habits, inactive lifestyles, tobacco smoking, and excessive drinking of alcohol—with the occurrence of the syndrome. Surprisingly, low levels of fruit and vegetable intake in the diet significantly add to the risk of MetS. The interplay of socio-economic status with lifestyle choice suggests that a properly coordinated initiative comprising nutritional education and public health measures could maximize the process of lifestyle decision-making. Thus, intervention for these modifiable risk factors, such as optimum lifestyle changes, has the potential to significantly lower the burden of MetS and its consequences, further establishing the critical role of these interventions in internal medicine (Cozma et al., 2018). Secondly, the psychological aspect of lifestyle changes cannot be overlooked. The introduction of vital changes in lifestyle is likely to require a shift in attitude and behavior, for which support systems and interventions that can help overcome barriers are necessary. Support schemes offering combined support, like nutritional counseling, behavioral therapy, and community support, are capable of enhancing compliance with lifestyle changes. Psychological aspects like motivation and self-efficacy have a significant influence on enhancing the success of such changes. Furthermore, the impact of cultural forces, including dietary and exercise orientations in society, is also a strong determinant in patient behavior. Coupled with tailored treatment, these combined approaches have the ability to allow patients to make informed choices that will lead to enduring health results. Consequently, the impact of lifestyle modification extends past mere nutritional adjustments into the realm of psychological and social dynamics, finally being an integrated scheme of health improvement in internal medicine for clinical nutrition and metabolism (Figure 11.13).

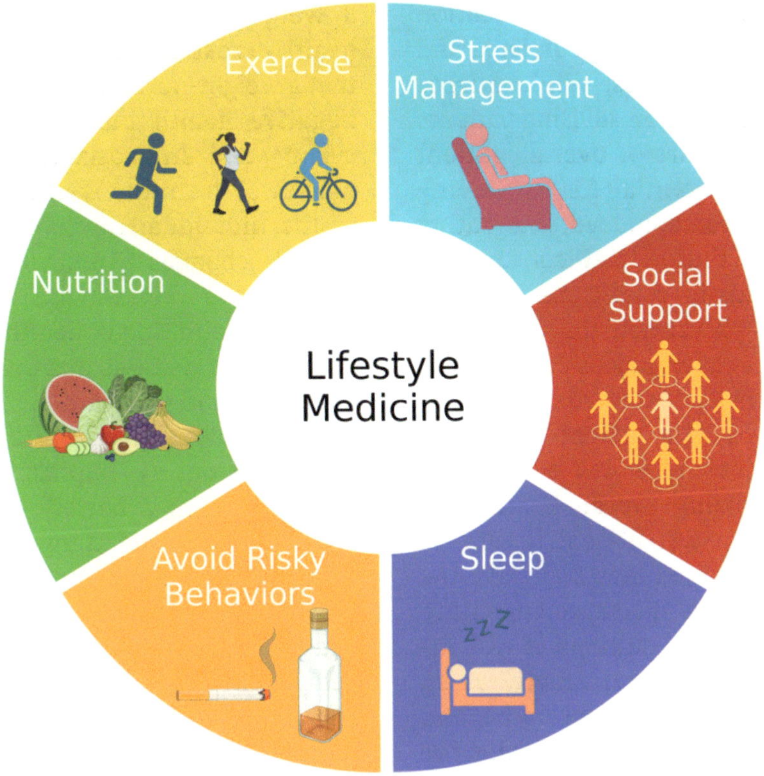

Figure 11.13. Lifestyle modifications play a pivotal role in managing various health conditions.

Source: https://www.researchgate.net/publication/372410795/figure/fig1/AS:11431281239280526@1714299815734/The-components-of-lifestyle-medicine-Lifestyle-medicine-focuses-on-six-pillars-of-a.tif.

11.5.1. Importance of Physical Activity

Exercise is a significant element in the prevention and treatment of chronic disease, which only serves to emphasize its utility in internal medicine. The current guidelines for exercise promote members of the public to undertake at least 30 minutes of moderate-intensity exercise on most days of the week. This is not simply a guideline, however, but rather a vital component of enhancing health outcomes and integrating into patient care practices. Understanding these guidelines is essential for health care professionals, particularly nurses, who are often in a position to counsel patients on lifestyle modifications. Evidence indicated that, while the majority of nurses possess knowledge of physical activity guidelines, priority assigned to physical activity counseling remains low compared to other patient needs. Interestingly enough, this difference also indicates a gap in the provision of holistic care that places equal emphasis on best lifestyle interventions as on traditional medical treatments (Bayles et al., 2012). Furthermore, disparity in confidence levels between healthcare providers in recommending physical activity impacts the health status of the patients. Evidence shows that baccalaureate-trained nurses are also more likely to adhere to physical activity guidelines compared to their master 's-educated peers, suggesting that this may impact practice patterns due to education level. Additionally, nurses who engage in regular physical activity themselves are also better informed about current guidelines. This association supports an argument for more training and education about physical activity in nursing curricula and continuing education courses. While nurses increasingly put more value on advising patients regarding exercise as part of overall patient care, there is more potential for improving the overall health outcome. Indeed, integrating physical activity into routine medical care not only controls immediate conditions but also fosters a culture of prevention that can avoid long-term healthcare costs (Bayles et al., 2012). Lastly, the transformation towards a weight-inclusive as opposed to a weight-normative model also reinforces the worth of exercise as a tool for maximizing overall health and well-being. Traditional weight-centric models have been found wanting in that they have the tendency to overlook the multifaceted nature of health and to stigmatize patients. A weight-inclusive model values physical activity as an approach to enhance health indicators beyond just the reduction of weight, considering the overall impacts of exercise, such as improved blood pressure and the decrease in the habit of binge eating. This is in regard to current public health models that emphasize health at any size and universalization of access to and attraction of physical activity for all individuals, irrespective of body weight. By placing a priority on participation in physical activity from this inclusive perspective, healthcare practitioners are in a better position to address the root causes of health disparities and assist various patient populations in the realization of their wellness aspirations.

11.5.2. Behavioral Changes for Better Nutrition

Initiating behavioral modification to improve nutrition is critical within the practice of internal medicine, specifically regarding the management of chronic illness and overall metabolic function. An important strategy is to transition away from a weight-normative approach, which focuses on weight loss as the chief marker of health, toward a weight-inclusive approach that promotes health across all sizes. Evidence has confirmed that a weight-normative paradigm is linked with negative health outcomes, including weight cycling and stigmatization, which ultimately take away from the well-being and motivation of the individual to change towards positive lifestyle changes (Annunziato et al., 2014). In contrast, the weight-inclusive model has a more inclusive definition of health, allowing for more holistic interventions that enhance physiological and psychological indices, for instance, by lowering blood pressure and reducing rates of depression. By emphasizing overall health, patients are in a better position to establish long-term lifestyle changes that will promote better nutrition. By appreciating the inherent inter-relationship between eating behaviors and food selection, health care providers can design interventions that address lifestyle and food choices. For instance, recognition of common precipitants of poor food choices, such as stress, fatigue, and environmental changes, can help individuals implement measures to buffer these factors. Episodic migraine studies highlight how stress and eating abnormalities can worsen illness, uncovering the complex link between diet and behavior (Marmura et al., 2018). Patient empowerment by monitoring eating habits and discovering triggers not only allows for heightened awareness of diet but also encourages positive health control. By focusing on personalized approaches involving stress management and dietary compliance, healthcare practitioners can facilitate significant, long-term modifications in diet. The diversion of focus away from traditional weight-reduction orthodoxy to behavioral and lifestyle changes also calls for educational initiatives among both patients and healthcare practitioners. Training sessions, educational resources, and public programs aimed at the dissemination of practical nutrition knowledge are all relevant instances. Such educational efforts must emphasize the value of balanced diets, increased physical activity, and emotional well-being as cornerstones of nutritional health. By raising awareness and tolerance of diverse body shapes and health states, healthcare professionals can decrease weight stigma while providing the public with the tools required for effective behavior change. Lastly, through coordinated education efforts, assistance, and by adopting a weight-inclusive paradigm, a platform is created for the development of better nutrition and the promotion of healthier lifestyles in varied populations (Annunziato et al., 2014) (Figure 11.14).

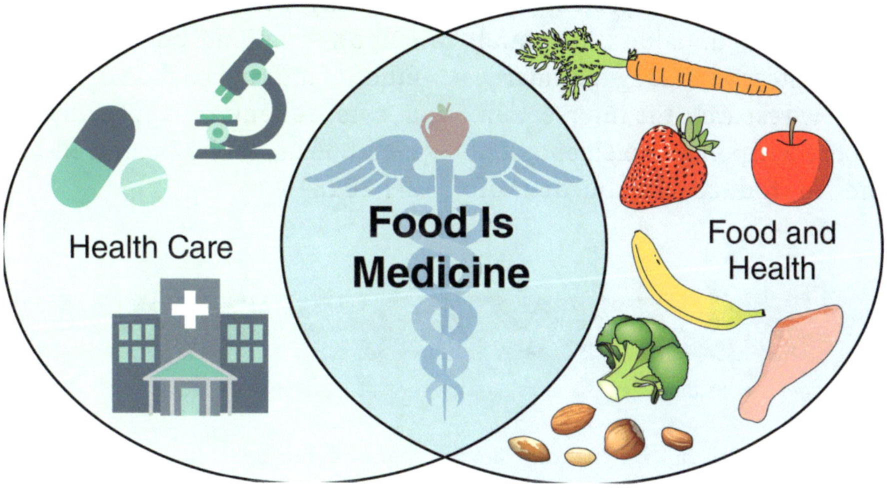

Figure 11.14. Implementing behavioral changes to enhance nutrition.

Source: https://www.ahajournals.org/cms/10.1161/CIR.0000000000001182/asset/1791ce0f-6911-49b0-84ea-de198c5e34fc/assets/graphic/cir.0000000000001182.fig01.jpg.

11.5.3. Role of Patient Education and Support

In the division of clinical nutrition and metabolism within internal medicine, patient education and assistance are the most important factors in achieving maximum health outcomes. Adequate patient education empowers them to obtain the information needed to make sound decisions about their diet, understand metabolic disorders, and manage chronic ailments. Education is highly emphasized, even more so considering the extent of obesity, hypertension, and diabetes—diseases that also overlap with dietary interventions. By raising awareness of the impact of food on their health, patients can understand the importance of sustainable lifestyle change. This education leads to self-efficacy, ultimately translating into improved compliance with medical instructions and dietary behavior aligned with clinical recommendations. Support also plays a complementary role to education by allowing for a healthcare setting that enables patient activation. Support systems, including health teams, family members, and community resources, help patients maintain confidence in their ability to control their own health. This is highly significant in cultures where health decisions are made communally. In conditions like cardiovascular and diabetes, supported patients who are given ongoing support will likely adhere to treatment and dietary recommendations more effectively, leading to better health outcomes.

The integration of culture-sensitive support mechanisms, especially for patient populations such as Saudi women—often affected by specific health problems—can optimize the efficacy of patient education interventions and healthcare delivery models, as recognized in current research findings (Clark et al., 2012). Second, the integration of education and support ensures a team-based approach in the provision of patient care, particularly among the elderly. Research indicates that policy to support patient self-management and care coordination is essential in enhancing health outcomes among the elderly. As discovered in new research, the intersection of education, support, and policy implementation has been found to reduce the burden of metabolic disease. For instance, initiatives in palliative care and empowerment of the family caregiver have proven to be crucial in addressing the comprehensive needs of the patients, so that they do feel valued and empowered to take part in decisions regarding their health care. Not only does this multi-component strategy empower patients but also harmonizes with the ethos of internal medicine—to value most highly a comprehensive appreciation of nutrition, metabolism, and overall well-being (Morton et al., 2015).

Test Your Knowledge

1. Why is physical activity considered an essential component in managing metabolic disorders such as obesity and type 2 diabetes?
2. What are two key behavioral changes that can support improved nutritional habits in patients with chronic diseases?
3. How does patient education and ongoing support contribute to the long-term success of nutritional interventions?

11.6. Challenges in Clinical Nutrition

Learning Outcome

1. Barriers to effective nutritional interventions
2. Cultural and socioeconomic factors
3. Addressing patient compliance and motivation

Among the challenges of clinical nutrition is effectively dealing with complex disorders such as polycystic ovary syndrome (PCOS). The endocrine condition, prevalent among women of reproductive age, carries several metabolic and dietary complexities complicating therapy. While PCOS pathogenesis is not yet definitely established, a combination of genetic and environmental components is said to be responsible for its occurrence. Given the condition's complex nature, interventions should address multiple symptoms at once, and thus it is extremely important to highlight a well-balanced diet as the first-line treatment. For example, studies point out that dietary changes can treat weight issues and thereby reduce insulin resistance and some related symptoms, such as hirsutism and infertility. Thus, the value of understanding the multietiologic nature of PCOS emphasizes the need for patient-individualized clinical nutritional strategies that consider individual patient profiles and their respective dietary requirements (Ghazeeri et al., 2021). Moreover, the integration of genomic nutritional profiling provides promising opportunities and regulatory challenges in the field of clinical nutrition. Nutrigenomics, the study of the effects of nutrients on gene expression, has been a new frontier in individualizing dietary recommendations to an individual's genetic profile, enabling clinicians to tailor nutrition to genetic tendencies. Such innovation holds promise, though there are overwhelming obstacles that prevent its adoption. The regulatory environment for nutrigenomic testing and its use in clinical settings is in flux, which could damp personalized nutrition interventions. Also, the price and access of genomic testing limit its broad application in heterogeneous populations of patients, complicating equity in medicine. Thus, the future of clinical nutrition must address these challenges while attempting to apply evidence-based, individualized care to improve patient outcomes in a reliable and equitable manner (Castle et al., 2007). The other key challenge is managing chronic diseases through nutritional interventions properly. Numerous chronic diseases, including diabetes, cardiovascular disease, and obesity, necessitate dietary changes that are frequently confronted by resistance from patients based on lifestyle habits, cultural beliefs, or unfamiliarity with the nutritional dynamics involved. Refusal or inability to make these healthier food choices has the potential to markedly interfere with treatment effectiveness, resulting in worsening health outcomes. Healthcare workers, therefore, must accord paramount importance to nutrition education and counseling and adopt measures that optimize patient participation and motivation. By fostering a supportive environment that is conducive to enabling patients to make correct dietary choices, healthcare professionals can deal with the behavioral as well as psychological aspects of diet adherence. Tackling socioeconomic factors influencing food availability and quality is also critical, since disparities can have a greater impact on nutritional status in high-risk populations. This multi-factorial approach is essential in overcoming the challenges of clinical nutrition (Ghazeeri et al., 2021) (Figure 11.15).

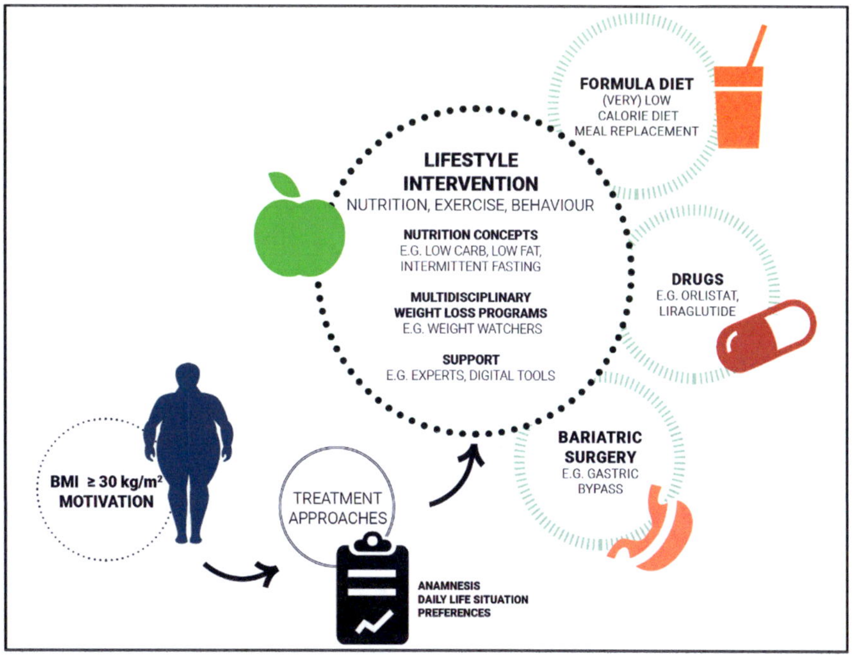

Figure 11.15. Challenges in clinical nutrition.

Source: https://pub.mdpi-res.com/nutrients/nutrients-14-00169/article_deploy/html/images/nutrients-14-00169-g001-550.jpg?1640870579.

11.6.1. Barriers to Effective Nutritional Interventions

The effectiveness of dietary interventions is often compromised by many barriers that can impede the implementation of dietary change. The most significant of these barriers is the lack of tailored nutritional advice individualized to patients' specific needs and wants. The majority of interventions are designed using a one-size-fits-all approach without considering the personal social, cultural, and economic determinants that influence eating behavior. Besides, health care providers may lack adequate nutrition training, resulting in a knowledge gap that reduces their ability to deliver effective counseling. This inexperience could make patient communication more difficult, which ultimately reduces the likelihood of adherence to recommended diet changes. Addressing such a barrier entails extensive training programs for health care providers to enhance their proficiency in nutrition counseling further and foster a more individualized approach to the treatment of patients. The other most important challenge is access to healthy food options, particularly in disadvantaged communities. Food deserts, with their low availability of healthy, affordable foods, pose significant challenges to effective nutritional interventions. In these areas, residents may have no choice but to consume processed foods high in sugars and unhealthy fats, which are usually convenient and less expensive than fresh vegetables and fruits. Furthermore, social determinants of health, such as income level, education, and access to transportation, greatly influence food choices. Without addressing these elements, nutritional interventions will never be fully effective in achieving their intended goals. Community organizations and policymakers must join forces in order to create better food environments for health and to make healthy options accessible to all populations that face these systemic impediments. Finally, psychological problems can contribute a lot to nutritional intervention compliance. Difficulty with motivation, self-efficacy, and emotional eating is common among most individuals and reduces the likelihood of changing eating habits. Inappropriate eating due to stress and anxiety, for instance, can occur, as can resistance to adopting a healthy diet due to low perceived ability to change. In addition, nutritional misinformation can further blur individuals' perceptions of what constitutes a healthy diet, leading to misperceptions and eventually degrading their ability to comply with prescribed interventions. In order to enhance the effectiveness of nutritional interventions, there is a need to incorporate behavioral interventions that address these psychological barriers. The incorporation of support systems such as peer mentoring and counseling can assist individuals to receive the support and resources they require to be able to deal with their problems and eat healthily effectively.

11.6.2. Cultural and Socioeconomic Factors

Socio-economic and cultural determinants play a crucial role in shaping health behaviors, particularly concerning nutrition and metabolism. These determinants can shape food choices and access to health care, as individuals from different cultures perceive food, health, and well-being differently. As an illustration, certain groups of individuals might prefer traditional ways of eating that significantly differ from conventional health guidelines. Socioeconomic status introduces another layer of complexity, with individuals in lower-income brackets potentially lacking access to fresh fruits and health foods. Therefore, the interaction of cultural beliefs and financial constraints exacerbates disparities in health outcomes, illustrating the complex matrix of forces that internal medicine physicians operate within when addressing clinical nutrition and metabolic health. Moreover, the early years of life are critical in establishing lifelong health behaviors and outcomes, which are directly linked with the prevailing socioeconomic conditions during childhood. The evidence indicates that socioeconomic adversity in early childhood could lead to adverse health and education later in life, perpetuating a poor health cycle for many generations (Sweeny K). Kids from lower socioeconomic backgrounds can have reduced exposure to nutrition education and limited access to physical activity, which can inhibit the child's overall development. With this in mind, prioritizing early intervention methods is vital for preventing such impacts, as preventive healthcare can significantly improve the course for those at risk. Knowledge of such dynamics enables healthcare practitioners to implement community-based interventions intended to make the environment healthier for future generations. In clinical nutrition, weight-centered models of health have been criticized regarding their effectiveness as well as their ethical acceptability. While most of the traditional methods have a tendency to place weight reduction as a central marker of health, more and more evidence favors the weight-inclusive model prioritizing the improvement of overall health and well-being rather than exclusive dependence on weight measurements (Annunziato et al., 2014). It favors acknowledgment of the various cultural and socioeconomic determinants of an individual's health experience in order to reduce stigmatization due to weight and promote equitable access to care. By focusing on overall measures of health and improving lifestyle variables separate from weight, clinicians can build a more supportive environment that addresses the underlying social determinants driving health disparities. In using this model, not only is patient care enhanced, but public health objectives are more aligned to build health equity between diverse populations (Figure 11.16).

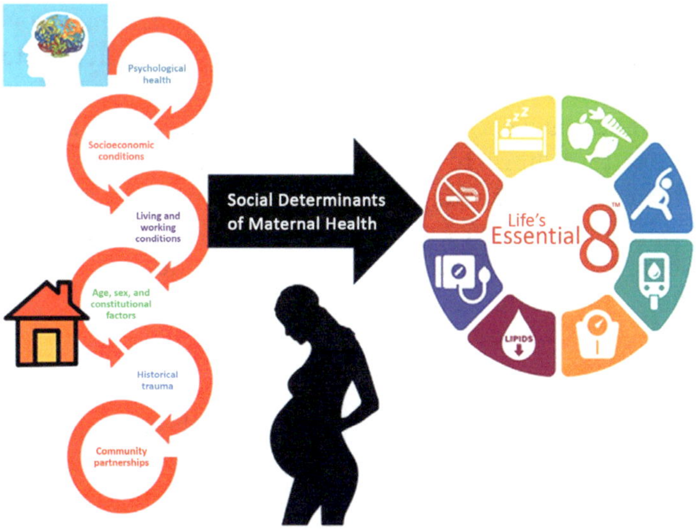

Figure 11.16. Cultural and socioeconomic factors.

Source: https://www.tandfonline.com/cms/asset/9c14d3eb-7d87-4015-ac8a-9d85d58b4ab5/whum_a_2310272_f0002_oc.jpg.

11.6.3. Addressing Patient Compliance and Motivation

Effective patient compliance with clinical nutrition and metabolism is essential for successful treatment of various health conditions, most notably chronic diseases such as obesity and diabetes. This demands an in-depth understanding of the determinants of patient motivation. Of particular relevance in this context is the relationship between physicians and patients, in which communication and trust are key to adherence to nutritional advice. A model of shared decision-making, engaging patients in making choices about their dietary habits, creates a sense of ownership of health. Additionally, using motivational interviewing techniques can enable practitioners to handle ambivalence and empower patients to take an active role in their desired health. By crafting this around the importance of informed decision-making and providing personalized dietary strategies, healthcare providers can enhance patient motivation leading to greater compliance and improved health. In addition to individual participation, the role of psychological and social factors in patient compliance cannot be overemphasized. As experience indicates, psychological health is an important factor in dietary compliance because stress, anxiety, and fear may all play a role in bad eating habits. To illustrate, patients awaiting liver transplants are more likely to have higher anxiety levels regarding undergoing the transplant, which can hurt their motivation to adhere to pre-transplant diet restrictions. Higher fear may be linked with avoidance behaviors, which are in turn associated with poorer quality of life and lower adherence to diet interventions (Cillo et al., 2017). Turning these emotional factors around with counseling and support systems can turn fears around and create a more positive outlook, thereby enhancing patients' motivation for compliance with nutritional suggestions and treatment. In addition, innovative interventions must be used to ensure long-term compliance and motivation of the patient with nutritional therapy. Increasing evidence indicates that technology, such as mobile technology and telemedicine services, holds the potential for advancing continued patient engagement. Such systems can monitor in real-time the intake of food and make instant feedback, making it possible for healthcare providers to modify recommendations based on personal trends. For instance, allowing patients to track their salivary nicotine levels using a device can assist with smoking cessation activity management, revealing hidden relationships between lifestyle and health impact (Alexescu et al., 2019). Permitting patients to view their nutrition journey instills accountability and reinforces healthy habits. Therefore, a multi-disciplinary approach that integrates technology, behavioral science, and emotional support can significantly improve patient compliance and motivation, ultimately yielding better outcomes in clinical nutrition and metabolism.

Test Your Knowledge

1. What are two common barriers that healthcare providers face when implementing effective nutritional interventions in clinical practice?
2. How can cultural and socioeconomic factors influence a patient's dietary habits and response to nutritional counseling?
3. What strategies can be used to improve patient motivation and compliance with nutritional recommendations?

SUMMARY

The interdependent relationships among clinical nutrition, internal medicine, and metabolism underscore the necessity of multidisciplinary treatment for metabolic and nutritional disorders. This kind of treatment is necessary not only in disease management but also in maintaining overall health outcomes. As new research determines, diseases such as polycystic ovary syndrome (PCOS) illustrate the way in which disequilibrium in metabolism has a significant influence on women's health. With attention to dietary adjustments, particularly in macronutrient content and physical activity, clinicians can more effectively treat the condition's symptoms. More understanding of the confluence of nutrition and endocrine function ultimately leads to improved patient education and treatment planning. Of equal concern is an appreciation that a one-size-fits-all diet prescription does not suffice in the clinical environment. Individualized nutritional interventions should consider each patient's metabolic and genetic profile to provide tailored care, encourage compliance, and maximize sustainability. Treatment of PCOS, for instance, must reverse insulin resistance and cardiovascular risk through a well-balanced diet supplemented with regular exercise. Current evidence supports a decrease in saturated fats combined with a focus on complex carbohydrates and restraint on proteins being conducive to metabolic health. By treating such subtle changes in diet initially, healthcare professionals can effectively address the complicated symptoms of disease like PCOS while promoting long-term health. Finally, ongoing research continues to shed light on the mechanisms behind the relationships between metabolism and diet, supporting the value of evidence-based practices in clinical settings. Future research will have to look at novel diet strategies and their related outcomes in diverse groups in order to better inform knowledge and treatment efficiency. Also, the use of technology such as GPS tracking during sports training underscores the need for precise measurement in assessing energy expenditure and performance. These procedures would find utility in clinical practice, offering insights for more efficient interventions. Overall, the establishment of the specialty of internal medicine through clinical nutrition and metabolism is contingent on the follow-through of research into practical application so that patient care can be holistic and evidence-based.

Integration of clinical nutrition into internal medicine has become increasingly core to the care of the complex relationship between food, metabolism, and overall health outcomes. One of the underlying principles of this practice is that an understanding of the notion that nutrition is not just adjunctive to medical treatment, but a cornerstone of disease management. Comprehensive nutritional assessment and tailored diet intervention can significantly improve patient outcomes, especially in diseases such as diabetes, cardiovascular disease, and obesity. Nutrition plays a paramount role when taking into consideration the intricate mechanisms through which specific food components may affect metabolism. This activity necessitates interdisciplinary planning on the part of healthcare professionals in order to devise and implement effective nutritional strategies that reinforce clinical goals. Ultimately, the growing awareness of nutrition's role reinforces the imperative for healthcare professionals to possess a good grasp of dietary principles (Ambrosetti et al., 2020). Furthermore, emerging evidence points to the significance of the microbiota-gut-brain axis when translated into clinical nutrition and metabolism. This dynamic relationship hints at the mechanisms through which gut health can influence a broad spectrum of physical and psychological states, suggesting that dietary choice can have profound consequences far beyond simple caloric intake. For instance, modulation of the microbiota of the gut through specific dietary patterns, such as increased intake of fiber, can enhance metabolic health and mitigate the threat of metabolic syndrome. particularly, the gut microbiomes effect on is to crucial neurobiological processes, connecting nutrition with mental health outcomes. With increasing evidence of the microbiome's involvement in the modulation of cognition and mood, medical professionals are compelled to incorporate dietary guidance that fosters an optimal gut microbiome (John et al., 2019). This systemic understanding of nutrition and its impact is priceless in designing wholesome treatment plans. In short, the evolving face of internal medicine demands a paradigm shift toward an integrated model of health that incorporates clinical nutrition and its interface with metabolic pathways. Key characteristics such as tailor-made dietary approaches, the role of the microbiota, and systemic effects of nutrition are key aspects for clinicians to consider. By embracing this multifaceted approach, health care professionals are better equipped to address the complexities of disease and the management of health. By a concentration on nutritional education and the incorporation of evidence-based dietetic management in clinical settings, not only will patient care be enhanced, but a more dynamic and responsive health care system as well. Hence, the integration of clinical nutrition into internal medicine is a step towards achieving optimal health outcomes and successful chronic disease management (Ambrosetti et al., 2020).

KEY TERMS FROM THIS CHAPTER

- Clinical Nutrition
- Metabolism
- Macronutrients
- Micronutrients
- Basal Metabolic Rate
- Energy Balance
- Malnutrition
- Obesity
- Body Mass Index
- Nutritional Assessment
- Enteral Nutrition
- Parenteral Nutrition
- Protein-Energy Malnutrition
- Electrolyte Balance
- Fluid Balance
- Insulin Resistance

CRITICAL THINKING QUESTIONS

1. **Which of the following is a classic feature of marasmus?**
   a. Edema
   b. Fatty liver
   c. Severe muscle wasting
   d. Moon face
2. **Which vitamin deficiency is commonly associated with chronic alcoholism?**
   a. Vitamin C
   b. Thiamine (Vitamin B1)
   c. Vitamin K
   d. Vitamin D
3. **Which laboratory marker is used to monitor long-term glycemic control?**
   a. Fasting glucose
   b. C-peptide
   c. Hemoglobin A1c
   d. Serum insulin
4. **Refeeding syndrome is most associated with which electrolyte abnormality?**
   a. Hypercalcemia
   b. Hypernatremia
   c. Hypophosphatemia
   d. Hyperkalemia
5. **What is the preferred route of nutritional support in a patient with a functioning gastrointestinal tract?**
   a. Intravenous dextrose
   b. Parenteral nutrition
   c. Enteral nutrition
   d. Sublingual supplements

Short Answer Questions

1. What are the common clinical signs of protein-energy malnutrition in hospitalized patients?
2. How is Body Mass Index (BMI) calculated, and what is the normal BMI range?
3. What is refeeding syndrome, and why is it a concern in malnourished patients starting nutritional therapy?
4. Which laboratory test is most commonly used to assess long-term glucose control in diabetic patients?
5. What is the difference between basal metabolic rate (BMR) and total energy expenditure (TEE)?
6. How does chronic inflammation affect nutritional status and metabolism in patients with chronic diseases?

Answers to Critical Thinking Questions

1. (c); 2. (b); 3. (c); 4. (c); 5. (c)

REFERENCES

1. Allergies, E. P. O. D. P. N. A. (2012). Scientific Opinion on the Tolerable Upper Intake Level of calcium. *EFSA Journal, 10*(7). https://doi.org/10.2903/j.efsa.2012.2814Adams, L. G., Bartges, J. W., Berent, A. C., Lulich, J. P., et al. (2016). ACVIM small animal consensus recommendations on the treatment and prevention of uroliths in dogs and cats. https://core.ac.uk/download/323070830.pdf (accessed on 17th July 2025).
2. Al-Dujaili, E., Good, G., & Tsang, C. (2016). Consumption of pomegranate juice attenuates exercise-induced oxidative stress, blood pressure and urinary cortisol/cortisone ratio in human adults. https://core.ac.uk/download/305121376.pdf (accessed on 17th July 2025).
3. Alexescu, T. G., Bordea, R., Boşca, B. A., Băbţan, A. M., et al. (2019). Insights into the pathogenesis of nicotine addiction. Could a salivary biosensor be useful in nicotine replacement therapy (NRT)? https://core.ac.uk/download/232440316.pdf (accessed on 17th July 2025).
4. Allan, P., Fiorino, G., Gatti, S., Gerasimidis, K., et al. (2017). Research gaps in diet and nutrition in inflammatory bowel disease. A topical review by D-ECCO Working Group (Dietitians of ECCO). https://core.ac.uk/download/84340703.pdf (accessed on 17th July 2025).
5. Alston, J. M., Parks, J. C., & Smith, A. D. (2025). Quantifying obesity in economic research: How misleading is the body mass index? https://core.ac.uk/download/pdf/6400779.pdf (accessed on 17th July 2025).
6. Ambrosetti, M., Abreu, A., Corrà, U., Davos, C. H., Hansen, D., Frederix, I., Iliou, M. C., et al. (2020). Secondary prevention through comprehensive cardiovascular rehabilitation: From knowledge to implementation. 2020 update. A position paper from the Secondary Prevention and Rehabilitation Section of the European Association of Preventive Cardiology. *European Journal of Preventive Cardiology, 28*, 460–495. https://doi.org/10.1177/2047487320913379 (accessed on 17th July 2025).
7. Annunziato, R. A., Burgard, D., Calogero, R. M., Danielsdottir, S., et al. (2014). The weight-inclusive vs. weight-normative approach to health: Evaluating the evidence for prioritizing well-being over weight. https://core.ac.uk/download/30708904.pdf (accessed on 17th July 2025).
8. Arble, D. M., Bass, J., Behn, C. D., Butler, M. P., et al. (2015). Impact of sleep and circadian disruption on energy balance and diabetes: A summary of workshop discussions. https://core.ac.uk/download/213087763.pdf (accessed on 17th July 2025).
9. Arefiev, Y., Chao, R., Chaudry, H., Klug, M. G., et al. (2017). Heme oxygenase induction suppresses hepatic hepcidin and rescues ferroportin and ferritin expression in obese mice. https://core.ac.uk/download/129592561.pdf (accessed on 17th July 2025).
10. Badiali, D., Bruno, G., Ribichini, E., Rossi, A. P., et al. (2019). Role of fiber in nutritional management of pancreatic diseases. https://core.ac.uk/download/231748461.pdf (accessed on 17th July 2025).
11. Bayles, C., Hoffman, L., Jakicic, J., Miketic, M., et al. (2012). Examination of acute care nurses' ability to engage in patient education related to physical activity as a health behavior. https://core.ac.uk/download/12212129.pdf (accessed on 17th July 2025).
12. Blatter, J. A. (2014). Folate status and asthma: An examination of the literature and implications for practice. https://core.ac.uk/download/33560581.pdf (accessed on 17th July 2025).

13. Blumenstein, I. U., Böhles, H., Goeters, C., Schulz, R. J., et al. (2009). Aminosäuren–Leitlinie Parenterale Ernährung, Kapitel 4. https://core.ac.uk/download/14527635.pdf (accessed on 17th July 2025).

14. Caesar, M., Crush, J., Drimie, S., Frayne, B., et al. (2011). No. 05: The HIV and urban food security nexus. https://core.ac.uk/download/157834898.pdf (accessed on 17th July 2025).

15. Castle, D. (2007). Genomic nutritional profiling: Innovation and regulation in nutrigenomics. https://core.ac.uk/download/28966982.pdf (accessed on 17th July 2025).

16. Choi, D. S., Yoo, H. J., Kang, H. J., Seo, J. A., Lim, K. I., Choi, K. M., Kim, N. H., et al. (2009). Prevalence of sarcopenia and sarcopenic obesity in Korean adults: The Korean Sarcopenic Obesity Study (KSOS). https://core.ac.uk/download/pdf/288318.pdf (accessed on 17th July 2025).

17. Cillo, U., Feltrin, A., Germani, G., Milo, C., et al. (2017). Courage and representations of death in patients who are waiting for a liver transplantation. https://core.ac.uk/download/84920833.pdf (accessed on 17th July 2025).

18. Clark, R., Rawas, H., Windsor, C., Yates, P., et al. (2012). Cultural challenges to secondary prevention: Implications for Saudi women. https://core.ac.uk/download/10909715.pdf (accessed on 17th July 2025).

19. Cozma, A., Daniel, M., Leucuta, D. C., Fodor, A., Muresan, M., et al. (2018). Unhealthy lifestyle and the risk of metabolic syndrome–The Romanian experience. https://core.ac.uk/download/216809662.pdf (accessed on 17th July 2025).

20. Cryan, J. F., O'Riordan, K. J., Cowan, C. S. M., Sandhu, K. V., Bastiaanssen, T. F. S., Boehme, M., Codagnone, M. G., et al. (2019). The microbiota-gut-brain axis. *Physiological Reviews, 99*, 1877–2013. https://doi.org/10.1152/physrev.00018.2018 (accessed on 17th July 2025).

21. Depauw, S., Heilmann, R. M., Hesta, M., Janssens, G. P. J., et al. (2014). Effect of diet type on serum and fecal concentration of S100/calgranulins in the captive *cheetah*. https://core.ac.uk/download/30645612.pdf (accessed on 17th July 2025).

22. Eijck, I., Groot, M., Kasteel, D., Kijlstra, A., et al. (2003). Analysis of black holes in our knowledge concerning animal health in the organic food production chain. https://core.ac.uk/download/10919416.pdf (accessed on 17th July 2025).

23. Eisengart, J. B., Lund, T. C., Miller, W. P., Orchard, P. J., et al. (2019). Biochemical and clinical response after umbilical cord blood transplant in a boy with early childhood-onset beta-mannosidosis. https://core.ac.uk/download/225130667.pdf (accessed on 17th July 2025).

24. Feldstein, A. E., Kharbanda, K. K., Kirpich, I. A., McClain, C. J., et al. (2018). Role of nutrition in alcoholic liver disease: Summary of the symposium at the ESBRA 2017 Congress. https://core.ac.uk/download/323064796.pdf (accessed on 17th July 2025).

25. Ghazeeri, G., Hmedeh, C., et al. (2021). Nutritional management in polycystic ovary syndrome: Challenges and opportunities. https://core.ac.uk/download/161103740.pdf (accessed on 17th July 2025).

26. Kinney, A. L. (2007). National scientific facilities and their science impact on non-biomedical research. http://arxiv.org/abs/0705.1797 (accessed on 17th July 2025).

27. Lampugnale, C. A. (2017). Surgical assessment of the geriatric oncology patient. https://open.bu.edu/bitstream/2144/26707/5/Lampugnale_bu_0017N_13146.pdf (accessed on 17th July 2025).

28. Lotrecchiano, G. R. (2013). Role and discipline relationships in a transdisciplinary biomedical team: Structuration, values override and context scaffolding. http://arxiv.org/abs/1308.1168 (accessed on 17th July 2025).
29. Mahmud, I., & Mbuya, N. (2016). Water, sanitation, hygiene, and nutrition in Bangladesh: Can building toilets affect children's growth? https://core.ac.uk/download/75783689.pdf (accessed on 17th July 2025).
30. Marmura, M. J. (2018). Triggers, protectors, and predictors in episodic migraine. https://core.ac.uk/download/213444199.pdf (accessed on 17th July 2025).
31. Maulder, P. S., & McDonald, K. (2018). The effects of morning preconditioning protocols on testosterone, cortisol and afternoon sprint cycling performance [conference presentation]. https://core.ac.uk/download/187724674.pdf (accessed on 17th July 2025).
32. Morton, S., & Dunn, W. (2015). Addressing the health needs of an aging America: New opportunities for evidence-based policy solutions. https://core.ac.uk/download/75783019.pdf (accessed on 17th July 2025).
33. N/A (2006). *Focal Spot, Spring 2006*. https://core.ac.uk/download/129069350.pdf (accessed on 17th July 2025).
34. Patel, N., Pandit, R., & Qumara, A. (2025). Attitude and practice of Indian clinicians on clinical usage of high protein supplementation in clinical recovery: A Pan India survey. *Indian Journal of Critical Care Medicine: Peer-reviewed, Official Publication of Indian Society of Critical Care Medicine, 29*, S248–S248. https://www.semanticscholar.org/paper/280eb7f5ccf740393b94f22977614a467a6b97d2 (accessed on 17th July 2025).
35. Sarmidi, M. R. (2012). Food is our medicine. https://core.ac.uk/download/11801185.pdf (accessed on 17th July 2025).
36. Sweeny, K. (2025). The influence of childhood circumstances on adult health. https://core.ac.uk/download/pdf/30672978.pdf (accessed on 17th July 2025).
37. Van der Merwe, F. H. (2018). GPS analysis of a team competing at a national Under 18 field hockey tournaments. https://core.ac.uk/download/187724717.pdf (accessed on 17th July 2025).
38. Wang, Y., Li, K., Dou, X., Bai, H., Zhao, X., Ma, X., Li, L., et al. (2019). Treatment of AECHB and severe hepatitis (liver failure). *Acute Exacerbation of Chronic Hepatitis B*. https://www.semanticscholar.org/paper/41400aa73017beb30fb722a888d1fee54ee07596 (accessed on 17th July 2025).
39. Weickert, M. O. (2012). Nutritional modulation of insulin resistance. https://core.ac.uk/download/18328007.pdf (accessed on 17th July 2025).
40. Wishart, D. S., Djoumbou-Feunang, Y., Marcu, A., Guo, A. C., Liang, K. Y. H., Vázquez-Fresno, R., Sajed, T., et al. (2017). *HMDB 4.0: The Human Metabolome Database for 2018. Nucleic Acids Research, 46*, D608–D617. https://doi.org/10.1093/nar/gkx1089 (accessed on 17th July 2025).

PREVENTIVE MEDICINE AND PUBLIC HEALTH IN INTERNAL MEDICINE

12

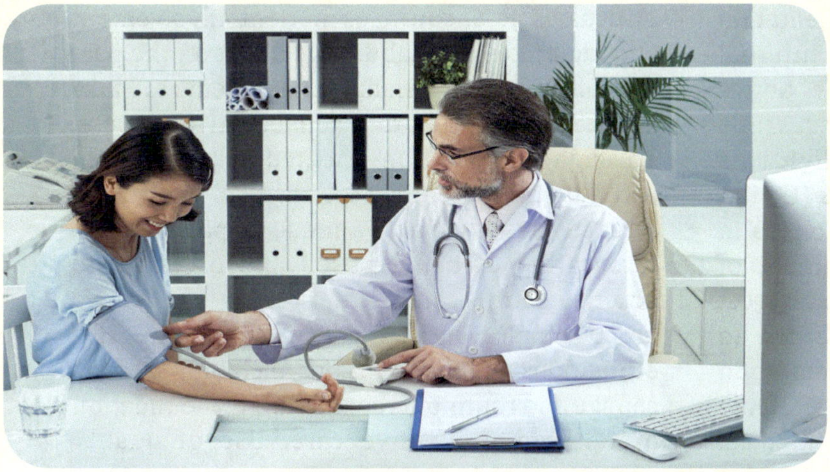

LEARNING OBJECTIVES

After studying this chapter, you will be able to:

1. Discuss the historical context of preventive medicine
2. Explain the role of internal medicine in preventive care
3. Understand public health policies and their impact
4. Know preventive medicine strategies
5. Discuss the challenges in implementing preventive medicine
6. Learn about future directions in preventive medicine

Introduction

In the arena of internal medicine, the role of preventive medicine and public health has become increasingly important in enhancing healthcare outcomes. Preventive medicine is based on proactive interventions that aim to prevent disease in the first place, and this plays a crucial role in combating the increasing burden of chronic diseases such as diabetes, cardiovascular disease, and obesity. The integration of preventive care not only reduces the expense of healthcare but also enhances the quality of life of patients, encouraging healthy living and minimizing the use of costly medical care. As the number of these diseases continues to rise, the intervention of health professionals in promoting preventive care becomes imperative. Through education and community engagement, internal medicine can effectively become a cornerstone of preventive care, foster healthier communities, and reduce health disparities. Despite medical science advancements, health disparities remain an issue for the delivery of healthcare. Various demographic factors, such as socioeconomic status and race, significantly influence the quality of patient care. Research demonstrates that disadvantaged groups are more likely to face barriers to preventive care, which leads to poorer health conditions and more untreated disease. For instance, studies indicate that minority communities are less likely to receive regular screening tests and preventive services, further exacerbating existing health disparities. These health disparities can be eradicated by having a deeper understanding of the sociocultural barriers still existing within healthcare systems. Through the implementation of specific policies and programs in internal medicine, doctors can eliminate the above inequities and provide equitable, accessible preventive health care to all individuals regardless of their demographic status (Collett et al., 2017). One of the effective strategies in preventive medicine is the establishment of specialized centers for education and direct care. For example, initiatives like the one to develop a Center of Preventive Medicine and Health Care at Sapienza University of Rome aim to meet the unique challenges of medical students and practitioners. This initiative recognizes that inappropriate lifestyle patterns and psychological stress can have a huge impact on people's health and functioning (Backhaus et al., 2017). By making available resources for preventive care and developing an enabling environment for health management, such centers can alleviate the adverse effect of such challenges. Additionally, they can serve as models for public health programs on a mass scale, highlighting the necessity to integrate preventive medicine into routine healthcare practice. With collective efforts and the application of new-age technologies, the practice of internal medicine can advance its preventive capabilities, eventually serving the greater cause of public health.

Definition of Preventive Medicine

Preventive medicine encompasses a broad range of measures to prevent disease and promote health. Compared with conventional treatment, which is reactive in nature in treating disease after it develops, preventive medicine is proactive. By intervening through vaccination, health education, screening, and counseling, preventive medicine aims at curbing risk factors associated with chronic diseases. By emphasizing early detection and lifestyle modification, preventive medicine not only curbs medical costs but also enhances patients' well-being. Preventive practice in internal medicine is even more critical as it encourages patient involvement and facilitates a collaborative effort on the part of healthcare professionals and patients to make maintenance of health a collaborative process. Through a prevention-oriented culture, health care has the potential to transform itself from a reactive to a proactive mode of patient care. Integrating evidence-based approaches into practice settings lies at the center of effective practice in preventive medicine. Comprehensive evaluations and interventions, including lifestyle change and routine screening, are the foundation of tailored preventive care. Use of quality improvement techniques by medical practices is crucial in creating health promotion-friendly environments. Primarily, active leadership, building team-based healing relationships, and enhanced access to care are key drivers that enable such techniques (Wagner et al., 2012). With such models, preventive medicine has the potential to transform healthcare delivery to shift the emphasis from treatment to prevention, resulting in healthier populations ultimately. Closing the gap between clinical guidelines and patient involvement maximizes responsiveness to preventive interventions, clearly showing the direct relationship between internal medicine and successful public health outcomes. Furthermore, the blending of traditional and non-conventional medicines (NCMs) adds a complex element to the debate about preventive medicine. Many people throughout the world utilize NCMs as a mode of therapy and prevention, showcasing the diversity of ways humans remain healthy. However, little effort has been directed towards studying the place of such practices within the broader context of preventive medicine and public health (Bukonda et al., 2013). Identification and integration of NCMs into the preventive care system would enhance the availability and accessibility of care, hence the enjoyment of the right to health by various populations. It is important to tackle the challenge posed by the dominance of conventional medicine to create an even more integrated health system, one that discovers and leverages the potential strengths of alternative health practices to promote public health and prevent disease (Figure 12.1).

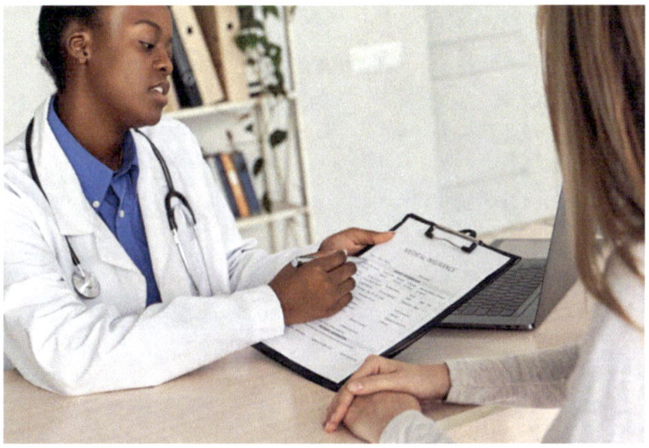

Figure 12.1. Physician discussing a medical report with a patient during a consultation.

Source: https://www.aucmed.edu/media/11516/preventative-medicine.jpg.

Importance of Public Health in Internal Medicine

The integration of public health concepts into internal medicine is essential to improving patient outcomes and population health. Internists, as the primary care physicians in most instances, are uniquely positioned to address the social determinants of health through incorporating preventive practices into their clinical practice. This model not only empowers patients to become active participants in the management of their health but also provides a proactive disease prevention model. By synchronizing their practice with public health programs, internists can do their part to slow the onset of chronic diseases, particularly among those populations most susceptible. Effective public health interventions, supported by evidence-based practice, have a major influence on shaping the clinical practices of internal medicine towards creating a healthy society overall. Reducing health disparities across groups is one of the most crucial functions of public health in internal medicine. Racial and ethnic health disparities in quality of care and access to care create significant barriers in achieving equitable health outcomes. Socioeconomic status and insurance status, not race and ethnicity, are the drivers of healthcare inequities (Jose, 2007) as per research studies. Internal medicine clinicians can increase access to care by identifying and addressing these barriers through targeted public health interventions. Moreover, it is essential to create cultural competency within the healthcare workforce to deliver care particularly tailored to address the needs of various patient populations and enhance the results of preventive medicine interventions. Secondly, the application of evidence-based public health (EBPH) is crucial to allow effective intervention in internal medicine. Leadership assistance in healthcare organizations can enhance the ability for EBPH, hence empowering practitioners with the proper tools to manage chronic diseases effectively. For instance, internal medicine units that emphasize evidence-informed practices are better positioned to mobilize resources more efficiently and ensure communication among providers, ultimately leading to improved patient health outcomes (Allen et al., 2018). This collaboration not only enables medical practitioners to apply data-driven methods but also allows for ongoing learning and adjustment as a reaction to changing public health needs. Generally, the integration of public health and internal medicine enables an extensive strategy for disease prevention and health promotion, critical to improving community health overall.

12.1. Historical Context of Preventive Medicine

Learning Outcome

1. Evolution of preventive medicine practices
2. Key milestones in public health initiatives
3. Impact of historical events on current practices

The history of preventive medicine is a rich painting shaped by social, scientific, and philosophical developments over centuries. From the 18th and 19th centuries, epidemiological studies highlighted the significance of environmental determinants to disease causation, particularly during cholera and smallpox epidemics. This was a watershed when public health turned into a professional field that was no longer merely about the cure of disease but prevention through improved sanitation, vaccines, and education. Interventions such as John Snow's tireless mapping of cholera outbreaks became the gold standard of how data were crucial in informing interventions in health. This assumption laid the foundation for the following preventive interventions, demonstrating that health outcomes could be optimized by controlling determinants that lay outside the individual sphere, an integral part of the preventive model of modern internal medicine. Along with shifting epidemiological knowledge, philosophical underpinnings for preventive medicine began to develop around integrative and holistic approaches. The evolution of complementary therapies, such as homeopathic medicine, introduced paradigms of alternative ideas based on the body's own ability to regulate itself and the importance of the internally regulated environment. This perspective was highly compatible with organic farming practices that emphasize preventive health, and it represented a shift towards a more human-oriented model of health care. The justification advanced by their advocates is that not only do such holistic therapies set out to minimize illness, but also general well-being through enhanced resistance to disease. Nevertheless, the integration of such therapy into conventional medicine is contentious and traditionally meets resistance based on established scientific standards. Such controversy highlights the necessity for expanded paradigms of study that can accommodate different healing ideologies without becoming divorced from the empirical foundation (Baars et al., 2003). This transition from traditional practices of preventive medicine to one that was formalized began in the 20th century with the establishment of schools of public health.

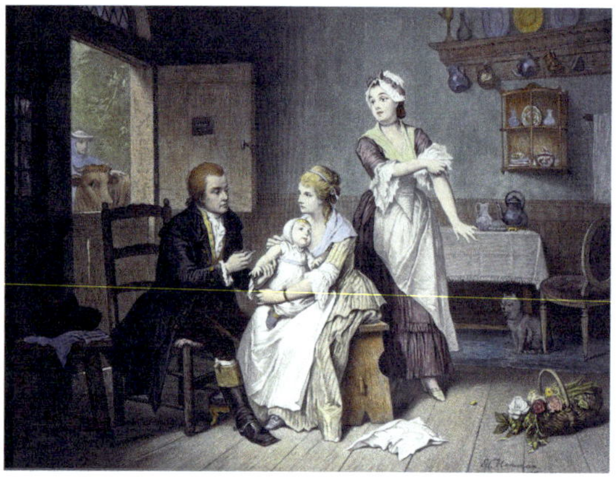

Figure 12.2. The historical context of preventive medicine.

Source: https://cdn.britannica.com/87/195187-050-69F3B576/Edward-Jenner-child-smallpox-engraving.jpg.

These institutes were developed with the intent of synthesizing existing knowledge and models for successful public health interventions, focusing on organizational and managerial systems that had the potential to affect effective health interventions. Today's research highlights the diligent analysis of such models to determine their strengths and weaknesses and enhance public health benefits (Goodall et al., 2011). As public health progresses, an understanding of the history of preventive medicine is essential for the effective incorporation of these strategies into internal medicine. This mixing of history and contemporary practice not only deepens knowledge of health promotion but also informs new methodologies in response to new health challenges on an increasingly complex global stage (Figure 12.2).

12.1.1. Evolution of Preventive Medicine Practices

The evolution of preventive medicine practice indicates a paradigmatic shift in the philosophy of healthcare, emphasizing anticipatory treatment over reactive therapy. Historically, medicine focused exclusively on symptom-focused treatment of disease as it arose, with little concern for underlying social and environmental determinants of health inequities. Over the span of a few decades, the development of evidence-based practice forced the shift towards prevention-driven healthcare. The application of data analytics to preventive interventions allows for customized treatment to enhance population health results significantly. This paradigm shift calls for coordination across all healthcare sectors, such as internal medicine, where treatment can be rendered more comprehensive by incorporating preventive care designed to lower the risk of chronic diseases. With these changes, contemporary preventive medicine practice today is more than ever influenced by quality incentive schemes that focus on increasing the level of care. These programs focus on improving specific health outcomes by linking financial incentives to the level of care provided. By looking at the prevalence, structure, and impact of such programs, it can be noted that not only are they targeted at quality improvement, but also address high-priority health problems in different populations. Looking at some specific initiatives, it can be noted that effective preventive medicine must have incentives tuned for quality improvement activities. Finally, such programs can be a good vehicle for fostering preventive medicine, thereby further improving overall patient care in internal medicine (Jon et al., 2007). Further, their fragmentation within the healthcare delivery system poses challenges that require strategic policy interventions. Their fragmentation creates inefficiencies in the effective implementation of preventive practices, calling for measures that encourage coordination among providers. Policy recommendations, including payment reform and regulation, are implemented to establish systems that support improved integration of care across settings. By addressing these system-level barriers, the healthcare system can increasingly enable the preventive interventions needed to manage chronic conditions and improve public health outcomes. With increased preventive medicine, these reforms become more critical to creating a more integrated, patient-centered health system with an added prevention focus and ultimately reducing the disease burden (Anne et al., 2008).

12.1.2. Key Milestones in Public Health Initiatives

Public health programs have long focused on significant milestones to improve health outcomes through preventive measures. Among the earliest milestones reached was the improvement of sanitation systems in the 19th century, which significantly reduced the spread of infectious diseases. This community-based public health initiative served as the foundation established, such as the implementation of vaccination programs. Vaccines, developed in the latter half of the 18th century, revolutionized public health by all but eradicating diseases like smallpox and drastically reducing cases of others, like polio and measles. Together, these efforts set the stage for organized public health initiatives that seek prevention over response, ultimately shifting the paradigm in internal medicine toward population management rather than the individual. One of the milestones of public health programs was achieved in the mid-20th century, with the development of comprehensive health education programs and the intensification of nutrition-based campaigns. These programs aimed to educate the masses with the knowledge to adopt healthier lifestyles and thereby reduce the prevalence of chronic conditions such as obesity, diabetes, and cardiovascular diseases. The activities of organizations that built quality infrastructure and applied innovative methods, as outlined by Len et al. (2009), were central to this instance. Not only did these intervention activities improve clinical preventive services, but they also facilitated the implementation of electronic health records, allowing for better tracking of health results. Through a focus on education and lifestyle modification, public health programs succeeded in having a direct influence over the practice of internal medicine and bringing about an increased consciousness of preventive health. Recent years have witnessed public health programs being redirected toward addressing emerging issues in the form of global health crises and health inequities in the population. The ongoing response to epidemics, such as the COVID-19 pandemic, underscores the greatest importance of resilient public health infrastructures with responsiveness and flexibility. Additional efforts towards enhanced health disparities highlight the importance of mainstreaming equity into public health measures. Occasional publications, such as the Iowa Department of Public Health newsletter presented in N/A (2011), are utilized to disseminate important information and encourage community participation. As a core part of preventive medicine, addressing the social determinants of health has come to the top of priorities. By reaffirming the interdependence between social determinants and health outcomes, public health is evolving to optimize the effectiveness of internal medicine through an integrated approach to health (Figure 12.3).

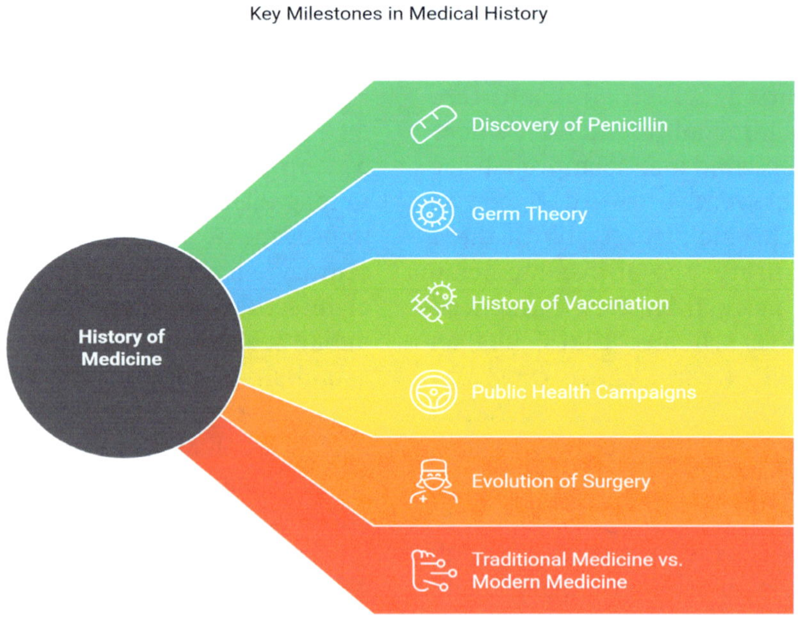

Figure 12.3. Key milestones in public health initiatives.

Source: https://wordpandit.com/wp-content/uploads/2025/01/Key-Milestones-in-Medical-History.png.

12.1.3. Impact of Historical Events on Current Practices

Preventive medicine and public health practice have been shaped significantly by past events, the most significant of which have been the discovery of vaccines. The smallpox vaccine revolutionized public health in the 18th century and demonstrated how vaccines can end infectious diseases. Such success was, however, accompanied by the tragic side effects of myths created about the vaccine that persisted over time. Vaccines were unfairly linked to autism by critics, mostly due to a discredited study, and only social media has made these falsehoods go further. The consequences of these previous falsehoods have been dire, with vaccination rates plummeting and outbreaks of diseases that were once all but gone. Refutation of such myths is essential in public health because it allows healthcare providers to present their information appropriately to parents and enable informed decision-making, and thereby safeguard children and optimize community health outcomes (Boom et al., 2018). Another essential element of history driving practice in internal medicine today is the integration of palliative care into standard medical practices. The realization that patients with terminal illnesses frequently experience avoidable pain has driven the evolution of multiprofessional palliative care teams. In the past, efforts were mainly directed at curative interventions while ignoring patients' physical, psychological, and spiritual requirements. With research uncovering the sheer magnitude of unremitting pain and psychological distress, a comprehensive approach became indubitable. Modern palliative care prioritizes the quality of life of the patient and the family, leading to better communication, greater satisfaction with care, and even a reduction in hospital costs. This shift has enriched internal medicine by emphasizing the necessity to respond to the comprehensive patient care needs and the aftermath of previous neglect in addressing severe diseases (Elk et al., 2017). The past public health occurrences have implications that extend beyond the immediate comprehension of community health patterns, too. The evolution of an awareness of herd immunity within vaccination practice has been directed by the prior spread of diseases like measles and pertussis, in which the mutual dependence of individual and public health was brought to light. Historical data indicating the return of such vaccine-preventable diseases due to declining vaccination rates, fueled by misinformation, has led to enhanced efforts to sensitize and educate the population. Public health initiatives are subsequently focused on building trust in vaccines through openness and widespread education, with a focus on their paramount role in protecting not just the individual but groups as well. These historical teachings highlight the need for ongoing advocacy in preventive medicine and for evolutionary public health interventions informed by lessons from past successes and failures (Boom et al., 2018).

Test Your Knowledge

1. How have preventive medicine practices evolved from ancient sanitation efforts to modern vaccination programs?
2. What are two key public health milestones that significantly improved population health outcomes (e.g., smallpox eradication, clean water access)?
3. How have historical events such as pandemics or industrialization shaped current preventive health strategies?

12.2. Role of Internal Medicine in Preventive Care

Learning Outcome

1. Preventive screenings and assessments
2. Chronic disease management strategies
3. Patient education and counseling

The position of internal medicine in preventive care is central to optimizing public health outcomes. Internists are best positioned to take a global view by prioritizing disease prevention through comprehensive patient assessments that place primacy on risk stratification. Through routine screening and diagnostic evaluation, internists can detect preclinical disease early, enabling interventions to reduce chronic disease burdens such as diabetes and hypertension. Second, the broad scope of internal medicine alerts physicians to the complexities of patients' medical histories, leading to personalized preventive care tailored to specific needs. Not only is this interactive process more likely to activate patients, but it also develops a preventive health culture that can yield dramatic improvements in the overall health of the population. Perhaps the most significant aspect of internal medicine preventive care is the coordination concept, or more precisely, through the formation of a patient-centered medical home. This is a care coordination model that is directed toward enhancing the continuity and quality of health services to patients by coordinating among various specialties. Through emphasis on provider communication and treatment plan coordination, internal medicine is better able to produce optimal health outcomes. As explicated by Ann et al. (2008), the implementation of such initiatives for medical homes demands a commitment to learning regarding patient needs and preferences, which ultimately results in improved chronic care management. Consequently, this integrated approach is essential to issues in public health due to the fact that it allows for more holistic interventions to patient-tailored risks as well as promotes preventive interventions that reduce healthcare expenses in the long term. Moreover, knowledge of health disparities is critical in the internal medicine practice of preventive care. Empirical evidence has revealed that socioeconomic status, insurance status, and language may influence access to and the quality of care (Jose, 2007). Internal medicine doctors are key players in identifying these disparities through their day-to-day interactions with diverse patients. By providing culturally sensitive care and advocating for equal access to medical care, internists can contribute significantly to increasing the level of public health. Internists' work is not only to cure disease but also to engage in community outreach and education programs that induce people to take back control of their health. This multi-component approach enhances the impact of prevention efforts and aligns with broader public health goals, strengthening the central role of internal medicine in the development of healthier communities (Figure 12.4).

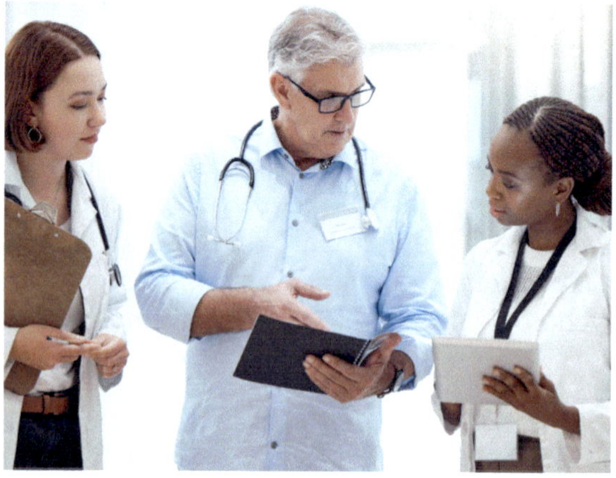

Figure 12.4. The role of internal medicine in preventive care.

Source: https://advancedmedicalgroupnj.com/wp-content/uploads/2024/12/role-of-internal-medicine-in-diabetes-prevention-1200x900.png.

12.2.1. Preventive Screenings and Assessments

Preventive examinations and tests are core aspects of an active healthcare strategy that aim to detect likely health threats while they are still in nascent stages. Through constant screenings, physicians can detect diseases such as diabetes, hypertension, and various types of cancer in their initial stages, which significantly enhances the efficacy of treatment and patient status. Critical to this effort is the use of standardized screening tools and guidelines that offer healthcare providers information on age-specific and risk-related screenings. Due to the significant inequalities noted between screening rates across differing racial and ethnic populations, targeted outreach must be employed to offer equal access to preventive interventions. These programs may fill gaps outlined in research, which indicated that non-Hispanic Blacks have 22% to 73% higher odds of receiving essential diabetes screenings compared to non-Hispanic Whites, ultimately supporting improved healthcare delivery among groups (Davis et al., 2018). Public health campaigns further pushing for early diagnosis and knowledge about a number of health risks can serve as additional impetus for preventive tests. Historically, the US healthcare system has failed to meet preventive health objectives, resulting in alarming national health statistics. Not only does this reflect the necessity for increased public awareness campaigns, but it also portends the possibilities of new solutions in preventive care. For instance, organizations like US. Preventive Medicine, Inc. is involved in establishing prevention in the healthcare system, demonstrating the value of early intervention in reducing the expense of chronic disease. By integrating preventive practice into routine medical care, healthcare systems can transform from a reactive to a proactive system, focusing on patient well-being and preventing long-term healthcare spending (Clarke et al., 2006). Further, the role of technology in constructing preventive screenings cannot be downplayed. With improved diagnostic equipment and greater telemedicine capabilities, healthcare providers now can reach underserved populations more effectively, avoiding constraints to accessing traditional healthcare. Remote screenings and assessments open doors for early intervention, particularly among populations that would otherwise put off routine check-ups due to logistical constraint or economic factors. These technological innovations not only facilitate the screening process but also empower individuals to take charge of their health through a culture of prevention. With the health system evolving continually, preventive tests and assessments remain paramount for improving public health and overall welfare (Clarke et al., 2006).

12.2.2. Chronic Disease Management Strategies

Effective management practices of chronic illnesses are an essential aspect of preventive medicine and public health in internal medicine, and they have the potential to revolutionize the course and effect of conditions such as diabetes, hypertension, and cardiovascular disease. Such management practices are a combination of patient education, coordination of care, and reinforcement for self-management. Through patient education regarding their illness, healthcare providers can strengthen adherence to therapy and lifestyle changes. Additionally, utilization of health information technology facilitates enhanced tracking of patient improvement and chronic illness data, enabling more personalized care plans. Shared resources between small and midsize practices, described in the research findings, can enhance utilization of these technologies as well as enhance overall care through consolidation of expertise and resources, particularly among rural populations (Anne-Marie et al., 2011). In addition, public health agency organizational structures play a pivotal role in ensuring proper chronic disease management. Endorsement by leadership is critical in establishing an environment where evidence-based public health (EBPH) strategies can thrive. Chronic disease prevention unit leaders must stress processes that improve information sharing between program areas, as well as maintain recruitment and retention of competent workers. This is particularly applicable since varying degrees of experience can shape the success of chronic disease programs. Training and technical support provided to employees both improve their knowledge and enable them to practice EBPH in addressing the community's immediate health issues. Thus, a responsibility to leadership-supported support is one of the strong determinants in the provision of effective chronic disease management programs (Allen et al., 2018). Beyond leadership within organizations, ongoing community engagement is critical to the efficiency of chronic disease management interventions. The formation of partnerships with local organizations and stakeholders is useful in outreach work and the dissemination of prevention and management resources to different population segments. Community-based initiatives focusing on physical activity, diet, and frequent health check-ups have been useful in reducing the prevalence of chronic diseases. Actions aimed at addressing social determinants of health, such as access to healthy food and safe play spaces, are essential in developing an environment to support changes in lifestyle. Such community interventions also have to be regularly evaluated and monitored so that best practices can be identified for translation to other settings. Lastly, an integrative plan that considers both health care and community resources will be required for best practice in the management of chronic diseases, furthering the goals of preventive medicine and public health in internal medicine (Figure 12.5).

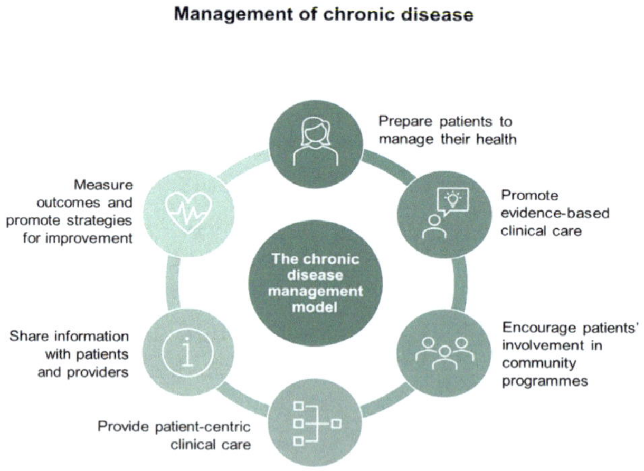

Figure 12.5. Chronic disease management strategies.

Source: https://neurotorium.org/wp-content/uploads/management-of-chronic-disease.jpg.

12.2.3. Patient Education and Counseling

Effective patient education and counseling are the building blocks of preventive medicine and public health, particularly within internal medicine practice. By offering education that enables patients to understand their health status and treatment options, healthcare providers can directly influence patients' outcomes. This is achieved through educating patients on preventive care such as immunizations, periodic screenings, and lifestyle modifications. Moreover, specialist counseling sessions can empower patients to take an active role in healthcare decision-making, thus promoting adherence to treatment regimens. As patients become more involved in managing their health, they usually experience greater motivation and reduced health disparities, particularly among underserved populations. Hence, integrating intensive patient education and counseling within the practice of medicine is essential to build a proactive approach towards health in consonance with public health objectives. The role of the healthcare professionals does not merely end with the dissemination of information; they must create an environment of empathy and interaction where patients are at liberty to express themselves about their health. Culturally adapted techniques of counseling can go a long way in enriching the patients' comprehension and acceptability of preventive measures. Given the multiracial mix of patients, healthcare providers need to take into account linguistic, cultural, and social differences when delivering education. The tailored approach not only ensures improved communication but also fosters patient-provider trust that is instrumental in determining treatment compliance and health outcomes. For instance, understanding cultural norms regarding health practice can inform the design of targeted educational interventions to engage patients and lead them to adopt recommended health behaviors and participation in prevention programs. Ultimately, successful patient counseling leads to quality of care improvement and serves as the foundation for public health action. Furthermore, the continually evolving nature of healthcare necessitates integrating digital tools and resources into patient education. Telehealth websites and web-based learning modules can reach into populations beyond those under routine care and extend counseling intervention visibility, including to geographically remote areas. From evidence over recent years, technology-supported patient education not only is convenient but also supports face-to-face contact. Notably, health practitioners must ensure that digital content is available and adaptable to cater to different patients' needs, including those of chronic disease management. For example, the application of digital platforms can enhance the effectiveness of educational interventions, particularly in managing diseases that involve rigorous lifestyle adjustments and persistent patient engagement. With the implementation of new learning styles, doctors will be able to more effectively advocate for preventive medicine principles, thereby improving health outcomes and fostering a culture of proactive health care in the population (Akhtar et al., 2025; Kim et al., 2025).

Test Your Knowledge

1. What is the role of preventive screenings (e.g., for hypertension, diabetes, and cancer) in early detection and intervention?
2. Why is patient education and counseling important in promoting long-term health behavior change and disease prevention?

12.3. Public Health Policies and Their Impact

Learning Outcome

1. Overview of major public health policies
2. Role of government in preventive health
3. Community health programs and initiatives

The development of public health policy plays an essential role in the preventive medicine climate and ultimately in health outcomes in the population. Effective public health policy has been crafted with respect to the complexity of healthcare delivery and incorporates dimensions that guarantee health equity and enhance access to care. Once such policies are implemented, they have the potential to lead to improved management of chronic conditions, reduction of health disparities, and increased care coordination among providers. The need for such coordination is embodied in the proposals aimed at changing healthcare payment systems and regulatory structures that have the potential to promote increased communication and cooperation among various healthcare settings (Anne et al., 2008). Therefore, as public health policy evolves, its impact is reflected in greater patient outcomes, augmented resource efficiency, and an overall more sustainable healthcare system. Public health programs focused on preventive programs are also particularly important in keeping the needs of specific groups, such as higher education students, in check. One such example is the project that has been conducted by the Center of Preventive Medicine and Health Care at Sapienza University of Rome, targeting health-related problems among medical students. Some of these problems are lifestyle hazards, including excessive tobacco use, unbalanced diets, and biological hazards like tuberculosis exposure (Backhaus et al., 2017). By implementing targeted programs that provide ambulatory care and health management, such programs can significantly enhance the welfare of students. Such a strategy not only improves the quality of life of students but also positively affects students' performance, illustrating the substantial impact that public policies designed to target specific populations can have on at-risk groups. As public health policies keep changing and adjusting to issues of our time, their success is not only determined by the approaches taken but also by the manner in which the populations they are intended to serve take them in. Through cooperation among stakeholders, including health organizations, learning institutions, and healthcare professionals, public health policies can be better tailored to respond to the particular needs of diverse communities. The impact of such policies is measured by whether or not they can help encourage positive health behaviors, increase the availability of healthcare resources, and increase community resilience to health hazards. As observed through many efforts, the crossroads of policy making and public participation ultimately determine the structure of preventive medicine, showing that well-crafted public health interventions have wide-ranging influences on determinants of individual and population well-being (Anne et al., 2008; Backhaus et al., 2017) (Figure 12.6).

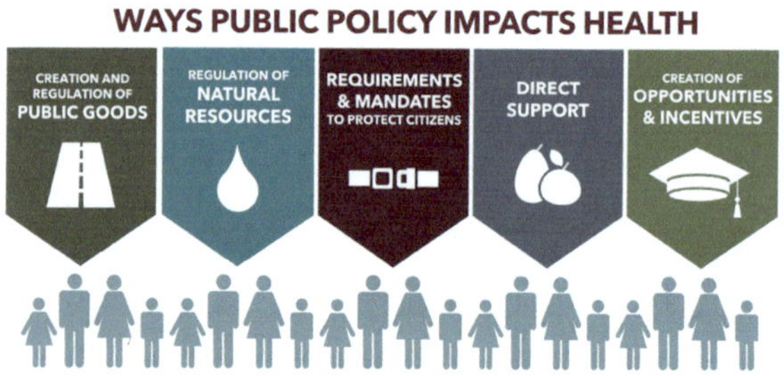

Figure 12.6. Public health policies and their impact.

Source: https://sycamoretn.org/wp-content/uploads/2017/05/5-ways-policy-impacts-health-e1532716467411.png.

12.3.1. Overview of Major Public Health Policies

United States public health policy has been shaped by many historical and contemporary forces that aim to promote population health and prevent disease. Significant policies often aim to reduce health disparities, improve access to care, and promote preventive services. One such instance is the Affordable Care Act (ACA), which expanded insurance coverage and paid for extra preventive services, thereby making necessary healthcare interventions more accessible. This trend towards preventive care can be considered part of a broader public health policy movement that recognizes the value of early intervention in reducing long-term healthcare costs and improving overall health outcomes. By implementing policies that facilitate regular screenings and immunizations, health authorities can, in effect, stem the prevalence of chronic illness and enhance community robustness. Such policies, then, are essential for internal medicine practitioners who also seek to improve healthcare outcomes through prevention. The place of preventive medicine within public policy is also exemplified by initiatives that target specific at-risk populations. For example, the establishment of the Center of Preventive Medicine and Health Care at Sapienza University underscores the importance of mitigating health threats for medical students. This move acknowledges the distinct challenges of these individuals, such as inappropriate lifestyle habits and pressures related to learning difficulties, which can negatively affect their health as well as scholastic performance. Through the provision of services like virtual medical consults and educational outreach, these centers aim to endow students with the capability to manage their health. Ultimately, these public health interventions not only improve individual health outcomes but also advance the overall cause of preventive medicine by fostering a culture of health literacy and self-management among emerging healthcare professionals (Backhaus et al., 2017). To offset the fragmentation of care that typically erodes strong public health interventions, comprehensive policy changes are needed. As noted in various analyses, proposals have been forthcoming for payment reform as well as for regulatory adjustments that emphasize coordination among providers and healthcare settings (Anne et al., 2008). They aim at dismantling the obstacles healthcare professionals face while delivering comprehensive care, promoting the streamlined delivery of healthcare. Continuity of care not only increases the effectiveness of health care systems but also improves the outcomes of patients, especially those suffering from chronic conditions that require frequent diagnosis and treatment. With the implementation of robust public health policies oriented towards care coordination, the ability to reduce healthcare expenditure and improve population health is significantly increased, underscoring the critical role that policy plays in preventive medicine within internal medicine.

12.3.2. Role of Government in Preventive Health

One of the most significant contributions the government has made to preventive health is developing systems that support a healthy delivery system of care. These systems help mitigate the fragmentation that is typically characteristic of health providers and institutions. The government's contribution also involves instituting policies that allow for coordinated care, therefore narrowing treatment gaps and providing individuals with full preventive care. Analysis of the current healthcare environment suggests an imperative need for reform in payment structures and regulatory structures. In embracing such reforms, the government can reinforce relationships among organizations in the healthcare sector, enhancing the overall quality and accessibility of preventive health care for the population. This approach not only helps in disease prevention but also aligns with broader public health aims for improving outcomes in health and reducing healthcare costs in the long term (Anne et al., 2008). Further, the government also plays a key role in promoting innovation in primary care to strengthen preventive health. Through legislation such as provisions of the 2010 health reform law, significant investment is placed in upgrading access and quality of primary care. The payment increase for Medicare and Medicaid is a calculated investment in the healthcare workforce that is essential to delivering preventive care. This comprehensive reform also encourages innovation in the delivery mode of care that can be attuned to the diverse needs of patient populations. By investing in training programs and retaining primary care practitioners, the government helps bridge preventive care gaps, such that individuals are not only healed from their ailments but also educated towards healthier lifestyles and preventive care (Lawlor et al., 2011). It is also evidenced by the government's role in public health campaigns, whose purpose is to educate and inform the masses on threats to health and prevention means. In designing programs that promote vaccinations, screenings, and health habit practices, the government acts as a formative force in fashioning community health practices. These types of campaigns are aimed at vulnerable populations that may be disproportionately affected by avoidable diseases, thus highlighting the government's commitment to health equity. Public health education also enables individuals to take ownership of their health, making preventive care rewarding and a priority. By implementing data-based approaches to assessing the health needs of populations, the government can make such outreach initiatives more accurate, so that preventive health communication can have a lasting effect on various groups, thus addressing the overall goals of public health in internal medicine (Figure 12.7).

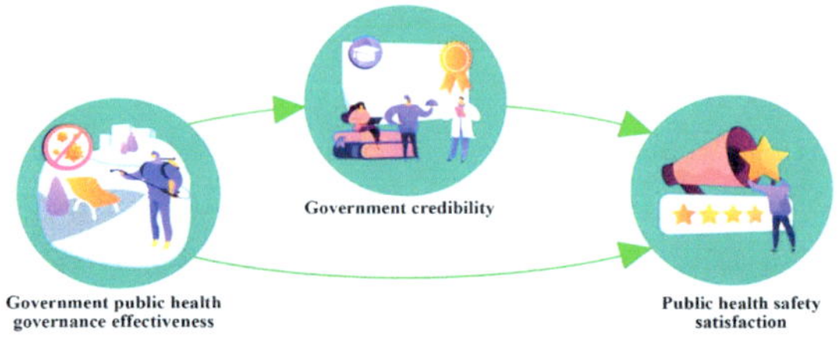

Figure 12.7. One of the most significant responsibilities of government in preventive health.

Source: https://media.licdn.com/dms/image/v2/D4D12AQFWAESlIX-enQ/article-cover_image-shrink_720_1280/article-cover_image-shrink_720_1280/0/1692677390250?e=2147483647&v=beta&t=zNnRMO1_-iMaU21S2Y6D7BFhk8aywtWBNpNJtVKSGEs.

12.3.3. Community Health Programs and Initiatives

The significance of community health interventions and programs cannot be overstated, as they play a key role in optimizing public health outcomes, particularly preventive care. The programs are aimed at intervening in numerous health problems at the level of communities, targeting social determinants of health that typically determine health disparities between communities. By establishing alliances among community organizations, health care providers, and local agencies, the initiatives aim to construct targeted interventions that resonate with the distinct needs of the population. For instance, programs in nutrition, physical activity, and mental health can have a significant effect on well-being in the community, moderating the effect of chronic disease that plagues underserved communities. As suggested by trends in health care spending, a shift toward supporting community health initiatives over costly medical interventions can yield benefits that extend far beyond the treatment of individual patients, sustaining the value of such an approach to public health policy. While the potential for better health outcomes through community initiatives is clear, the fiscal constraints governing public health funding too frequently stifle their achievement. A significant portion of America's healthcare expenditures is not improving health for the population, primarily due to exorbitant prices and administrative inefficiencies (Fielding et al., 2017). Wastage of this money diverts resources away from those that are required for social determinants of health, resulting in a decrease of investments in essential public health and social programs. To take just one example, California dropped its General Fund expenditures on public health from 34.8% in 1990 to 21.4% in 2014, despite increasing healthcare expenditures. These patterns illustrate a disconcerting trend away from prevention that would avoid health crises and promote long-term community well-being. Redirecting money from excessive medical expenditures to current community health initiatives would not only enhance outcomes but also have a stunning economic payoff, ultimately benefiting taxpayers and communities too. Besides, evaluating and rewarding community health initiatives plays an essential role in determining if they are successful and sustainable. Quality incentive programs offer an avenue for measuring and enhancing the performance of health programs in terms of understandable measures of success (Jon et al., 2007). By focusing on measurable indicators of health outcomes—such as declines in hospitalization rates or increases in high school students' graduation rates—such programs are able to obtain the funding and support required to extend their reach and impact. For example, the redirection of resources to preventive care has been shown to reduce the prevalence of chronic disease and improve overall health equity. Additionally, applying a rigorous process of assessment and feedback guarantees that community health programs are responsive and flexible to the changing health landscape, with a climate that may enable the co-existence of preventive medicine and public health practice. Ultimately, incorporating community health programs into the broader healthcare system is very promising to enhance population health and avoid illness (Figure 12.8).

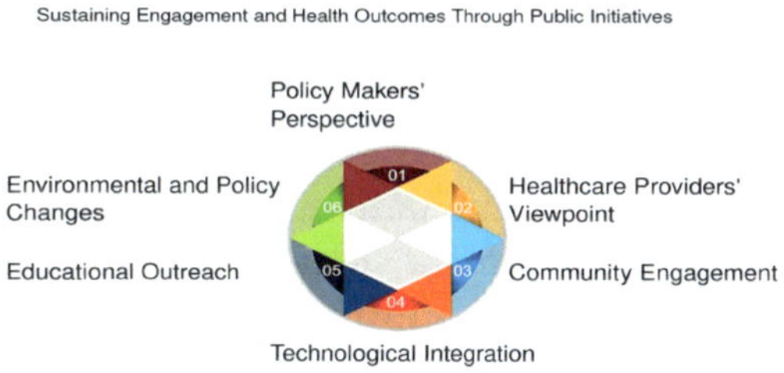

Figure 12.8. The significance of community health programs and initiatives.

Source: https://fastercapital.co/i/Community-engagement--Public-Health-Initiatives--Healthy-Communities--The-Contribution-of-Public-Health-Initiatives-to-Engagement--Sustaining-Engagement-and-Health-Outcomes-Through-Public-Initiatives.webp.

Test Your Knowledge

1. What are two major public health policies that have significantly contributed to disease prevention and health promotion at the population level?
2. How does the government contribute to preventive healthcare through legislation, funding, and health campaigns?
3. What is the role of community health programs in addressing local health issues and improving access to preventive services?

12.4. Preventive Medicine Strategies

Learning Outcome

1. Vaccination programs and their importance
2. Lifestyle modifications and behavioral interventions
3. Screening guidelines for various populations

Intervention through preventive medicine practices is critical to reversing the increasing demand for chronic disorders in internal medicine. By adopting proactive health practices, healthcare providers can reduce the incidence and prevalence of lifestyle-related diseases such as cardiovascular disease, diabetes, and obesity. Preventive practices include periodic screenings, vaccinations, and patient education regarding feasible lifestyle alternatives. The reconfiguration of health practice into patient-centered medical homes is a model for a successful approach in which active leadership is a crucial element. Medical homes prioritize continuous and team-based healing relationships, allowing for whole-person care that is individualized. The implementation of these models builds a culture that focuses on preventive care and fosters improved overall health results, mirroring the significant impact of systematic preventive measures on public health programs (Wagner et al., 2012). In addition to patient-centered models of care, the integration of evidence-based public health (EBPH) practices is essential for enhancing population health. By adopting a systematic method of applying research results to inform public health decision-making, EBPH is a foundation for successful preventive intervention at the community level. It is not merely a case of identifying health hazards and inequities but taking steps to actively counteract them by direct intervention. In a review of a study that measured determinants facilitating EBPH in chronic disease prevention departments, leadership support was identified as playing a critical role in establishing an evidence-informed practice environment (Allen et al., 2018). This finding suggests the requirement of public health leaders to promote EBPH processes so that health departments are capable of helping staff justify their preventive health programs and establish complementary partnerships that can enhance community health responses. Furthermore, the success of preventive medicine strategies depends on effective coordination among healthcare practitioners, public health agencies, and community stakeholders. This interdisciplinary approach enables a comprehensive understanding of health determinants and the implementation of person-focused interventions addressing heterogeneous populations. As an illustration, physical activity, nutrition, and mental well-being efforts not only play a part in managing individual risk factors but also promote healthier surroundings. Public health personnel contribute further by providing training and technical assistance to gain skills necessary to be effective in working with communities. However, issues such as financial uncertainties and staff turnover must be addressed for the sustainability of these efforts, underlining the importance of leadership strength and committed structures that support sustained preventive efforts in public health and internal medicine (Allen et al., 2018) (Figure 12.9).

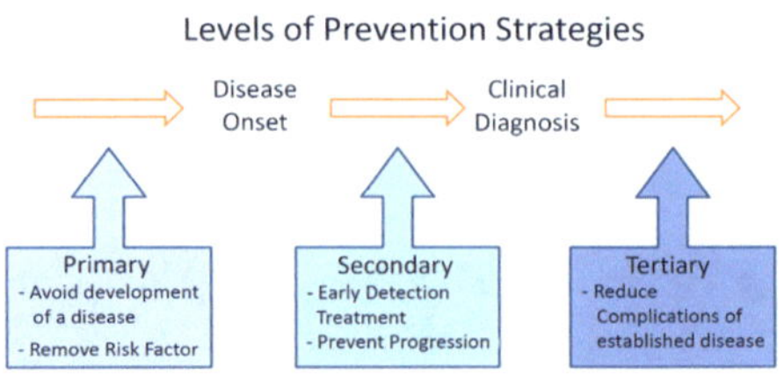

Figure 12.9. The adoption of preventive medicine strategies.

Source: https://bpb-us-w2.wpmucdn.com/edblogs.columbia.edu/dist/3/817/files/2017/04/prevention_strategy-1nr9qp0.jpg.

12.4.1. Vaccination Programs and Their Importance

Immunization campaigns are at the heart of the cosmos of preventive medicine and public health, even more in the practice of internal medicine. They not only safeguard people from vaccine-preventable diseases but also achieve community-wide immunity, or herd immunity. This herd immunity occurs when a high proportion of the population has been vaccinated, thereby reducing the overall prevalence of disease, which serves to safeguard the unvaccinated and individuals with weakened immunity. By a dramatic reduction in infectious disease incidence, vaccination interventions assist in minimizing health care costs associated with emergency department care and hospital stays that ultimately fortify the health care system. Furthermore, keeping a healthy population lowers the risk of pandemic outbreaks and encourages stability in society, ranking the importance of such programs topmost in today's public health initiatives. Beyond their protective functions, vaccination programs are valuable learning materials for public health literacy. As people interact with vaccine programs, they become more aware of the broader context of preventive care and the benefits of early interventions. Health insurance literacy also comes into play, affecting how inclined people are to take advantage of preventive services. Research indicates that many people may be unaware of the benefit attached to their health coverage, for instance, the provision of recommended preventive services such as immunizations, resulting in underutilization of these life-saving practices (Goold et al., 2018). Efforts to enhance health insurance literacy through vaccination outreach can affect enrollment rates in these programs and contribute to improved public health outcomes while ensuring that more people gain access to available preventive services. Furthermore, the success of vaccination programs relies on coordination among healthcare providers, public health practitioners, and community-based agencies. These partnerships enable effective communication and information provision as well as resource delivery to targeted groups, hence avoiding barriers to vaccine access such as geographic, economic, or educational disparities. Targeted interventions, for example, outreach campaigns within disadvantaged groups, can improve vaccine uptake and equitable access to healthcare, maintaining the principle that public health should be inclusive and representative of all groups. With concerted action, healthcare stakeholders can make vaccination programs sustainable and effective, ultimately safeguarding the population's health. Further, ongoing research and collaboration on future infectious diseases serve even better to validate the importance of vaccination as a preventive measure in averting future public health crises (Bourhy et al., 2012) (Figure 12.10).

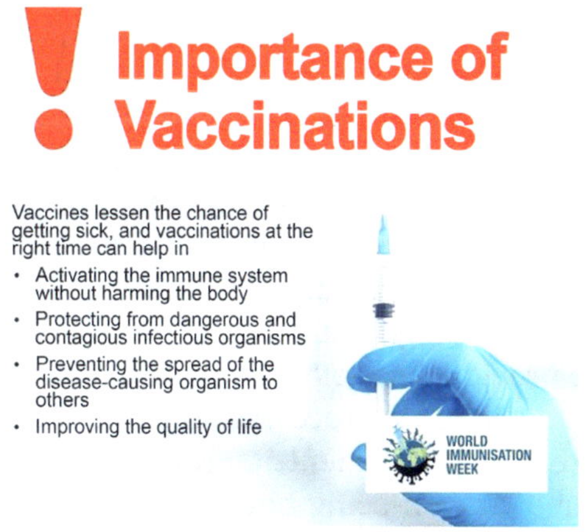

Figure 12.10. Vaccination programs and their importance.

Source: https://lirp.cdn-website.com/69c0b277/dms3rep/multi/opt/Importance+of+vaccinations+-+WIW-640w.jpg.

12.4.2. Lifestyle Modifications and Behavioral Interventions

In the past few years, lifestyle change and behavior intervention have been given significant importance in the realm of preventive medicine and public health. These behavior interventions target various health behaviors, including diet, exercise, and stress management, which are important for the prevention of chronic diseases such as diabetes and cardiovascular disease. Evidence shows that engaged patients with lifestyle change have improved overall health outcomes, lower healthcare expenses, and improved quality of life. Additionally, self-management-focused interventions have been shown to be effective in enabling individuals to incorporate healthier behavior and sustain the same in the long run, as seen in various studies addressing the intersection of mental and physical health outcomes (N/A, 2011). Thus, the use of behavioral interventions in clinical practice is important in addressing the complex needs of a diverse population of patients. The creation of digital health technologies provides a new avenue for bringing about lifestyle change among patients, especially from underprivileged groups. Research has established that one can modify digital diabetes prevention programs for low-income groups and that these patients are receptive to such interventions despite challenges of digital literacy and access (Fontil et al., 2016). By modifying educational content to be culturally adapted and readable, health care providers can effectively engage patients in their well-being processes. Such modifications not only allow patients to regain control over their own well-being but also equip clinicians with adequate means of delivering personalized care. In the end, integrating technology into behavioral interventions holds the promise of enhancing health literacy and promoting sustained lifestyle modification among vulnerable populations. Healthcare professionals also have a critical role in facilitating lifestyle modification and behavioral interventions. Successful communication and support by clinicians can significantly influence patient compliance and motivation regarding prescribed lifestyle change. Motivational interviewing and cultural care have the prospect of bridging the gap between intention and action among patients. Clinicians who have been trained in these interventions are also more likely to identify facilitators of change and to come up with interventions in light of such recognition, providing a conducive environment for patient support. Integrating these approaches not only enhances the effectiveness of health promotion interventions but also aligns with the overall goal of preventive medicine: optimizing public health outcomes through a patient-centered approach (Fontil et al., 2016; N/A, 2011). Hence, incorporating lifestyle modification into routine care is critical to enhance the objectives of preventive medicine and optimize population health (Figure 12.11).

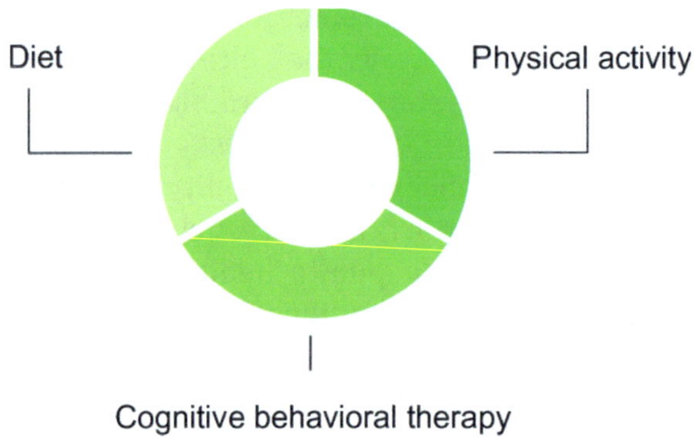

Figure 12.11. Lifestyle modifications and behavioral interventions.

Source: https://www.researchgate.net/profile/Riccardo-Dalle-Grave/publication/257757050/figure/fig1/AS:601628080082975@1520450720816/Principal-components-of-lifestyle-modification-programs.png.

12.4.3. Screening Guidelines for Various Populations

Screening protocols in preventive care are essential in addressing the health needs of different populations. Their success depends on their tailored application, which encompasses the population's unique characteristics. As the disparities in access to and quality of care expand, culturally sensitive screening measures are more relevant than ever. Research has identified that both socioeconomic status and race exert significant influences on whether or not appropriate screenings are performed for patients, indicating systemic disparities in the delivery of care. For instance, studies have shown that African American patients tend to be under-screened for vaccinations and hypertension compared to Caucasian patients, and guidelines that account for these disparities are necessary (Collett et al., 2017). With an emphasis on these disparities, directed recommendations for screening are key to closing the public health gap and narrowing the disparities in preventive care. Integrating equity-focused strategies into guidelines for screening not only enhances health outcomes but also develops a more equitable healthcare environment. Results report that the obstacles to access faced by minority and low-income patients—e.g., limited access to specialists, physician biases, and geographic limitations—are all significant predictors of their potential to achieve access to timely screenings (Carlson et al., 2016). Directed screening practices that account for such obstacles are important in increasing disadvantaged populations' access to healthcare. Some interventions that can be employed include community outreach to educate underserved populations about the importance of preventive care and mobilizing resources to make screening more accessible. Through the incorporation of equity into the provision of care, health systems can enhance the quality of preventive services and also work towards eradicating health disparities that cut across different demographic groups. Furthermore, the necessity of continuous monitoring and fine-tuning of screening guidelines is also of top priority in an ever-evolving health setting. As new evidence arises about the efficacy of screenings on different populations, doctors must remain vigilant about revising their practices. This is particularly necessary with the changing demographics and transforming dynamics of diseases. Advances in technology and data analytics enable more tailored population health management, with responses to screening protocols made possible in real time. Ensuring that the screening guidelines are formulated on the most recent available evidence and that they meet the diverse needs of the population will not only enhance preventive care but also help patients assume responsibility for their health. Through an active, equity-focused approach to screening guidelines, the practice of internal medicine can take significant strides toward the promotion of health equity and the best possible well-being of all patients.

Test Your Knowledge

1. Why are vaccination programs considered a cornerstone of public health, and how do they contribute to herd immunity?
2. What are two effective lifestyle or behavioral interventions recommended to reduce the risk of chronic diseases such as diabetes or heart disease?
3. How do screening guidelines vary among different populations, and why is age, risk level, or gender considered in screening recommendations?

12.5. Challenges in Implementing Preventive Medicine

Learning Outcome

1. Barriers to accessing preventive care
2. Socioeconomic factors affecting health outcomes
3. Resistance to change in patient behavior

Preventive medicine is constrained by interconnected problems stemming from systemic flaws in the healthcare system. The most significant obstacle is the failure to appropriately integrate prevention paradigms into routine clinical practice, particularly primary care. The majority of healthcare workers are typically bogged down by acute care demands, which leaves them little time to prioritize prevention. As outlined in the provisions of the 2010 health reform law, efforts to improve primary care have been made through enhanced Medicare and Medicaid reimbursement and innovation in care delivery, but these measures in isolation cannot guarantee a cultural shift toward preventive medicine. Clinicians must operate in an environment that, at times, puts short-term patient problems before long-term health strategies, making promotion of preventive health interventions challenging for both health workers and patients (Lawlor et al., 2011). Budget constraints are also a significant consideration in keeping preventive medicine in check. Even while a great deal of documentation exists regarding the potential cost savings that can be achieved by preventive interventions, the initial investment needed to introduce them effectively deters healthcare systems from deploying such programs. The quality incentive programs have acted as a tool in connecting these two variables by making sure higher quality care is delivered, and costs are concurrently contained. The effectiveness of these programs is, however, dependent on careful design and implementation. The current situation reflects substantial variation in the measurement and perception of these incentives, leading to variation in effectiveness and actual improvement in patient outcomes (Jon et al., 2007). Thus, the stakeholders in the healthcare system must critically analyze the financial and structural barriers that hinder the growth of preventive medicine. Finally, public opinion and patient participation are key factors in the successful implementation of preventive medicine interventions.

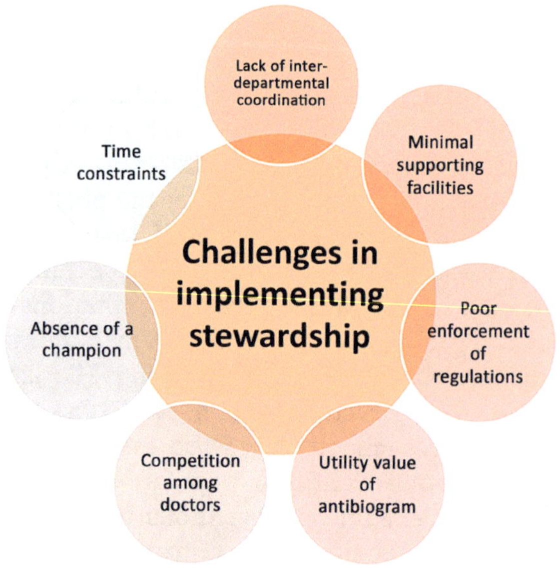

Figure 12.12. Challenges in implementing preventive medicine.

Source: https://www.frontiersin.org/files/Articles/493904/fpubh-08-493904-HTML/image_m/fpubh-08-493904-g003.jpg.

A majority of the people are ignorant of the benefits of preventive health interventions or doubt their usefulness and therefore will not seek preventive services. The culture works to enhance the difficulties in developing an aggressive approach to managing health. In order for preventive medicine to work, there needs to be educational programs that explain the significance and role of preventive care.

These campaigns have to aim towards bringing about a paradigm shift where patients do not merely view preventive measures as appendages but as focal points of health maintenance. Engaging patients in such discussions can modify attitudes and behavior, thereby creating a solid foundation for systemic changes necessary for preventive medicine to succeed in both public and internal medicine (Figure 12.12).

12.5.1. Barriers to Accessing Preventive Care

Preventive care access obstacles are multifaceted, involving issues related to systemic difficulties in the provision of healthcare and the socio-economic position of populations. Chronic diseases are a significant obstacle due to their skewing within demographic categories. For example, studies have established that African-American women have higher rates of incidence of chronic pain conditions compared to their non-Hispanic White counterparts. This, combined with the prevalence of such conditions as breast and cervical cancer, means an extreme disparity in the provision of preventive care. The chronic arthritic pain of joints prevalent in these women tends to raise competing demands upon their resources and time, ultimately equating to decreased odds of accessing essential preventive treatments, such as pap smears and mammograms. These inequalities necessitate particular interventions designed to increase the continuity and scope of care provided to vulnerable populations (Anderson et al., 2012). The second critical impediment is language and communication in the health sector. Differences in languages could lead to miscommunication or an inability to comprehend the importance of preventive services. For non-native English speakers, the inability to communicate effectively with health care providers can be a significant obstacle to accessing the health care system. This is not only an obstacle to possibly accessing preventive care but also a contributor to racial and ethnic health disparities. Provision of adequate resources towards facilitating language access is essential in ensuring all patients, regardless of their linguistic status, understand and can effectively utilize preventive services (Piotrowski et al., 2003). Closing these language gaps is thus pivotal in developing an equitable health care environment. Further, socio-economic factors such as income, educational attainment, and health insurance coverage pose ubiquitous barriers to access to preventive care. Patients of lower socio-economic groups often face financial constraints that prevent access to routine care, including preventive screening. Being asked to pay for services, coupled with not having health insurance, worsens their situation and leads to a delay in diagnosis and increased morbidity. Educational disparities may also affect perceptions of the importance of preventive care as well as available services. They may lack adequate information about preventive care, thereby perpetuating the cycle of not receiving necessary health screenings. Resolving socio-economic issues requires system-level changes in public health policy to enhance access to low-cost care and educational programs that promote preventive health awareness (Anderson et al., 2012).

12.5.2. Socioeconomic Factors Affecting Health Outcomes

Socioeconomic determinants play a central role in influencing health outcomes and access to healthcare services. Individuals of low socioeconomic status are likely to face significant barriers that disrupt optimal health. These barriers include a shortage of finances, which restricts opportunities for access to healthy food, affordable accommodation, and proper medical care. Further, educational deficits lead to low health literacy, which confuses patients about the complexity of the healthcare system. Without the cultural component of competence among health care providers, as is the focus of research with the Tool for Assessing Cultural Competence

Training (TACCT), these issues are exacerbated, resulting in miscommunication and substandard care for disenfranchised populations. Lastly, resolution of such socioeconomic determinants is essential to the realization of equal health outcomes and the provision of preventive health measures being duly executed among populations (Jernigan et al., 2016). In addition, one's place of residence also plays an important role in one's health behavior and health. It has been shown that living in a neighborhood with poor provision of recreational facilities and safe spaces may lead to a sedentary lifestyle. This sitting culture is generally linked with a variety of unfavorable health outcomes, such as obesity and cardiovascular diseases. Compounding the issue, the health-related effects of physical inactivity are shaped by a variety of factors such as socioeconomic status, which determines opportunities for physical activity. An understanding of such complex relations is imperative in designing suitable public health interventions to encourage active living. These results may be supported with cultural and socioeconomic information to inform niche interventions that consider not just physical health but also system-level barriers within diverse groups (Alves et al., 2019). Finally, the alignment of socioeconomic determinants and health outcomes also stresses the need for targeted public health interventions. For instance, preventive medical care mindful of socioeconomic status can actually enhance the provision of health programs. By developing culturally sensitive and accessible interventions throughout socioeconomic levels, healthcare professionals can establish an environment conducive to improved health outcomes. Additionally, by emphasizing community-based approaches and collaboration, the access-to-healthcare gap and the health-literacy gap can be addressed, leading to sustainable behavioral and health changes. These types of projects must include ongoing observation and adjustment of strategy to accommodate evolving community needs, a process that not only improves health but also directly addresses the inequities created by socioeconomic status (Jernigan et al., 2016) (Figure 12.13).

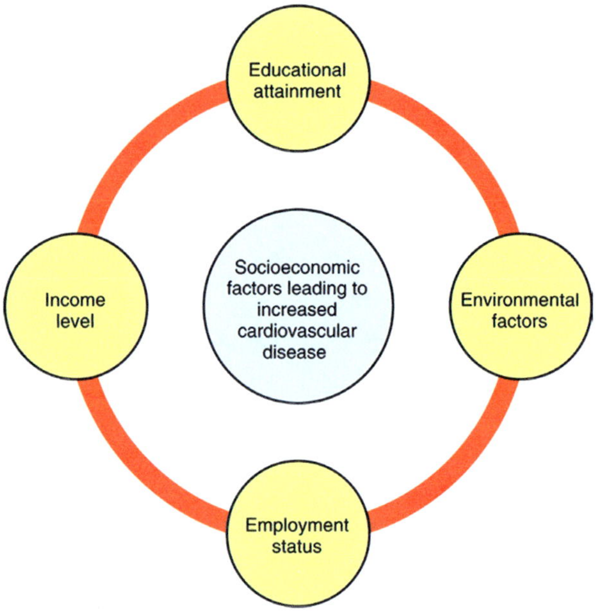

Figure 12.13. Socioeconomic factors affecting health outcomes.

Source: https://www.ahajournals.org/cms/10.1161/CIRCULATIONAHA.117.029652/asset/fe134b30-0ad1-47b3-a183-4b042aa20bd5/assets/images/large/2166fig01.jpg.

12.5.3. Resistance to Change in Patient Behavior

Resistance to change in patient behavior is one of the biggest barriers to effective preventive medicine and public health policy in internal medicine. Healthcare professionals need to understand the determinants of resistance to change in psychology and social contexts as they prepare to implement changes in patients' behavior. The patients are often resistant to lifestyle change, such as the consumption of healthier food or constant physical exercise, primarily due to habits deeply ingrained in them and the lack of immediate incentives. Patient behavior changes are often met with suspicion because, most of the time, individuals perceive no tangible benefits arising from the alteration of their habits. This suggests the necessity for healthcare professionals not merely to instruct, but also to persuade and facilitate incremental behavior change through tailor-made interventions that resonate with every patient's individual circumstances and beliefs. Additionally, the efficacy of interventions such as Screening and Brief Intervention (SBI) can be diminished by healthcare professionals' own resistance to change. Practice programs that seek to enhance the ability of practitioners to facilitate behavioral change in patient populations show that even when there is a willingness to utilize educational material, there is a gap in wanting to promote such practices among colleagues. This uncertainty is a twofold problem: not only can the healthcare professionals themselves be unsure of adopting new practices, but this in itself affects their ability to persuade patients to act in similar ways. Proper evidence shows that education and training can facilitate confidence in using evidence-based methods and, therefore, overcome resistance. But creating a culture within healthcare settings that promotes continuous learning and adaptability is still one to be addressed at the institutional level (Coogle et al., 2015). Finally, cultural competence for healthcare is part of dispelling resistance barriers to patient behavioral change. As more diverse populations increase to become the dominant population in patients, cultural sensitivity is more important. Cultural competence training equips healthcare providers with invaluable skills that enhance their effectiveness in communicating with patients of varying backgrounds. Evidence has shown that such training has a positive impact on the attitude and behavior of medical trainees towards improved patient interaction. Despite this, widespread heterogeneity in the application and execution of cultural competence interventions suggests greater comprehensive and uniform methods are needed. Through a focus on cultural humility and the social determinants of health, practitioners can develop more trusting relationships with patients and, therefore, reduce resistance to prescribed lifestyle change. By this approach, patients are not only empowered but also align with greater public health initiatives in constructing sustained health behavior change (Jernigan et al., 2016) (Figure 12.14).

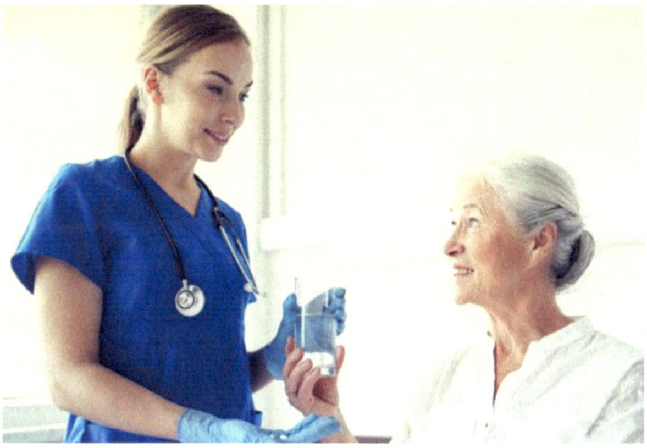

Figure 12.14. Resistance to change in patient behavior.

Source: https://www.touchpointmed.com/sites/default/files/styles/max_650x650/public/2021-07/How-ADCs-Reduced-Fear-and-Anxiety-in-Nurses.jpg?itok=RO8n5_Lp.

Test Your Knowledge

1. What are two common barriers that prevent individuals from accessing preventive healthcare services?
2. How do socioeconomic factors such as income and education level influence health outcomes and access to preventive care?
3. What are some reasons patients may resist making lifestyle changes, even when aware of health risks, and how can providers address this resistance?

12.6. Future Directions in Preventive Medicine

Learning Outcome

1. Innovations in technology and health monitoring
2. Integration of genomics in preventive strategies
3. Collaborative approaches in public health

The path of preventive medicine is increasingly guided by the need for a primary care paradigm emphasizing patient-centered practice and integrated health systems. This calls for innovative models of strategy that propel the delivery of care while driving meaningful patient activation. As elaborated in contemporary models, for instance, models that demand reorganization of practices into patient-centered medical homes, central concepts center on activated leadership, quality improvement strategy, and persistent team-based healing relationships. Emphasizing these factors, the guidelines towards preventive medicine in the future will likely entail a concerted endeavor at creating health systems that conform to patient experiences and outcomes, finally affecting improved public health outcomes. With the adoption of such tenets, the potential to close gaps in the existing health care system is realized, thereby optimizing the efficacy of preventive interventions and improving patient care standards (Wagner et al., 2012). Moreover, the intersection of technology and data analysis will revolutionize preventive medicine in a way that supports personalized health strategies and targeted interventions. The convergence of big data, artificial intelligence, and wearable health technologies enables clinicians to monitor patients before they fall ill, creating the potential for early interventions to decelerate the progression of chronic diseases. Preventive medicine's future directions will likely leverage these advances to refine the accuracy of risk stratification, so that clinicians can tailor interventions to personal risk profiles. In addition, policy frameworks promoting care innovation, such as the healthcare reform law, have identified will be important for setting new preventive service norms. Such initiatives can foster the development of the workforce in primary care and make preventive interventions evidence-based as well as universally available (Lawlor et al., 2011). Finally, as preventive medicine evolves, addressing the social determinants of health is one of the top priorities. Understanding how socioeconomic status, education, and living conditions affect health outcomes will be the prime driver of the interventions to reduce health disparities. Future preventive measures will need to involve interdisciplinary coordination among public health professionals, health practitioners, and community organizations to develop comprehensive models that account for these determinants. These concerted efforts will enable preventive medicine not only to be kept outside clinical settings but also incorporated into the community structure, promoting health equity and overall public health. By engaging directly with these broader societal issues, the field of preventive medicine can better position itself towards the ultimate goal of building a healthier population through proactive, inclusive action (Figure 12.15).

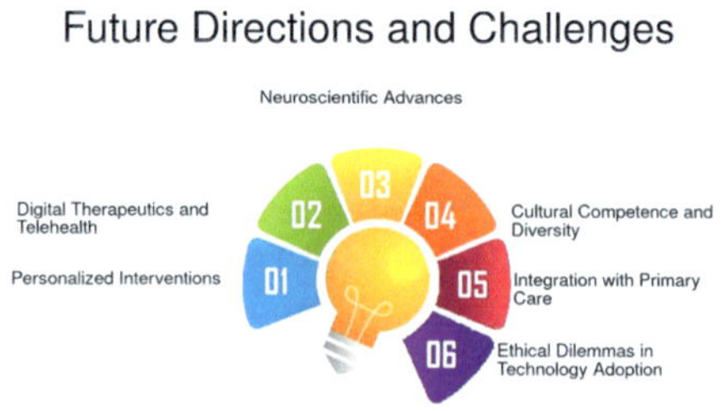

Figure 12.15. Future directions in preventive medicine.

Source: https://fastercapital.co/i/Behavioral-therapy-innovation-Revolutionizing-Mental-Health--Innovations-in-Behavioral-Therapy--Future-Directions-and-Challenges.webp.

12.6.1. Innovations in Technology and Health Monitoring

The integration of technology into health monitoring is a landmark innovation in preventive care. Emerging technologies such as cell phone-based health apps, wearable health sensors, and telemedicine platforms are transforming patient interaction with healthcare providers and self-management of chronic illness. They facilitate around-the-clock monitoring of health through tracking of the vital measures such as heart rate, blood glucose levels, and exercise. Thus, patients become active stakeholders in managing their health, a fundamental factor in ensuring timely detection and early intervention. Technology advancements not only increase patient engagement but also provide increased access to health services, particularly for the poor, thereby developing an equitable approach to public health. Data analysis is also important in maximizing the effectiveness of health monitoring technologies. By collecting and analyzing large volumes of health-related data, physicians can identify patterns and predict potential health risks. This anticipatory process permits the implementation of focused preventive measures, enabling more tailored approaches to care. Of special note is how technological innovation in big data analysis can inform public health initiatives by tracking disease outbreaks and evaluating the effectiveness of prevention measures on a community basis. Using these technologies, healthcare workers can maximize health outcomes while reducing healthcare expenditures, underscoring the need to incorporate revolutionary practices into internal medicine. The intersection of policy transformation and technology is instrumental to securing the proper execution of innovations in monitoring health. Ineffective care coordination between healthcare sites is fundamental to making these advances comprehensively, as in policy guidance for technical changes and infrastructure development to enhance healthcare provision (Anne et al., 2008). Delivery of primary and chronic care has been reorganized at the state level in order to advance leadership, payment incentives, and monitoring mechanisms for improving care quality while enabling small practices (Anne et al., 2010). By closing policy gaps, health systems are better able to leverage technological progress to amplify its benefits for prevention and, ultimately, for healthier populations and greater health equity.

12.6.2. Integration of Genomics in Preventive Strategies

The integration of genomics in prevention policy is a paradigm shift for preventive medicine and public health. Knowledge of genetic risk factors for diseases allows health care providers to identify at-risk populations more accurately and use preventive interventions accordingly. For instance, genomic data can be used to guide lifestyle modifications, screening, and early interventions for diabetes or cardiovascular disease. But this integration has not been effortless. A survey of European Public Health Association members revealed that even with an overall positive inclination towards the use of genetic testing in public health, professionals lack the knowledge required to implement these measures successfully (Baccolini et al., 2020). Additionally, concerns remain about the diversion of funds away from other social determinants of health, and it is implied that the way towards successful genomic integration must be carefully tread. In order to effectively take advantage of the potential of genomic data, there needs to be a solid framework for public health genomics education and practice. The current situation indicates a broad knowledge gap among public health workers, with a majority of them underestimating the potential of genomics to impact preventive interventions. Specifically, as low as 28.9% of surveyed members named conditions for which there is evidence of supporting genetic testing appropriately, indicating a need for targeted educational programs (Baccolini et al., 2020). These programs can build an informed health workforce capable of integrating genomic information into daily preventive care. Such integration not only enhances the precision of health interventions but also promotes a more focused approach, enabling healthcare providers to effectively address their patients' unique genetic profiles. The vision of P4 medicine—personalized, predictive, preventive, and participatory—continues to emphasize strategic incorporation of genomics into preventive care. As technology advances continuously, it is becoming more and more possible to scrutinize patient-specific data and tailor interventions that would substantially reduce disease incidence and improve quality of life. However, the promotion of P4 medicine is still a contentious issue since supportive evidence is still in the process of maturation. Concerns about overdiagnosis and overtreatment remain, suggesting that genomic incorporation, while promising, should be approached with caution. Public health challenges of today necessitate a paradigm change in the sense that genomic technologies are being combined with holistic prevention approaches so that benefits eclipse drawbacks. Thenceforth, a balanced assessment of interventions and resources will be required to realize genomics' full potential in the context of preventive medicine and public health (Figure 12.16).

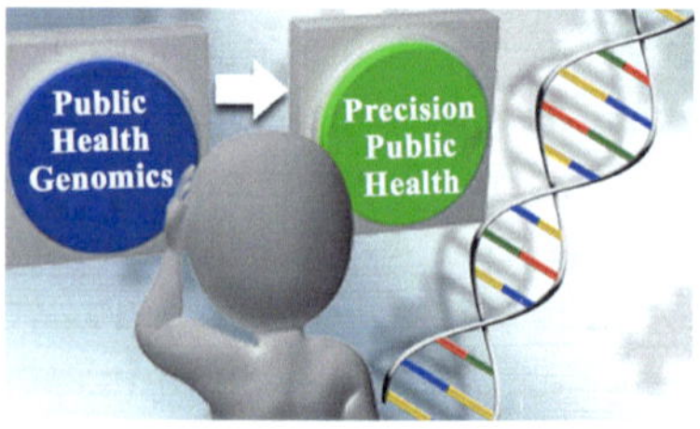

Figure 12.16. Integration of genomics in preventive strategies.

Source: https://blogs.cdc.gov/genomics/wp-content/uploads/sites/20/2019/02/2019-02_blog_PHG_next2.jpg.

12.6.3. Collaborative Approaches in Public Health

Interprofessional practice in public health has gained added prominence as the central mechanism for addressing the multidimensionality of issues presented by preventive medicine and internal medicine. The multidimensionality of health conditions—typically requiring a mix of social and medical interventions—requires a workgroup-based strategy that emphasizes integration across sectors of health care. By advancing partnerships between health care providers, community organizations, and agencies of public health, collaborative practice can be applied to enhance the continuum of care. Synthesizing several perspectives leads to more holistic models of treatment that address not only physical conditions but also the social determinants of health and the psychological determinants of health. Holistic approaches are necessary to advance patient outcomes, particularly in individuals with comorbid disorders, where restricted medical care is not sufficient. Lastly, collaboration not only improves the quality of care provided but also improves the resilience of public health systems to new and emerging health risks. Good cooperation in public health also significantly relies on the application of health information technology, which serves as a platform for resource sharing and coordination of care. Through the common digital platforms, health professionals can monitor patient health data in real-time, enhancing response capabilities for urgent needs and smooth transitions of care. Inter-disciplinary communication and patient activation through self-management are improved by the linking of health information systems. As outlined in literature already in existence, enhancing models of resource sharing in small and midsize practices significantly empowers such providers to deliver quality care despite insufficient financial or human resources (Anne-Marie et al., 2011). Through the creation of networks that share information and pool resources, collaborative approaches enhance efficiency and the provision of preventive care, thereby improving public health outcomes at the community level. Furthermore, such inter-sectoral public health collaborations can have improved policy implications that reshape the landscape of preventive medicine. For instance, collaborations can advocate for legislative changes that facilitate increased adoption of integrated models of care to provide systematic integration of mental health services with physical health interventions. This integration is especially vital with respect to the shocking number of patients who are affected by both medical and mental conditions, which has been linked with increased death rates and healthcare system expenses (N/A, 2011). By addressing both sides under an integrated system, public health interventions can be sure to deliver comprehensive, evidence-based care tailored to each patient's specific requirements. Therefore, collaborative approaches can redefine measures of success in public health, including not just short-term medical outcomes but also long-term quality-of-life improvements and the community's overall resilience.

Test Your Knowledge

1. How are wearable health technologies and remote monitoring devices transforming preventive healthcare?
2. In what ways can genomic data be integrated into personalized preventive strategies for chronic diseases?
3. Why are interdisciplinary and community-based collaborations essential for the future of public health prevention efforts?

SUMMARY

The integration of preventive medicine and public health into internal medicine reflects a paradigm shift towards prevention and health promotion. By emphasizing evidence-based practice, health practitioners can now deal with chronic diseases that disproportionately afflict different population groups. Intersectoral approaches to strengthening the public health infrastructure, as documented in the literature, highlight the importance of leadership commitment in promoting evidence-informed public health. Such support not only encourages competency growth among public health practitioners but also encourages efficient collaboration that maximizes the expansion of preventive interventions to communities. Leadership involvement ensures that practitioners are sufficiently empowered to use evidence-based practices, thereby maximizing overall health outcomes and reducing morbidity from chronic diseases (Allen et al., 2018). Also, consideration of health disparities is necessary in understanding the complexity of healthcare delivery. Scientists have identified long-standing inequalities in the provision of preventive interventions, notably between ethnic minorities and those from lower socioeconomic groups. These are accounted for by many factors, including caregiver healthcare recommendation bias, as shown in studies of Physician Assistant decision-making. The study recognizes significant variations in screening behavior across a patient's race, thereby indicating the need for intervention aimed at equitable provision of healthcare (Collett et al., 2017). Ultimately, the disparities have to be addressed to design effective public health measures that do not underserve any demographic. To reinforce the achievements in preventive medicine, continuous evaluation and modification of healthcare policies are important. Engagement of stakeholders like policymakers and community leaders can foster a culture of adoption of innovative preventive health practices. Using evidence-based information and considerations for population needs, healthcare systems can structure interventions that are appealing to diverse communities. Apart from addressing present disparities, this integrative strategy also encourages active participation in health maintenance. In conclusion, the future of internal medicine must align closely with public health principles that prioritize preventive interventions as the mainstay of promoting health equity and an enduring health status in all populations (Allen et al., 2018; Collett et al., 2017).

The incorporation of preventive medicine and public health procedures within internal medicine is essential to the improvement of patient care outcomes. A fundamental building block is an understanding of the key change concepts that are utilized to transform medical practices towards patient-centered medical homes. These concepts are centered on engaged leadership and utilizing quality improvement methodologies. By facilitating continuous, team-oriented healing relationships and expanded access to care, physicians can systematically advance patient engagement and outcomes. This approach integrates preventive care initiatives with regular medical practice, allowing for a greater understanding of patient needs and sustained health. Such foundations not only optimize patient experience but also facilitate expanded use of preventive interventions within internal medicine. As healthcare delivery systems fragment, the need for new policy solutions to enhance care coordination becomes clear. The successful integration of preventive medicine into public health relies upon filling existing gaps among providers and locations of care. Payment reform, regulatory reform, and building the healthcare infrastructure are the most important strategies for integrating fragmented services. These proposals highlight the necessity of reframing healthcare provision into an integrated system where preventive practices can be more realized. Internal medicine, with its focus on care coordination, can transition from disease treatment alone to disease prevention, thereby bringing in a more sustainable public health system. In addition, applying these practices in preventive medicine promotes a culture of health that benefits communities. A coordinated care strategy can enhance education and awareness of disease prevention and have profound implications for public health overall. Internal medicine clinicians can implement team-based models of care to provide individualized interventions targeting specific population health issues. Such an approach, grounded in the principles outlined in the concepts of change above, empowers patients with comprehensive support for health care. As internal medicine practice evolves, embracing these preventive methods and public health programs will not only promote the health of individual patients but also that of healthier communities overall, reinforcing the functional synergy between preventive medicine and public health in the practice of internal medicine.

KEY TERMS FROM THIS CHAPTER

- Preventive Medicine
- Primary Prevention
- Health Promotion
- Screening
- Lifestyle Modification
- Communicable Diseases
- Occupational Health
- Community Medicine
- Public Health
- Secondary Prevention
- Disease Prevention
- Immunization
- Non-Communicable Diseases
- Environmental Health
- Health Education
- Health Policy

CRITICAL THINKING QUESTIONS

1. **Which of the following is an example of primary prevention?**
   a. Mammography screening for breast cancer
   b. Statin therapy after myocardial infarction
   c. Vaccination against hepatitis B
   d. Rehabilitation after stroke
2. **The most effective public health measure to reduce smoking rates is:**
   a. Free nicotine patches
   b. Mass media campaigns
   c. Increasing tobacco taxes
   d. School-based education
3. **Which of the following is a modifiable risk factor for cardiovascular disease?**
   a. Age
   b. Gender
   c. Family history
   d. Smoking
4. **What is the goal of secondary prevention?**
   a. Prevent disease recurrence
   b. Detect disease early and treat to prevent progression
   c. Prevent risk factor exposure
   d. Rehabilitate after complications occur
5. **Body mass index (BMI) is used primarily to assess:**
   a. Nutritional intake
   b. Cardiovascular endurance
   c. Obesity and weight-related risk
   d. Basal metabolic rate

Short Answer Questions

1. What are the three levels of disease prevention, and how do they differ?
2. Why is vaccination considered a critical tool in preventive medicine?
3. What is the role of screening programs in internal medicine (e.g., for hypertension, diabetes, or cancer)?
4. How does smoking cessation impact the risk of cardiovascular and pulmonary diseases?
5. What is the purpose of health education in promoting preventive healthcare behaviors?
6. How do public health policies (e.g., sugar tax, tobacco control laws) contribute to disease prevention?

Answers to Critical Thinking Questions

1. (c); 2. (c); 3. (d); 4. (b); 5. (c)

REFERENCES

1. Akhtar, S. O., Raza, A. A., Abdullah, Y., & Samadi, A. (2025). Exploring the role of consanguinity in thalassemia prevalence in Pakistan: an in-depth analysis of genetic and cultural factors affecting public health. *Annals of Medicine and Surgery*, *87*(7), 4222–4228. https://doi.org/10.1097/ms9.0000000000003404Allen, P., Bass, K., Best, L. A., Brownson, R. C., et al. (2018). Lessons learned in promoting evidence-based public health: Perspectives from managers in state public health departments. https://core.ac.uk/download/287887998.pdf (accessed on 17th July 2025).
2. Alves, S., Bento, T., Cid, L., Machado, M. F., et al. (2019). Ejercicio físico y estilo de vida sedentario: consecuencias para la salud. https://core.ac.uk/download/286590210.pdf (accessed on 17th July 2025).
3. Anderson, J., Purdy, C., Ransom, A., Tumiel-Berhalter, L., et al. (2012). Racial disparities in cancer screening among women with chronic joint pain. https://digitalscholarship.unlv.edu/cgi/viewcontent.cgi?article=1031&context=jhdrp (accessed on 17th July 2025).
4. Audet, A. M. J., Fryer, A. K., & Doty, M. M. (2011). Sharing resources: Opportunities for smaller primary care practices to increase their capacity for patient care. https://core.ac.uk/download/71358935.pdf (accessed on 17th July 2025).
5. Baars, E., Baars, T., de Bruin, A., et al. (2003). Desk study on homeopathy in organic livestock farming: Principles, obstacles and recommendations for practice and research. https://core.ac.uk/download/10920251.pdf (accessed on 17th July 2025).
6. Baccolini, V., Barnhoorn, F., D'Andrea, E., de Vito, C., et al. (2020). Genomics knowledge and attitudes among European public health professionals: Results of a cross-sectional survey. https://core.ac.uk/download/323191909.pdf (accessed on 17th July 2025).
7. Backhaus, I., Chiappetta, M., Cocchiara, R., Cottarelli, G., et al. (2017). Preventive medicine center and health care for students of medicine and health professions at the Sapienza University of Rome: A research protocol. https://core.ac.uk/download/188833343.pdf (accessed on 17th July 2025).
8. Boom, J. A., Cunningham, R. M., & McGee, L. U. (2018). Vaccine myths: Setting the record straight. https://core.ac.uk/download/212897181.pdf (accessed on 17th July 2025).
9. Bourhy, H., Gaidet, N., & Molia, S. (2012). Mission to Indonesia to participate in the 1st Indonesia-France Seminar in Medicine & Public Health and investigate potential collaborations on animal health: 2nd–9th of November 2012. http://agritrop.cirad.fr/567354/1/document_567354.pdf (accessed on 17th July 2025).
10. Bukonda, N. K. Z., Chastonay, P., Mpinga, E. K., Kandala, N. B., et al. (2013). Traditional/alternative medicines and the right to health: Key elements for a convention on global health. https://core.ac.uk/download/16663861.pdf (accessed on 17th July 2025).
11. Carlson, C., Sholk, J., Nanni, J., Peterson, K., Smith, L. A., & Bhavaraju, N. (2016). Breaking the barriers to specialty care: Practical ideas to improve health equity and reduce cost–Ensuring high-quality specialty care. https://core.ac.uk/download/75785771.pdf (accessed on 17th July 2025).
12. Christianson, J. B., Sutherland, K., & Leatherman, S. (2007). Paying for quality: Understanding and assessing physician pay-for-performance initiatives. https://core.ac.uk/download/71346847.pdf (accessed on 17th July 2025).

13. Clarke, J. L., & Meiris, D. (2006). Preventive medicine: A cure for the healthcare crisis. https://core.ac.uk/download/46965275.pdf (accessed on 17th July 2025).
14. Collett, D. A., & Tyler, K. M. (2017). The effects of patient characteristics on clinician's adherence to preventive practice guidelines. https://digitalscholarship.unlv.edu/cgi/viewcontent.cgi?article=1470&context=jhdrp (accessed on 17th July 2025).
15. Coogle, C. L., & Owens, M. G. (2015). Screening and brief intervention for alcohol misuse in older adults: Training outcomes among physicians and other healthcare practitioners in community-based settings. https://core.ac.uk/download/215483536.pdf (accessed on 17th July 2025).
16. Davis, M. E., Mahabaleshwarkar, R., Spencer, M. D., Taylor, Y. J., et al. (2018). Racial/ethnic disparities in diabetes care and outcomes: A mixed methods study. https://digitalscholarship.unlv.edu/cgi/viewcontent.cgi?article=1748&context=jhdrp (accessed on 17th July 2025).
17. Elk, R. (2017). The need for culturally-based palliative care programs for African American patients at end-of-life. https://core.ac.uk/download/132289944.pdf (accessed on 17th July 2025).
18. Escarce, J. J. (2007). Racial and ethnic disparities in access to and quality of health care. https://core.ac.uk/download/71346896.pdf (accessed on 17th July 2025).
19. Fielding, J. E., Tran, L. D., & Zimmerman, F. J. (2017). Public health and the economy could be served by reallocating medical expenditures to social programs. https://core.ac.uk/download/286729126.pdf (accessed on 17th July 2025).
20. Fontil, V., Gibson, E., Lyles, C. R., McDermott, K., et al. (2016). Adaptation and feasibility study of a digital health program to prevent diabetes among low-income patients: Results from a partnership between a digital health company and an academic research team. https://core.ac.uk/download/323073202.pdf (accessed on 17th July 2025).
21. Gauthier, A. K., Shih, A., McCarthy, D., Davis, K., Nuzum, R., & Schoenbaum, S. C. (2008). Organizing the U.S. health care delivery system for high performance. https://core.ac.uk/download/71353608.pdf (accessed on 17th July 2025).
22. Gauthier, A. K., Sims-Kastelein, K., Takach, M., & Kaye, N. (2010). Strengthening primary and chronic care: State innovations to transform and link small practices. https://core.ac.uk/download/71355266.pdf (accessed on 17th July 2025).
23. Goodall, D., Lombardo, C., & Steven, A. (2011). Models for schools of public health: A scoping review and synthesis of existing evidence. https://core.ac.uk/download/5900218.pdf (accessed on 17th July 2025).
24. Goold, S. D., Kieffer, E. C., Kullgren, J. T., Politi, M. C., et al. (2018). Association between health insurance literacy and avoidance of health care services owing to cost. https://core.ac.uk/download/287888076.pdf (accessed on 17th July 2025).
25. Green, S., & Vogt, H. (2016). Personalizing medicine *in silico* and *in socio*. https://core.ac.uk/download/160113419.pdf (accessed on 17th July 2025).
26. Jernigan, V. B. (2016). An examination of cultural competence training in US medical education guided by the Tool for Assessing Cultural Competence Training. https://digitalscholarship.unlv.edu/cgi/viewcontent.cgi?article=1426&context=jhdrp (accessed on 17th July 2025).

27. Lawlor, G., Abrams, M., Nuzum, R., & Mika, S. (2011). Realizing health reform's potential: How the Affordable Care Act will strengthen primary care and benefit patients, providers, and payers. https://core.ac.uk/download/71354230.pdf (accessed on 17th July 2025).

28. N/A. (2011). *Access Update, June 2011.* https://core.ac.uk/download/11353864.pdf (accessed on 17th July 2025).

29. N/A. (2011). *Mental Disorders and Medical Comorbidity.* https://core.ac.uk/download/71353251.pdf (accessed on 17th July 2025).

30. Nichols, L. M., & Emswiler, T. (2009). *Baylor Health Care System: High-Performance Integrated Health Care.* https://core.ac.uk/download/71349488.pdf (accessed on 17th July 2025).

31. O'Malley, A. S., Peikes, D., Pham, H. H., Maxfield, M., & Ginsburg, P. B. (2008). Making medical homes work: Moving from concept to practice. https://core.ac.uk/download/71352896.pdf (accessed on 17th July 2025).

32. Wagner, E., Sugarman, J. R., Phillips, K., Coleman, K., & Reid, R. J. (2012). Guiding transformation: How medical practices can become patient-centered medical homes. https://core.ac.uk/download/71358341.pdf (accessed on 17th July 2025).

INDEX

A

Adherence 36, 37, 52
Adult illnesses 140
Adult medicine 345
Advanced Life Support 305, 339
Airway Management 339
Allergy 139, 140, 141, 146, 147, 153, 155, 156, 157, 162, 164, 166, 167, 169
Amenorrhea 300
Anaphylaxis 149, 150, 167
Anemia 28, 72, 73, 134
Antenatal Care 300
Antibody 167
Antigen 167
Anxiety Disorder 64, 65
Artificial intelligence (AI) 206, 220
Autoimmune Disease 28
Autosomal Dominant 232
Autosomal Recessive 232

B

Basal Metabolic Rate 374
Behavioral medicine 35, 36, 37, 38
Behavioral services 36
Beyond developments 174
Biopsy 134
Bipolar Disorder 64
B Lymphocyte 167
Body Mass Index 374, 375
Bone 243, 268

C

Cachexia 134
Cardiac Arrest 339
Cardiac disease 242
Cartilage 268
Cervix 301
Chemotherapy 134
Chromosome 232
Chronic disease management 345, 346, 374
Chronic diseases 71, 72, 75, 78, 85, 88, 94, 98
Clinical information 174
clinical manifestations 142
Clinical Nutrition 345, 347, 353, 368, 374
Clinical practice guidelines 174
Cognitive Impairment 99
Collaboration 306
Communicable Diseases 407
Community Medicine 407
Complex health 71, 73, 80, 101
Complexity 241, 243, 247, 257, 267
Comprehensive geriatric assessment (CGA) 72, 81, 83, 100
Computer-aided orthopedic surgery (CAOS) 244
Contemporary 176
Critical Care 305, 306, 307, 334, 339
cultural change 106
Cytokine 167

D

Delirium 99
Delusion 64, 65
Dementia 77, 99, 100, 102
Depression 48, 64
Diabetes Mellitus 28
Diagnostic capabilities 174, 186, 187
Diagnostic equipment 174
Disease 206, 207, 208, 209, 211, 212, 213, 214, 215, 216, 218, 219, 220, 221, 222, 223, 224, 226, 227, 229, 231, 232, 233
Disease Prevention 407
Disease transmission 175, 179, 182, 184, 199
Dislocation 268
Distant territories 176
Dysmenorrhea 300
Dysphagia 99

E

ecological changes 175, 178
Ecological resilience 175, 203
Effective communication 141
Electrolyte Balance 374
Emergency departments (EDs) 306, 325
Emergency medicine 305, 306, 307, 308, 309, 310, 311, 312, 313, 314, 315, 317, 318, 319, 320, 321, 322, 323, 324, 325, 326, 327, 328, 329, 330, 331, 332, 333, 334, 335, 336, 337, 338, 339, 340
Emergency physicians (Eps) 305
Emotional 71, 75, 77, 78, 80, 82, 89, 90, 91, 92, 97
Endometriosis 287
Energy Balance 374
Enteral Nutrition 374
Environmental Health 407
Epigenetics 232, 235
Erythema 28, 29

F

Falls 99
Fertilization 300
Fluid Balance 374
Foreign pathogens 176
Fracture 249, 268
Frailty 81, 99

G

Gene 217, 221, 225, 229, 232
Genome 208, 209, 210, 211, 231, 232, 236
Genomic medicine 206, 213, 220, 236
Genotype 232
Geriatric internal medicine 71
Geriatric medicine 71, 73, 75
Geriatrics 88, 91, 99
Geriatric syndromes 72, 73, 94
Global pandemics 176
Gynecologic medicine 273, 274, 275, 277, 278, 286, 287, 288, 292, 295, 297, 298, 299
Gynecology 273, 274, 275, 276, 277, 278, 279, 283, 284, 288, 289, 291, 292, 293, 296, 298, 300, 304

H

Hallucination 64
Healthcare 1, 2, 4, 5, 8, 13, 14, 15, 17, 20, 21, 22, 24, 25, 28, 30, 31, 32, 205, 206, 207, 208, 212, 216, 219, 220, 221, 222, 223, 226, 228, 231, 232, 234, 236, 237
Healthcare arena 305
Healthcare professionals 72, 75, 80, 81, 85, 86, 87, 91, 92, 95, 98, 240, 268
Healthcare system 71, 73, 74, 93
Health challenges 175, 177, 190
Health disparities 379, 380, 381, 384, 386, 389, 390, 391, 392, 397, 399, 402, 406
Health Education 407
Health hazards 72
Health professionals 175, 176, 188
Health Promotion 407
Health system 241
Hemodynamic Monitoring 339
Herbalism 176
Histamine 147, 148, 167
Holistic approach 174, 176, 192
Human anatomy 239
Human Metabolome Database (HMDB) 346
Hypersensitivity 167

I

Illnesses 1, 2, 3, 4, 5, 6, 7, 8, 12, 15, 16, 17
Immediate health 174
Immune-mediated disorders 139
Immune system 139, 141, 143, 145, 147, 148, 149, 150, 151, 154, 155, 156, 158, 159, 160, 163, 164, 169
Immunity 158, 167
Immunization 395, 407
Immunoglobulin E 145, 147, 158, 160, 167, 169
Immunological disorders 140, 142
Immunology 139, 140, 141, 142, 143, 144, 146, 147, 150, 151, 152, 155, 157, 158, 160, 162, 163, 164
Immunotherapy 125, 134
Implantation 300
Incontinence 99
Infectious disease 175, 181, 182, 185, 188, 189, 192, 193, 197, 198, 199, 200
Informed decisions 1, 20
Inheritance 214, 232
Innovative solutions 174, 198
Insulin Resistance 374
Integrated health system 381
Intensive care units (ICUs) 307, 308
Internal medicine 1, 2, 3, 4, 5, 6, 7, 8, 9, 11, 12, 13, 14, 15, 16, 17, 18, 19, 20, 21, 23, 24, 25, 26, 27, 28, 29, 31, 32, 35, 36, 37, 38, 39, 40, 41, 42, 43, 44, 45, 46, 47, 48, 49, 50, 51, 52, 53, 54, 55, 56, 57, 58, 59, 60, 61, 62, 139, 140, 141, 142
Internet of Medical Things (IoMT) 206, 236

J

Joint 242, 245, 256, 268

L

Labor 279, 281, 282, 300
Lifestyle Modification 407
Ligament 268

M

Macronutrients 374
Malabsorption 28
Malnutrition 99, 356, 357, 374
Mast Cell 167
Mechanical Ventilation 339
Medical management 71
Medical Nutrition Therapy 361, 363
Medical professionals 105, 131
Medicine training 139, 140
Mendelian Disorder 232
Menopause 300
Menstrual Cycle 300
Mental health 35, 36, 37, 38, 39, 40, 41, 42, 43, 44, 45, 46, 47, 48, 50, 51, 52, 53, 54, 55, 56, 57, 58, 59, 60, 61, 62, 66, 67, 68, 69
Mental illnesses 37, 38, 40, 42, 45, 48, 51, 58, 61
Mental Status Examination 64
Metabolic Syndrome 28, 357
Metabolism 345, 346, 347, 348, 349, 350, 351, 352, 353, 354, 355, 356, 361, 363, 364, 367, 368, 370, 371, 372, 373, 374, 375
Metastasis 134
Microaggressions 35, 36
Micronutrients 374
Miscommunication 306, 312
Misjudgment 306
Mobility Impairment 99
Modern healthcare 73
multidisciplinary palliative tumor board (MPTB) 105
Multifaceted approach 71
Muscle 268
Musculoskeletal 239, 240, 241, 242, 243, 244, 245, 246, 247, 248, 249, 250, 251, 252, 253, 255, 256, 257, 258, 259, 260, 261, 262, 263, 264, 265, 266, 267, 268, 270, 272
Musculoskeletal medicine 240, 241
Musculoskeletal System 242, 268
Mutation 232
Myofascial pelvic pain (MFPP) 242

N

nanotechnology 2, 19, 26, 30
Neurotransmitter 64
Neutropenia 134
Non-Communicable Diseases 407

Non-conventional medicines (NCMs) 380
Nutritional Assessment 349, 352, 374
Nutritional Deficiency 28

O

Obesity 356, 357, 374, 377
Obligation 347
Obsessive-Compulsive Disorder 64
Obstetric 273, 274, 275, 276, 277, 278, 279, 280, 282, 284, 285, 286, 287, 289, 290, 291, 292, 294, 295, 296, 297, 298, 299, 300, 302, 304
Obstetrics 273, 274, 275, 276, 277, 278, 279, 280, 284, 288, 289, 291, 292, 293, 294, 296, 298, 300
Occupational Health 407
Oncologists 106, 107, 108, 109, 110, 111, 114, 116, 117, 119, 125, 130, 133
Oncology 105, 106, 107, 108, 109, 110, 111, 112, 113, 114, 116, 117, 118, 119, 120, 121, 122, 123, 124, 125, 126, 127, 128, 129, 130, 131, 132, 133, 134, 136, 137, 138
Orthopedic management 240, 252
Orthopedic medical 239, 244
Orthopedic medicine 239, 240, 242, 243, 245, 246, 250, 251, 252, 253, 255, 257, 258, 259, 260, 263, 265, 266, 267
Orthopedic patients 240, 259
Orthopedics 268
Osteoarthritis 242, 246, 247, 248, 268
Osteoporosis 99, 268
Ovulation 300

P

Pain management 240, 256, 267, 271
Pain mechanisms 240, 267
Palliative care 105, 106, 107, 108, 109, 110, 111, 112, 113, 114, 115, 116, 117, 118, 119, 120, 121, 122, 123, 124, 125, 126, 127, 128, 129, 130, 131, 132, 133, 134, 135, 136, 137, 138
Palliative Care 91, 105, 108, 112, 113, 120, 128, 129, 134, 137, 138
Palliative medicine 106, 137, 138
Parenteral Nutrition 374
Parturition 300
pathology 173
Patient care 174, 177, 188, 189, 192
Patient-centred care 274
Patient-needs-oriented 106
Peculiar health 173
Perimenopausal 274
Personal information 207, 226
Pharmacogenomics 220, 222, 223, 234, 235
Phenotype 232
Physiological function 242
Polycystic 275, 287, 301
Polymorphism 232
Polypharmacy 84, 85, 99, 100, 101, 103
Postnatal Care 300
Postoperative delirium 74
Postsurgical recovery 240
Post-Traumatic Stress Disorder 64
Potential barriers 174
Pregnancy 286, 287, 288, 300
Prehospital services 306
Pressure Ulcer 99
Preventive Medicine 379, 380, 382, 383, 387, 390, 391, 394, 398, 402, 407
Primary Prevention 407
Procedural sedation and analgesia (PSA) 307
Prognosis 37
Protein-Energy Malnutrition 374
Pruritus 28
Psychiatric 36, 37, 38, 39, 40, 41, 44, 45, 46, 47, 49, 51, 52, 53, 54, 55, 56, 57, 58, 59, 61, 62, 65, 67, 68, 69
Psychological 35, 36, 37, 38, 40, 41, 42, 44, 47, 48, 49, 50, 51, 52, 53, 54, 55, 57, 60, 67, 68
Psychopharmacology 55, 56, 64
Psychosis 64
Public Health 379, 381, 383, 384, 390, 391, 403, 404, 407, 409

Q

Quality improvement 380, 383, 402, 406
Quantify resilience 175

R

Radiotherapy 134

Rehabilitation 246, 259
Resuscitation 339
Rheumatoid Arthritis 248, 268

S

Sarcopenia 99
Schizophrenia 64, 65
Screening 394, 396, 401, 407, 410
Secondary Prevention 407
Sepsis 25, 339
Shock 339
Skin diseases 3, 4, 5, 6, 7, 8, 9, 10, 14, 15, 17, 19, 20, 21, 22, 24, 25, 27
Skin manifestations 1, 10, 29
Sleep medicine 36
Social health 38
Societal attitudes 274, 295, 298
Sociocultural contexts 175
Sprain 268
Staging 134
Substance Use Disorder 64
Sympathetic 106
Syndrome illustrates 240
Systemic Lupus Erythematosus 28

T

Targeted Therapy 134, 137
Tendon 268
Therapy 380, 382, 383, 387, 402, 408
Thrombocytopenia 134
T Lymphocyte 167
Trauma 318, 339, 340, 344
Treatment 205, 206, 207, 208, 209, 210, 211, 212, 213, 214, 216, 219, 220, 221, 222, 224, 227, 228, 229, 230, 231, 233, 236
Treatment effectiveness 36
Treatment efficacy 2
Tropical medicine 174, 175, 176, 177, 178, 179, 180, 185, 186, 187, 188, 189, 193, 195, 196, 197, 199
Tumor Marker 134

U

Unique healthcare 71
Universal growth 347
Urticaria 28, 29

V

Vaccine policy 175
Vasculitis 28

W

Whole genome sequencing (WGS) 205, 228

X

X-Linked Disorder 232